# Monte Carlo in Heavy Charged Particle Therapy

This book explores the current difficulties and unsolved problems in the field of particle therapy and, after analysing them, discusses how (and if) innovative Monte Carlo approaches can be used to solve them.

Each book chapter is dedicated to a different sub-discipline, including multi-ion treatments, flash-radiotherapy, laser-accelerated beams, nanoparticles effects, binary reactions to enhance radiobiology, and space-related issues. This is the first book able to provide a comprehensive insight into this exciting field and the growing use of Monte Carlo in medical physics.

It will be of interest to graduate students in medicine and medical physics, in addition to researchers and clinical staff.

**Key Features:**
- Explores the exciting and interdisciplinary topic of Monte Carlo in particle therapy and medicine.
- Addresses common challenges in the field.
- Edited by an authority on the subject, with chapter contributions from specialists.

**Pablo Cirrone** is a medical physicist and researcher at the Laboratori Nazionali del Sud of INFN, Italy, where he supports and coordinates various experimental groups. Dr. Cirrone is an expert in the use of proton and ion in radiation treatment and of absolute and relative dosimetry in electron, photon and ion beam. He is an expert in the development and test of detectors for medical applications, of the production and use of laser-driven beams for medical and multidisciplinary applications and recipient of the Michael Gotein Award. He is active on many scientific committees and organizes national and international conferences.

**Giada Petringa** is a researcher at the Laboratori Nazionali del Sud of INFN, Italy. Dr. Petringa has a professional experience in the field of Monte Carlo simulations for medical applications, dosimetry, microdosimetry, and diagnostics with conventional and laser-driven proton beams. In 2019 she had a MSCA-IF-2019 (Marie Sklodowska-Curie Actions-Individual Fellowship) grant funded by the European Community in the framework of the H2020 program. She is a member of the Editorial Board of the international journal Physica Medica - European Journal of Medical. She organized more than fifteen international Geant4 Schools. She is an official member of the Geant4 code Collaboration at CERN since 2019. She is a code developer, and she collaborates to maintain two of the official examples of the code.

# Monte Carlo in Heavy Charged Particle Therapy

## New Challenges in Ion Therapy

Edited by Pablo Cirrone and Giada Petringa

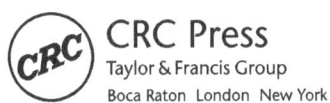

**CRC Press**
Taylor & Francis Group
Boca Raton London New York

CRC Press is an imprint of the
Taylor & Francis Group, an **informa** business

Designed cover image: Shutterstock_ 752346715

First edition published 2024
by CRC Press
6000 Broken Sound Parkway NW, Suite 300, Boca Raton, FL 33487-2742

and by CRC Press
4 Park Square, Milton Park, Abingdon, Oxon, OX14 4RN

*CRC Press is an imprint of Taylor & Francis Group, LLC*

© 2024 selection and editorial matter, Pablo Cirrone and Giada Petringa; individual chapters, the contributors

**Library of Congress Cataloging-in-Publication Data**

Names: Cirrone, Pablo, editor. | Petringa, Giada, editor.
Title: Monte Carlo in heavy charged particle therapy : new challenges in
ion therapy / edited by Pablo Cirrone and Giada Petringa.
Description: First edition. | Boca Raton, FL : CRC Press, 2024. |
Series: Series in medical physics and biomedical engineering | Includes
bibliographical references and index. |
Summary: "This book explores the current difficulties and unsolved problems in the
field of particle therapy and, after analysing them, discusses how (and if) innovative
Monte Carlo approaches can be used to solve them. Each book chapter is dedicated
to a different sub-discipline, including multi-ion treatments, flash-radiotherapy,
laser-accelerated beams, nanoparticles effects, binary reactions to enhance
radiobiology, and space-related issues. This is the first book able to provide a
comprehensive insight into this exciting field and the growing use of Monte Carlo
in medical physics. It will be of interest to graduate students in medicine and medical
physics, in addition to researchers and clinical staff"-- Provided by publisher.
Identifiers: LCCN 2023021860 | ISBN 9780367897161 (hardback)
| ISBN 9781032562742 (paperback) | ISBN 9781003023920 (ebook)
Subjects: LCSH: Medical physics--Mathematics. | Monte Carlo method.
Classification: LCC R905 .M658 2024 | DDC 610.1/53--dc23/eng/20230823
LC record available at https://lccn.loc.gov/2023021860

ISBN: 978-0-367-89716-1 (hbk)
ISBN: 978-1-032-56274-2 (pbk)
ISBN: 978-1-003-02392-0 (ebk)

DOI: 10.1201/9781003023920

Typeset in font CMR10
by KnowledgeWorks Global Ltd.

# Contents

# About the Series

The *Series in Medical Physics and Biomedical Engineering* describes the applications of physical sciences, engineering, and mathematics in medicine and clinical research.

The series seeks (but is not restricted to) publications in the following topics:

- Artificial organs
- Assistive technology
- Bioinformatics
- Bioinstrumentation
- Biomaterials
- Biomechanics
- Biomedical engineering
- Clinical engineering
- Imaging
- Implants
- Medical computing and mathematics
- Medical/surgical devices

- Patient monitoring
- Physiological measurement
- Prosthetics
- Radiation protection, health physics, and dosimetry
- Regulatory issues
- Rehabilitation engineering
- Sports medicine
- Systems physiology
- Telemedicine
- Tissue engineering
- Treatment

The *Series in Medical Physics and Biomedical Engineering* is an interna- tional series that meets the need for up-to-date texts in this rapidly developing field. Books in the series range in level from introductory graduate textbooks and practical handbooks to more advanced expositions of current research.

The *Series in Medical Physics and Biomedical Engineering* is the official book series of the International Organization for Medical Physics.

# Preface

Computer simulations are applied in many areas of research and development. They can save time by avoiding cumbersome experiments, create potential scenarios that are difficult to create experimentally or, most importantly, allow the determination of quantities that can not be measured directly. Monte Carlo methods utilized in economy (e.g., to predict market behavior), meteorology (e.g., to predict weather patterns), mathematics (e.g., to solve differential equations), physics (e.g., to predict detector response), and many other fields. Solving problems using Monte Carlo is typically slower compared to the use of analytical algorithms but the efficiency of the latter is more impacted by the complexity of the problem at hand.

The idea to use stochastic sampling arguably started with the French naturalist Georges-Louis Leclerc, Comte de Buffon, in the 18th century and a random method was already used to calculate the properties of the newly discovered neutron in 1930. Nevertheless, the beginning of the modern Monte Carlo method in physics was in the 1940s when the term "Monte Carlo" was introduced as a code name in Los Alamos for neutron transport simulations. As many of the early work was classified, the first publication entitled "The Monte Carlo Method" didn't appear until 1949. Subsequently, the Monte Carlo method found applications in solving various physics problems, e.g., to design equipment and to interpret experimental results. Mainly due to high-energy physicists entering the field of medical physics, the Monte Carlo method eventually started to play a role in addressing radiation transport problems in radiation therapy. Monte Carlo simulations were first widely applied for electron transport simulations. It became feasible to simulate particle tracking of charged particles in reasonable time scales with the advent of the condensed history algorithm in the 1960s, thus paving the way of its use not only in photon and neutron transport but also for heavy charged particles.

Monte Carlo simulations have played a huge role particularly in advancing ion therapy where more precise dose delivery also demanded more accurate methods to predict dose distributions in patients. While in the beginning the focus was on investigating particle transmission and dose deposition as well as dosimetry by assessing ion chamber response, the area of Monte Carlo simulations has grown significantly in recent years. This makes this book very timely as it outlines current applications as well as challenges in state-of-the-art Monte Carlo for ion therapy.

After an introduction into physics models (Chapter 1), current dosimetry applications are being described (Chapter 2). While clinical dosimetry still plays a large role in medical physics, as in the early days of Monte Carlo, new concepts are now being studied such as innovative dose verification and imaging applications. These have not only helped to improve precision in radiation therapy but also to validate Monte Carlo methods and the underlying physics models. Arguably the most important advancement in the field of Monte Carlo in the last few years has been its expansion into the world of biology and chemistry as demonstrated in Chapters 3–5 of this book. The goal of these simulations is to provide a link from physics interactions to observed biological endpoints. The expanding potential and capabilities of Monte Carlo often comes at a price. Efficiency of Monte Carlo simulations have been a major concern throughout its history. Some current efforts to address these challenges are described ins Chapter 6.

In summary, this book provides an excellent overview of current topics and applications of Monte Carlo simulations in ion therapy and will provide an important reference for researchers and students.

# The International Organization for Medical Physics

The International Organization for Medical Physics (IOMP) represents over 18,000 medical physicists worldwide and has a membership of 80 national and 6 regional organizations, together with a number of corporate members. Individual medical physicists of all national member organizations are also automatically members.

The mission of IOMP is to advance medical physics practice worldwide by disseminating scientific and technical information, fostering the educational and professional development of medical physics and promoting the highest quality medical physics services for patients.

A World Congress on Medical Physics and Biomedical Engineering is held every three years in cooperation with International Federation for Medical and Biological Engineering (IFMBE) and International Union for Physics and Engineering Sciences in Medicine (IUPESM). A regionally based international conference, the International Congress of Medical Physics (ICMP) is held between world congresses. IOMP also sponsors international conferences, workshops and courses.

The IOMP has several programmes to assist medical physicists in developing countries. The joint IOMP Library Programme supports 75 active libraries in 43 developing countries, and the Used Equipment Programme coordinates equipment donations. The Travel Assistance Programme provides a limited number of grants to enable physicists to attend the world congresses.

IOMP co-sponsors the *Journal of Applied Clinical Medical Physics*. The IOMP publishes, twice a year, an electronic bulletin, *Medical Physics World*. IOMP also publishes e-Zine, an electronic news letter about six times a year. IOMP has an agreement with Taylor & Francis for the publication of the *Medical Physics and Biomedical Engineering* series of textbooks. IOMP members receive a discount.

IOMP collaborates with international organizations, such as the World Health Organizations (WHO), the International Atomic Energy Agency (IAEA), and other international professional bodies such as the International Radiation Protection Association (IRPA) and the International Commission on Radiological Protection (ICRP), to promote the development of medical physics and the safe use of radiation and medical devices.

Guidance on education, training and professional development of medical physicists is issued by IOMP, which is collaborating with other professional organizations in development of a professional certification system for medical physicists that can be implemented on a global basis.

The IOMP website (www.iomp.org) contains information on all the activities of the IOMP, policy statements 1 and 2 and the "IOMP: Review and Way Forward" which outlines all the activities of IOMP and plans for the future.

# 1 The Monte Carlo method and its application to heavily charged particle therapy

*Vladimir Ivanchenko*
CERN, European Organization for Nuclear Research, Geneva, Switzerland

*Luciano Pandola*
Istituto Nazionale di Fisica Nucleare (INFN) Laboratori Nazionali del Sud (LNS), Catania, Italy

## CONTENTS

The name "Monte Carlo" defines a class of methods which provide numerical solutions to complex problems by employing random numbers. This approach is best suited to treat the evolution and the behavior of complex systems made by a large number of individual components: while the behavior of each component is known, the evolution of the system as a whole depends on a huge number of correlated parameters, so that analytic or approximate solutions are unfeasible. In order to describe the system, a viable solution consists in simulating the evolution of the system by following its elementary components: the procedure is then repeated iteratively, making use of random numbers, until the convergence is achieved. The proper convergence to the average for a large number $N$ of iterations is guaranteed by the Law of Large Numbers. Provided that the underlying probability density function has a finite variance, the Monte Carlo estimate of the average converges to the true value as the well-known $1/\sqrt{N}$ law from the Central Limit Theorem.

While the idea of using random numbers for solving complex problems dates back to the XVII century, the actual implementation of the modern Monte Carlo method took place only when computers came into the play, in the '40. The name itself, Monte Carlo, comes after the city in Monaco hosting a world-renowned casino, which is the undisputed reign of random numbers. The name was coined by John von Neumann who also pioneered, together with Stanislaw Ulam and Nicholas

DOI: 10.1201/9781003023920-1

Metropolis, the foundations and the development of the technique initially used for the complex calculations required for the design of nuclear weapons in Los Alamos [40, 39, 12, 13]. Monte Carlo techniques are nowadays used in a large variety of applications in mathematics and physics, especially for those problems whose complexity stems from the interaction and correlation of many variables and are hence not affordable with standard analytical methods. Typical applications are found in many-body quantum theory, statistical physics, and radiation transport, but also in completely different domains, such as social sciences, economy, genetics, and epidemiology. While the method makes intrinsically use of random numbers, its applicability is not limited to probabilistic problems, as quantum physics and radiation transport, but also includes purely deterministic problems, like numerical integration.

In the following of this contribution, the focus is given to the application of the Monte Carlo techniques for radiation transport and radiation-matter interaction, i.e. to evaluate the effect (dose, energy deposit, etc.) of a given radiation field impinging on a system. While the interactions of particles are governed by the known laws of physics, the complexity of the problem, which is also due to the existence of different materials and of geometric boundaries, makes any analytic solution impossible.

## 1.1   MONTE CARLO SIMULATION OF PARTICLE INTERACTIONS

The interaction of a primary particle of kinetic energy $E$ within a material can be described by a total cross section $\sigma(E)$. As usually particles can undergo many different interactions with matter (e.g. Compton scattering and photoelectric effect for $\gamma$-rays), the total cross section is expressed as the summation of all individual contributions $\sigma_i$,

$$\sigma = \sum_i \sigma_i. \tag{1.1}$$

The interactions are mutually exclusive (i.e. only one of them can take place in a given position), and the outcomes of each kind are random variables with probability $p_i = \sigma_i/\sigma$. The distance $s$ between two subsequent interactions in the material is a continuous random variable distributed according to an exponential distribution, whose average is

$$\langle s \rangle = \frac{1}{N\sigma}, \tag{1.2}$$

with $N$ being the number of atoms per unit volume. As it is expected, the average distance between subsequent interactions, which is called *step*, gets shortest when the material is denser and/or the cross section is higher. The average distance $\langle s \rangle$ depends on the particle, on its energy, and on the material. The actual step length $s$ can be sampled according to an exponential distribution having mean $\langle s \rangle$. Another random number is then drawn to select which of the competing interactions takes place at the end of the step, based on the probabilities $p_i$.

For most processes, as for instance Compton or Rayleigh scattering, the particle emerging after the interaction has a different energy $E'$ and direction than the initial one. The new energy and direction are described by a (double) differential distribution $\frac{d^2\sigma}{dE'd\Omega}$: this distribution is in principle known from physics, and it is a characteristic of the specific interaction type. The interaction can potentially cause the disappearance of the primary particle (e.g. photoelectric effect) and/or the emission of secondary particles. This basic tracking algorithm, which involves the sampling of a step length and of a subsequent interaction, is repeated iteratively until the primary particle and all possible secondaries are fully transported: the entire sequence is called a *history*. Following the general Monte Carlo approach, many histories are generated in order to evaluate the average behavior of the system, with statistical uncertainty scaling as $1/\sqrt{N}$.

A variety of codes are available which implement the Monte Carlo algorithm for radiation transport in materials. In medical physics applications, the following codes are often used EGS [43, 34],

FLUKA [24, 14], Geant4 [1], MCNPX [18], and Penelope [9]. Those codes differ for the particles being transported[1], the energy range of applicability, the programming language (FORTRAN vs. C++), and the distribution format. Geant4 is a general-purpose toolkit for the Monte Carlo simulation of the interactions of particles with matter: it is developed and maintained by the international Geant4 collaboration, written in C++, and regularly released as a free software under a very permissive license [26]. Geant4 is capable to transport leptons, hadrons, ions, and $\gamma$-rays within a wide energy range of applicability and implements a large set of alternative/complementary physics models to describe the interactions.

In the following, the usage of Geant4 as a Monte Carlo tool for proton therapy and hadron therapy applications will be discussed. The simulation of the interaction of protons and nuclei with matter for medical applications requires the detailed modeling of both electromagnetic interactions and hadronic interactions. While the former is mainly responsible for the slow down, spatial displacement, and production of secondary electrons within the material being traversed, the latter account for nuclear interactions, such as the fragmentation of the projectile and target nuclei. After a general introduction about the Geant4 structure and the philosophy for physics modeling given in Sect. 1.2. Sects. 1.3 and 1.4 are devoted to the description of the electromagnetic and hadronic processes, respectively.

## 1.2 GEANT4 AND PHYSICS MODELING

The Geant4 toolkit is based on the object-oriented approach, which means that interactions of the components are managed via abstract C++ interfaces. The most important interfaces will be shown below using small-caps fonts. The general scheme of Geant4 and the toolkit design are described in the major Geant4 publications [1, 3, 4].

A geometry of a setup is modeled as a set of geometrical volumes filled by materials. The geometry parameters are defined at the initialization phase of Geant4. Geometry description includes shape, dimension, position, and rotation of components. Material definition includes density, temperature, pressure, and list of atoms (elements) with their partial densities. Each Geant4 element includes a list of isotopes with their abundances.

Geant4 physics is initialized after geometry. Before a run is started, all particles and physics processes are initialized. Every Geant4 particle is associated to a class (G4ParticleDefinition) which holds the static parameters, such as name, mass, charge, and various quantum numbers. For sampling of physics a G4DynamicParticle is introduced which includes: G4ParticleDefinition, four-momentum, and polarization of the particle. For tracking in the setup, a G4Track object is used, which includes: G4DynamicParticle, position, and state of the track. For the simulation of physical interactions, each particle must be associated with a set of physics processes, each implemented according to the G4VProcess abstract interface. In Geant4, there are several types of physics processes:

- Transportation – particles are transported through the volumes of the geometry setup, which can possibly host electromagnetic fields;
- Decay – unstable particles may decay in flight or at rest. Radioactive decay describes $\alpha$, $\beta$, and $\gamma$ radioactivity of unstable isotopes;
- Electromagnetic – $\gamma$-rays, electrons, and all charged particles interact with atomic electrons and atomic nuclei via electromagnetic interactions;
- Hadronic – particles interact with atomic nuclei via strong forces providing elastic scattering, excitation, or fragmentation of the nucleus;
- Optical – absorption, refraction, and other processes of transportation of optical photons.

---

[1]For instance, EGS and Penelope are devoted to $e^{\pm}$ and $\gamma$-rays, and MCNPX is specialized for neutrons.

In order to define the appropriate physics models to be considered in the simulation, the users can use either one of the predefined Physics Lists or create a custom Physics List object. A set of reference Physics Lists is provided by the Geant4 Collaboration, which cover a number of common use-cases. These reference Physics Lists undergo regular validations and can be used in many user applications directly.

The Geant4 simulation is performed as a series of "events." Each event starts from the creation of one or several initial G4Track objects. Each G4Track is transported separately via geometry step by step. At each step, energy deposition is sampled for charged particles. The step length may be defined by the crossing of a volume boundary, by the decay of an unstable particle, by the total energy loss of a charged particle, or by one of the possible interactions which the particle can undergo. All types of interactions are treated via abstract interfaces in a similar way. A random number generator is used to decide which interaction happens, as described in Sect. 10.1. As the outcome of an interaction, the initial track may be killed, and a set of secondary tracks may be created, which are added to the list of tracks for transportation. A track is eventually killed if the particle loses all its kinetic energy and has no decay or interactions at rest, or if it leaves the so-called world volume, which includes the whole geometry of the application. The event is completed when all tracks are fully transported via the setup. There are user hooks allowing access to information on each step or track of a particle during simulation. This is needed to score quantities of interest. Some scoring is built-in in the toolkit and can be used without the addition of extra user C++ classes.

## 1.3   ELECTROMAGNETIC INTERACTIONS

### 1.3.1   THE MIXED MONTE CARLO APPROACH

The detailed simulation of all individual interactions in matter becomes computationally unfeasible when the number of interactions per track grows above a few hundreds. The limitation is particularly severe for charged particles, whose cross sections for elastic and inelastic scattering are much larger than for neutral particles, such as $\gamma$-rays: this causes the steps between subsequent interactions to be extremely short. The most viable solution is to employ a condensed history Monte Carlo, in which the global effect of multiple interactions on the track (e.g. kinetic energy, direction, and position) is calculated in a single and sufficiently long step. The cumulative effect of the individual interactions on the track is evaluated statistically throughout a longer step, thus allowing for a substantial reduction of the computing load. When the condensed step contains more than 10 or 20 individual interactions, the conditions of the Central Limit Theorem are typically fulfilled, and the cumulative effects can be sampled from Gaussian distributions. Therefore, the computation is reduced to the evaluation of the first and the second moments for the probability density functions that are involved, namely energy loss by inelastic collisions or displacement and change of direction by elastic collisions. This is, for instance, the scope of Multiple Coulomb Scattering (MCS) models (Molière [41, 11], Goudsmit and Saunderson [28], Lewis [36]), which describe in a statistical way the cumulative effect of many Single Coulomb Scattering (SCS) interactions [33, 32, 17].

While a purely condensed approach is computationally much more convenient than a detailed approach, it is often less precise, especially in terms of spatial distributions and in the vicinity of volume boundaries. A compromise between the two requirements, i.e. precision and computing performance, can be achieved by the mixed Monte Carlo approach. In this scheme, a threshold is set (e.g. on energy loss or scattering angle), so that all individual interactions whose effect is smaller than the threshold ("soft interactions") are simulated by a condensed Monte Carlo, while interactions above thresholds ("hard interactions") are simulated using the detailed approach. In fact, for charged particles, the probability of soft events is typically much higher than of hard events: the mean number of hard events per track, and hence the number of steps to be computed during the tracking, gets low enough to allow for a detailed simulation. On the other hand, the cumulative effect of the large number of soft interactions which takes place between each pair of consecutive hard interactions can be accurately described by the statistical approach of a condensed Monte Carlo. The relative balance between the hard and soft interactions can be changed by adjusting the thresholds, in a customizable trade-off between precision (= detailed simulation) and computing performance (= condensed simulation).

Geant4 supports the mixed Monte Carlo approach by defining different "actions" in the basic interface G4VProcess from which all physics processes inherit from: the PostStep and the AtRest actions implement the detailed simulation, while the AlongStep action implements the condensed simulation of the sub-threshold interactions. The discrete actions of all processes are in competition, i.e. only one of them takes place at the end of the step, while the AlongStep actions co-work: the status (kinetic energy, position, direction) of the particle being tracked is updated according to the global effect of *all* condensed processes. All actions of all processes can limit the length of the step: each action proposes a step length – based on the process that it describes, on the cross section and on the material – and the shortest one is eventually selected [27]. The AlongStep actions can limit the step length in order to avoid that the continuous contribution gets too large with respect to the potential PostStep effect. The Geant4 processes that do not implement AlongStep actions are always simulated as fully detailed ("discrete").

The threshold which is used to separate the detailed regime from the condensed regime for the energy loss processes in Geant4 is defined by the user as a cut-in-range $R$: secondary particles are generated from the process and tracked by Geant4 only if they are able to travel for at least a distance $R$. All secondaries having a range shorter than $R$ are taken as "soft": they are not tracked individually and their global effect is accounted in the AlongStep contribution. The minimum kinetic energy which is required to travel a distance $R$ depends on the particle type and on the material which is being crossed. A special treatment is applied when the particle is closer than $R$ to a volume boundary: in this case, a secondary sub-threshold emission can be generated. At the initialization time, Geant4 takes care to convert the user-defined cut-in-range $R$ into energy thresholds $W_0$ for all applicable particles (i.e. those having at least one process with the AlongStep action) and in all materials which are used in the geometry. As an additional feature to optimize the computing performance, Geant4 supports the definition of different cuts-in-range in different regions of the geometry (G4Region).

As anticipated above, the relative balance between the hard and soft interactions can be changed by adjusting the thresholds in a customizable trade-off between precision and computing performance. An example is displayed in Figure 1.1, which shows the mean energy deposit from a 5-MeV electron in a water layer of 1 cm thickness, calculated by Geant4 for different values of the cut-in-range $R$. The lower panel of the figure shows the relative CPU time, normalized to the configuration $R = 100$ mm. The simulations run with high $R$ overestimate the energy deposit by approximately 3%, as they suppress the production of energetic secondaries and hence miss possible escape effects. However, the results of the simulation are remarkably stable as long as the cut-in-range is reasonably short. Furthermore, calculations run with very small $R$ produce the same results, but at the unnecessary cost of a much longer CPU time: the calculation run with $R = 0.1$ μm gives the same mean energy deposition as one with $R = 0.1$ mm, but it takes ×100 longer CPU time. In general, intermediate values of $R$ represent the optimal compromise which allows to get physically correct results within a reasonable computing time. The optimal cut could, however, depend on the specific observable under investigation and on the required precision. For instance, Figure 1.2 shows the angular displacement of the electrons of the simulation above after having crossed the 1-cm water layer: a comparison is made between the configuration with $R = 1$ cm (which overestimates the mean energy release) and the optimal configuration with $R = 100$ μm (which is slower by a factor of $\sim 2$). The simulation with $R = 1$ cm overestimates the fraction of large-angle events and underestimates the small-angle ones: as visible from the ratio in the lower panel, the difference is of the order of a few percent.

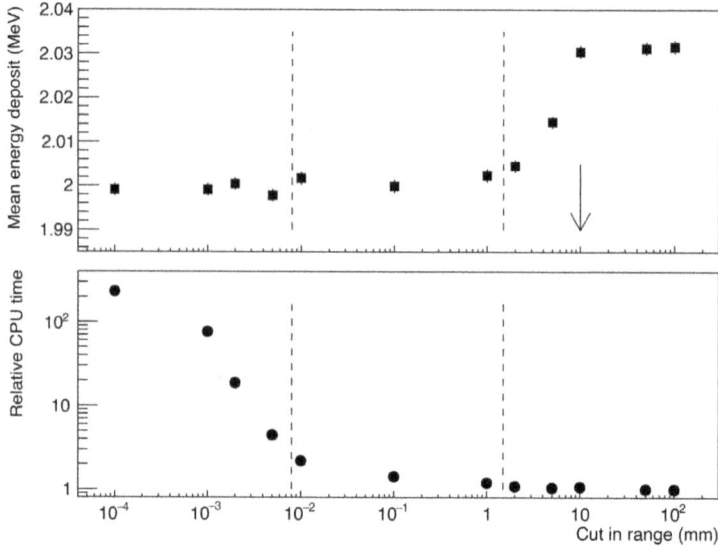

**Figure 1.1** *Upper panel:* mean energy deposit in a 1-cm thick water layer produced by a 5-MeV electron, calculated by Geant4 with different values of the cut-in-range $R$. Each simulation is performed with $10^8$ histories and with the electromagnetic models of the G4EmStandardPhysics_option4 constructor of Geant4 (see Sect. 1.3.2 for details). Statistical uncertainties are included, but they are typically smaller than the size of the marker. The arrow marks the physical dimension of the water layer. *Lower panel:* relative CPU time taken to produce the results of the upper panel for different values of $R$, normalized with respect to the calculation at $R = 100$ mm. The vertical dashed lines indicate the optimal configurations of the cut-in-range, which guarantee physically correct results within a reasonable computing time.

### 1.3.2 $\gamma$-RAY AND ELECTRON TRANSPORT

The electromagnetic interactions of electrons, positrons, and $\gamma$-rays are handled by the electromagnetic package of Geant4. Following the general philosophy of Geant4, multiple models are available to describe the same physics process: they have different characteristics in terms of precision, CPU performance and energy range of applicability. Three complete sets of electromagnetic models are available in Geant4 [1, 6, 4, 31, 7]:

1. the "standard" models are tailored to LHC applications [5];
2. the "Livermore" models (only $\gamma$-rays and electrons) employ a data-driven tracking approach using the EPDL [22] and EEDL [46] data libraries from Livermore. They also account for fluorescence and atomic effects, hence allowing for increased accuracy at low energy, but they are more CPU-intensive with respect to the standard models [20];
3. the "Penelope" models, which derive from the re-implementation of the original low-energy analytical models of the FORTRAN code Penelope [9]; the models are applicable to $\gamma$-rays, electrons, and positrons and are also tailored to low-energy applications.

Models from these sets may be combined for energy range and detector regions. Additional specialized model exists for high-energy applications, for polarized particles, or for specific high-precision simulations, e.g. full relativistic description of Compton scattering [19]; molecular interference effects in $\gamma$-ray elastic scattering [45]; $\gamma$-ray elastic interactions with combined Rayleigh, nuclear Thomson, and Delbrück scattering [44]. The Geant4 interface supports the usage of different

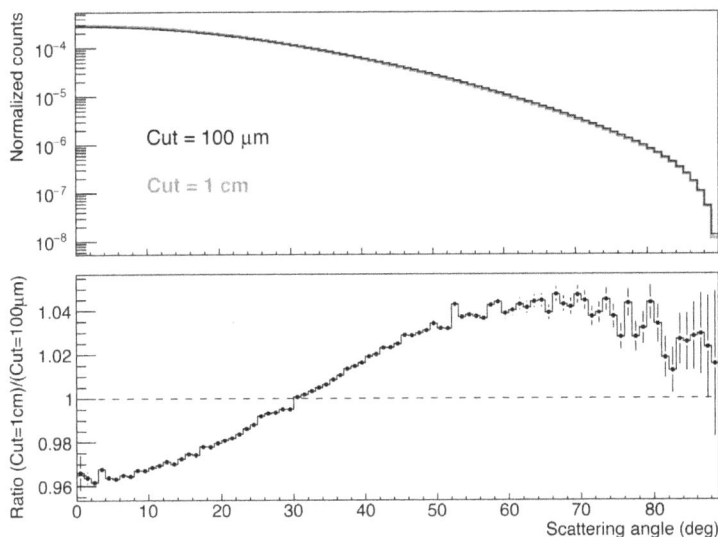

**Figure 1.2**   *Upper panel:* distribution of the angular displacement of 5-MeV electrons after crossing a 1-cm thick layer of water. Two simulations were performed, each with $10^8$ histories and with the same physics models as in Figure 1.1, having two different cuts-in-range $R$: 100 μm (thin black line) and 1 cm (thick gray line). The cut $R = 100$ μm corresponds to the optimal configuration of Figure 1.1. *Lower panel:* ratio (R = 1 cm)/R(100 μm) between the two distributions of the upper panel, with statistical uncertainties. See text for more details.

models in different energy ranges in order to achieve an optimal balance between precision and CPU performance.

Due to the much lower cross section, which causes mean free paths of the order of > mm in solid materials, γ-rays can always be treated with a fully detailed approach: all γ-ray processes implement the PostStep action only. Four processes are available for γ-rays: Rayleigh scattering, Compton scattering, photoelectric effect, and $e^\pm$ production. As mentioned above, each process can be described by many alternative models, some of which are specialized to account for polarization. The γ-ray models of Geant4 are extensively validated in Ref. [21] and were successfully used for medical applications [7].

Interactions of $e^\pm$ cannot be efficiently handled by a fully detailed approach[2] and are described in Geant4 using the mixed approach described in Sect. 1.3.1. Two main energy loss processes are available (G4eIonisation for ionization and G4eBremsstrahlung for bremsstrahlung), which implement the AlongStep action for the soft emission and the PostStep action for the hard emission. The bremsstrahlung models can be customized by alternative angular generators for the emitted photons. The sampling of the continuous (AlongStep) energy loss for an $e^\pm$ of kinetic energy $E$ is based on the calculation of the average *stopping power*[3], restricted to interactions below the

---

[2]Dedicated fully-detailed models (i.e. without the continuous energy loss component) are available for very specific applications in which it is critical that secondary electrons are generated down to very low energies. In Geant4, pure discrete ionization models are available for liquid water (in the framework of the Geant4-DNA extension [29]) and for silicon and other semiconductor materials, for microelectronics applications [48, 49].

[3]Historically, the name "stopping power" indicates the mean energy loss per unit length in a material.

threshold $W_0$

$$S_s(E) = N \sum_i \int_0^{W_0} W \frac{d\sigma_i}{dW}(E)dW \tag{1.3}$$

and of the *straggling*

$$\Omega_s^2(E) = N \sum_i \int_0^{W_0} W^2 \frac{d\sigma_i}{dW}(E)dW. \tag{1.4}$$

where $N$ is the number density of the material being traversed and $d\sigma_i/dW$ is the differential cross section of the $i$-th interaction for the emission of a secondary of energy $W$. The summations account for the fact that all AlongStep processes (e.g. ionization and bremsstrahlung) co-work to the cumulative energy loss. Given the step length $s$, the total energy loss $W$ along the step is distributed with mean

$$\langle W \rangle = S_s(E) \cdot s \tag{1.5}$$

and variance

$$\text{var}(W) = \Omega_s^2(E) \cdot s. \tag{1.6}$$

During the Monte Carlo tracking, the energy loss in each step is randomly sampled according to a Gaussian distribution of mean $\langle W \rangle$ and variance $\text{var}(W)$: as the step is usually long enough to contain a large number of soft interactions, the Central Limit Theorem applies. For relatively short steps, the energy loss distribution is far from a Gaussian, and a dedicated model is applied.

As for the case of $\gamma$-rays, multiple models are available, which are tailored to different energy ranges and application domains. Two processes are available to describe the Coulomb scattering of $e^\pm$, with either multiple scattering (MSC) approach (G4eMultipleScattering) [32] or with the more CPU-demanding single scattering approach (G4ColumbScattering). Models available for MCS are G4UrbanMscModel, G4WentzelVIModel and G4GoudsmitSaundersonModel, the latter being the most accurate for $e^\pm$ below 100 MeV [8, 4, 32, 33]. The model available for single Coulomb scattering is G4eSingleScatteringModel [41, 17]. A pure discrete process is available to describe the positron annihilation, G4eplusAnnihilation.

Geant4 provides several physics list constructors for the electromagnetic interactions, which are tailored to specific applications or domains, for an optimized trade-off between precision and CPU performance. The constructors implement different mixtures of the electromagnetic models used for each process and possibly provide custom parameters within each model, as for instance the range factor of the MSC model [32]. The constructor G4EmStandardPhysics_option4 is the one that is regarded as the most precise combination of the electromagnetic physics models available in Geant4. Other less CPU-demanding constructors that are suitable for proton therapy and medical physics applications [7] are G4EmLivermorePhysics, G4EmPenelopePhysics, and G4EmStandardPhysics_option3. The electromagnetic processes for $e^\pm$ and $\gamma$-rays are complemented by lepto-nuclear and gamma-nuclear processes, describing the interaction of leptons and $\gamma$-rays with nuclei, respectively. For that, the constructor G4EmExtraPhysics is available in Geant4 as a ready-for-the-use physics list component.

### 1.3.3 PROTONS AND HEAVY IONS TRANSPORT

The hadron and ion transport are critical for many Monte Carlo applications. There are about 40 quasi-stable hadrons with different mass and charge and about 3000 known isotopes. Some of these isotopes exist in nature, while others are unstable: they only are produced as a result of nuclear reactions, and they have various radioactive decay channels. For accurate simulations, a detailed transport of all kinds of hadrons and ions is usually required. For medical applications, proton and ion fragmentation is an important process, as it affects the radiation field in the patient's body, in a variety of treatment equipments, and in the elements of the room. The optimization of a treatment plan for proton or ion beams requires the precise calculation of the dose map, by means of a detailed simulation of primary and secondary particles, also including neutron transport and radioactive decay of unstable isotopes.

Models describing most of the hadrons and ions interactions are available in Geant4. The main electromagnetic interactions are ionization and elastic scattering in the Coulomb field of atoms. These interactions are implemented using the condensed history approach described in the Sect. 1.3.1. By default, elastic scattering is simulated as multiple elastic scattering at a macroscopic simulation step [32], and inelastic interaction as a continuous ionization process with energy loss at a step (AlongStep) and the production of secondary electrons above the threshold (PostStep). For protons, the ionization process in Geant4 is described by the classical Bethe-Bloch formula above 2 MeV with density effect and shell corrections [2]. Below 2 MeV, atomic shell corrections become larger than the main Bethe-Bloch term and stopping power parameterizations are used based on evaluated data [10, 47]. Recently, new accurate parameterizations of stopping powers in liquid water and air were published [30], which are also available in Geant4.

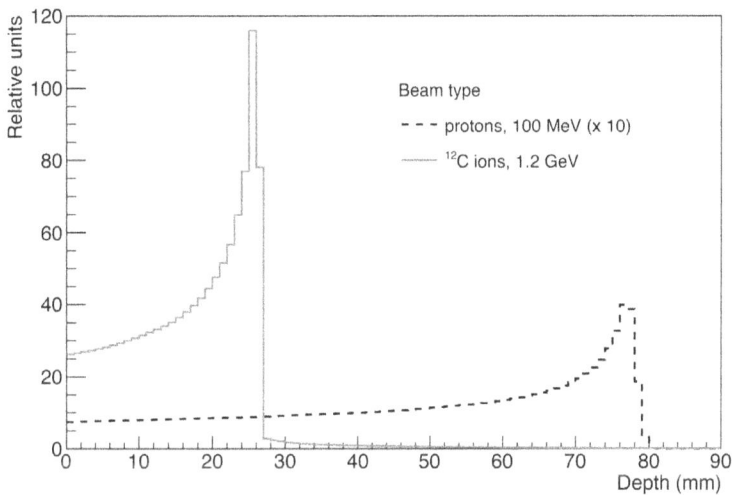

**Figure 1.3**   Profile of dose deposition vs. penetration depth in water for a beam of 100 MeV protons (black dashed) and of 1.2 GeV $^{12}$C ions (gray solid), from a Geant4 simulation using the electromagnetic models from the `G4EmStandardPhysics_option4` constructor and the Binary cascade hadronic models (see Sect. 1.4.2). The proton dose deposition is scaled by a factor of 10, for better visibility. The main structure at the end of the particle range is the Bragg peak. For the carbon beam, the dose deposition at depths deeper than the Bragg peak is due to lighter ions produced by fragmentation.

The stopping power of a proton produces a prominent Bragg peak at low energies (see Figure 1.3). This peak corresponds to the situation when the proton velocity is comparable to the typical velocity of the atomic electrons. In such conditions, the proton transfers much more energy per unit length than in the case of high energy. The Bragg peak is used as a key design feature for proton therapy facilities. It is possible to have a high radiation field in a tumor but relatively limited radiation in the surrounding healthy organs. For this purpose, special filters are installed at proton medical beam lines, which allow to tune the energy of protons according to the individual treatment plan for each patient. The proton facilities are available in many countries all over the world.

In the case of light ions, like an $\alpha$ particle ($^4$He) or a carbon ion $^{12}$C, the Bragg peak of ionization is even more prominent than for protons. This property is used at carbon ion treatment facilities, which are technically more demanding. For a long time, facilities constructed in Japan have been leading the field. For the accurate simulation of ion Bragg peak, nuclear fragmentation should be taken into account. Elastic and inelastic cross sections of light ions are significantly higher than that of protons, which provides a higher and longer fragmentation tail downstream the Bragg peak and higher radiation field upstream the Bragg peak (Figure 1.3). In the case of carbon therapy, a much stronger radiation field is created inside the Bragg peak but, at the same time, a significantly higher radiation field also exists upstream and downstream: therefore, the treatment plan must take into account possible radiation effect on healthy organs more carefully than in the case of the proton therapy. So, accurate simulation of medical beam irradiation requires accurate description both of electromagnetic and hadronic interactions. The existence of the fragmentation tail limits the practical possibility of using beams of ions heavier than carbon for therapy.

## 1.4   NUCLEAR INTERACTIONS

For a number of common use-cases in medical physics, all relevant electromagnetic and nuclear processes are required, including the detailed description of neutron production and transport. In the Geant4 toolkit, there are sub-libraries for hadronic cross sections and for generators of final particles. Such sub-division provides independent development and validation of the software components responsible for the simulation of hadronic interactions.

### 1.4.1   HADRONIC CROSS SECTIONS

The cross sections used in Geant4 are either based on theoretical models or on open-source evaluated databases. The largest Geant4 data set includes various neutron cross sections at energies below 20 MeV. It is derived from the Evaluated Nuclear Structure Data File (ENSDF) [42] and includes elastic scattering, inelastic interactions, capture, and partial neutron cross sections for various target isotopes. In the cases where the highest tracking accuracy is required, the interaction cross sections for low-energy protons and light ions are also derived from the evaluated data of the ENSDF database [42] or from the calculations included in the TENDL data library, based on the TALYS nuclear model [35].

Hadron-nucleon cross sections are parameterized in a wide energy range from the threshold to very high asymptotic energies. A Glauber-Gribov formalism is used at high energy to compute the interaction cross section of a hadron on any target nucleus, allowing to derive hadron/ion cross section using hadron-proton and hadron-neutron elementary cross sections [4].

### 1.4.2   NUCLEAR FRAGMENTATION

Hadron/ion nuclear fragmentation process includes several stages. If the energy of the hadron projectile is above a few GeV, the strong interaction of the projectile with the target produces new quarks and antiquarks, which form a string of secondary hadrons via quark hadronization. These hadrons and excited nucleons can have re-scattering on nucleons of the target and leave the nucleus. The process of re-scattering of hadrons and nucleons can also take place when the energy of the projectile is below the threshold for the string formation. So, in both cases, a similar nuclear cascade happens. In the Geant4 toolkit there are three main models providing simulation of this cascade: the Bertini cascade [50], the Binary cascade [25], and INCLXX [38]. These models are applicable for energies from zero to a few GeV. Depending on projectile energy and the reaction their results and performance may be different. For example, the Binary cascade is recommended for proton, neutron, and ion projectiles below 2 GeV. See Ref. [4, 7] for a detailed description of the properties and features of the three cascade models available in Geant4.

As a result of emission of hadrons and nucleons for the target, the residual nucleus remains in excited state. The nuclear de-excitation and the radioactive decay modules of Geant4 are in charge for the simulation of the subsequent nuclear de-excitation. Low-energy neutrons, $\gamma$-rays, and light ions produced in these processes are responsible for the formation of the radiation field due to the fragmentation process. Quantitative comparisons of the different Geant4 cascade models in reproducing experimental fragmentation data are given several references, as Refs. [7, 16, 37, 23, 15].

For the case of proton therapy, the fragmentation tail (Figure 1.3) is relatively small and produced mainly by neutrons. For carbon ion therapy, the tail is significantly larger due to the production of light ions, which have smaller electric charge and correspondingly smaller ionization loss. These light ions have longer ranges in the target than the initial carbon ion.

Physics of hadronic nuclear interactions is complex. For this reason, Geant4 provides many sub-models for the simulation of various aspects of such interactions. Conservation of electric charge, baryon number, and energy are the main requirements for simulation of the nuclear fragmentation. Successful models are based on general theory, particle phenomenology, and parameterization of experimental data.

### 1.4.3  RADIOACTIVE DECAY

Hadronic interactions within the target material can produce stable or unstable daughter nuclei. The delayed decay of short-lived nuclei generates additional radiation, which can potentially produce an extra energy deposit. A specific process of Geant4, G4RadioactiveDecay is in charge to handle the radioactive decay of unstable nuclei, according to the half-lives, the decay modes, the $Q$-values, and the branching ratios provided by database files based on the ENSDF [42]. The process supports $\alpha$, $\beta^+$, $\beta^-$ emission, and electron capture (EC), and the time of the final state is sampled according to the decay half-life. If the daughter nucleus of a decay is in an excited state, the prompt nuclear de-excitation is simulated by the G4PhotoEvaporation module, which makes use of database files from the ENSDF, containing the relevant data of the nuclear data levels. The photon evaporation model accounts for timing, for $\gamma$-ray cascades (potentially including the angular correlation, by enabling the corresponding flag), and for internal electron conversion.

### REFERENCES

1. S. Agostinelli et al. GEANT4–a simulation toolkit. *Nucl. Instrum. Meth. A*, 506:250–303, 2003.
2. S. P. Ahlen. Theoretical and experimental aspects of the energy loss of relativistic heavily ionizing particles. *Rev. Mod. Phys.*, 52:121–173, Jan 1980.
3. J. Allison et al. Geant4 developments and applications. *IEEE Trans. Nucl. Sci.*, 53:270, 2006.
4. J. Allison et al. Recent developments in Geant4. *Nucl. Instrum. Meth. A*, 835:186–225, 2016.
5. J. Apostolakis, A. Bagulya, S. Elles, V. N. Ivanchenko, O. Kadri, M. Maire, and L. Urban. The performance of the Geant4 standard EM package for LHC and other applications. *J. Phys. Conf. Ser.*, 119:032004, 2008.
6. J. Apostolakis et al. Progress in Geant4 electromagnetic physics modelling and validation. *J. Phys. Conf. Ser.*, 664(7):072021, 2015.
7. P. Arce et al. Report on G4-Med, a Geant4 benchmarking system for medical physics applications developed by the Geant4 Medical Simulation Benchmarking Group. *Med. Phys.*, 48(1):19–56, 2021.
8. A. Bagulya et al. Recent progress of GEANT4 electromagnetic physics for LHC and other applications. *J. Phys. Conf. Ser.*, 898(4):042032, 2017.
9. J. Baró, J. Sempau, J. M. Fernández-Varea, and F. Salvat. PENELOPE: An algorithm for Monte Carlo simulation of the penetration and energy loss of electrons and positrons in matter. *Nucl. Instrum. Meth. B*, 100(1):31–46, 1995.
10. M. J. Berger, M. Inokuti, H. H. Andersen, H. Bichsel, D. Powers, S . M. Seltzer, D . Thwaites, and D. E. Watt. Report 49. *J. Int. Comm. Radiat. Units Meas.*, os25(2):NP–NP, 04 2016.
11. H. A. Bethe. Molière's theory of multiple scattering. *Phys. Rev.*, 89:1256–1266, Mar 1953.

12. A. F. Bielajew. History of Monte Carlo. In *Monte Carlo Techniques in Radiation Therapy*. CRC Press, 1st edition, 2013.
13. A. F. Bielajew. Fundamentals of the Monte Carlo method for neutral and charged particle transport. 2001.
14. T. T. Böhlen, F. Cerutti, M. P. W. Chin, A. Fassò, A. Ferrari, P. G. Ortega, A. Mairani, P. R. Sala, G. Smirnov, and V. Vlachoudis. The FLUKA Code: Developments and Challenges for High Energy and Medical Applications. *Nucl. Data Sheets*, 120:211–214, 2014.
15. T. T. Böhlen, F. Cerutti, M. Dosanjh, A. Ferrari, I. Gudowska, A. Mairani, and J. M. Quesada. Benchmarking nuclear models of FLUKA and GEANT4 for carbon ion therapy . *Phys. Med. Biol.*, 55:5833–5847, 2010.
16. D. Bolst et al. Validation of Geant4 fragmentation for Heavy Ion Therapy. *Nucl. Instrum. Meth. A*, 869:68–75, 2017.
17. M. J. Boschini, C. Consolandi, M. Gervasi, S. Giani, D. Grandi, V. Ivanchenko, P. Nieminen, S. Pensotti, P. G. Rancoita, and M. Tacconi. An expression for the Mott cross section of electrons and positrons on nuclei with Z up to 118. *Rad. Phys. Chem.*, 90:39–66, 2013.
18. F. Brown, B. Kiedrowski, and J. Bull. MCNP - A General N-Particle Transport Code, Version 5. Technical report, 2003.
19. J. M. C. Brown, M. R. Dimmock, J. E. Gillam, and D. M. Paganin. A low energy bound atomic electron Compton scattering model for Geant4. *Nucl. Instrum. Meth. B*, 338:77–88, 2014.
20. S. Chauvie et al. Geant4 low energy electromagnetic physics. In *2004 IEEE Nuclear Science Symposium and Medical Imaging Conference*, number 3, pages 1881–1885, 2004.
21. G. A. P. Cirrone, G. Cuttone, F. Di Rosa, L. Pandola, F. Romano, and Q. Zhang. Validation of the Geant4 electromagnetic photon cross-sections for elements and compounds. *Nucl. Instrum. Meth. A*, 618:315–322, 2010.
22. D. Cullen, J. H. Hubbel, and L. Kissel. The Evaluated Photon Data Library (EPDL). Lawrence Livermore National Laboratory, Report UCRL-50400, vol. 6, 1997.
23. M. De Napoli et al. Carbon fragmentation measurements and validation of the Geant4 nuclear reaction models for hadrontherapy. *Phys. Med. Biol.*, 57:7651, 2012.
24. A. Ferrari, P. R. Sala, A. Fassò, and J. Ranft. FLUKA: a multi-particle transport code. Technical report, 2005.
25. G. Folger, V. N. Ivanchenko, and J. P. Wellisch. The Binary Cascade. *Eur. Phys. J. A*, 21:407–417, 2004.
26. Geant4 Collaboration. Geant4 License. https://geant4.web.cern.ch/license.
27. Geant4 Collaboration. Geant4 Physics Reference Manual. http://cern.ch/geant4-userdoc/UsersGuides/PhysicsReferenceManual/html/index.html, 2021.
28. S. Goudsmit and J. L. Saunderson. Multiple scattering of electrons. *Phys. Rev.*, 57:24–29, Jan 1940.
29. S. Incerti et al. The Geant4-DNA Project. *Int. J. Model. Simul. Sci. Comput.*, 01(02):157–178, 2010.
30. International Commission on Radiation Units & Measurements. ICRU Report 90: Key Data for Ionizing-Radiation Dosimetry: Measurement Standards and Applications. https://journals.sagepub.com/toc/crua/14/1, 2014.
31. V. Ivanchenko et al. Geant4 electromagnetic physics progress. *EPJ Web Conf.*, 245:02009, 2020.
32. V. N. Ivanchenko, O. Kadri, M. Maire, and L. Urban. Geant4 models for simulation of multiple scattering. *J. Phys. Conf. Ser.*, 219:032045, 2010.
33. O. Kadri, V. Ivanchenko, F. Gharbi, and A. Trabelsi. Incorporation of the Goudsmit-Saunderson electron transport theory in the Geant4 Monte Carlo code. *Nucl. Instr. Meth. B*, 267(23-24):3624–3632, Dec 2009.

34. I. Kawrakow. Accurate condensed history Monte Carlo simulation of electron transport. I. EGSnrc, the new EGS4 version. *Med. Phys.*, 27(3):485–498, 2000.
35. A. J. Koning, J. S. Rochman, J. Sublet, N. Dzysiuk, M. Fleming, and S. van der Marck. TENDL: Complete Nuclear Data Library for Innovative Nuclear Science and Technology. *Nucl. Data Sheets*, 155:1–55, 2019.
36. H. W. Lewis. Multiple scattering in an infinite medium. *Phys. Rev.*, 78:526–529, Jun 1950.
37. C. Mancini Terracciano et al. Validation of Geant4 nuclear reaction models for hadron therapy and preliminary results with BLOB. *IFMBE Proceedings*, 68/1:675, 2018.
38. D. Mancusi, A. Boudard, J. Cugnon, J.-C. David, P. Kaitaniemi, and S. Leray. Extension of the Liège intranuclear-cascade model to reactions induced by light nuclei. *Phys. Rev. C*, 90(5):054602, 2014.
39. N. Metropolis, A. W. Rosenbluth, M. N. Rosenbluth, A. H. Teller, and E. Teller. Equation of state calculations by fast computing machines. *J. Chem. Phys.*, 21(6):1087–1092, 1953.
40. N. Metropolis and S. Ulam. The Monte Carlo Method. *J. Am. Stat. Assoc.*, 44(247):335–341, 1949.
41. G. Molière. Theorie der Streuung schneller geladener Teilchen. I. Einzelstreuung am abgeschirmten Coulomb-Feld. II. Mehrfach- und Vielfachstreuung. *Z. Naturforsch., A*, 2:133–145, 1947.
42. National Nuclear Data Center. Evaluated Nuclear Structure Data Files (ENSDF). `https://www.nndc.bnl.gov/ensdf`.
43. W. R. Nelson and D.W.O. Rogers. Structure and operation of the EGS4 code system. In: Jenkins, T. M., Nelson, W. R., Rindi, A. (eds) Monte Carlo Transport of Electrons and Photons. Ettore Majorana International Science Series, vol 38. Springer, Boston, MA. https://doi.org/10.1007/978-1-4613-1059-4_12
44. M. Omer and R. Hajima. Including Delbrück scattering in GEANT4. *Nucl. Instrum. Meth. B*, 405:43–49, 2017.
45. G. Paternò, P. Cardarelli, A. Contillo, M. Gambaccini, and A. Taibi. Geant4 implementation of inter-atomic interference effect in small-angle coherent x-ray scattering for materials of medical interest. *Physica Medica*, 51:64–70, 2018.
46. S. T. Perkins et al. Tables and graphs of electron-interaction cross sections from 10 eV to 100 GeV derived from the LLNL evaluated electron data library (EEDL), $Z = 1 - 100$. Lawrence Livermore National Laboratory, Report UCRL-50400, vol. 31, 1997.
47. R. M. Sternheimer, M. J. Berger, and S. M. Seltzer. Density effect for the ionization loss of charged particles in various substances. *At. Data and Nucl. Data Tables.*, 30:261–271, 1984.
48. A. Valentin, M. Raine, M. Gaillardin, and P. Paillet. Geant4 physics processes for microdosimetry simulation: Very low energy electromagnetic models for protons and heavy ions in silicon. *Nucl. Instrum. Meth. B*, 287:124–129, 2012.
49. A. Valentin, M. Raine, J.-E. Sauvestre, M. Gaillardin, and P. Paillet. Geant4 physics processes for microdosimetry simulation: Very low energy electromagnetic models for electrons in silicon. *Nucl. Instrum. Meth. B*, 288:66–73, 2012.
50. D. H. Wright and M. H. Kelsey. The Geant4 Bertini Cascade. *Nucl. Instrum. Meth. A*, 804:175–188, 2015.

# 2 Applications of Monte Carlo calculations in clinical dosimetry of proton and ion beams

*Kilian-Simon Baumann*
University of Applied Sciences, Giessen, Germany
University Hospital Giessen-Marburg, Marburg, Germany
Marburg Ion-Beam Therapy Center, Marburg, Germany Marburg, Germany

*Jorg Wuff*
West German Proton Therapy Centre Essen, Essen, Germany
University Hospital Essen, Essen, Germany
West German Cancer Center (WTZ), Essen, Germany

*Carles Gomà*
Hospital Clínic de Barcelona, Barcelona, Spain

## CONTENTS

## 2.1   INTRODUCTION TO CLINICAL DOSIMETRY

Monte Carlo (MC) simulations of radiation transport in matter have multiple applications in radiation dosimetry of proton and ion beams[1]. MC calculations can be used to quantify the different response of detectors in different radiation beam qualities – e.g. $^{60}$Co radiation typically used for calibration versus proton (or ion) beams. MC calculations can also be used to correct for the limitations of commercially-available detectors to accurately determine necessary quantities for beam data commissioning. For example, to correct for the finite size of large-area plane-parallel ionization chambers used to measure integrated depth-dose curves [2, 3, 4].

---

[1] It was recommended by IAEA and ICRU [1] to call any nuclei with an atomic number equal to, or smaller than, that of neon (Z=10) a light ion. Throughout this text the term "ion" is used for all ions heavier than protons.

DOI: 10.1201/9781003023920-2

However, in the context of clinical dosimetry, MC simulations play possibly the most important role in the field of beam monitor chamber calibration, since it is needed for the calculation of key quantities in calorimetry, Faraday cup dosimetry and ionization chamber-based reference dosimetry.

In water calorimetry, MC calculations have been used to determine fluence perturbations, e.g. by the glass or PMMA vessels containing high-purity water. In graphite calorimetry, the conversion from dose-to-graphite to dose-to-water is supported by MC calculations to determine the required water-to-graphite stopping-power ratios (see section 2.2), fluence perturbation and further corrections [5, 6].

Faraday cup dosimetry was the method traditionally used for beam monitor chamber calibration in proton beams. In this case, MC calculations are needed to convert the integrated fluence of particles determined by the Faraday cup to (integrated) absorbed dose-to-water at the depth of interest [7, 8].

Nowadays, however, ionization chamber-based dosimetry is the most-widely used method for beam monitor chamber calibration in clinical proton and ion beams. Because of its paramount importance, this chapter will focus on the application of MC calculations in air-filled ionization chamber dosimetry.

## 2.2 THEORY

The principles of ionization chamber-based radiation dosimetry are based on the cavity theory [9]. Cavity theories study the relationship between the absorbed dose in a homogeneous cavity inside a homogeneous medium ($D_{cav}$) and the absorbed dose at a point in the medium in the absence of the cavity ($D_m$). The Bragg–Gray theory states that, if

1. The size of the cavity is small compared to the range of the charged particles that cross it, so that the cavity does not perturb the fluence of charged particles in the medium, and
2. The absorbed dose in the cavity is deposited only by the charged particles that cross it,

then $D_m = D_{cav} \cdot s_{m,cav}$, where $s_{m,cav}$ is the so-called *Bragg–Gray medium-to-cavity stopping-power ratio*, which may be expressed as [9]

$$s_{m,cav} = \frac{\sum_i \int_0^{E_{max}} \Phi_m^i(E)\,(S_{el}(E)/\rho)_m^i\,dE}{\sum_i \int_0^{E_{max}} \Phi_m^i(E)\,(S_{el}(E)/\rho)_{cav}^i\,dE}, \tag{2.1}$$

where $i$ runs over all the charged particle types that contribute to the absorbed dose in the cavity, except for secondary electrons; $\Phi_m^i(E)$ is the distribution of the fluence with respect to the (kinetic) energy of the $i$-th particle type in the medium; and $(S_{el}/\rho)^i$ is the unrestricted mass electronic stopping power of the $i$-th particle type. Note that the Bragg–Gray theory assumes that secondary electrons deposit all their energy locally.

The Spencer–Attix cavity theory [10] is a refinement of the Bragg–Gray theory. It takes into account the fact that secondary electrons do not deposit all their energy locally. Hence, the parameter $\Delta$ is introduced which defines the mean energy of the electrons that have a sufficient range to cross (i.e. escape) the cavity. For proton and ion beams, the *Spencer–Attix medium-to-cavity stopping-power ratio* may be expressed as [11, 12]

$$s_{m,cav} = \frac{\sum_i \int_{E_{cut}^i}^{E_{max}} \Phi_m^i(E)\,(L_\Delta(E)/\rho)_m^i\,dE + \Phi_m^i(E_{cut}^i)\,(S_{el}(E_{cut}^i)/\rho)_m^i\,E_{cut}^i}{\sum_i \int_{E_{cut}^i}^{E_{max}} \Phi_m^i(E)\,(L_\Delta(E)/\rho)_{cav}^i\,dE + \Phi_m^i(E_{cut}^i)\,(S_{el}(E_{cut}^i)/\rho)_{cav}^i\,E_{cut}^i}, \tag{2.2}$$

where $i$ runs over all the charged particle types that contribute to the absorbed dose in the cavity (including secondary electrons); $E_{cut}^i$ is the cut-off energy of the $i$-th particle type; and $(L_\Delta/\rho)^i$ is the restricted mass electronic stopping power of the $i$-th particle type. Typically, $E_{cut}^i$ is defined as the mean energy of the $i$-th particle type with a sufficient residual range to cross the cavity (i.e. for electrons, $E_{cut} = \Delta$).

In practice, however, air-filled ionization chambers do not fulfill Bragg–Gray conditions within the level of accuracy needed in radiation therapy. In particular, they do not fulfill the requirement that the cavity should not perturb the fluence of charged particles in the medium. For the particular case of clinical ion beams, one could assume that, on a first approximation, this requirement is fulfilled by protons and ions (as they undergo little scattering); but certainly not by the secondary electrons resulting from inelastic electromagnetic interactions. Therefore, to keep using the cavity theory formalism, the concept of *perturbation correction factor* or simply *perturbation factor*, $p$, is introduced, so that the relationship between the absorbed dose in the medium and the absorbed dose in the cavity is expressed as

$$D_m = D_{cav} \cdot s_{m,cav} \cdot p \tag{2.3}$$

where the factor $p$ accounts for any fluence perturbation introduced by the cavity. Historically, the global perturbation factor of a given detector, $p$, has been assumed to be the product of different and independent perturbation factors, $p_i$, i.e. $p = \prod p_i$. Typical perturbation factors of ionization chambers used in the dosimetry of external radiotherapy beams are $p_{cav}$, $p_{cel}$, $p_{dis}$ and $p_{wall}$, which take into account that the cavity, the central electrode and the wall of the ionization chamber are not equivalent to the medium and, hence, are perturbing the fluence – see Ref. [13] for a detailed definition of these terms.

When the fluence of charged particles in both the medium and the cavity is known – as it is possible by means of MC calculations – it is possible to calculate the global perturbation factor of a detector, making an investigation of individual perturbation factors unnecessary [14]. Furthemore, if the fluence of charged particles in both the medium and the detector cavity is known, it is also needless to split the proportionality between $D_m$ and $D_{cav}$ in two factors: $s_{m,cav}$ and $p$. That is, the relationship between the absorbed dose in the medium and the absorbed dose in the cavity may be expressed as [15]

$$D_m = D_{cav} \cdot f \tag{2.4}$$

where $f = s_{m,cav} \cdot p$ is an ionization chamber-specific factor.

Theoretically, one could calculate the absorbed dose in the cavity of an air-filled ionization chamber from first principles

$$\bar{D}_{air} = \frac{Q}{V \cdot \rho_{air}} \cdot \frac{W_{air}}{e}, \tag{2.5}$$

where $Q$ is the electric charge created in the cavity, $V$ is the sensitive volume of the ionization chamber, $\rho_{air}$ is the mass density of air, $e$ is the charge of the electron and $W_{air}$ is the mean energy needed to create an ion pair in air.

In practice, however, the sensitive volume of the ionization chambers typically used in radiotherapy beams is not known with sufficient accuracy. Thus, in order to determine the absorbed dose-to-air, or directly to water, with sufficient accuracy, one has to fall back on the calibration of ionization chambers in a reference beam quality ($Q_0$), typically $^{60}$Co radiation. To transfer the calibration factor from the calibration beam quality to the user beam quality ($Q$), one needs the so-called *beam quality correction factor* ($k_{Q,Q_0}$) – note that, when the reference quality is $^{60}$Co radiation, the subscript $Q_0$ in $k_{Q,Q_0}$ is typically omitted – which may be calculated either indirectly as [16]

$$k_Q = \frac{s_{w,air,Q}}{s_{w,air,Q_0}} \cdot \frac{W_{air,Q}}{W_{air,Q_0}} \cdot \frac{p_Q}{p_{Q_0}} \tag{2.6}$$

or directly, by means of MC simulation, as [15]:

$$k_Q = \frac{f_Q}{f_{Q_0}} \cdot \frac{W_{\mathrm{air},Q}}{W_{\mathrm{air},Q_0}} = \frac{(D_{\mathrm{w}}/\bar{D}_{\mathrm{air}})_Q}{(D_{\mathrm{w}}/\bar{D}_{\mathrm{air}})_{Q_0}} \cdot \frac{W_{\mathrm{air},Q}}{W_{\mathrm{air},Q_0}}. \tag{2.7}$$

where $f$ is the ionization chamber-specific (and beam quality-dependent) factor defined in eq. 2.4, that establishes the proportionality between the absorbed dose-to-water at the reference point of measurement in the absence of the detector ($D_{\mathrm{w}}$) and the average absorbed dose-to-air in the ionization chamber sensitive volume ($\bar{D}_{\mathrm{air}}$).

## 2.3  CODES OF PRACTICE

There is consensus on the required accuracy for the delivery of absorbed dose to a clinical target in the order of 3-5% [13]. The determination of absorbed dose in a reference dosimetry setup is just one source of uncertainty, but a significant contributor to this and should ideally be performed with an uncertainty of 1% or even less. To achieve such low uncertainty the need for a standardized procedure (i.e. "dosimetry protocol" or "code of practice – CoP") for the determination of absorbed dose in proton and ion beams was recognized since the early days of radiation therapy.

The first of those dosimetry protocols for proton and ion beams (ECHED, AAPM-TG16) recommended the use of calorimeters [17] and Faraday cups [18] while ionization chambers were considered as secondary choice dosimeters. The ICRU 59 report [19] took later into account that concepts of reference dosimetry with calibrated ionization chambers are much easier to establish. In fact, ionization chambers are still the most widespread commercially available type of detectors in a clinical setting. The TRS-398 CoP published in 2000 by IAEA [13] was solely based on calibrated ionization chambers, traceable to national standards of absorbed dose-to-water and allowed the harmonization for dosimetry of photon, electron, proton and carbon ion beams. Following the TRS-398 CoP, the absorbed dose-to-water $D_{\mathrm{w},Q}$ at a beam quality $Q$ using air-filled ionization chambers can be determined by:

$$D_{\mathrm{w},Q} = M_Q \cdot N_{D,\mathrm{w},Q_0} \cdot k_{Q,Q_0} \tag{2.8}$$

where $M_Q$ is the chamber reading corrected for influence quantities, other than beam quality – e.g. air temperature and pressure, $N_{D,\mathrm{w},Q_0}$ is the chamber-specific calibration factor determined at the reference beam quality $Q_0$, and $k_{Q,Q_0}$ (or $k_Q$ in the case of $^{60}$Co radiation being the beam quality $Q_0$) is the beam quality correction factor.

TRS-398 first recommendation was to use calorimeters to determine the beam quality correction factors $k_Q$ for each individual chamber in each individual therapy beam. It was clear that this route is difficult to establish in clinical practice since, on the one hand, calibration laboratories normally have no access to clinical proton and carbon ion beams, and, on the other hand, for most clinics it is not feasible to perform calorimetry. Hence, the calculation of $k_Q$ factors (see also section 2.5.1) was considered the most practical approach and tabulated values for a variety of chambers are provided in the TRS-398 CoP. The tabulations apply for a defined set of reference conditions, i.e. phantom depth, phantom material, field-size, etc. and give $k_Q$ values as a function of chamber type and in case of protons as a function of beam quality $Q$, which specifies the user beam in terms of residual range. TRS-398 CoP contains a thorough uncertainty analysis on the determination of $D_{\mathrm{w}}$ which amounts to 2.1-2.5% for protons and 3.8-4.1% for ion beams. A major contribution of this uncertainty can be traced to $k_Q$ values (table 2.1).

The general concepts of TRS-398 CoP were adopted in ICRU report 78 [20] for protons and later in ICRU report 93 for light ion beam therapy [21], the latter adding a re-evaluation on $W_{\mathrm{air}}/e$. The national German protocol DIN6801-1 [22] also inherited the TRS-398 CoP concepts. A more explicit consideration of the effective point of measurement (EPOM) is given in DIN6801-1 following the analytical and MC-based calculations of Ref. [23]. The measurement within a solid phantom with the use of MC derived fluence correction factors [24] is allowed in this protocol and the use of

**Table 2.1**

**Uncertainty estimation for the determination of absorbed dose-to-water with a $^{60}$Co-calibrated ionization chamber for proton and ion beams following TRS-398 CoP. All values are given as relative standard uncertainty in %. For proton and carbon ion beams two values are given: the left value applies to cylindrical ionization chambers, the right one applies to plane-parallel ionization chambers.**

|                                            | protons    | ions      |
|--------------------------------------------|------------|-----------|
| $s_{w,air}$                                | 1.1        | 2.1       |
| assignment of $s_{w,air}$ to beam quality  | 0.4        | —         |
| $W_{air}/e$                                | 0.5        | 1.5       |
| Combined standard uncertainty in $p_Q$     | 1.1/ 1.7   | 1.0/ 1.8  |
| Combined standard uncertainty in $k_Q$     | 1.7/ 2.1   | 2.8/ 3.2  |
| Combined standard uncertainty in $D_{w,Q}$ | 2.1/ 2.5   | 3.8/ 4.1  |

more recent MC calculations for the perturbation correction factor $p_{Co}$ in $^{60}$Co radiation is the basis of tabulated $k_Q$ values.

Although a revision of TRS-398 CoP is underway, the concept stayed and still – twenty years after the first publication – the chamber-specific beam quality correction factors remain a major source of uncertainties for ion beams. For primary photon beams it has been demonstrated that the MC calculated $k_Q$ factors in conjunction with calorimetric measurements helped to decrease the $k_Q$ factor standard uncertainty approaching 0.4% [25], superseding the approximations made in the original TRS-398 CoP which led to 1%. This sets the expectation for MC calculations in proton and ion beam dosimetry, where a similar uncertainty is ultimately desired.

## 2.4   MONTE CARLO CODES

The relevant MC codes and systems for dosimetry are developed by large university and research institutions and resulting collaborations amongst them. In the case of proton and ion beams, the general-purpose codes, capable of simulating the electromagnetic and nuclear interactions of primary and secondary particles in the energy range for therapy down to a few keV (or eV of thermal neutrons), are suitable in general.

Nowadays various general-purpose codes are available to the research community with flexible geometry packages and physics processes and models the user can adjust. The latter is required to ensure the accurate simulation of transport in the often small regions of a radiation detector model. The codes typically used in ionization chamber simulations are Geant4 with the toolkits TOPAS and GATE [26, 27, 28], FLUKA [29] and PENH [30, 31, 32].

In the coupled photon/electron codes the calculation of ionization chamber response has historically been considered the classical challenge and limited the available codes for this specific task with low uncertainty to EGSnrc [33] and PENELOPE [31]. The modeling of multiple Coulomb scattering in an efficient condensed-history algorithm is one of the functionalities that any modern MC general purpose code provides. The proper and stable implementation for ionization chamber response calculations is however crucial, as handling the boundary crossing for the density change between the ionization chamber cavity and the surrounding may lead to artifacts. The magnitude of these artifacts depends on the code-specific implementations, but also on the user's choice e.g. of cut-off energies. The behavior of the MC code under such conditions can be tested objectively by means of the so-called Fano test. In a MC calculation, conditions of charged particle equilibrium (CPE) can be established which lead – as long as the local cross sections are uniform – to a constant fluence throughout the simulation geometry, independent of local density. A geometry with a low-density cavity surrounded by e.g. structures of higher density such as chamber wall or water phantom can be created and the expected result for the calculation determined. This concept has been applied to proton beams for the FLUKA code [34], Geant4 and PENH [35, 36].

The accuracy of hadronic nuclear interaction models on the other hand remains a challenge and it is specific to each available MC code [37]. There is currently no ultimate ground truth available to benchmark the results against. Hence, it remains an uncertainty to be considered in the calculated ionization chamber response.

## 2.5    IONIZATION CHAMBER-BASED DOSIMETRY (REFERENCE DOSIMETRY)

### 2.5.1    INDIRECT CALCULATION

Traditionally, $k_Q$ factors have been calculated using eq. 2.6. The reason for that is that perturbation correction factors in proton and carbon ion beams were unknown and, hence, assumed to be unity. This indirect approach was the one used in IAEA TRS-398 CoP.

#### 2.5.1.1    Water-to-air stopping-power ratios

With the assumption of perturbation factors equal to unity for proton and carbon ion beams, the role of MC simulations focuses on the calculation of water-to-air stopping-power ratios. In particular, MC simulations are used to calculate the fluence (differential in energy) of charged particles in water, $\Phi_w(E)$, entering in equations 2.1 and 2.2. In turn, for a given particle type, the fluence is calculated as

$$\Phi = \frac{\sum l}{V}, \tag{2.9}$$

where $\sum l$ is the sum of the track lengths of all the particles of the same type in the scoring volume $V$. Besides, restricted and unrestricted electronic stopping powers ($L_\Delta$ and $S_{el}$) are typically taken from international consensus data, such as ICRU 90 Report [38].

There are two ways of calculating the water-to-air stopping-power ratios. The "offline" method uses MC simulations only to obtain $\Phi(E)$ for all charged particles in water as well as in the scoring volume, and the calculation of $s_{w,air}$ is performed afterwards (i.e. offline) by computing the integral in equations 2.1 or 2.2. On the other hand, the "online" method computes $s_{w,air}$ directly in the MC code. That is, for each charged particle entering the scoring volume, its contribution to the fluence (i.e. track length per unit volume) is directly multiplied by the ratio of restricted (or unrestricted) electronic stopping powers, yielding directly the particle contribution to $s_{w,air}$ [39]. The online method has the advantage that it avoids any possible influence of the energy binning used to score the fluence – although this effect is negligible when a sufficiently dense energy binning is used for the offline calculation [12].

For proton beams, the water-to-air stopping-power ratios are relatively constant with depth until they increase steeply at the end of range – see Figure 2.1(left). The peak-to-entrance ratio decreases with increasing energy. This is due to range straggling, which makes the proton energy spectrum at the Bragg peak region much broader for higher energies. It is important to point out that Bragg–Gray $s_{w,air}$ values are systematically 0.5–0.6% lower than Spencer–Attix $s_{w,air}$ values [39, 11]. The reason is that the former do not account for the contribution of particles other than protons that have a sufficient energy to cross or escape the cavity (which are mainly secondary electrons).

For carbon ion beams, the water-to-air stopping-power ratios increase slowly with depth in the entrance region, they peak sharply at the Bragg peak region, and they fall and remain relatively constant in the fragmentation tail region – see Figure 2.1(right). As for protons, the peak-to-entrance ratio decreases with increasing energy due to range straggling, and so does the peak-to-tail ratio. For both proton and carbon ion beams, the main source of uncertainty in the $s_{w,air}$ values is the uncertainty in the mean excitation energy of water ($I_w$) (and air) used in the computation of electronic stopping powers [33, 38].

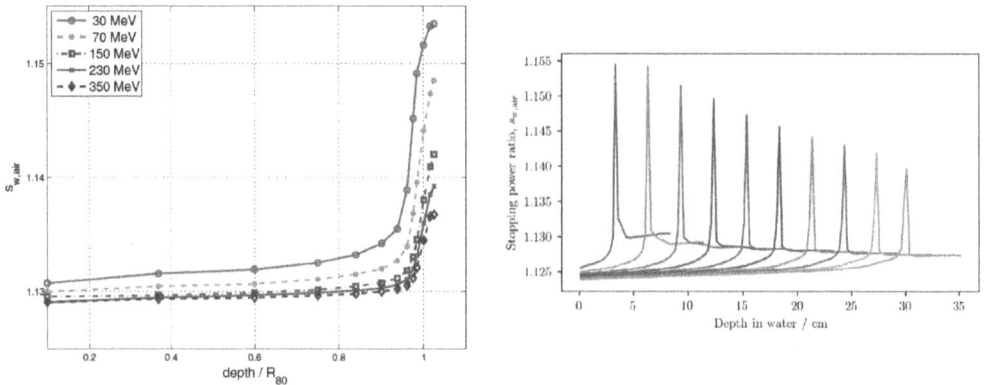

**Figure 2.1**    Left: Spencer–Attix $s_{w,air}$ values as a function of depth in terms of the $R_{90}$ for proton beams of initial energies from 30 to 350 MeV (taken from [12]). Right: Bragg–Gray $s_{w,air}$ values as a function of depth for carbon ion beams with a range in water between 3 and 30 cm (taken from [40]).

#### 2.5.1.2    $W_{air}$

A key component entering directly in the MC calculation of beam quality correction factors is the mean energy needed to create an ion pair in dry air ($W_{air}$) (eq. 2.6). ICRU 90 [38] recommends a value of $34.44 \pm 0.14$ eV for proton beams and $34.71 \pm 0.52$ eV for carbon ions, based on the comparison of ionization chamber dosimetry and calorimetry. It is worth pointing out that, due to the lack of data at that time, this comparison assumes perturbation correction factors equal to unity [8] – an assumption compensated for by an increased uncertainty. Since then, several publications have shown that, at least for proton beams, perturbation correction factors may be significantly different than unity. This recent data on perturbation factors could lead to a more accurate and precise estimation of $W_{air}$, at least for proton beams.

### 2.5.2    DIRECT CALCULATION

#### 2.5.2.1    Monte Carlo calculated $k_Q$ factors

The direct calculation of beam quality correction factors using MC simulations is an efficient and more accurate alternative to the indirect calculation. Using blueprints, the ionization chamber geometry needs to be modeled as accurately as possible in the MC code. For the modeling, the correct dimensions as well as material definitions like composition, mass density and mean ionization potential $I$ used to calculate the electronic stopping powers have to be considered. In order to determine $k_Q$ factors following equation 2.7, the dose values $D_w$ and $\bar{D}_{air}$ have to be calculated at the beam qualities $Q$ and $Q_0$. If the reference beam quality $Q_0$ is $^{60}$Co radiation, corresponding consensus $f_{Q_0}$ factors have already been published [25]. For the calculation of $D_w$, the absorbed dose-to-water in a reference volume positioned at the measurement depth within the water phantom has to be determined. Since $D_w$ is a punctual quantity, this volume should be as small as possible. However, in order to guarantee a reasonable computing time the volume cannot be infinitely small. Hence, the user has to increase this volume in a way that the average dose stays constant. E.g. in broad photon and proton beams some authors have used a disk with a diameter in the order of 1 cm and a height in beam direction of 250 µm positioned with its center at the measurement depth. To calculate $\bar{D}_{air}$

the absorbed dose in the air-filled cavity has to be determined. This can be achieved either by directly scoring the dose-to-air in the cavity or by scoring the deposited energy within the cavity and subsequently deriving the dose by dividing the deposited energy by the mass of the cavity.

Especially for the calculation of $\bar{D}_{air}$, the simulations have to be carried out as detailed as possible due to the complex geometry and possible large differences in mass densities between the individual constructive details of the chamber – e.g. graphite in the chamber wall and air in the cavity. In particular, the production rate and range of secondary electrons highly depends on the atomic composition and mass density of the material. Hence, to avoid fluence artifacts, the production threshold for secondary particles has to be set as low as reasonable possible. Most commonly a threshold in the order of 1 keV to 10 keV is chosen. Additionally, the length of a condensed history step has to be adjusted to be smaller than the dimensions of the constructive details of the chamber. However, the more accurate the simulation, the longer the computing time. Hence, it is convenient to conduct these detailed simulations only within the region of interest – in this case the chamber geometry – and a surrounding envelope as shown in Figure 2.2. In the residual geometry – in this case the residual water phantom – larger production cuts and longer condensed history steps can be applied. The envelope surrounding the chamber geometry guarantees that the particle fluence inside the chamber is not perturbed by the larger production cuts applied outside the envelope and, hence, should be large enough. A possible approach is to choose the thickness to be at least the *continuous slowing down approximation range* $R_{CSDA}$ corresponding to the production cut applied outside the envelope multiplied with a safety factor of 1.2.

Concerning the dimensions of the water phantom, it should be larger than the applied proton beam by at least 5 cm to all four sides and by at least 5 g cm$^{-2}$ longer than the maximum measurement depth. However, for simulations of proton beams, the water phantom might be shorter since backscattering can be considered negligible.

In the updated version of the TRS-398 CoP, MC calculated $f_Q$ factors are included in the derivation of $k_Q$ factors in clinical proton beams. So far, PENH, Geant4, and FLUKA have been used to calculate $f_Q$ and $k_Q$ factors for several plane-parallel and cylindrical ionization chambers in clinical proton beams [42, 35, 43, 44, 45, 46]. All codes were able to calculate $k_Q$ factors in agreement with experimental data on the 1.5% level [47, 48, 49].

In Figure 2.3 MC calculated $k_Q$ factors for two exemplary ionization chambers are shown for protons: the cylindrical NE 2571 Farmer chamber and the plane-parallel NACP-02. Additionally, the corresponding $k_Q$ factors as calculated following the TRS-398 CoP in the version from 2000 [13] are shown. A fit through the MC calculated $k_Q$ factors is given as well. The fit for the NE 2571 chamber only includes energies of 150 MeV or higher as explained later in this chapter.

Concerning the comparison between the different MC codes it can be seen that they lead to comparable results for low and medium energies with deviations of $\sim$1.2% at maximum. However, larger differences of up to 2.0% can be observed for higher energies while PENH leads to the largest $k_Q$ factors and FLUKA to the smallest ones. Correspondingly, the uncertainty of the fit increases with energy. The divergence between the codes at high energies might be due to the fact that different nuclear interaction models are implemented in the various MC codes whereas the impact of these nuclear interactions increases with energy. Unfortunately, experimental data for $k_Q$ factors for this energy regime are available only for two cylindrical ionization chambers [49], whereas the results of the MC codes agree with the experimental values within one standard uncertainty.

While $k_Q$ shows almost no dependency on energy for the plane-parallel chamber, it is strongly pronounced for cylindrical chambers where $k_Q$ increases for decreasing energy. The reason is that, following the TRS-398 CoP, cylindrical chambers are placed with their symmetry axis at the measurement depth and not with their effective point of measurement (EPOM). The effective point of measurement accounts for the displacement of the surrounding medium by the chamber and is defined as the point in water where the particle fluence is the same as in the air cavity of the chamber [50, 22, 23]. Typically, the effective point of measurement is positioned between the

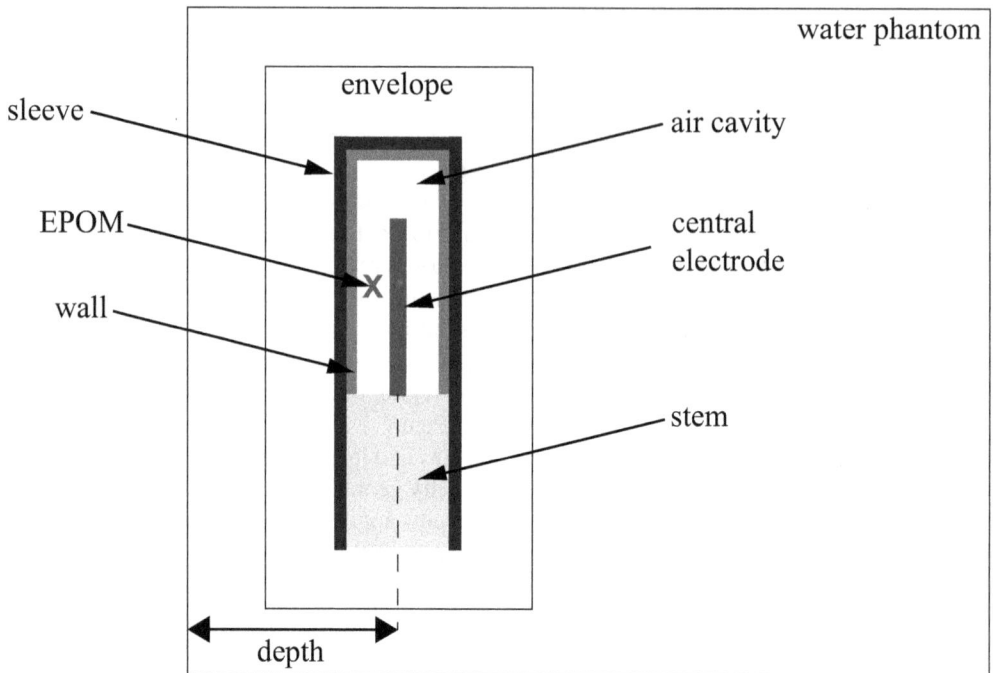

**Figure 2.2**   Scheme of a cylindrical ionization chamber and the corresponding simulation set-up for MC calculation of $k_Q$ factors. The beam is coming from the left. The effective point of measurement (EPOM) is marked by a cross.

central electrode and chamber wall within the air cavity [50, 22] (see Figure 2.2). If the chamber is placed with its EPOM at the measurement depth, the $k_Q$ factor is independent on energy as shown in Figure 2.3. The difference in $k_Q$ factors for both placements is almost negligible for energies of 150 MeV or higher. As a result, in the upcoming version of the TRS-398 CoP cylindrical chambers will only be proposed for high energies starting from 150 MeV which is also the reason why the fit of MC calculated $k_Q$ factors includes only these energies. Note that the energy dependence of $k_Q$ is not present for plane-parallel chambers since they are positioned with their EPOM at the measurement depth. For plane-parallel chambers the EPOM is positioned at the center of the inner surface of the chamber's entrance window.

Concerning the comparison of MC calculated $k_Q$ factors with the values tabulated in the TRS-398 CoP in the version from 2000 [13] it can be seen that, for the plane-parallel chamber, an agreement on the 1% level is achieved for low and medium energies. For high energies larger deviations of up to 2% are present while especially the values calculated with FLUKA are smaller. The agreement between the TRS-398 CoP values and the MC calculated fit is better than 1% for all energies. For the cylindrical chamber larger deviations between the TRS-398 CoP and individual MC values of up to 2.8% are present for both low and high energies while the deviations for low energies are due to the fact that the EPOM is not considered in the TRS-398 CoP. The deviations for high energies might be due to the fact that the perturbation correction factor $p_Q$ is approximated to be unity in the TRS-398 CoP while especially for high energies the chamber wall leads to a fluence perturbation as discussed in the next chapter. The difference between the TRS-398 CoP values and the fit of MC calculated $k_Q$ factors is up to 2%.

Since MC codes are under constant further development, especially concerning the improvement of underlying physics models, different version of a MC code might lead to significantly different

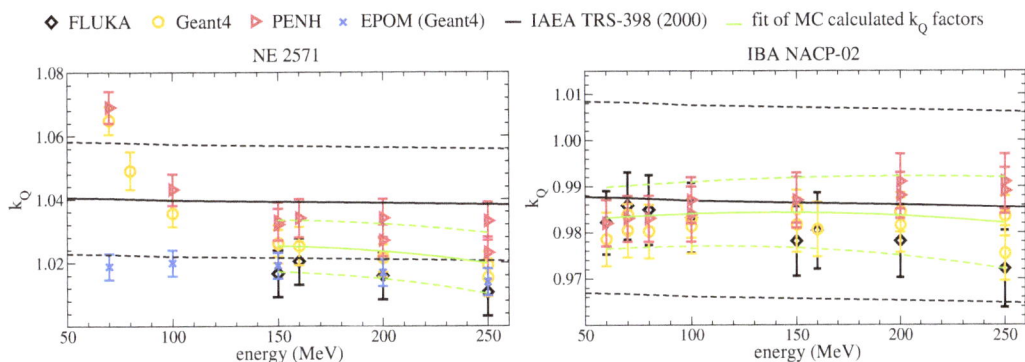

**Figure 2.3**  MC calculated $k_Q$ factors for monoenergetic proton beams as a function of initial proton energy for the codes FLUKA, Geant4 and PENH. The error bars correspond to one standard uncertainty. The solid black line represents the $k_Q$ factors as calculated according to the TRS-398 CoP from 2000 [13]. In dashed lines the corresponding uncertainties (k = 1) of the TRS values are shown. The solid green line depicts a fit through the MC calculated $k_Q$ factors with corresponding uncertainties (k = 1) in dashed lines. For the NE 2571 chamber the fit only includes energies of 150 MeV or higher.

results when calculating $f_Q$ or $k_Q$ factors. In Figure 2.4 the $f_Q$ factors for two exemplary ionization chambers for high energies are shown for different versions of the MC code Geant4. The differences between both versions are up to 0.9%.

### 2.5.2.2  Monte Carlo calculated perturbation correction factors

Several MC-based studies investigated different aspects of perturbation effects, e.g. the perturbation induced by the chamber wall [51, 52]. Individual perturbation correction factors in clinical proton beams for ionization chambers were recently calculated using Geant4 and FLUKA [34, 45, 53]. In order to determine perturbation correction factors the chamber has to be modeled in the MC code and the dose absorbed in the air cavity has to be calculated as described before. Subsequently, constructive details of the chamber are being removed step by step and after each step the dose absorbed in the air cavity is calculated (compare Figure 2.5). By comparing the dose values the individual perturbation corrections factors can be determined. In a last step, the dose absorbed to water in a reference volume has to be calculated. Using this method, the perturbation factors for the central electrode $p_{cel}$, chamber stem $p_{stem}$, sleeve $p_{sleeve}$, wall $p_{wall}$, and the product of $p_{cav} \cdot p_{dis} \cdot s_{w,air}$ can be determined. The product of $p_{cav} \cdot p_{dis} \cdot s_{w,air}$ takes into account that the chamber cavity consists of air ($s_{w,air}$) compared to the surrounding medium water in which the dose shall be determined, that the chamber has finite dimensions ($p_{cav}$) and also leads to a displacement of the surrounding medium ($p_{dis}$).

Exemplary perturbation correction factors for one cylindrical and one plane-parallel ionization chamber are shown in Figure 2.6. For the cylindrical ionization chamber, the perturbation correction factors $p_{cel}$, $p_{stem}$ and $p_{sleeve}$ are close to unity and show no significant dependency on energy. The product of the perturbation correction factors $p_{cav} \cdot p_{dis}$ is larger than unity and shows a pronounced dependency on energy: For low energies it is larger and decreases with increasing energy. The reason is that, following the TRS-398 CoP, the EPOM is not considered. The perturbation correction factor $p_{wall}$ is smaller than and significantly different from unity. The reason is that secondary particles, especially alpha particles and other fragments from nuclear interactions, that are scattered from the chamber wall into the air cavity lead to an overresponse of the chamber and hence a perturbation

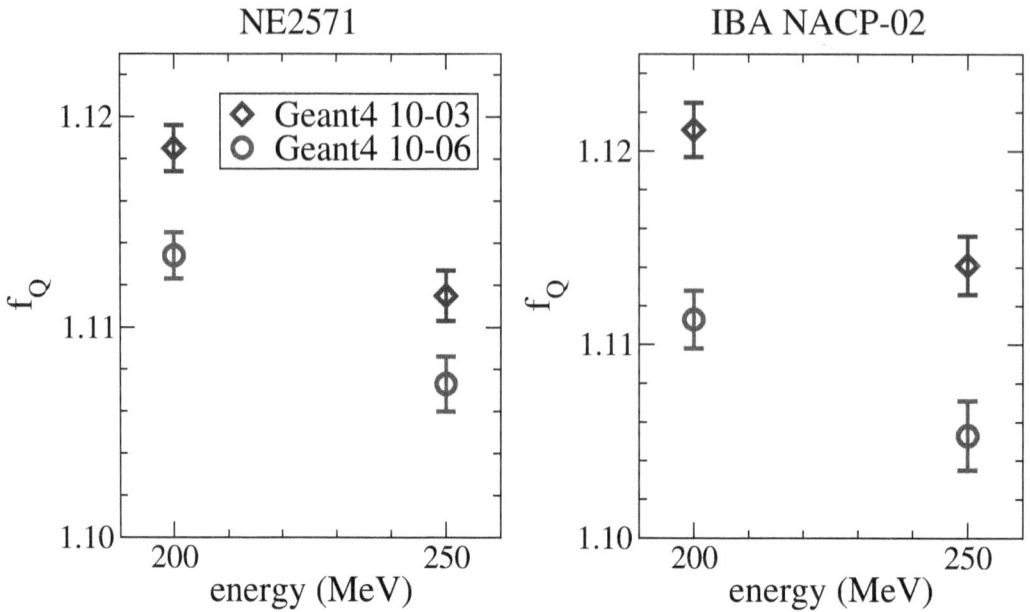

**Figure 2.4** The influence of different versions of the MC code Geant4 on the calculation of $f_Q$ factors for high energies.

correction factor smaller than unity.[2] The deviation of $p_{wall}$ from unity is larger the thicker the chamber wall. The total perturbation correction factor $p_Q$ depends on energy and follows the course of $p_{cav} \cdot p_{dis}$. For small energies it is larger than unity, for high energies it is smaller than unity. The largest deviation of $p_Q$ from unity is 2.0%. In the upcoming version of the TRS-398 CoP cylindrical chambers will be recommended for energies of at least 150 MeV. For this energy regime the average deviation of $p_Q$ from unity is 0.9% and the maximum deviation is 1.5%.

For the plane-parallel ionization chamber fewer perturbation correction factors can be calculated due to a less complex geometry of the chamber type. While the perturbation correction factor $p_{cav}$ is larger than unity, the factor $p_{wall}$ is smaller than unity. The resulting total perturbation correction factor $p_Q$ is smaller than unity, as well, with a maximum deviation from unity of 1.3%.

In general, perturbation correction factors of ionization chambers in proton beams can be significantly different from unity – in contrast to the assumption from the TRS-398 CoP. This is an explanation for the discrepancy between MC calculated $k_Q$ factors and the values tabulated in the TRS-398 CoP as shown in Figure 2.3: For chambers and energies where the total perturbation correction factor $p_Q$ is significantly different from unity, the deviation between the MC calculated $k_Q$ factors and the values from the TRS-398 CoP is larger.

## 2.6  FUTURE CHALLENGES IN MONTE CARLO-BASED DOSIMETRY

Since MC simulations are well-established for clinical dosimetry applications, the use of these simulations will further increase in the future. Not only due to a cost reduction of computing power, MC simulations will get more and more interesting in the clinical routine, e.g. as a support of QA measurements. However, it has to be kept in mind that all MC generated results depend on the usage of each code and the code itself. On the one hand, the modeling of an air-filled ionization chamber in a MC code does not only depend on the accuracy of the blueprint the user has at hand and the user's

---

[2]Note that it might also be that these particles are produced in water and less particles are stopped by the chamber wall.

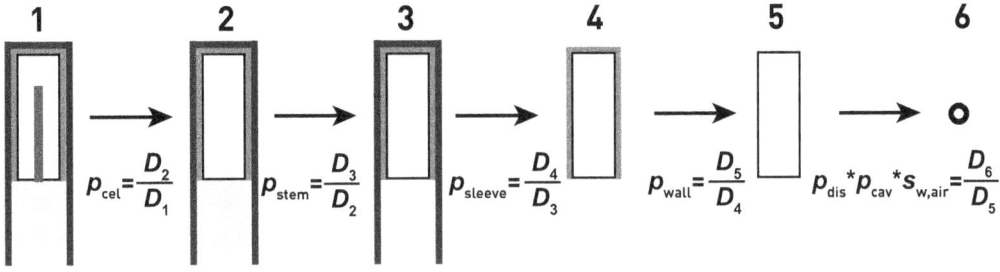

**Figure 2.5**  Schematic description of the determination of perturbation correction factors for cylindrical air-filled ionization chambers. The perturbation correction factors are derived by comparing the dose values calculated in the air-filled cavities while specific constructive details are missing (steps 1 to 5) and the absorbed dose-to-water calculated in a water-filled reference volume (step 6). The dose $D_i$ is the dose absorbed in the cavity in step $i$ (taken from [53]).

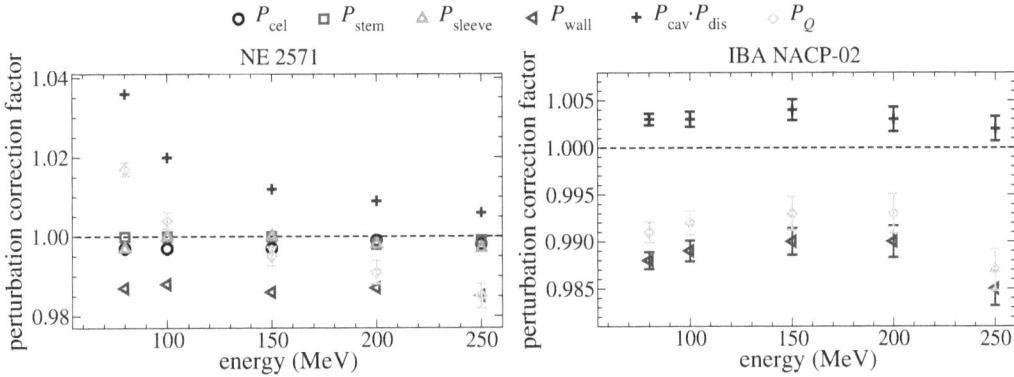

**Figure 2.6**  Perturbation correction factors for cylindrical and plane-parallel ionization chambers as a function of initial proton energy. The error bars correspond to one standard deviation. For data points where the error bars are smaller than the symbol size none are depicted. A dashed line is used to visualize $p = 1$ (taken from [53]).

ability to translate this blueprint into a chamber geometry using the predefined geometry components provided by the MC code. It also depends crucially on the definition of the materials installed in the chamber concerning mass density, the ionization potential and other material characteristics like the composition of a compound material.

On the other hand, the accuracy of the MC simulations depends on the physical models implemented in the code. This becomes especially apparent when looking at the $k_Q$ factors at high energies calculated with different MC codes as it seems that different models describing the nuclear interactions lead to different results. Hence, a future challenge for the improvement of MC calculated quantities will be to reduce type-B uncertainties, e.g. by enhancing the accuracy of nuclear interaction models. One possibility to achieve this is by measuring nuclear reaction cross sections [54, 55]. In general, the user of MC codes has to keep in mind that improvements of the underlying physics models can lead to different results in the calculation of dosimetric quantities.

Further challenges lie in the consideration of the possible death volume within the air-filled cavity in the presence of a guard ring [56]. This guard ring is used to apply an electric field in order to prevent that secondary particles scattering from the chamber stem into the air-cavity distort the measured charge. In MC simulations this death volume is not taken into account which might influence the calculation of $f_Q$ and, hence, $k_Q$ factors. Since the amount of secondary particles being scattered from the chamber stem into the cavity is small in proton beams – which correlates to a perturbation correction factor $p_{stem}$ being close to unity – this effect might be negligible as shown by Ref. [44].

## REFERENCES

1. A. Wambersie, P. Deluca, P. Andreo, and J. Hendry, "Light" or heavy" ions : a debate of terminology?," *Radiotherapy and Oncology*, vol. 73, p. iiii, 2004. Carbon-Ion Therapy.
2. M. T. Gillin, N. Sahoo, M. Bues, G. Ciangaru, G. Sawakuchi, F. Poenish, B. Arjomandy, C. Martin, U. Titt, K. Suzuki, A. R. Smith, and X. R. Zhu, "Commissioning of the discrete spot scanning proton beam delivery system at the University of Texas M.D. Anderson Cancer Center, Proton Therapy Center, Houston," *Medical Physics*, vol. 37, no. 1, pp. 154–63, 2010.
3. B. Clasie, N. Depauw, M. Fransen, C. Gomà, H. R. Panahandeh, J. Seco, J. B. Flanz, and H. Kooy, "Golden beam data for proton pencil-beam scanning," *Physics in Medicine and Biology*, vol. 57, no. 5, pp. 1147–58, 2012.
4. C. Gomà, S. Safai, and S. Vörös, "Reference dosimetry of proton pencil beams based on dose-area product: a proof of concept," *Physics in Medicine and Biology*, vol. 62, no. 12, pp. 4991–5005, 2017.
5. H. Palmans, "Monte carlo calculations for proton and ion beam dosimetry," in *Monte Carlo Techniques in Radiation Therapy* (F. V. Joao Seco, ed.), pp. 185–199, CRC Press, Taylor & Francis Group, 2013.
6. L. Petrie, S. Galer, D. Shipley, and H. Palmans, "Monte carlo calculated correction factors for the npl proton calorimeter," *Radiation Physics and Chemistry*, vol. 140, pp. 383–385, 2017. 2nd International Conference on Dosimetry and its Applications (ICDA-2) University of Surrey, Guildford, United Kingdom, 3-8 July 2016.
7. C. Gomà, S. Lorentini, D. Meer, and S. Safai, "Proton beam monitor chamber calibration," *Physics in Medicine and Biology*, vol. 59, no. 17, pp. 4961–71, 2014.
8. C. Gomà, S. Lorentini, D. Meer, and S. Safai, "Reply to comment on 'proton beam monitor chamber calibration'," *Physics in Medicine and Biology*, vol. 61, no. 17, pp. 6494–601, 2016.
9. F. H. Attix, *Introduction to radiological physics and radiation dosimetry*. Mörlanbach: Wiley-VCH, 1986.
10. A. Nahum, "Water/air mass stopping power ratios for megavoltage photon and electron beams," *Physics in Medicine and Biology*, vol. 23, no. 5, pp. 24–38, 1978.
11. R. F. Laitano and M. Rosetti, "Proton stopping powers averaged over beam energy spectra," *Physics in Medicine and Biology*, vol. 45, no. 10, pp. 3025–43, 2000.
12. C. Gomà, P. Andreo, and J. Sempau, "Spencer–attix water/medium stopping-power ratios for the dosimetry of proton pencil beams," *Physics in Medicine and Biology*, vol. 58, no. 8, pp. 2509–22, 2013.
13. P. Andreo, D. T. Burns, K. Hohlfeld, M. S. Huq, T. Kanai, F. Laitano, V. G. Smythe, and S. Vynckier, "Absorbed dose determination in external beam radiotherapy. An international code of practice for dosimetry based on standards of absorbed dose to water," Technical Reports Series No. 398, International Atomic Energy Agency, 2000.
14. A. E. Nahum, "Perturbation effects in dosimetry: Part I. Kilovoltage x-rays and electrons," *Physics in Medicine and Biology*, vol. 41, no. 9, pp. 1531–80, 1996.
15. J. Sempau, P. Andreo, J. Aldana, J. Mazurier, and F. Salvat, "Electron beam quality correction factors for plane-parallel ionization chambers: Monte Carlo calculations using the PENELOPE system," *Physics in Medicine and Biology*, vol. 49, no. 18, pp. 4427–44, 2004.

16. P. Andreo, J. Wulff, D. T. Burns, and H. Palmans, "Consistency in reference radiotherapy dosimetry: resolution of an apparent conundrum when $^{60}$Co is the reference quality for charged-particle and photon beams," *Physics in Medicine and Biology*, vol. 58, no. 19, pp. 6593–621, 2013.

17. S. Vynckier, D. Bonnett, and D. Jones, "Code of practice for clinical proton dosimetry," *Radiotherapy and Oncology*, vol. 20, no. 1, pp. 53–63, 1991.

18. J. T. Leyman, G. T. Y. Chen, P. Fessenden, M. Goitein, J. C. Mcdonald, and A. F. Smith, "Protocol for Heavy Charged-Particle Therapy Beam Dosimetry," A Report of Task Group 20 Radiation Therapy (New York, USA), American Association of Physicists in Medicine, 1986.

19. L. Verhey, H. Blattman, P. M. Deluca, and D. Miller, "Clinical Proton Dosimetry Part I: Beam Production, Beam Delivery and Measurement of Absorbed Dose," ICRU Report 59, International Commission on Radiation Units and Measurements, 1998.

20. D. T. L. Jones, H. D. Suit, Y. Akine, G. Goitein, N. Kanematsu, R. L. Maughan, T. Tatsuzaki, H. Tsuijii, and S. M. Vatnitsky, "Prescribing, Recording, and Reporting Proton-Beam Therapy," *Journal of the ICRU*, vol. 7, no. 2, 2007.

21. O. Jäkel, "Icru report 93: Prescribing, recording, and reporting light ion beam therapy," *Journal of the ICRU*, vol. 16, 2019.

22. "Dosismessverfahren nach der Sondenmethode für Protonen- und Ionenstrahlung – Teil 1: Ionisationskammern," DIN 6801-1, Normenausschuss Radiologie (NAR) im DIN, 2019.

23. H. Palmans, "Perturbation factors for cylindrical ionization chambers in proton beams. Part i: corrections for gradients," *Physics in Medicine and Biology*, vol. 51, no. 14, pp. 3483–501, 2006.

24. H. Palmans, J. E. Symons, J.-M. Denis, E. A. de Kock, D. T. L. Jones, and S. Vynckier, "Fluence correction factors in plastic phantoms for clinical proton beams," *Physics in Medicine and Biology*, vol. 47, pp. 3055–3071, aug 2002.

25. P. Andreo, D. T. Burns, R. P. Kapsch, M. McEwen, S. Vatnitsky, C. E. Andersen, F. Ballester, J. Borbinha, F. Delaunay, P. Francescon, M. D. Hanlon, L. Mirzakhanian, B. Muir, J. Ojala, C. P. Oliver, M. Pimpinella, M. Pinto, L. A. de Prez, J. Seuntjens, L. Sommier, P. Teles, J. Tikkanen, J. Vijande, and K. Zink, "Determination of consensus k q values for megavoltage photon beams for the update of IAEA TRS-398," *Physics in Medicine & Biology*, vol. 65, p. 095011, may 2020.

26. S. Agostinelli, J. Allison, K. Amako, J. Apostolakis, H. Araujo, P. Arce, M. Asai, D. Axen, S. Banerjee, G. Barrand, F. Behner, L. Bellagamba, J. Boudreau, L. Broglia, A. Brunengo, H. Burkhardt, S. Chauvie, J. Chuma, R. Chytracek, G. Cooperman, G. Cosmo, P. Degtyarenko, A. Dell'Acqua, G. Depaola, D. Dietrich, R. Enami, A. Feliciello, C. Ferguson, H. Fesefeldt, G. Folger, F. Foppiano, A. Forti, S. Garelli, S. Giani, R. Giannitrapani, D. Gibin, J. G. Cadenas, I. González, G. G. Abril, G. Greeniaus, W. Greiner, V. Grichine, A. Grossheim, S. Guatelli, P. Gumplinger, R. Hamatsu, K. Hashimoto, H. Hasui, A. Heikkinen, A. Howard, V. Ivanchenko, A. Johnson, F. Jones, J. Kallenbach, N. Kanaya, M. Kawabata, Y. Kawabata, M. Kawaguti, S. Kelner, P. Kent, A. Kimura, T. Kodama, R. Kokoulin, M. Kossov, H. Kurashige, E. Lamanna, T. Lampén, V. Lara, V. Lefebure, F. Lei, M. Liendl, W. Lockman, F. Longo, S. Magni, M. Maire, E. Medernach, K. Minamimoto, P. M. de Freitas, Y. Morita, K. Murakami, M. Nagamatu, R. Nartallo, P. Nieminen, T. Nishimura, K. Ohtsubo, M. Okamura, S. O'Neale, Y. Oohata, K. Paech, J. Perl, A. Pfeiffer, M. Pia, F. Ranjard, A. Rybin, S. Sadilov, E. D. Salvo, G. Santin, T. Sasaki, N. Savvas, Y. Sawada, S. Scherer, S. Sei, V. Sirotenko, D. Smith, N. Starkov, H. Stoecker, J. Sulkimo, M. Takahata, S. Tanaka, E. Tcherniaev, E. S. Tehrani, M. Tropeano, P. Truscott, H. Uno, L. Urban, P. Urban, M. Verderi, A. Walkden, W. Wander, H. Weber, J. Wellisch, T. Wenaus, D. Williams, D. Wright, T. Yamada, H. Yoshida, and D. Zschiesche, "Geant4—a simulation toolkit," *Nuclear Instruments and Methods in Physics Research A*, vol. 506, no. 3, pp. 250–303, 2003.

27. J. Perl, J. Shin, J. Schumann, B. Faddegon, and H. Paganetti, "TOPAS: an innovative proton Monte Carlo platform for research and clinical applications," *Medical Physics*, vol. 39, no. 11, pp. 6818–37, 2012.

28. S. Jan, D. Benoit, E. Becheva, T. Carlier, F. Cassol, P. Descourt, T. Frisson, L. Grevillot, L. Guigues, L. Maigne, C. Morel, Y. Perrot, N. Rehfeld, D. Sarrut, D. R. Schaart, S. Stute, U. Pietrzyk, D. Visvikis, N. Zahra, and I. Buvat, "GATE v6: a major enhancement of the GATE simulation platform enabling modelling of CT and radiotherapy," *Physics in Medicine and Biology*, vol. 56, pp. 881–901, jan 2011.

29. T. Böhlen, F. Cerutti, M. Chin, A. Fassò, A. Ferrari, P. Ortega, A. Mairani, P. Sala, G. Smirnov, and V. Vlachoudis, "The FLUKA code: Developments and challenges for high energy and medical applications," *Nuclear Data Sheets*, vol. 120, pp. 211–214, 2014.

30. F. Salvat, "A generic algorithm for Monte Carlo simulation of proton transport," *Nuclear Instruments and Methods in Physics Research B*, vol. 316, pp. 144–159, 2013.

31. F. Salvat, PENELOPE-2014: *A code system for Monte Carlo simulation of electron and photon transport*. Nuclear Energy Agency, 2014.

32. F. Salvat and J. M. Quesada, "Nuclear effects in proton transport and dose calculations," *Nuclear Instruments and Methods in Physics Research Section B: Beam Interactions with Materials and Atoms*, vol. 475, pp. 49–62, 2020.

33. I. Kawrakow, E. Mainegra-Hing, D. Rogers, F. Tessier, and B. Walters, *The EGSnrc Code System: Monte Carlo simulation of electron and photon transport. Technical Report PIRS-701*. National Research Council Canada, 2017.

34. A. Lourenço, H. Bouchard, S. Galer, G. Royle, and H. Palmans, "The influence of nuclear interactions on ionization chamber perturbation factors in proton beams: Fluka simulations supported by a fano test," *Medical Physics*, vol. 46, no. 2, pp. 885–891, 2019.

35. J. Wulff, K.-S. Baumann, N. Verbeek, C. Bäumer, B. Timmermann, and K. Zink, "TOPAS/Geant4 configuration for ionization chamber calculations in proton beams," *Physics in Medicine and Biology*, vol. 63, no. 11, p. 115013, 2018.

36. E. Sterpin, J. Sorriaux, K. Souris, S. Vynckier, and H. Bouchard, "A Fano cavity test for Monte Carlo proton transport algorithms," *Medical Physics*, vol. 41, no. 1, p. 11706, 2014.

37. S. Muraro, G. Battistoni, and A. Kraan, "Challenges in monte carlo simulations as clinical and research tool in particle therapy: A review," *Frontiers in Physics*, vol. 8, p. 391, 2020.

38. S. M. Seltzer, J. M. Fernández-Varea, P. Andreo, P. M. Bergstrom, D. T. Burns, I. Krajcar Bronić, C. K. Ross, and F. Salvat, "Key data for ionizing-radiation dosimetry: measurement standards and applications. ICRU Report 90," *Journal of the ICRU*, vol. 14, pp. 1–110, 2016.

39. J. Medin and P. Andreo, "Monte Carlo calculated stopping-power ratios, water/air, for clinical proton dosimetry (50-250 MeV)," *Physics in Medicine and Biology*, vol. 42, no. 1, pp. 89–105, 1997.

40. L. N. Burigo and S. Greilich, "Impact of new ICRU 90 key data on stopping-power ratios and beam quality correction factors for carbon ion beams," *Physics in Medicine and Biology*, vol. 64, no. 19, p. 195005, 2019.

41. K. Henkner, N. Bassler, N. Sobolevsky, and O. Jäckel, "Monte Carlo simulations on the water-to-air stopping power ratio for carbon ion dosimetry," *Medical Physics*, vol. 36, no. 4, pp. 1230–5, 2009.

42. C. Gomà, P. Andreo, and J. Sempau, "Monte Carlo calculation of beam quality correction factors in proton beams using detailed simulation of ionization chambers," *Physics in Medicine and Biology*, vol. 61, no. 6, pp. 2389–406, 2016.

43. C. Gomà and E. Sterpin, "Monte carlo calculation of beam quality correction factors in proton beams using PENH," *Physics in Medicine and Biology*, vol. 64, no. 18, p. 185009, 2019.

44. K.-S. Baumann, S. Kaupa, C. Bach, R. Engenhart-Cabillic, and K. Zink, "Monte carlo calculation of beam quality correction factors in proton beams using TOPAS/GEANT4," *Physics in Medicine and Biology*, vol. 65, no. 5, p. 055015, 2020.

45. J. Kretschemer, A. Dulkys, L. Brodbek, T. S. Stelljes, H. K. Looe, and B. Poppe, "Monte Carlo simulated beam quality and perturbation correction factors for ionization chambers in monoenergetic proton beams," *Medical Physics*, vol. 47, no. 11, pp. 5890–5905, 2020.

46. K.-S. Baumann, L. Derksen, M. Witt, J. Burg, R. Engenhart-Cabillic, and K. Zink, "Monte carlo calculation of beam quality correction factors in proton beams using fluka," *Physics in Medicine and Biology*, vol. 66, 2021.

47. J. Medin, C. K. Ross, N. V. Klassen, H. Palmans, E. Grusell, and J.-E. Grindborg, "Experimental determination of beam quality factors, $k_q$, for two types of Farmer chamber in a 10 MV photon and a 175 MeV proton beam," *Physics in Medicine and Biology*, vol. 51, no. 6, pp. 1503–21, 2006.

48. J. Medin, "Implementation of water calorimetry in a 180 MeV scanned pulsed proton beam including an experimental determination of $k_q$ for a Farmer chamber," *Physics in Medicine and Biology*, vol. 55, no. 12, pp. 3287–98, 2010.

49. J. Medin, P. Andreo, and H. Palmans, "Experimental determination of kq factors for two types of ionization chambers in scanned proton beams," *Physics in Medicine & Biology*, 2022.

50. "Dosismessverfahren nach derSondenmethode für Photonen- und Elektronenstrahlung – Teil 2: Dosimetrie hochenergetischer Photonen- und Elektronenstrahlung mit Ionisationskammern," DIN 6800-2, Normenausschuss Radiologie (NAR) im DIN, 2006.

51. H. Palmans and F. Verhaegen, "Monte Carlo study of fluence perturbation effects on cavity dose response in clinical proton beams," *Physics in Medicine and Biology*, vol. 43, no. 1, pp. 65–89, 1998.

52. H. Palmans, "Secondary electron perturbations in farmer type ion chambers for clinical proton beams," in *Standards, Applications and Quality Assurance in Medical Radiation Dosimetry (IDOS)*, (Vienna), pp. 309–17, International Atomic Energy Agency, 2011.

53. K.-S. Baumann, S. Kaupa, C. Bach, R. Engenhart-Cabillic, and K. Zink, "Monte carlo calculation of perturbation correction factors for air-filled ionization chambers in clinical proton beams using topas/geant4," *Zeitschrift für Medizinische Physik*, vol. 31, no. 2, pp. 175–191, 2021.

54. F. Horst, C. Schuy, U. Weber, K.-T. Brinkmann, and K. Zink, "Measurement of charge- and mass-changing cross sections for $^4$He $+^{12}$C collisions in the energy range 80–220 mev/u for applications in ion beam therapy," *Physical Review C*, vol. 96, p. 024624, Aug 2017.

55. F. Horst, G. Aricò, K.-T. Brinkmann, S. Brons, A. Ferrari, T. Haberer, A. Mairani, K. Parodi, C.-A. Reidel, U. Weber, K. Zink, and C. Schuy, "Measurement of $^4$He charge- and mass-changing cross sections on h, c, o, and si targets in the energy range 70–220 mev/u for radiation transport calculations in ion-beam therapy," *Physical Review C*, vol. 99, p. 014603, Jan 2019.

56. S. Pojtinger, R.-P. Kapsch, O. S. Dohm, and D. Thorwarth, "A finite element method for the determination of the relative response of ionization chambers in MR-linacs: simulation and experimental validation up to 1.5 t," *Physics in Medicine & Biology*, vol. 64, no. 13, p. 135011, 2019.

# 3 Solving range uncertainties with gamma prompt/ charged particle prompt

*Marco Pinto*
Ludwig-Maximilians-University of Munich, Munich, Germany

*Vincenzo Patera*
Sapienza University of Rome, Rome, Italy

## CONTENTS

## 3.1 PROMPT-GAMMA RADIATION

### 3.1.1 REQUESTS ON A RANGE MONITOR DEVICE EXPLOITING PG RADIATION

Ion range monitoring exploiting PG radiation poses considerable challenges. The broad energy spectrum of the PG radiation up to 10 MeV makes developing PG cameras particularly difficult due to the extensive energy range and the relatively high energy (see Figure 3.1). As comparison, positron emission tomography (PET) monitoring operates by detecting 511-keV events in coincidence. A PET scanner for ion range monitoring has challenges, but the energy is well defined and relatively low compared to PG monitoring. Some research groups exploit the PG characteristic emission from specific transitions for ion range monitoring, making the target energy well defined. However, the energy continues to be relatively high, typically above 4 MeV. The PG spectroscopy section below covers this topic. Another challenge is related to the nature of this radiation: prompt radiation. PG radiation is generally emitted in less than a nanosecond, forcing its detection at irradiation time. Conversely, PET monitoring is not typically performed while the beam is being delivered, even for the case of in-beam PET modality which is usually achieved using the delayed radiation emitted in-between spills [7]. There are exceptions (e.g. [58]) but they are not the norm in terms of PET monitoring. Acquiring events when the beam is effectively on forces the system to deal with high

DOI: 10.1201/9781003023920-3

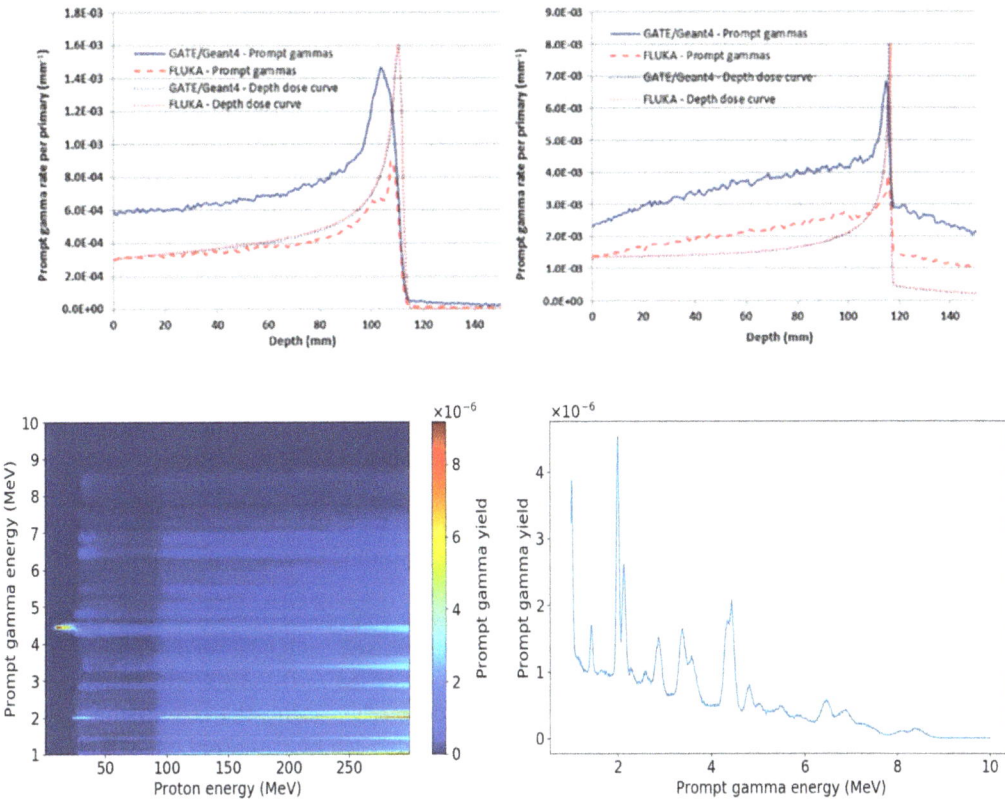

**Figure 3.1** Simulated profiles of PG radiation exiting a PMMA phantom obtained using GATE/Geant4 and FLUKA for a 134-MeV proton beam (top left) and 260-AMeV carbon ion beam (top right). Incident proton energy as a function of simulated PG radiation energy (bottom left) and PG energy spectrum for a 150-MeV proton beam (bottom right). Top figures from [52] and bottom figures from [45].

background levels. While PET monitoring avoids such a background, PG monitoring must always deal with it. The most straightforward approach used ever since the infancy of PG monitoring to partially tackle the background is to apply energy thresholds (sometimes also referred to as energy windows and energy selection) on the events detected (e.g. [33, 35, 60]). The rationale is that scattered photons and photons originating from neutron capture tend to have lower energies than PG [35]. The energy threshold strategy should not be confused with PG spectroscopy. The former tries to remove unwanted (i.e. not correlated to ion range) background events from the data, while the latter uses the photons of well-defined energy from specific transitions to assess ion range. To what extent using energy thresholds removes valuable information is still unclear. For example, exploiting low-energy photons from bremsstrahlung has been proposed as an ion range monitoring technique for both proton [70, 3] and carbon ion [71] therapies. A significant component of the research in this field relies on Monte Carlo simulations.

Regarding imaging needs, in theory, ion range monitoring to assess ion range shifts only requires a PG signal along the beam axis, hence a 1D distribution or profile (see Figure 3.1). Several approaches only provide 1D information, even though volumetric data can be retrieved by placing several detectors around the patient. Other techniques can intrinsically provide volumetric imaging, such as Compton cameras. Retrieving volumetric imaging while performing ion range monitoring can potentially improve the monitoring outcome in the presence of high lateral inhomogeneities [6]. However, more research is required to identify the cases where this is worthwhile, and Monte Carlo simulations are an invaluable tool to support addressing this question.

Another topic where Monte Carlo simulations can provide input is understanding the information obtained with PG radiation and how it correlates to dose delivery quality. Janssen et al. [25] published a simulation study in which they assessed the correlation between the inflexion point of the falloff near the end of the range in the PG distribution and parameters like mass density, phantom diameter, and detector acceptance angle. They also looked at how beam energy, time-of-flight, energy thresholds used for PG signal analysis, and elemental composition affect the accuracy of the range retrieval from the PG information.

Furthermore, if multiple ion range monitoring approaches are available, it is reasonable to consider that some can yield better monitoring outcomes than others. In this regard, Moteabbed et al. [36] made a comprehensive Monte Carlo study comparing PET and PG monitoring from the radiation emission perspective. They reported that PG emission exhibits significantly higher gamma production rates for all cases studied than PET. However, when considering detection technologies, the effects of detector acceptance and efficiency may hold PET superior in terms of the amplitude of the detected signal, depending on the future development of PG detection technology [36]. When considering specific cases, they also found that PG emission could benefit small tumors in the presence of high tissue heterogeneities.

Monte Carlo simulations also assist in developing data analysis and automatic shift detection algorithms, new approaches to using PG information better, and analytical prediction algorithms. Gueth et al. [19] proposed a machine learning approach based on Monte Carlo simulations to detect discrepancies between planned and delivered dose when using PG information. Tian et al. [63, 62, 61] developed a method in which a treatment plan can be optimized using high-weight spots, i.e. spots with a significantly higher number of protons, which increases the quality of PG monitoring outcomes on those spots. They found that this can be safely done without compromising the treatment quality by using Monte Carlo simulations. Pinto et al. [45] published a study where they extended the filtering approach of Parodi and Bortfeld [39] to PG monitoring. The original work [39] considered PET monitoring, and the extension to PG monitoring relied heavily on Monte Carlo simulations to obtain expected PG spatial distributions and PG energy spectra considering elemental composition. Finally, Schumann et al. [54] used the same framework of Parodi and Bortfeld [39] to reconstruct the delivered dose based on PG distributions.

PG radiation emission follows distinct nuclear channels that depend on the target considered. By analysing the PG signal from specific energies, it is possible to estimate the elemental composition of the irradiated tissues, namely carbon and oxygen (e.g. [49, 27, 23]). Even though this type of usage of PG radiation information is not directly correlated to ion range (it can still be indirectly correlated if analyzed adequately, as is the case discussed in the section PG spectroscopy), it paves the way to a better understanding of the irradiated tissues and thus better tissue parameters to use in ion dose calculations. Paganetti [38] estimated that the conversion from computed tomography data to tissue could add a range uncertainty up to 0.5%, while the uncertainty on the mean excitation energy of tissues could add 1.5%. Reducing this type of uncertainty potentially leads to higher tumor conformality by reducing the associated safety margins in the treatment plan.

## 3.1.2    COLLIMATED GAMMA CAMERA

Collimated cameras for PG monitoring have been considered the most straightforward implementation of range monitoring exploiting PG radiation. This type of camera employs a detection system and a mechanical collimator that ensures spatial correlation between detected and emitted events (see Figure 3.2). From an image processing point of view, this solution is also straightforward since no image reconstruction is required. It is important to stress that a "collimated gamma camera" in

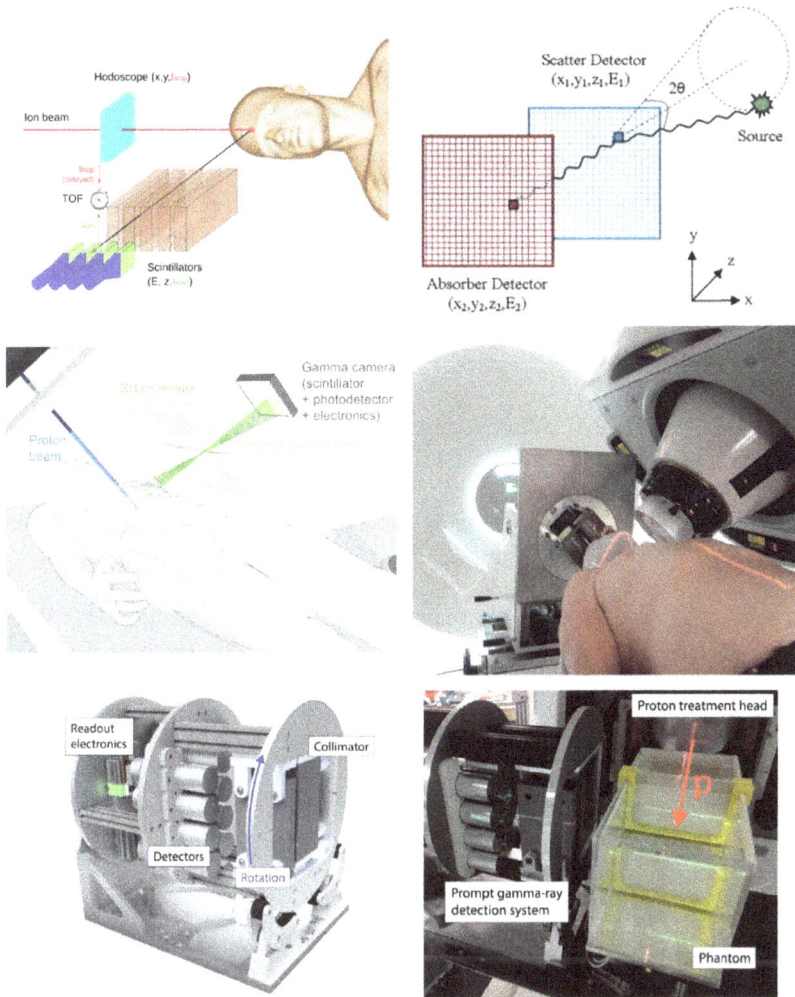

**Figure 3.2** Top left: multi-slit collimated camera principle with an array of detectors, a multi-slit collimator and a hodoscope to tag the incoming protons as an option for TOF (from [46]). Top right: the principle of a Compton camera with one scatter detector and one absorber. The cone of interaction is obtained with the location and energy information in both detectors (from [21]). Middle left: the principle of the knife-edge slit camera with a single slit camera and the detection system (from [41]). Middle right: a picture of the first clinical study with one patient using a knife-edge slit camera (from [51]). Bottom (from [23]): 3D model of the clinical prototype system for PG spectroscopy (left) and a picture of the experimental setup in a gantry treatment room using a phantom (right).

this context is a device relying solely on spatial information using a collimator with many openings, referred to as a multi-slit, multi-slab, or multi-parallel slit collimator. Ideally, this type of camera has a field of view (FOV) covering the entire ion range inside the patient, facilitating the range assessment due to the signal rise at the entrance. Other solutions exist that use mechanical collimation but include other techniques to achieve range monitoring or use a collimator with a single slit. An example of the former is the PG monitoring using spectroscopic information, while the latter is the knife-edge slit camera. Both cases are discussed in a separate section. However, one has to distinguish between a single-slit PG camera approach and experiments using single-slit collimator setups. Research and development of PG collimated cameras generally start with simplified experimental setups using single-slit collimators and moving the target phantom. Such a strategy allows for more flexibility (e.g. changing slit opening width), a better understanding of fundamental questions (e.g. no events from neighboring slits), and lower research costs before building a multi-slit camera.

A collimated camera tends to be bulky and heavy due to the collimator. The broad energy spectrum extending up to 10 MeV requires a thick collimator to maximize the emission-detection position correlation by constraining the angular acceptance. Coarser collimation inevitably leads to lower correlation, translating into PG profiles with a less sharp PG falloff at the end of the ion range. However, even though finer collimation does improve the PG falloff contrast, the amount of signal is considerably reduced. Ultimately, this increases the noise in the detection of the PG signal.

Moreover, events associated with neutrons, namely photons created after neutron interactions with the high atomic number materials used for the collimators (typically lead or tungsten), create a considerable background (see Figure 3.3). In some fields, signal-to-noise ratio (SNR) and signal-to-background ratio (SBR) can be interchangeable. However, the two ratios can have different definitions when considering PG monitoring using collimated cameras. SNR relates the mean value of the signal to its variance, and it is governed by counting statistics, namely Poisson statistics. In contrast, SBR relates the PG signal to events not correlated to the range.

Furthermore, the usual quantity of interest in PG range monitoring is the shift of the PG distribution shift compared to a prediction and not the vertex of the detected events since a PG distribution shift correlates to an ion range shift. For example, diagnostic nuclear medicine has a different aim: gamma cameras create images showing the spatial distributions of some radionuclides. The change in focus from localising a vertex to estimating a distribution shift reduces the importance of the spatial resolution of the camera. It also introduces a different quantity: precision in finding ion range shifts (hereafter referred to as precision). Conceptually, a gamma camera used for scintigraphy resembles a PG camera. Both use a collimator and have a detection system. However, the former is used in a scenario with well-known energy defined by the radionuclide imaged and no background (at least background as considered in the PG monitoring field). The choice of the collimator for a given gamma scan is a compromise between spatial resolution and sensitivity. The relationship between the two quantities is often clear, and it can be estimated with analytical expressions based on geometrical considerations and photon energy (e.g. [20]). For a PG camera, the relation between SNR, SBR and precision is far from trivial. The design optimization, testing, and validation of PG cameras is a cumbersome process regularly employing Monte Carlo tools (e.g. [56, 44]).

Monte Carlo simulations are not only indispensable to designing a full-scale PG monitoring system, but they also provide invaluable information when preparing experimental setups. Beam time availability can be scarce, and its costs can be substantial. Therefore, beam time preparation requires careful planning. The first experimental prototype for detecting PG radiation in particle therapy was developed by Min et al. in 2006 [33], but not without previous Monte Carlo simulations. Seo et al. [55] implemented a simulation framework based on MCNPX [40] and FLUKA [1] to compare neutron moderator materials for the construction of the PG camera. The authors compared two materials and how that choice impacts the SBR with a changing distance between the PG camera and phantom. The simulation study of Seo et al. [55] was crucial to serve as input for Min et al. [33] to build the experimental prototype.

Similarly to Min et al. [33] with the decision on the neutron moderator material, Biegun et al. [4] made a Monte Carlo simulation study assessing the impact of including time-of-flight (TOF) information to reject events associated with neutrons. They showed that considering TOF in a PG camera can reduce the background associated with neutrons by more than 99%. This study was vital to deciding on pursuing years of research to implement demanding TOF technology in a PG

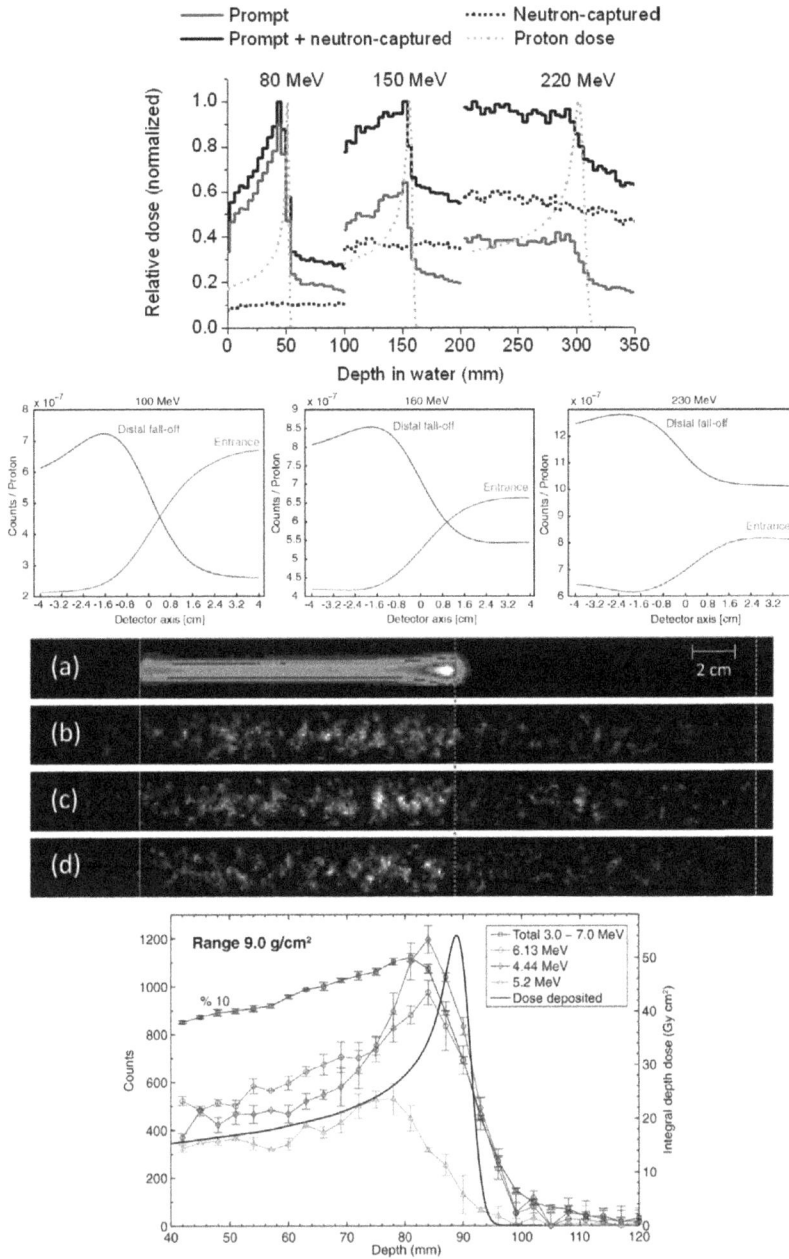

**Figure 3.3** Examples of distributions after different PG monitoring methods. First row: PG profiles obtained with a multi-slit collimator camera and for three proton energies. PG signal, events associated with neutrons and proton dose are depicted (from [34]). Second row: PG profiles reconstructed after detection with a knife-edge slit camera for three proton energies. Each energy case shows the PG detection at the phantom entrance and PG falloff (from [41]). Third row: dose distribution (a) and three PG distributions from a Compton camera. The case shown in (b) is the PG radiation measured for a 150-MeV proton beam, while (c) and (d) depict the PG distributions with the range shifted by 3 mm and 5 mm, respectively (from [47]). Fourth row: PG distributions after data selection using the PG spectroscopy approach. The plot shows the dose deposited, the total PG distribution with a 3 to 7 MeV energy threshold, and the PG profiles obtained by selecting the gamma lines at 4.44 MeV, 5.2 MeV and 6.13 MeV (from [65]).

camera. That decision culminated with the work of Cambraia Lopes et al. [31], where the authors compared the performance of a knife-edge slit camera clinical prototype with and without TOF. The SBR was improved by a factor of 3 when using TOF. A knife-edge slit camera is a particular type of collimated PG camera employing a collimator with a single slit, and since it is the only type of collimated PG camera that has been clinically tested so far, it will have a section on its own.

In the development of collimated PG cameras, the simulation studies of Polf et al. [48] and Pinto et al. [44] are also noteworthy. Polf et al. [48] assessed the effects of detector size and distance from the patient when detecting PG radiation. Their Monte Carlo study looked into several aspects affecting PG detection. They then proposed an analytical expression of the PG detection rate as a function of distance from the isocenter, detector size and proton energy used to guide the design and usage of clinical PG imaging detectors. In turn, Pinto et al. [44] used Monte Carlo simulations to optimize a multi-slit camera by considering how the precision is affected by the different geometrical parameters of the camera. In the end, the authors proposed three different designs based on different endpoints. Using the wealth of Monte Carlo simulation data needed for the optimization, the authors also developed a model describing the correlation between the different parameters for the proposed designs, thus allowing for a fast recalculation of the expected precision if one or more geometrical parameters are different in an experimental setting. For example, for one of the optimized designs, the PG camera would need to have its collimator entrance placed at 322.3 mm from the beam axis, and there may be situations where such a distance may not be possible.

### 3.1.3   KNIFE-EDGE SLIT CAMERA

A knife-edge slit camera is a collimated PG camera with a single slit collimator shaped like a knife-edge (see Figure 3.2). The rationale behind this type of collimator is to act as a pinhole collimator, a commonly used collimator in diagnostic nuclear medicine when good spatial resolution and magnification are of interest at the cost of sensitivity. A typical application is thyroid imaging, where the anatomical structure is smaller than the field of view and potentially with small lesions to assess. From all the PG monitoring modalities, the knife-edge slit camera was the first design utilized with patients for both passive [51] (see Figure 3.2) and active proton beam delivery [69].

The first proposal for the application collimator of this kind in a PG camera was made by Bom et al. [5]. The authors relied on Monte Carlo simulations to perform a feasibility study on such a novel solution, which showed that a precision lower than 1 mm could be achieved with this approach. A comprehensive study from Smeets et al. [56] was published shortly after, which can arguably be viewed as a seminal work in the field of PG monitoring. Smeets et al. is a work mixing Monte Carlo simulations and experimental work. The authors reported on the feasibility, development, and experimental test of a knife-edge slit camera, starting from fundamental research, such as expected signal, background and precision for several clinically relevant proton energies, and data selection and analysis approaches. The work ends with the construction, validation and test in clinical conditions of said device.

A knife-edge slit camera offers advantages compared to a PG camera based on a multi-slit collimator. When comparing performances, a knife-edge slit camera exhibits higher efficiency by collecting more PG signal and generally expressing a more favorable SNR [57]. Typically, higher efficiency leads to more reliable information on the range, which is more noticeable at lower doses. Moreover, from a practical point of view, the knife-edge slit camera tends to have a considerably smaller footprint, likely allowing for easier integration in a treatment room where mechanical and weight constraints matter.

However, there are also drawbacks to using a knife-edge slit camera. The first and foremost drawback is related to the concept itself. Since there is only one slit, the camera can only monitor the expected end-of-range position with a limited camera FOV. Furthermore, since it relies on a single slit, its width is significantly larger when compared to the case of a slit in a multi-slit collimator camera. Consequently, the knife-edge slit camera yields a poor spatial resolution, and the entire PG signal within the FOV is blurred (see Figure 3.3). The poor spatial resolution does not necessarily affect the detection of ion range shifts since the shift retrieval aims at estimating a difference and not an absolute position. Nonetheless, it impacts the methods used for such retrieval, and any added information one could obtain with a higher spatial resolution is lost, namely PG signal differences when crossing various tissues. This loss of information can affect the retrieval of the detected ion range shifts since comparing two distributions with well-defined high gradient regions tends to yield higher confidence levels.

Regarding the limited FOV of the knife-edge slit camera, Gueth et al. [19] used machine learning algorithms to detect discrepancies of 5 mm between planned and delivered doses, and they found that using the entire distribution leads to better specificity and sensitivity than when just using the PG falloff region. This algorithm tries to look for patterns (features) in the PG signal data of the entire beam. If something happens along the beam path that introduces an ion range shift, the algorithm may detect it from some feature proximal to the falloff.

The knife-edge slit camera also suffers from geometrical artefacts due to parallax effects [43]. The signal less affected is at the center of the camera, hence the need to align the camera to the expected ion range positions. The implication is that conceivably the camera can only reliably monitor spots within a given depth, likely disregarding most of the spots in the irradiation field. The same applies to the limited camera FOV (if no camera repositioning during treatment is planned).

Monte Carlo simulations have been of paramount importance for the research and development of the knife-edge slit camera. As addressed above, Bom et al. and Smeets et al. launched the initial seed with the first feasibility studies. However, several studies have been published since then, many relying on Monte Carlo simulations. Janssens et al. [26] made a sensitivity study of PG imaging in heterogeneous anatomies. They also proposed a fast analytical algorithm for PG distribution prediction based on pre-computed tables from Monte Carlo simulations, extended and validated by Sterpin et al. [59].

### 3.1.4  COMPTON CAMERA

Compton cameras exploit the principles of Compton scattering to determine the source of the event. The most straightforward design has one scatterer and one absorber. Ideally, the photon is scattered in the former and absorbed in the latter. By assuming complete absorption of the photon in the absorber and by knowing the scattering angle between the scatterer and absorber, it is possible to create a cone whose surface defines the possible locations from where the photon originated. This process mimics the principle of collimation; therefore, Compton cameras employ so-called electronic collimation. In one scatterer and one absorber design (see Figure 3.2), it is assumed that the photon is fully absorbed to determine its energy; otherwise, the cone will be wrongly estimated. This limitation can be reduced by considering more than one scattering interaction of the photon [42, 50, 32, 37], thus removing the need for complete absorption. Monte Carlo simulations play a critical role in optimising the designs regardless of single or double scattering approaches, namely in the scenario of ion range monitoring involving the detection of high-energy photons. Optimization of the materials used, the number of scatterers, and distances between elements and dimensions can be addressed using Monte Carlo simulations. Roellinghoff et al. [53] published a study analysing the potentialities of a single-scattering Compton camera. Richard et al. [50] proposed a double scattering design using a stack of silicon detectors to act as scatters. Kormoll et al. [28] studied the performance of some Compton camera designs for proton therapy monitoring, where they found that a design comprising cadmium zinc telluride (CdZnTe) layers as scatterers and a lutetium oxyorthosilicate (LSO) scintillator as an absorber could be a good candidate. Llosá et al. [30] developed a double lanthanum bromide (LaBr3) scintillator (one crystal as scatterer and one as absorber) Compton camera prototype after several simulation studies, with promising experimental results for point-like sources.

### 3.1.5   PG SPECTROSCOPY

PG spectroscopy in this context is the approach proposed by Verburg et al. [65], where energy and time information from PG detection are used for ion range monitoring purposes. The authors introduced a novel concept using the magnitude of discrete gamma lines to estimate the proton range. This concept was considerably extended in the work of Verburg and Seco [66] with the publication of the detailed analysis workflow to determine proton ranges. By constructing PG profiles along the beam path using the data from single gamma lines and employing models derived from differential cross sections, the authors obtained absolute proton range measurements with a single slit device (see Figure 3.3). The fundamental research for this approach relied on Monte Carlo simulations to find the relations between gamma lines and how range can be determined. This project began with a comprehensive simulation study of Verburg et al. [67], in which an extensive assessment of cross sectional data from several Monte Carlo tools was carried out.

Although both use a single-slit collimator, a clear distinction should be made between the knife-edge slit camera and PG spectroscopy. The former assesses proton range shifts with respect to a reference coordinate system. The proton range is thus relative. On the other hand, PG spectroscopy uses models based on cross sections of the different nuclear channels to pinpoint where the proton is in its path. Hence, an absolute range assessment. Collimated and Compton cameras also yield absolute proton range, provided both the PG entrance and falloff are considered. An absolute proton range can be inferred by determining where the PG signal starts (i.e. entrance of the patient) and where it ends (i.e. near the end of the range). Nevertheless, only PG spectroscopy directly measures it with the aid of models and a single measuring point in the beam path.

Hueso-González et al. [23] reported a full-scale clinical prototype based on PG spectroscopy, including all the workflow steps (see Figure 3.2). The authors also demonstrated PG spectroscopy's capability to determine the elemental composition and density of irradiated materials using experimental data. For a delivered dose of 0.9 Gy, the authors reported a mean proton range precision per spot of 1.1 mm at a 95% confidence level when considering the aggregation of neighboring spots.

### 3.1.6   UNCOLLIMATED APPROACHES: PG TIMING AND PG PEAK INTEGRATION

Two uncollimated approaches using PG information for proton range monitoring have been proposed: PG timing (PGT) and PG peak integration (PGPI). Both methods are built around TOF information but with some key differences.

PG timing was first introduced by Golnik et al. [18], and it correlates the average and width of the PG time spectrum with the proton transit time inside the patient. Protons with a longer range must travel a longer path, continuously emitting PG radiation. Consequently, the PG peak will be broader for longer ranges and exhibit a distinct peak shift towards longer times. In the first feasibility study [18], the authors stated that proton range variations of at least 2 mm are expected to be detectable with this technique. As with most of the research involving PG radiation, the development of this technique relied heavily on Monte Carlo simulations to assess its feasibility. Further research on this method, including experimental measurements of PGT data with increasingly complex phantoms, has been published [22, 68]. The promising results support the usefulness of using this technique in a clinical environment, provided some caveats are addressed, such as challenges with background, calibration to the initial proton energy and the time structure of the proton beam.

PG peak integration uses the same PG time spectrum as PGT, but it correlates the integral of the PG peak in the TOF spectrum to deviations between planned and delivered dose [29]. Monte Carlo simulations and experiments show it is possible to detect proton ranges of 3 mm under some circumstances. Even though this method can detect range shifts, it is not its primary goal since it may not be precise enough compared to other approaches. The authors state that their goal is to have a simple and cost-effective monitoring system to detect treatment deviations, particularly severe overdosage cases [29].

## 3.2   CHARGED PARTICLES

The emission profile of the photons emitted by the beam has a favorable shape to provide information about the entire path of the hadron beam. However the exploitation of photon radiation requires the use of collimation, mechanical or electronic, to estimate the origin of the photon itself. A unavoidable drawback of the collimation is to reduce the collected statistic of several order of magnitudes. On the other hand the photons are not the only particles emitted by beam during the treatment since the proton nuclear interactions produce a sizeable number of neutrons and light ions, in particular protons.

During its path inside the tissue a non negligible fraction of the beam interacts with the patient nuclei and both projectile (if the beam is a carbon ion) and the target can undergo a fragmentation process. This physics process is scarcely known at this energy mainly because of the lack of data. As a consequence, the nuclear model that are embedded in the MC code are often based on higher energy model extrapolated to the energy of interest of the particle therapy. The few measurements of this process showed that fragments produced are peaked in the forward region and mostly contained within few degrees of the beam axis, with the exception of protons and neutrons, that represent the largest sample and show tails at large emission angles and energies.

The flux of charged fragments produced increase rapidly with the charge of the beam. In case of carbon therapy the emission is quite large and moreover the fragments have enough energy to escape the patient, so they can be used as a possible source of information about the path of beam in the patient.

Up to now methods using the secondary charged particles has been proposed and tested in carbon therapy to monitor beam range, beam transverse position and the morphological changes of the patient between fractions.

The use of charged tracks (mainly protons) has a clear advantage from the detection point of view with respect to photons. The efficiency detection with a standard tracking device can be close to unity and the angular resolution of tracker detectors allows a very good determination of the particle direction outside the patient. There are some drawbacks that compensates the quoted advantages: the cross section for the production of the secondary protons increase with the beam energy. This implies an anticorrelation of the charged production yield with respect to the dose release, since as the beam loses energy travelling toward the Brag Peak it increase the dose release but emits less and less protons. A unfavorable consequence is that the emission of charged secondary decreases as the beam approaches to the Bragg Peak [10].

Another critical aspect of the use of the charged particles is their interaction with the patient tissue: they lose energy continuously while they cross the patient tissue, so they need a minimum of kinetic energy to escape, and this minimum depends from the path length crossed to exit the patient. Another effect typical of the charged particle is that they suffer multiple scattering when they cross materials. The multiple scattering changes the direction of the emitted fragments at the exit of the patient with respect to its original direction at the emission, and the effect is larger for low-energy protons. All these features point out that the most useful part of charged radiation that can be used outside of the patient as source of information for monitoring purpose is the higher energy component. Must be remarked that for the energy of the emitted protons holds the same law that rules the proton emission yield: the higher the energy of the beam the higher the emitted proton energy.

Considering the angular distribution of the protons a correlation can be found with the emission energy and the emission abundance: the secondary protons emitted at large angle with respect to the beam have less energy and are less abundant with respect to the protons emitted in the same direction of the beam.

The features of secondary fragments escaping from the patient, and that can be used for monitoring purpose, do not depend only on nuclear interaction of the beam, but are also dependent on the tissue material that both the beam and the secondaries cross. The patient morphology has a double

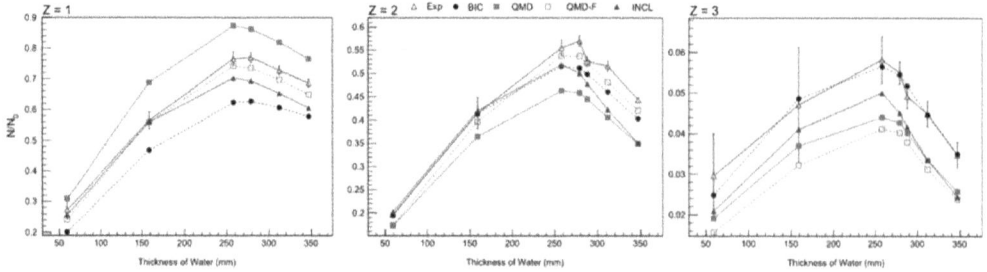

**Figure 3.4** Comparison between the different Geant4 nuclear interaction model and the experimental fragment yields for H, He, Li production for different thicknesses of water [9].

role: the fragmentation probability of the carbon beam is directly proportional to the density of the crossed tissue (for instance, the secondary production is higher in bone then in a muscle) but is also enhanced by target material with high atomic number. The effect of the material on the charged secondaries is related with the amount of tissue these protons have to cross to escape the patient and reach detector. Depending from the geometry and size of the patient and on the type of tissue crossed, the threshold kinetic energy needed to exit from the patient changes. As a consequence, since the kinetic energy distribution of the charge secondary produced is rapidly dropping with the energy, the amount of charged secondary emerging from the patient is highly dependent on the patient geometry.

### 3.2.1 REQUESTS ON A RANGE MONITOR DEVICE EXPLOITING CHARGED PARTICLES EMISSION

The complex dependency of the secondary flux on many parameters (physics and morphology) makes the MC a unique tool. The MC can be fundamental not only in the design and optimization phase of the monitor device construction, but is often indispensable also in the operation of the device.

In general nowadays there is a fair agreement between data and MC as far as the total production cross section is concerned. In Figure 3.4 a comparison between the fragment yields of different nuclear interaction model of GEANT4 and data is reported.

On the other hand in literature there are very few measurement [24] of differential cross section with respect to the energy and the angle of emission of the charged secondary, in particular for the energies and the targets of interest in carbon therapy. This lack of knowledge has an impact on the accuracy of the MC prediction of the flux [64, 9] and of the features of the charged secondaries. Nowadays simulation code as G4 or FLUKA can hardly reach the 10% precision level in the simulation of the protons escaping from the patient in a treatment, but on the contrary can be safely used as driving guide in the design and in the operation of the monitor devices.

Extracting beam information from this charged secondary population is quite simple in case of active scanning beam delivery. With this delivery system the direction of each pencil beam that irradiates the patient is well known from the dose delivery, in particular the transverse position and the direction of the beam defines the pencil beam direction in the space. The IVI [15] method (Interaction Vertex Imaging) matches the pencil beam direction information with the charged track line of flight reconstructed from a tracking detector. The method assumes that the point of minimum approach (PCA) of these two lines in the space is the emission point of the charged secondary. From clear geometrical reason the resolution of this method is linearly dependent from the minimum distance between the detector and the pencil beam.

There are several sources of unaccuracy of the IVI method. The first is purely geometric: even if the direction of the beam is very well known, the beam spot has a finite transverse size of the order of few mm and for the PCA determination only the reference pencil beam direction is considered. The size of this effect is inversely proportional to the tangent of the detection angle with respect to the beam. This effect prevent to adopt a detection setup with detector placed at small angle where the flux and the energy of the emitted protons is higher. On top of that the choice of very small detection angle is not fully compatible with a realistic clinical setup, due to the possible geometrical interference with the patient positioning.

Another important source of unaccuracy stems from the reconstruction of the secondary proton: usually for standard tracking detector, the very good angular and position resolution on the reconstructed track is spoiled by the multiple scattering of protons inside the patient. Actually, the main source of uncertainty on the point of minimum approach is due to the deviation of the proton track exiting from the patient with respect to the exact emission direction due to the multiple scattering, that is minimum for high energy protons usually emitted at small angle.

A trade off must be found between the quoted effects, geometry and multiple scattering, and some experiments [12, 17] showed that in principle, using solid state tracking devices at 30 degrees with respect to the beam direction, the distal edge of the beam could be estimated with an accuracy of 1.3 mm. in a very simple geometry.

Coming to the design of a device for beam monitoring for active scanning carbon therapy, two beam parameters are of great importance: the fluence of the single pencil beam and the time structure of the pencil beam delivery. These parameters have direct impact on the statistic that can be collected and on the related monitoring accuracy. In a standard $^{12}C$ treatment delivering 2 Gy dose per fraction, each pencil beam is made of $5 \times 10^4$ to $5 \times 10^5$ carbon ions, with the higher statistic is for the pencil beams having the BP in the tumor distal region. A typical fraction of irradiation can be made of $10^5$ pencil beams, each one with time delivery of 10 ms. With this number the flux of charged protons escaping the patient and impinging on a detector reaches $10^6$ Hz/sr at 60 degrees [11] and rapidly increase at lower angles. At this rate the dead time of the detector can be a serious issue and can be a limiting factor to collect enough statistic, in particular at lower angles.

A possible detection setup can rely on a large acceptance tracking detector placed at large angle with respect to the beam axis. In [13] MC studies is quoted that a detection angle of 60 degree can be an effective trade off between the reconstruction geometry that prefers large angles and the statistic collection and the MS that both suggest low detection angle.

In particular at angle larger than $60^0$ the point of minimal approach can be determined with reasonable accuracy and with resolution that is independent from the beam spot size. In the same paper is reported that going to at $90^0$ angle would decrease the proton flux of factor $\simeq 4$.

Summarizing the main requests on a monitor device that uses the charged secondary are mainly a large active area to integrate statistics and a low acquisition dead time to deal with the high secondary instantaneous rate. As far the angular resolution is concerned, no extreme performance are required( order or slightly better than tenth of mrad) due to the dominating contribution of the multiple scattering on the reconstruction accuracy.

### 3.2.2 THE BEAM RANGE MONITORING

An example of the accuracy achievable with this method on the beam range monitoring is given in Figure 3.5. Exploiting the IVI method the authors [8] easily detected the difference in the longitudinal vertex distribution of ö12C beam with 297.8 and 293.5 MeV/u, clearly indicating that this method can achieve good resolution of the beam range determination if enough statistic is collected. Must be remarked that this proof-of-principle experiment has been carried out using a $10^7$ incident carbon ions, a much larger statistic with respect to a standard pencil beam used in a treatment.

The right panel of Figure 3.6 [12] shows the details of the possible different methods of monitoring the beam range: i) a linear fit can be done to the fall-off region of the emission point distribution and the point corresponding at a given height of this linear fit (usually 50% of the linear fit range) can be used as range parameter. ii) Two linear fit are done to the fall-off and to the tail of the distribution

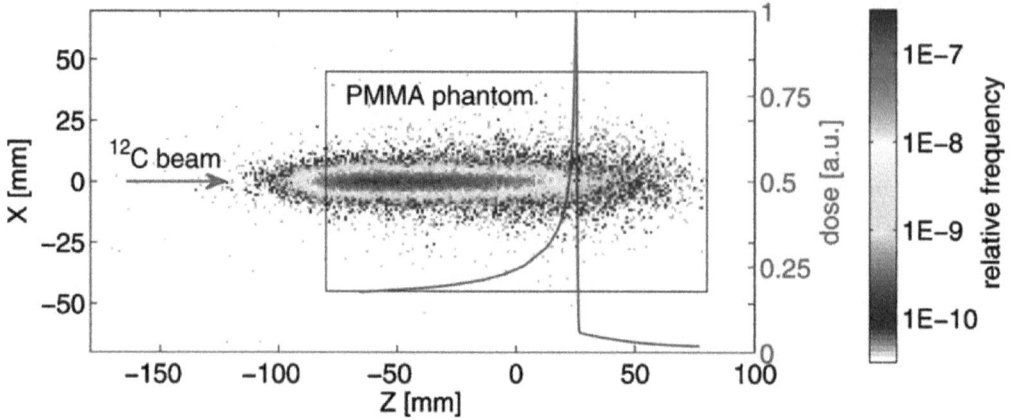

**Figure 3.5** Distribution of the track back-projections for $5 \times 10^4$ measured secondary charged particles. The dimensions of the cylindrical PMMA phantom are illustrated by the rectangle (view from the side). The origin of the coordinate system is aligned with the center of the phantom which was placed in the isocenter. The carbon ion beam was directed along the Z-axis. The depth dose distribution measured in water and scaled to the phantom WEPL is superimposed. Due to experimental limitations, the depth dose distribution could be measured only for water depths greater than 20 mm. Initial carbon ion beam parameters: E = 250.08 MeV/u, FWHM = 4.3 mm [12].

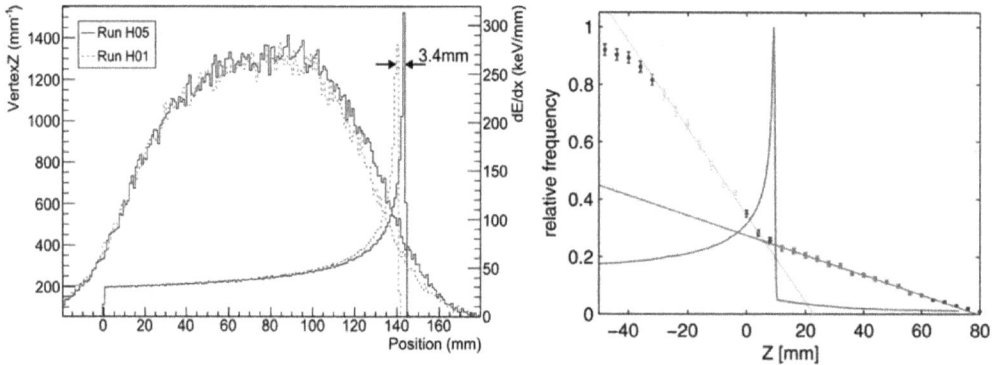

**Figure 3.6** Left panel: Longitudinal vertex distributions and corresponding dose distribution for run H05 at an energy of 297.8 MeV/u and run H01 at an energy of 293.5 MeV/u. These distributions were obtained with $10^7$ incident carbon ions [8]. Right Panel: linear fits to the distal fall-off to obtain the position of the slope change. The depth dose curve of the primary beam is illustrated in ref [12].

and the crossing of the two lines can be taken as range evaluation. Of course these possible range estimators need to be calibrate with respect to the effective BP position. The role of the MC is crucial in this calibration, because the charged secondary production depends not only on the electronic density but also on the atomic mass number of the material crossed by the beam, and then cannot be easily expressed in terms of water equivalent path lenght. Thus the experimental calibration versus water or PMMA phantom is not going to represent accurately the real treatment situation, while a MC simulation based on the true CT of the patient could provide an accurate calibration.

## 3.2.3 THE INTER-FRACTIONAL MONITORING

The charged secondaries can be used a source of information not only about the beam path in the patient, but also on the patient itself. The monitoring of the changes in the patient morphology during the many fractions of a treatment is crucial. In fact the patient, also due to the effects of the treatment, it's likely to change mass and shape during the treatment that can last a month, and this variation can spoil the accuracy of the treatment. Usually the standard procedure is to make additional CTs and to adapt TPS along the treatment, but after how many fraction this replanning is needed is something that is left to the doctor intuition. Such a doctor decision is made even more difficult since usually internal morphology changes are not clearly seen from outside the patient.

The flux of charged secondary can be exploited to identify the occurrence of such morphological changes inside the patient by comparing the reconstructed emission maps of the charged secondary acquired during each treatment fractions. As the fragment production yield is correlated to the tissue density, it is possible to identify morphological changes in the tissues crossed by the beams studying the inter-fraction differences in the shape of the secondary fragment emission map.

The charged secondary that can be detected outside the patient provide information about the material crossed by the beam, since the secondary proton production is largely dependent by this material, and the comparison of the emission 3D map that are acquired in different fraction can spot a change of morphology as change of charged emission This technique has been tested in a clinical trial at CNAO [2]. The monitoring device was a charged particle detector composed of eight tracker planes made of plastic scintillating fibers fixed by means of an aluminum frame (Dose Profiler). Each fiber plane has a section of $19.2 \times 19.2$ cm$^2$ and is made up of two orthogonal layers of 384 fibers (length of 19.2 cm). The two orthogonal layers allow to have a two-dimensional view along the x and y axis respectively and to reconstruct the 3D path of the proton inside the detector.

The FLUKA MC code was used to simulate the interactions of all the primary ions foreseen in the Treatment Planning System. The beam nozzle and the RS were included in the setup accordingly to the measurements performed in the CNAO treatment room. The full DP mechanical and read-out details were implemented in the Monte Carlo simulation. The optical cross-talk between the fibers, the energy resolution and the layer detection efficiency were also taken into account to reproduce the experimental conditions. The simulation was used also to evaluate the spatial accuracy on the emission point that is of the order of 7mm, mainly due to the multiple scattering.

An example of the results achieved is reported in Figure 3.7. A patient affected by Adenoid Cystic Carcinoma, that underwent a re-evaluation CT imaging session after the first eight fractions were delivered, was used to check the method. CT1 and CT2 correspond to the scans before and after eight fractions, respectively. The 3D map of the emission point reconstructed by the DP at the frst and at the eighth fraction have been compared with the method of gamma index. The point on space where the two map are different, in the sense of not passing the gamma index test, are reported in the rightmost panel and precisely correspond to the region of the CT where a modification in the patient can be identified.

To check this result the full two fraction have been simulated using FLUKA. The plan used for the simulation study consists of $\simeq 33 \times 10^3$ Pencil Beams (PB), with kinetic energy in the range between 126 MeV/u and 278 MeV/u (57 slices), and a number of ions shot in each PB in the range between $10^3$ and $10^5$. The CTV volume is $5 \times 10 \times 10 cm^3$. The same plan was simulated considering the two different CT and then the emission maps where compared, confirming the identification of the region with a morphology change. The same simulation has been used to check that the statistical fluctuation of the detected charged secondary, in case of same patient CT, cannot give rise to a signal faking a morphological change.

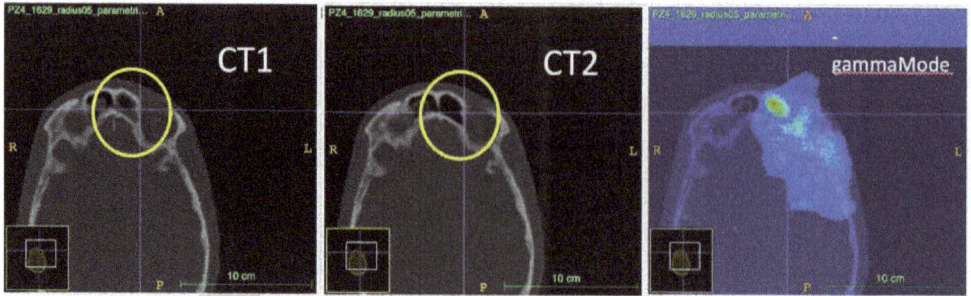

**Figure 3.7** Comparison between the CTs of a patient corresponding to first fraction (CT1) and to 13 days later during the treatment (CT2). The circle spots the morphology modification. The rightmost panel shows the gamma test between the charged emission 3D map corresponding to the 2 CTs, where the geometrical position of the change is clearly identified.

### 3.2.4 THE BEAM TRANSVERSE POSITION MONITORING

The charged production vertexes lie in a thin cylinder whose axis is the nominal direction of the pencil beam and the radius is given by the convolution of the initial beam spot size and the effect of the beam multiple scattering.

This experimental signature can be used to monitor the beam position in the plane orthogonal to its flight direction, providing an online feedback that can be used to cross-check that provided from the beam transverse position monitor chambers [12]. The beam transverse position is extracted from the secondary charged directions reconstructed by a tracking monitoring device in the plane orthogonal to the primary beam direction.

To associate the secondary detected to the correct pencil beam the time information are used, comparing the time of the secondary detection with the delivery time of the pencil beam. The technique has been applied with good results [16] to a phantom irradiate with carbon ion at HIT center. A carbon-ion treatment plan was used to treat a $100cm\ddot{o}3$ tumor volume in the center of an Alderson head phantom and two silicon pixel detectors based on the Timepix3 technology were used to detect and to track outgoing secondary ions. The average of the projection of the reconstructed tracks in the transverse plane at the isocenter provides the information of the pencil beam position in this plane.

In Figure 3.8 the comparison between the pencil beam position detected by the secondary tracks and the reference position is reported. The monitored position follows clearly the pencil beam movement in time. A resolution of the order of 2 mm is reported on the x direction, while the other transverse coordinate has worse resolution due to the setup geometry.

A similar technique has been applied using the same device during a real patient treatment [14]. For each pencil beam that must be monitored, the projections in the plane (xy) orthogonal to the beam direction of the charged secondary directions is computed and then filled in a 2D histogram, representing the track density in the transverse plane. The pencil beam position is then identified by the maximum density point in the histogram, where there is the accumulation point of all the tracks.

A FLUKA simulation was used to optimize the filtering procedure to smooth the statistical fluctuation due to a low number of reconstructed tracks. The MC takes into account the reconstruction resolution of the proton emission point in the transverse plane, the beam spot size, the geometry of the monitor device. Such an optimization in the reported paper suggested the use of a 2D gaussian filter with a $\sigma$ of 1.0 cm is applied to the 2D track density histogram.

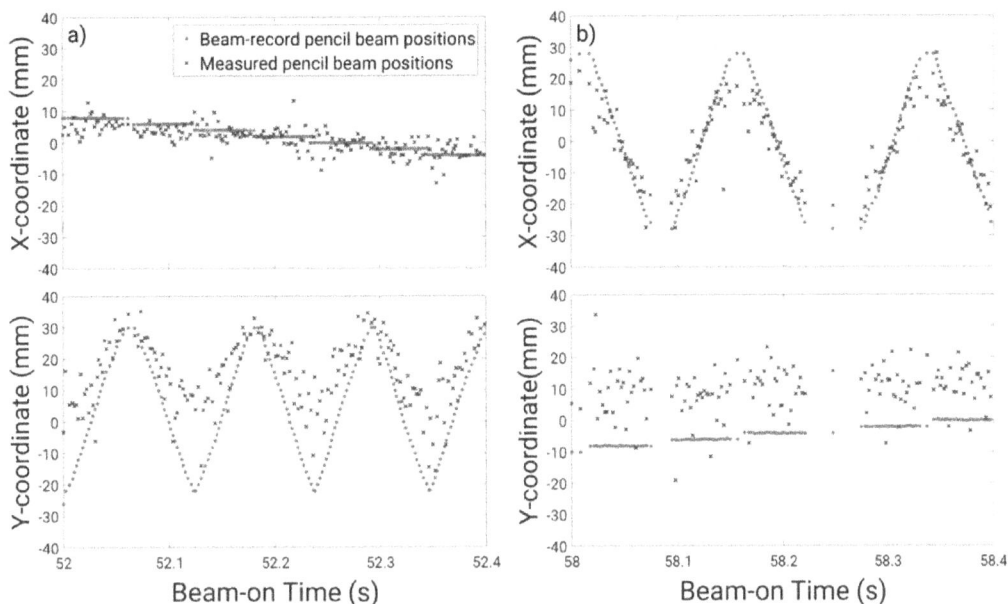

**Figure 3.8** Comparison of the measured beam spot positions (crosses) with respect to the beam spot positions (points) from the beam-record file. (a) Main beam scanning direction in X coordinate (top) while the movement of the secondary scanning direction is in Y coordinate (bottom), for the energy layer 11. (b) Main beam scanning direction in Y coordinate (bottom) while the movement of the secondary scanning direction is in X coordinate (top), for the energy layer 12 [16].

The resolution of course depends on the detector and the geometry of the setup (the monitor device was at 60 cm from isocenter), and in the reported paper is given by $\sigma = (4.9 \pm 0.1)/\sqrt{(N_t)}$ cm where $N_t$ is the number of the detected charged secondary of the pencil beam. In the reported treatment the average number of track was 60, for a resolution of the order of 6 mm.

## REFERENCES

1. A. Fasso A. Ferrari, P.R. Sala and J. Ranft. *FLUKA: a multi-particle transport code*, 2005. CERN-2005-10, INFN/TC05/11, SLAC-R-773.
2. M. Fischettiet al. Inter-fractional monitoring of 12c ions treatments: results from a clinical trial at the cnao facility. *Sci Rep*, page 20735, 2020.
3. Koki Ando, Mitsutaka Yamaguchi, Seiichi Yamamoto, Toshiyuki Toshito, and Naoki Kawachi. Development of a low-energy x-ray camera for the imaging of secondary electron bremsstrahlung x-ray emitted during proton irradiation for range estimation. 62(12):5006–5020.
4. Aleksandra K Biegun, Enrica Seravalli, Patrícia Cambraia Lopes, Ilaria Rinaldi, Marco Pinto, David C Oxley, Peter Dendooven, Frank Verhaegen, Katia Parodi, Paulo Crespo, and Dennis R Schaart. Time-of-flight neutron rejection to improve prompt gamma imaging for proton range verification: a simulation study. 57(20):6429–6444.
5. Victor Bom, Leila Joulaeizadeh, and Freek Beekman. Real-time prompt gamma monitoring in spot-scanning proton therapy using imaging through a knife-edge-shaped slit. 57(2):297–308.
6. E Draeger, D Mackin, S Peterson, H Chen, S Avery, S Beddar, and J C Polf. 3d prompt gamma imaging for proton beam range verification. 63(3):035019.
7. W Enghardt, P Crespo, F Fiedler, R Hinz, K Parodi, J Pawelke, and F Pönisch. Charged hadron tumour therapy monitoring by means of PET. 525(1):284–288.

8. C. Finck et al. Study for online range monitoring with the interaction vertex imaging method. *Phys. Med. Biol.*, page 9220, 2017.

9. D. Bolst et al. *Nucl Instrum Meth A*, page 68,75, 2017.

10. E. Haettner et al. Experimental study of nuclear fragmentation of 200 and 400 mev/u (12)c ions in water for applications in particle therapy. *Phys. Med. Biol.*, pages 486–487, 2013.

11. G.Traini et al. Review and performance of the dose profiler, a particle therapy treatments online monitor. *Physica Medica*, pages 84,93, 2019.

12. K. Gwosch et al. Non-invasive monitoring of therapeutic carbon ion beams in a homogeneous phantom by tracking of secondary ions. *Phys. Med. Biol.*, page 3755, 2013.

13. L. Piersanti et al. Measurement of charged particle yields from pmma irradiated by a 220 mev/u (12)c beam. *Phys. Med. Biol.*, page 1857, 2014.

14. M. Toppi et al. Paprica: The pair production imaging chamber—proof of principle. *Front. of Phys.*, page 568139, 2021.

15. P. Enriquet et al. Interaction vertex imaging (ivi) for carbon ion therapy monitoring: a feasibility study. *Phys. Med. Biol.*, 2012.

16. R. Felix-Bautista et al. *Phys. Med. Biol.*, page 175019, 2019.

17. T. Gaa et al. Visualization of air and metal inhomogeneities in phantoms irradiated by carbon ion beams using prompt secondary ions. *Physica Medica*, page 140, 147, 2017.

18. Christian Golnik, Fernando Hueso-González, Andreas Müller, Peter Dendooven, Wolfgang Enghardt, Fine Fiedler, Thomas Kormoll, Katja Roemer, Johannes Petzoldt, Andreas Wagner, and Guntram Pausch. Range assessment in particle therapy based on prompt Îş-ray timing measurements. 59(18):5399–5422.

19. P. Gueth, D. Dauvergne, N. Freud, J. M. Létang, C. Ray, E. Testa, and D. Sarrut. Machine learning-based patient specific prompt-gamma dose monitoring in proton therapy. 58(13):4563.

20. D. L. Gunter. Collimator design for nuclear medicine. In *Emission Tomography: The Fundamentals of PET and SPECT*, chapter 8, page 153– 168. Elsevier Academic, 2004.

21. L. J. Harkness, P. Arce, D. S. Judson, A. J. Boston, H. C. Boston, J. R. Cresswell, J. Dormand, M. Jones, P. J. Nolan, J. A. Sampson, D. P. Scraggs, A. Sweeney, I. Lazarus, and J. Simpson. A Compton camera application for the GAMOS GEANT4-based framework. 671:29–39.

22. Fernando Hueso-González, Wolfgang Enghardt, Fine Fiedler, Christian Golnik, Guillaume Janssens, Johannes Petzoldt, Damien Prieels, Marlen Priegnitz, Katja E Römer, Julien Smeets, François Vander Stappen, Andreas Wagner, and Guntram Pausch. First test of the prompt gamma ray timing method with heterogeneous targets at a clinical proton therapy facility. 60(16):6247–6272.

23. Fernando Hueso-González, Moritz Rabe, Thomas A Ruggieri, Thomas Bortfeld, and Joost M Verburg. A full-scale clinical prototype for proton range verification using prompt gamma-ray spectroscopy. 63(18):185019.

24. et al. J. Dudouet. Double differential fragmentation cross sections measurements of 95 mev/u 12c on thin targets for hadrontherapy. *Phys Rev C*, page 024606, 2013.

25. FMFC Janssen, G. Landry, P. Cambraia Lopes, G. Dedes, J. Smeets, D. R. Schaart, K. Parodi, and F. Verhaegen. Factors influencing the accuracy of beam range estimation in proton therapy using prompt gamma emission. 59(15):4427.

26. Guillaume Janssens, Julien Smeets, François Vander Stappen, Damien Prieels, Enrico Clementel, Eugen-Lucian Hotoiu, and Edmond Sterpin. Sensitivity study of prompt gamma imaging of scanned beam proton therapy in heterogeneous anatomies.

27. Laurent Kelleter, Aleksandra Wrońska, Judith Besuglow, Adam Konefał, Karim Laihem, Johannes Leidner, Andrzej Magiera, Katia Parodi, Katarzyna Rusiecka, Achim Stahl, and Thomas Tessonnier. Spectroscopic study of prompt-gamma emission for range verification in proton therapy. 34:7–17.

28. T. Kormoll, F. Fiedler, S. Schöne, J. Wüstemann, K. Zuber, and W. Enghardt. A Compton imager for in-vivo dosimetry of proton beams—a design study. 626-627:114–119.

29. J. Krimmer, G. Angellier, L. Balleyguier, D. Dauvergne, N. Freud, J. Hérault, J. M. Létang, H. Mathez, M. Pinto, E. Testa, and Y. Zoccarato. A cost-effective monitoring technique in particle therapy via uncollimated prompt gamma peak integration. 110(15):154102.

30. G. Llosá, J. Cabello, S. Callier, J.E. Gillam, C. Lacasta, M. Rafecas, L. Raux, C. Solaz, V. Stankova, C. de La Taille, M. Trovato, and J. Barrio. First Compton telescope prototype based on continuous LaBr3-SiPM detectors. 718:130–133.

31. Patricia Cambraia Lopes, Enrico Clementel, Paulo Crespo, Sebastien Henrotin, Jan Huizenga, Guillaume Janssens, Katia Parodi, Damien Prieels, Frauke Roellinghoff, Julien Smeets, Frederic Stichelbaut, and Dennis R. Schaart. Time-resolved imaging of prompt-gamma rays for proton range verification using a knife-edge slit camera based on digital photon counters. 60(15):6063.

32. Dennis Mackin, Steve Peterson, Sam Beddar, and Jerimy Polf. Evaluation of a stochastic reconstruction algorithm for use in Compton camera imaging and beam range verification from secondary gamma emission during proton therapy. 57(11):3537.

33. Chul-Hee Min, Chan Hyeong Kim, Min-Young Youn, and Jong-Won Kim. Prompt gamma measurements for locating the dose falloff region in the proton therapy. 89(18):183517.

34. Chul Hee Min, Han Rim Lee, Chan Hyeong Kim, and Se Byeong Lee. Development of array-type prompt gamma measurement system for in vivo range verification in proton therapy. 39(4):2100–2107.

35. Chul Hee Min, Jang Guen Park, So Hyun An, and Chan Hyeong Kim. Determination of optimal energy window for measurement of prompt gammas from proton beam by monte carlo simulations. 45:28–31.

36. M Moteabbed, S España, and H Paganetti. Monte Carlo patient study on the comparison of prompt gamma and PET imaging for range verification in proton therapy. 56(4):1063–1082.

37. P. G. Ortega, I. Torres-Espallardo, F. Cerutti, A. Ferrari, J. E. Gillam, C. Lacasta, G. Llosá, J. F. Oliver, P. R. Sala, P. Solevi, and M. Rafecas. Noise evaluation of Compton camera imaging for proton therapy. 60(5):1845.

38. Harald Paganetti. Range uncertainties in proton therapy and the role of monte Carlo simulations. 57(11):R99.

39. Katia Parodi and Thomas Bortfeld. A filtering approach based on gaussian–powerlaw convolutions for local PET verification of proton radiotherapy. 51(8):1991.

40. D.B. Pelowitz. *MCNPX Users Manual Version 2.7.0*, 2011. LA-CP-11-00438.

41. I Perali, A Celani, L Bombelli, C Fiorini, F Camera, E Clementel, S Henrotin, G Janssens, D Prieels, F Roellinghoff, J Smeets, F Stichelbaut, and F Vander Stappen. Prompt gamma imaging of proton pencil beams at clinical dose rate. 59(19):5849–5871.

42. S W Peterson, D Robertson, and J Polf. Optimizing a three-stage Compton camera for measuring prompt gamma rays emitted during proton radiotherapy. 55(22):6841–6856.

43. Johannes Petzoldt, Guillaume Janssens, Lena Nenoff, Christian Richter, and Julien Smeets. Correction of geometrical effects of a knife-edge slit camera for prompt gamma-based range verification in proton therapy. 2(4):25.

44. M. Pinto, D. Dauvergne, N. Freud, J. Krimmer, J. M. Letang, C. Ray, F. Roellinghoff, and E. Testa. Design optimisation of a TOF-based collimated camera prototype for online hadron-therapy monitoring. 59(24):7653.

45. M Pinto, K Kröniger, J Bauer, R Nilsson, E Traneus, and K Parodi. A filtering approach for PET and PG predictions in a proton treatment planning system. 65(9):095014.

46. Marco Pinto. *Modelling and simulation of physics processes for in-beam imaging in hadron-therapy*. PhD thesis, Université Claude Bernard Lyon 1, 2014.

47. Jerimy C Polf, Stephen Avery, Dennis S Mackin, and Sam Beddar. Imaging of prompt gamma rays emitted during delivery of clinical proton beams with a compton camera: feasibility studies for range verification. 60(18):7085–7099.

48. Jerimy C. Polf, Dennis Mackin, Eunsin Lee, Stephen Avery, and Sam Beddar. Detecting prompt gamma emission during proton therapy: the effects of detector size and distance from the patient. 59(9):2325.

49. Jerimy C. Polf, Rajesh Panthi, Dennis S. Mackin, Matt McCleskey, Antti Saastamoinen, Brian T. Roeder, and Sam Beddar. Measurement of characteristic prompt gamma rays emitted from oxygen and carbon in tissue-equivalent samples during proton beam irradiation. 58(17):5821.

50. M. Richard, M. Chevallier, D. Dauvergne, N. Freud, P. Henriquet, F. Le Foulher, J. M. Letang, G. Montarou, C. Ray, F. Roellinghoff, E. Testa, M. Testa, and A. H. Walenta. Design guidelines for a double scattering Compton camera for prompt-Îş imaging during ion beam therapy: A monte carlo simulation study. 58(1):87–94.

51. Christian Richter, Guntram Pausch, Steffen Barczyk, Marlen Priegnitz, Isabell Keitz, Julia Thiele, Julien Smeets, Francois Vander Stappen, Luca Bombelli, Carlo Fiorini, Lucian Hotoiu, Irene Perali, Damien Prieels, Wolfgang Enghardt, and Michael Baumann. First clinical application of a prompt gamma based in vivo proton range verification system.

52. C Robert, G Dedes, G Battistoni, T T Böhlen, I Buvat, F Cerutti, M P W Chin, A Ferrari, P Gueth, C Kurz, L Lestand, A Mairani, G Montarou, R Nicolini, P G Ortega, K Parodi, Y Prezado, P R Sala, D Sarrut, and E Testa. Distributions of secondary particles in proton and carbon-ion therapy: a comparison between GATE/Geant4 and FLUKA Monte Carlo codes. 58(9):2879–2899.

53. F. Roellinghoff, M.-H. Richard, M. Chevallier, J. Constanzo, D. Dauvergne, N. Freud, P. Henriquet, F. Le Foulher, J.M. Létang, G. Montarou, C. Ray, E. Testa, M. Testa, and A.H. Walenta. Design of a Compton camera for 3D prompt-gamma imaging during ion beam therapy. 648:S20–S23.

54. A Schumann, M Priegnitz, S Schoene, W Enghardt, H Rohling, and F Fiedler. From prompt gamma distribution to dose: a novel approach combining an evolutionary algorithm and filtering based on gaussian-powerlaw convolutions. 61(19):6919–6934.

55. Kyu Seo, Chan Kim, and Jong Kim. Comparison of titanium hydride (TiH2) and paraffin as neutron moderator material in a prompt gamma scanning system. 48(4):5.

56. J Smeets, F Roellinghoff, D Prieels, F Stichelbaut, A Benilov, P Busca, C Fiorini, R Peloso, M Basilavecchia, T Frizzi, J C Dehaes, and A Dubus. Prompt gamma imaging with a slit camera for real-time range control in proton therapy. 57(11):3371–3405.

57. Julien Smeets, Frauke Roellinghoff, Guillaume Janssens, Irene Perali, Andrea Celani, Carlo Fiorini, Nicolas Freud, Etienne Testa, and Damien Prieels. Experimental comparison of knife-edge and multi-parallel slit collimators for prompt gamma imaging of proton pencil beams. 6.

58. G Sportelli, N Belcari, N Camarlinghi, G A P Cirrone, G Cuttone, S Ferretti, A Kraan, J E Ortuño, F Romano, A Santos, K Straub, A Tramontana, A Del Guerra, and V Rosso. First full-beam PET acquisitions in proton therapy with a modular dual-head dedicated system. 59(1):43–60.

59. E. Sterpin, G. Janssens, J. Smeets, François Vander Stappen, D. Prieels, Marlen Priegnitz, Irene Perali, and S. Vynckier. Analytical computation of prompt gamma ray emission and detection for proton range verification. 60(12):4915.

60. E. Testa, M. Bajard, M. Chevallier, D. Dauvergne, F. Le Foulher, N. Freud, J.-M. Létang, J.-C. Poizat, C. Ray, and M. Testa. Monitoring the bragg peak location of 73 MeV‚àïu carbon ions by means of prompt Îş-ray measurements. 93(9):093506.

61. Liheng Tian, Ze Huang, Guillaume Janssens, Guillaume Landry, George Dedes, Florian Kamp, Claus Belka, Marco Pinto, and Katia Parodi. Accounting for prompt gamma emission and detection for range verification in proton therapy treatment planning. 66(5):055005.

62. Liheng Tian, Guillaume Landry, George Dedes, Marco Pinto, Florian Kamp, Claus Belka, and Katia Parodi. A new treatment planning approach accounting for prompt gamma range verification and interfractional anatomical changes. 65(9):095005.

63. Liheng Tian, Guillaume Landry, Georgios Dedes, Florian Kamp, Marco Pinto, Katharina Niepel, Claus Belka, and Katia Parodi. Toward a new treatment planning approach accounting for in vivo proton range verification. 63(21):215025.

64. et al. T.T. Bohlen. Benchmarking nuclear models of fluka and geant4 for carbon ion therapy. *Phys. Med. Biol.*, page 5833, 2010.

65. Joost M Verburg, Kent Riley, Thomas Bortfeld, and Joao Seco. Energy- and time-resolved detection of prompt gamma-rays for proton range verification. 58(20):L37–L49.

66. Joost M. Verburg and Joao Seco. Proton range verification through prompt gamma-ray spectroscopy. 59(23):7089.

67. Joost M Verburg, Helen A Shih, and Joao Seco. Simulation of prompt gamma-ray emission during proton radiotherapy. 57(17):5459–5472.

68. Theresa Werner, Jonathan Berthold, Fernando Hueso-González, Toni Koegler, Johannes Petzoldt, Katja Roemer, Christian Richter, Andreas Rinscheid, Arno Straessner, Wolfgang Enghardt, and Guntram Pausch. Processing of prompt gamma-ray timing data for proton range measurements at a clinical beam delivery. 64(10):105023.

69. Yunhe Xie, El Hassane Bentefour, Guillaume Janssens, Julien Smeets, François Vander Stappen, Lucian Hotoiu, Lingshu Yin, Derek Dolney, Stephen Avery, Fionnbarr O'Grady, Damien Prieels, James McDonough, Timothy D. Solberg, Robert A. Lustig, Alexander Lin, and Boon-Keng K. Teo. Prompt gamma imaging for in vivo range verification of pencil beam scanning proton therapy. 99(1):210–218.

70. Mitsutaka Yamaguchi, Yuto Nagao, Koki Ando, Seiichi Yamamoto, Toshiyuki Toshito, Jun Kataoka, and Naoki Kawachi. Secondary-electron-bremsstrahlung imaging for proton therapy. 833:199–207.

71. Mitsutaka Yamaguchi, Kota Torikai, Naoki Kawachi, Hirofumi Shimada, Takahiro Satoh, Yuto Nagao, Shu Fujimaki, Motohide Kokubun, Shin Watanabe, Tadayuki Takahashi, Kazuo Arakawa, Tomihiro Kamiya, and Takashi Nakano. Beam range estimation by measuring bremsstrahlung. 57(10):2843–2856.

# 4 Macroscopic and microscopic calculation approaches for LET calculations

*M.A. Cortes-Giraldo*
Universidad de Sevilla, Seville, Spain

*A. Bertolet*
Massachusetts General Hospital and Harvard Medical School, Boston, MA, USA

*A. Baratto-Roldan*
CERN, European Organization for Nuclear Research, Geneva, Switzerland

*A. Carabe*
Hampton University Proton Therapy Institute, Hampton University, Hampton, VA, USA

## CONTENTS

## 4.1 THE CONCEPT OF LET AND ITS AVERAGES

Linear energy transfer (LET) is a non-stochastic quantity which has become key nowadays in radiation therapy, especially in particle therapy. The biological effect of a ionizing radiation on living matter is usually quantified by the radiobiological effectiveness (RBE), defined as the dose need to cause a given damage by a reference radiation (typically a $^{60}$Co source) over the radiation under study. For charged particle beams, the RBE depends on physical properties of the beam, such as dose, dose rate, and beam LET, and on biological properties of the irradiated tissue or organ. Among them, the RBE dependence with respect to the LET has been widely studied to develop phenomenological models based on the LET ([1, 2, 3]). Further, some institutions have incorporated the calculation of LET distributions into the treatment planning system (TPS) software to include radiobiological optimization in their treatment plans.

The LET is strongly related with the stopping power, but we must treat their differences with special care. According to the ICRU report 85 ([4]), for charged particles of a given type and energy,

DOI: 10.1201/9781003023920-4

the LET or *restricted linear electronic* stopping power, $L_\Delta$, of a material, is given by

$$L_\Delta = \frac{dE_\Delta}{dl} \, , \qquad (4.1)$$

where $dE_\Delta$ is the mean energy lost by the charged particle due to electronic interactions along a distance $dl$, excluding the kinetic energy carried by secondary electrons released with initial kinetic energy equal or greater than $\Delta$. The LET is usually expressed in keV/μm in particle therapy, sometimes in MeV/mm or MeV/cm, whereas the subscript $\Delta$ is expressed in eV (i.e., $L_{250}$ means LET restricted to 250 eV).

According to this, $L_\Delta$ can be also calculated by

$$L_\Delta = S_{el} - \frac{d\overline{E}_{e,\,\Delta}}{dl} \, , \qquad (4.2)$$

where $S_{el}$ is the linear *electronic* stopping power, and $d\overline{E}_{e,\,\Delta}$ is the mean sum of the kinetic energies of all the electrons released with initial kinetic energy greater than $\Delta$ by the charged particle along a trajectory length $dl$. This expression gives a more explicit view on the energy balance to consider when calculated LET. The LET is a magnitude thought to estimate the *local* energy deposition per unit path length by excluding the electrons released with a kinetic energy larger than a given threshold. One limiting case is $L_0$, which excludes the kinetic energy of *all* the electrons released to medium; thus $L_0$ accounts for the mean energy lost by the charged particle per unit path length due to electronic excitation plus the energy expended to overcome the binding energy of each interaction producing ionization. In other words, $L_0$ includes the energy loss of the charged particle due to electronic collisions which is not converted into kinetic energy of secondary electrons.

All the electrons released can be included by considering the formal limit $\Delta \to \infty$, used often in particle therapy. In such a case $L_\infty = S_{el}$, where $L_\infty$ is known as *unrestricted* LET. The subscript $\infty$ is frequently dropped, so that in many works the unrestricted LET is simply referred as "LET," being the term "restricted LET" used for cases with a finite $\Delta$-value. As for the linear stopping power of a material for particles of a given type and energy, we recall that it is the result of the sum of three terms: *electronic*, *nuclear*, and *radiative*; at typical particle therapy energies, the electronic term is much larger than the sum of the other two.

Another type of restriction, sometimes applied to LET, is of spatial kind. The LET can be also calculated applying a *radial* restriction around the ion track core. If so, it is usually represented by $LET_r$ or $L_r$. ([5])

Typically, the radiation field incoming at a given elementary volume in the material $dV$, centered around a point given by r, is composed by particles of different types and energies; this results on having a distribution of LET values at $dV$. This introduces the need of calculating an average value at $dV$ to obtain an effective LET with which the biological effect is estimated. There are two ways of averaging, namely track average LET, represented by $\overline{L}_{\Delta,\,T}$ or LETt, and dose average LET, represented by by $\overline{L}_{\Delta,\,D}$ or LETd. ([5])

Track average LET at a given point is given by

$$\overline{L}_{\Delta,\,T}(\mathrm{r}) = \int_0^\infty L_\Delta \, t\,(L_\Delta;\mathrm{r}) \, dL_\Delta \, , \qquad (4.3)$$

where $t\,(L_\Delta;\mathrm{r})$ is the normalized track length distribution at r as function of $L_\Delta$, i.e., $t\,(L_\Delta;\mathrm{r})\,dL_\Delta$ represents the fraction of track lengths with LET value between $L_\Delta$ and $L_\Delta + dL_\Delta$ observed in the elementary volume $dV$ centered at r. Similarly, dose average LET at r is given by

$$\overline{L}_{\Delta,\,D}(\mathrm{r}) = \int_0^\infty L_\Delta \, d\,(L_\Delta;\mathrm{r}) \, dL_\Delta \, , \qquad (4.4)$$

where $d(L_\Delta;r)$ is the normalized dose distribution at r as function of $L_\Delta$, i.e., $d(L_\Delta)\,dL_\Delta$ represents the fraction of dose absorbed at LET value between $L_\Delta$ and $L_\Delta+dL_\Delta$ observed in the elementary volume $dV$ centered at r. It can be shown that both distributions are related as follows

$$d(L_\Delta;r) = \frac{L_\Delta\, t(L_\Delta;r)}{\overline{L}_{\Delta,\,T}(r)} \,. \tag{4.5}$$

Considering the relation between fluence and path lengths described within an elementary volume $dV$ ([48, 4]), and a change of integration variable from $L_\Delta$ to the energy of the charged particle $E$, the averages expressed in (3) and (4) can be rewritten as follows

$$\overline{L}_{\Delta,T}(r) = \frac{\int_0^\infty \phi_E(r)\, L_\Delta(E;r)\, dE}{\int_0^\infty \phi_E(r)\, dE} \,, \tag{4.6}$$

$$\overline{L}_{\Delta,D}(r) = \frac{\int_0^\infty \phi_E(r)\, L_\Delta^2(E;r)\, dE}{\int_0^\infty \phi_E(r)\, L_\Delta(E;r)\, dE} \,, \tag{4.7}$$

Where $L_\Delta(E;r)$ is the LET distribution in terms of $E$ at r, and $\phi_E(r) \equiv d\phi(r)/dE$ is the spectral fluence of particles at $dV$ due to charged particles of the same type at energies between $E$ and $E+dE$, thus $\int_0^\infty \phi_E(r)\, dE \equiv \Phi(r)$ is the total fluence of charged particles of the same kind at r.

Finally, it can be shown that $\overline{L}_{\Delta,D}(r) \geq \overline{L}_{\Delta,T}(r)$, where the equality holds only for the case of having a constant $L_\Delta(E;r)$ distribution (i.e., independent of the particle energy). In the context of particle therapy, this is only achieved by having at r a pure monoenergetic radiation field composed by particles of the same kind. ([6])

## 4.2   SCORING STRATEGIES FOR DIRECT COMPUTATION OF AVERAGE LET

In Monte Carlo calculations for particle therapy, average LET distributions are often calculated. But the translation of equations (3)-(4) or (6)-(7) into scorers in a Monte Carlo code must be handled with care, especially as for dose average LET, as discussed in next paragraphs. For simplicity, let us focus on the calculation of average *unrestricted* LET, i.e. $\overline{L}_{\infty,D}$. Thus, the LET will be understood hereinafter as unrestricted unless otherwise stated, so that the subscript $\Delta \to \infty$ will be dropped to ease notation.

Let us consider a simple case of calculation of average LET distribution. Let us assume a primary beam composed by charged particles (e.g. protons) in which each primary defines an independent history (named *event* in Geant4), and the beam irradiates a phantom modeled with a voxelized geometry. After simulating $N$ independent histories, we focus on the calculation of both averages of LET at an arbitrary voxel centered at $r_i$, $\overline{L}_D(r_i)$. Since, during the simulation, the energy deposition and energy lost by a charged particle can be obtained, the most intuitive translation of (6)-(7) to a Monte Carlo scorer, which we name technique (I), probably is

$$\overline{L}_{T,(I)}(r) = \frac{\int_{n=1}^N \int_{s=1}^{S_n} \omega_n \left(\frac{\varepsilon_{sn}}{l_{sn}}\right) l_{sn}}{\int_{n=1}^N \int_{s=1}^{S_n} \omega_n\, l_{sn}} = \frac{\int_{n=1}^N \int_{s=1}^{S_n} \omega_n\, \varepsilon_{sn}}{\int_{n=1}^N \int_{s=1}^{S_n} \omega_n\, l_{sn}} \tag{4.8}$$

$$\overline{L}_{D,(I)}(r) = \frac{\int_{n=1}^N \int_{s=1}^{S_n} \omega_n \left(\frac{\varepsilon_{sn}}{l_{sn}}\right) \varepsilon_{sn}}{\int_{n=1}^N \int_{s=1}^{S_n} \omega_n\, \varepsilon_{sn}} = \frac{\int_{n=1}^N \int_{s=1}^{S_n} \omega_n\, \frac{\varepsilon_{sn}^2}{l_{sn}}}{\int_{n=1}^N \int_{s=1}^{S_n} \omega_n\, \varepsilon_{sn}} \tag{4.9}$$

where the index $n \in [1,N]$ is the history number (known as *event* in Geant4 terminology), the index $s$ is the $s$-th step described by a charged particle of the selected type under study in the volume centered at r so that at the $n$-th history the number of calculated steps is $S_n$, $\varepsilon_{sn}$ and $l_{sn}$ are the energy lost due to electronic collisions and step length, respectively, calculated for a charged particle of the type of interest at the $s$-th step of the $n$-th history, and $\omega_n$ is the statistical weight of the $n$-th primary. This technique was one of the first methods used in proton therapy ([7, 8]) but it has been proved to be prone to give biased values depending on the level of detail of the voxelized geometry and on the threshold set to track secondary electrons. ([9, 10])

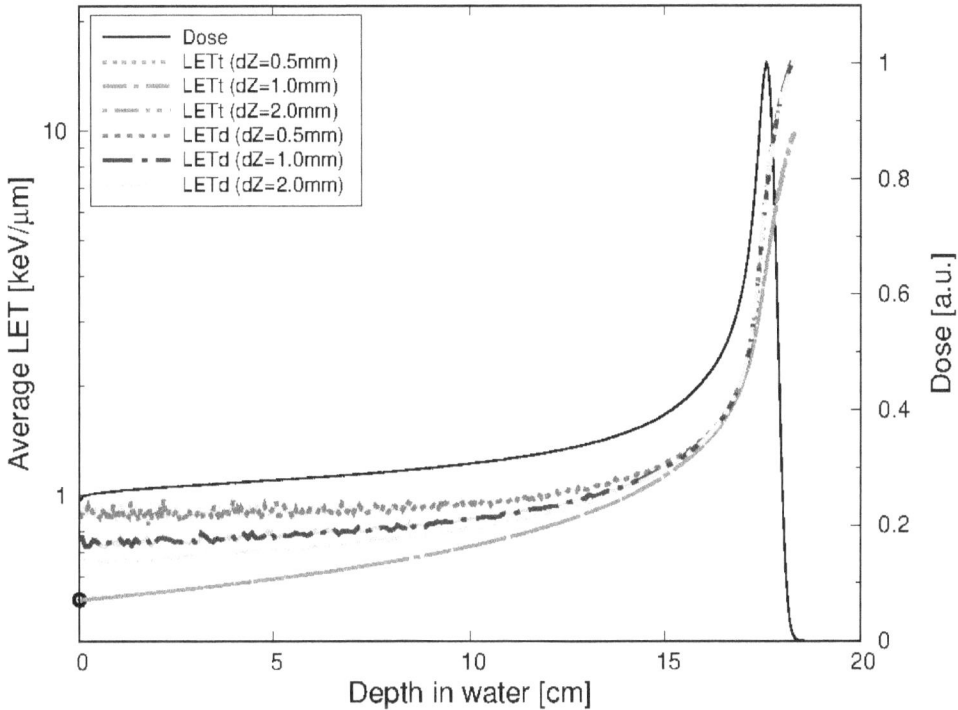

**Figure 4.1**   Track- and dose average LET curves calculated with equations (8)–(9), i.e. method "A" described in ([9]), for a 160-MeV monoenergetic proton beam irradiating a water tank. The thickness of the scoring cells varied between 0.5 and 2.0 mm.

Figure 4.1 shows the results provided by average LET scorers implementing equations (8) and (9) for track- and dose average LET, respectively, calculated with the Geant4 toolkit ([11, 12, 13]), version 10.6.3, for a proton beam irradiating a cylindrical water tank, similarly as done by [9]. The proton beam was monoenergetic, 160 MeV, having a 2D Gaussian profile with $\sigma = 8.5$ mm. The water tank was divided into voxels following its cylindrical symmetry; the size of the voxels along the $z$-axis was varied from 0.5 to 2.0 mm, whereas the radial size was always 5 mm. The reference physics list QGSP_BIC_HP_EMZ was used with a production threshold of secondary particles set to 0.1 mm. The calculations shown correspond to the voxels placed along the central axis. Although no significant differences are observed for the track average LET calculations, the dose average LET values increase as the voxel size decreases, which is a behavior not desirable according to the properties of the LET. The main reason lies in the fact of having steps with artificially short lengths due to voxel boundary crossing, which introduces spurious "high-LET" steps into the average, as shown and discussed by [9]. In addition, the value of the production threshold of secondary particles has also an impact on the dose average LET calculated using this technique, again biasing the calculation to higher values as the production threshold value decreases. ([9, 10]). In addition, track- and dose average LET should converge at the entrance of the tank ($z = 0$), according to the fact that the incident beam is monoenergetic; this is not observed either in the figure.

To calculate appropriately dose average LET values, [9] proposed another scoring technique, named method "C" in the paper and here called technique (II), given by

$$\overline{L}_{D,(II)}(r) = \frac{\int_{n=1}^{N} \int_{s=1}^{S_n} \omega_n L_{sn} \varepsilon_{sn}}{\int_{n=1}^{N} \int_{s=1}^{S_n} \omega_n \varepsilon_{sn}}, \qquad (4.10)$$

where $L_{sn}$ is the LET obtained by interpolation of pre-calculated data tables for the specific combination of travelling particle, kinetic energy and material given at the step $s$ of particle $n$. With this method, the LET calculated at each step depends only on the particle-material combination mentioned, which is the minimum information needed to calculate the *mean* energy lost per unit path length; thus, the calculation does not depend on the step length nor on the production threshold of secondaries anymore. As for the kinetic energy of a given step, the arithmetic mean between the initial and final kinetic energy seems to be the best choice, especially if the LET value changes abruptly with the kinetic energy of the travelling particle. Analogously, technique (II) applied for the track average LET becomes

$$\overline{L}_{T,(II)}(r) = \frac{\int_{n=1}^{N} \int_{s=1}^{S_n} \omega_n L_{sn} l_{sn}}{\int_{n=1}^{N} \int_{s=1}^{S_n} \omega_n l_{sn}}. \qquad (4.11)$$

Figure 4.2 shows the track- and dose average calculation obtained for this technique (II) for the same cases as shown in Figure 4.1. Clearly, track- and dose average LET values show no dependence on the voxel grid considered. Moreover, both averages fulfill the property stated previously, $\overline{L}_D(r) \geq \overline{L}_T(r)$, as both averages converge at the beam entrance ($z = 0$), where the beam is monoenergetic, and diverge as the beam penetrates in the water tank because of energy straggling, being the dose average LET larger than the track average LET (see inset). Further, the value of the average LET at the entrance tend to the electronic linear stopping power obtained from ICRU Report 90 data ([14]) for protons in water at 160 MeV, 0.52 keV/μm, which is clearly missed by the dose average LET calculated at entrance with technique (I). Thus, the use of technique (II) is strongly recommended for the calculation of dose average LET calculations. As for track average LET, both techniques give similar results although the convergence and numerical stability of the calculations carried out with technique (II) is superior. Thus, we can conclude that technique (II) must be the choice to calculate both LET averages. For these reasons, technique (II) has been implemented by several groups ([15, 16, 17, 18])

Some technical aspects to note about the scorers defined by equations (10)-(11) are the following:

1. At a given step, the kinetic energy of the particle changes from the initial to the final point. Using the initial kinetic energy to retrieve the LET representative of the step may be an acceptable simplification where the gradient of LET vs energy is not important within the energy range covered in a simulation (in particle therapy, this means not covering very low energies). But in general, it is a good idea to calculate the arithmetic mean between the initial and final kinetic energy at each step, especially in cases where the final kinetic energy is equal to, or close to zero.

2. Because of the previous point, it is important to carry out the calculation with steps calculated due to electromagnetic interactions only. Steps defined by hadronic interactions may terminate the tracking of the particle, in which case the final kinetic energy could be assumed to be zero; however, this energy change was not produced by electromagnetic collisions. It is true that this filter does not have a significant impact at typical particle therapy scenarios, as the probability of having a step defined by hadronic interactions is much smaller than those defined by electromagnetic interactions. But in scenarios with higher energies and ion masses including this filter may impact the result.

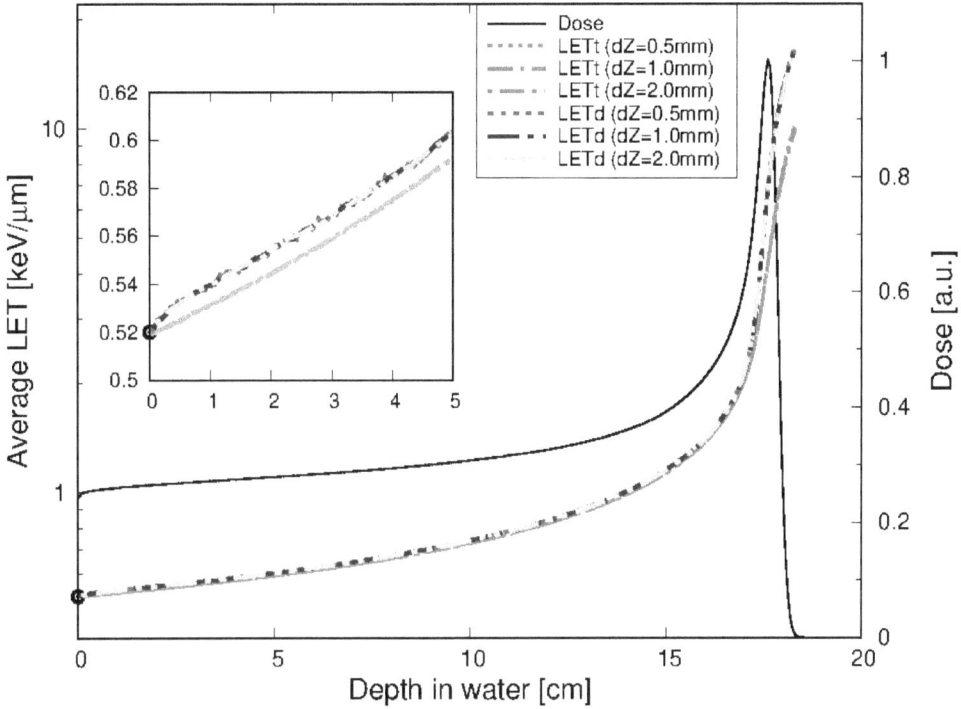

**Figure 4.2** Track- and dose average LET curves calculated with equations (10)-(11), i.e. method "C" described in ([9]), for a 160-MeV monoenergetic proton beam irradiating a water tank. The thickness of the scoring cells varied between 0.5 and 2.0 mm. The inset zooms the depth interval from 0 to 5 cm to highlight the convergence of both LET averages at the entrance surface, where the proton beam is purely monoenergetic.

3. The calculation of the energy loss due to electronic collisions, weighting factor $\varepsilon_{sn}$, must be done considering if the LET calculated is restricted or not. For unrestricted LET, $\varepsilon_{sn}$ can be obtained by sum of the energy deposition along the step (this is energy lost due to "soft" electromagnetic collisions) and the kinetic energy transferred to the secondary electrons released at the end of the step (energy lost due to a "hard" collision). For restricted LET, then the secondary electrons released with kinetic energy higher than the threshold $\Delta$ considered must be discarded.
4. For both averages, scoring of the numerator has to be done separate from the scoring of the denominator until the end of the simulation, as the quotient has to be calculated once numerator and denominator sums have been calculated.

Other techniques used to calculate average LET are based on the calculation of the spectral fluence at each voxel, so that an LET value is associated with each energy bin ([6]). This approach is a direct translation of equations (6)–(7) and is mostly used in analytical calculations. In these calculations, the bin width used to calculate the spectral fluence must be small enough to consider the LET is constant for each bin. This is key for low energies, where the gradient of LET vs particle energy is larger.

Despite dose average LET is a quantity widely used in proton therapy for RBE calculations ([2, 19, 20, 21, 22]) some issues have been raised on the inclusion of secondary particles, especially in proton therapy, into the calculation of the dose average LET. Along their path, clinical proton

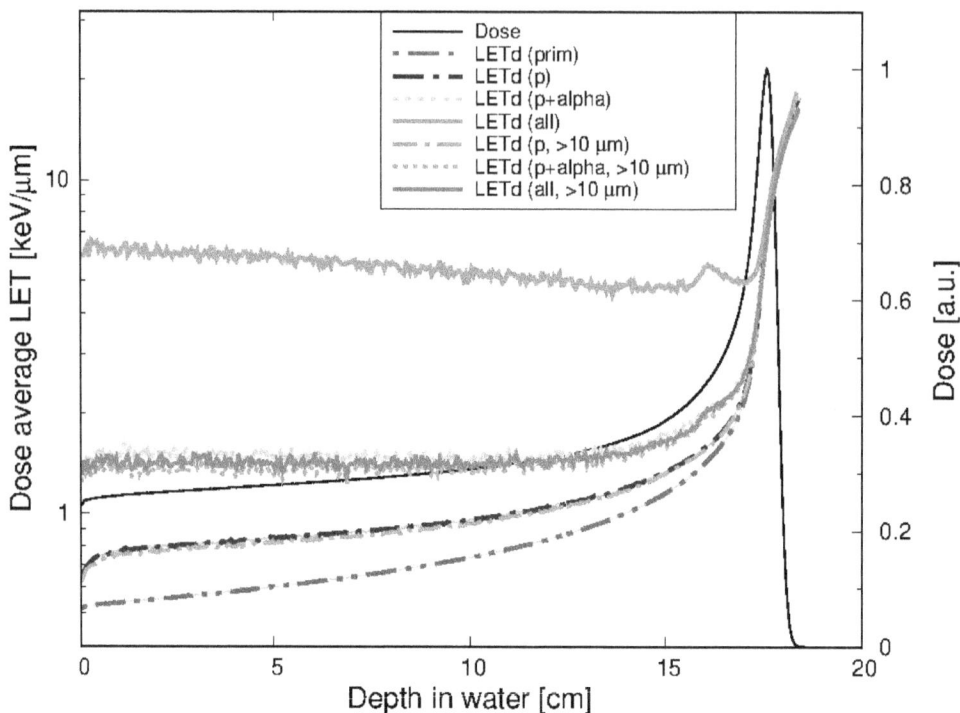

**Figure 4.3**  Dose average LET curves calculated with equations (10)-(11), i.e. method "C" described in ([9]), for a 160-MeV monoenergetic proton beam irradiating a water tank; scoring cell thickness was 0.5 mm. Various secondary particle species were incorporated into the calculation of the dose average LET curves as indicated at the legend.

beams produce secondary ions of very short range, typically smaller than cell dimensions, which biological role is not clear. However, secondary ions introduce very high LET terms into the average, changing drastically its value ([23, 24]). Figure 4.3 illustrates this by comparing the dose average LET obtained including secondary protons, alphas, and ions, respectively, into the calculation. Clearly, the dose average LET values depend on the type of secondary particles considered into the average. Actually, the inclusion of secondary ions heavier than alpha particles produces a drastic increase on the dose average LET, despite their ranges are typically smaller than 10 microns. This is illustrated by the change observed when excluding steps smaller than 10 microns from the dose average calculation (see gray lines in Figure 4.3), in which case the dose average LET calculated including all ion species into the average converges to that calculated considering the contribution of protons and alphas only. This sensitivity to the type of secondary ions included into the average shows a particular limitation of using a "global" dose average LET as quantity to characterize the radiation beam quality ([25]). As a consequence, it has been suggested that more accurate descriptions are needed when reporting average LET distributions for RBE calculations (Kalholm et al. 2021). Thus, whether secondary ions should be included into the calculation of dose average LET for clinical proton beams is an issue which remains unclear and open due to the issues described above and the fact that it has been observed that the biological effect produced by various ion beams at same LET depends on the ion type as well ([26]).

## 4.3  CONNECTION BETWEEN LET AND MICRODOSIMETRIC QUANTITIES

Another approach to assess the radiation field quality is based on the theory of microdosimetry. In one of its approaches to assess biological damage induced by ionizing radiation is based on the analysis of the microscopic patterns of the interactions by which the energy is deposited. This analysis can be done by calculating the distribution of energy imparted to critical cell structures, usually modeled as *sites*. Contrary to LET, microdosimetry quantities are stochastic but measurable.

Indeed, the analog to LET in microdosimetry is the *lineal energy*, $y = \varepsilon_s/\bar{l}$, where $\varepsilon_s$ is the energy imparted to the site per single ion track, and $\bar{l}$ is the mean chord length of the site; for example, if the site is a sphere with radius $R$, then $\bar{l} = (4/3)R$.

Both averages of the LET can be written in terms of microdosimetry quantities (Kellerer 1985). For the track average LET, it is verified that

$$\bar{L}_{s,T} = \bar{y}_F \,, \tag{4.12}$$

where $\bar{y}_F = y = \varepsilon_s/\bar{l}$ is the frequency-mean lineal energy, and the subscript $s$ denotes that the LET calculated with this method is *restricted* by the site size. This restriction is somewhat similar to the radial restriction mentioned above, but not exactly the same.

The relation of the dose average LET with microdosimetric quantities is more complex, as it involves the variance of various magnitudes which characterize the irradiation incident to a site, namely, the LET variability of each incident ion, distribution of path lengths of ion trajectories within the site and variability of the energy imparted to the site per track (energy straggling). The computation of the latter is especially complicated due to the finite range of secondary electrons, which introduces the need of considering the escape and influx of these electrons, which needs to be assessed with Monte Carlo simulations. It can be shown that (Kellerer 1985)

$$\bar{L}_{s,D} = \bar{y}_D \frac{\bar{l}_F}{\bar{l}_D} - \frac{\delta_2}{\bar{l}_D} \,, \tag{4.13}$$

where $\bar{y}_D = y^2/\langle y \rangle$ is the dose-mean lineal energy, $\bar{l}_D = l^2/\langle l \rangle$ is the weighted-average of chord lengths $l$ described by the ion tracks, $\bar{l}_F = \langle l \rangle$ is the frequency-average of chord lengths, and $\delta_2$ is the weighted-average of the energy imparted to the site per individual collision $\varepsilon_c$, i.e. $\delta_2 = \varepsilon_c^2/\langle \varepsilon_c \rangle$.

Thus, LET restricted to site dimensions can be calculated from track structure Monte Carlo simulation. Among the quantities involved, $\delta_2$ is the most challenging one as it requires to identify with a numerical tag each electron shower emerging directly from the ion track, so that each energy exchange occurring in the site can be associated to a single electron shower using this tag. ([9, 22, 27]; Baratto-Roldán et al. 2021)

This connection is especially useful to carry out simultaneous calculations of restricted LET and microdosimetric quantities in TPSs in order to provide various approaches for RBE calculations. With this purpose, Bertolet et al. proposed recently a simplification of (13) for the limit of protons crossing sites small enough to consider their stopping power constant, but large enough to neglect secondary electron outflux. ([28]) In such a case,

$$\bar{L}_{s,D} = \frac{\overline{\overline{\varepsilon_s(E)}}}{\bar{s}} \left( 1 + \frac{\sigma_{\bar{\varepsilon}_s}^2}{\left(\overline{\overline{\varepsilon_s(E)}}\right)^2} \right) \,, \tag{4.14}$$

where $\overline{\overline{\varepsilon_s(E)}}$ is the average of the mean energy imparted per event $\overline{\varepsilon_s}(E)$ calculated as function of the proton energy $E$, $\bar{s}$ is the mean path (or segment) length described by protons, and $\sigma_{\bar{\varepsilon}_s}^2$ is the variance of the distribution of mean energy imparted per event. Under these conditions, the number of quantities needed to calculate either microscopic and macroscopic quantities is lower than in the general case, simplifying the calculations.

## 4.4  IMPLEMENTATION IN TREATMENT PLANNING SYSTEMS

Radiation therapy treatments are patient-wisely tailored to account for the geometric characteristics of every individual. To this goal, TPS are utilized. While commercially available TPSs for proton therapy focus on the distribution of dose throughout the patient, there have recently been multiple attempts to incorporate the calculation of LET distributions into these systems. Ideally, TPSs should not only provide forward calculations to evaluate both dose and LET distributions but also use this information to inverse-optimize plans, a process in which multiple iterations are typically involved. Therefore, TPS-based calculations need to be not only accurate, but also as fast as possible. The available approaches to accomplish this can be split apart into two general categories: (a) Monte Carlo-based; and (b) analytical algorithms.

Monte Carlo-based calculations rely on the simulation of proton tracks to score the complete spectrum of LET (i.e., the LET of each track) in a voxel-by-voxel basis. To make calculation times affordable in the clinical routine, these simulations normally are performed under simplified physics, thus considering only the dominant processes involved in the interaction between protons and matter. Also, most of the secondary particles produced after nuclear interactions can be neglected for a faster performance. For example, RayStation (RaySearch Laboratories AB, Stockholm, Sweden) incorporates a Monte Carlo dose engine able to compute LET distributions for primary protons, secondary protons, deuterons and alpha particles ([29]), disregarding processes such as nuclear absorption and multiple scattering. A special scoring system is used in voxels near the end of the particle range to account for effects, consisting of dividing the path of the particle inside the voxel in a maximum of 90 logarithmic steps in terms of kinetic energy, and sampling the stopping power according to this division. Another major vendor in proton radiotherapy, Varian Medical Systems, has equipped their TPS, with AcurosPT, a Monte Carlo engine to calculate dose distributions ([30]). However, to date, AcurosPT does not provide LET calculations. Other in-house approaches have been also published along the last years. A direct implementation of Cortés-Giraldo and Carabe scoring method "C" is presented in MCsquare ([15]), a fast, open-source Monte Carlo code which can be integrated with other tools for planning ([31]) or secondary dose calculation check ([32]). As increased computational speed is required, other approaches are based on the use of GPU instead of CPU to process Monte Carlo simulations, such as gPMC ([33, 34]), Fred ([35]) or the GPU-based code developed by Beltran and colleagues ([36, 37]).

On the other hand, analytical algorithms prioritize computational speed over accuracy. Analytical algorithms employ models of the quantity to be calculated, e.g., dose and/or LET, instead of obtaining them from the explicit transport of the particles. As of today, due to the relative high number of beams used in proton therapy and the corresponding computational burden, analytical methods remain as the most employed in inverse-optimization problems. Because of the ballistic properties of protons, the main approach traditionally utilized is the so-called convolution-superposition pencil beam algorithm, which decomposes a broad beam into narrow beamlets, whose contributions can be treated independently and eventually superposed. This approach usually provides clinically acceptable accuracy in most of scenarios, although major deviations can be found, particularly in cases with complex geometries ([38]). Analogously to dose, beamlet-wise LET models are analytical functions of the depth and lateral position with respect to the beam axis that are usually fitted against Monte Carlo simplistic simulations in liquid water ([39]). As it happens with the Monte Carlo approaches themselves, the physics, i.e., processes and secondary particles- included in this modeling processes varies from author to author. There is, therefore, a trade-off between the complexity of these functions and the speed of the calculations. FoCa is an in-house TPS that offers analytical LET calculation disregarding the lateral dependence of LET ([40, 41]), focusing only on the LET at the beamlet central axis as also done at the Institut Curie ([42]). Other authors have refined this approach by using more complex functions to model the lateral shape of the proton LET behavior in water ([43, 44]). A different approach has been developed as an external script for Eclipse (Varian Medical Systems, Palo Alto, CA), consisting of modeling the spectral fluence of a beamlet instead of the LET itself ([45]). This way, both dose ([46]) and LET can be obtained as indirect products of the spectral fluence. Also, microdosimetric calculations can be performed simultaneously ([22]).

## REFERENCES

1. Wilkens, J. J., and U. Oelfke. 2004. "A Phenomenological Model for the Relative Biological Effectiveness in Therapeutic Proton Beams." Physics in Medicine and Biology 49 (13): 2811–25. https://doi.org/10.1088/0031-9155/49/13/004.
2. Carabe, Alejandro, Maryam Moteabbed, Nicolas Depauw, Jan Schuemann, and Harald Paganetti. 2012. "Range Uncertainty in Proton Therapy Due to Variable Biological Effectiveness." Physics in Medicine and Biology 57 (5): 1159–72. https://doi.org/10.1088/0031-9155/57/5/1159.
3. Wedenberg, Minna, Bengt K Lind, and Björn Hårdemark. 2013. "A Model for the Relative Biological Effectiveness of Protons: The Tissue Specific Parameter $\alpha$ / $\beta$ of Photons Is a Predictor for the Sensitivity to LET Changes." Acta Oncologica 52 (3): 580–88. https://doi.org/10.3109/0284186X.2012.705892.
4. ———. 2011. "ICRU Report 85: Fundamental Quantities and Units for Ionizing Radiation (Revised)." Journal of the ICRU 11 (1): 32. http://jicru.oxfordjournals.org/%5Cnhttp://jicru.oxfordjournals.org/cgi/doi/10.1093/jicru/ndr004.
5. ICRU. 1970. "ICRU Report 16: Linear Energy Transfer." Journal of the International Commission on Radiation Units and Measurements os9 (1): 62.
6. Kempe, Johanna, Irena Gudowska, and Anders Brahme. 2006. "Depth Absorbed Dose and LET Distributions of Therapeutic H1, He4, Li7, and C12 Beams." Medical Physics 34 (1): 183–92. https://doi.org/10.1118/1.2400621.
7. Grassberger, C., and H. Paganetti. 2011. "Elevated LET Components in Clinical Proton Beams." Physics in Medicine and Biology 56 (20): 6677–91. https://doi.org/10.1088/0031-9155/56/20/011.
8. Romano, F, G A P Cirrone, G Cuttone, F Di Rosa, S E Mazzaglia, I Petrovic, A Ristic Fira, and A Varisano. 2014. "A Monte Carlo Study for the Calculation of the Average Linear Energy Transfer (LET) Distributions for a Clinical Proton Beam Line and a Radiobiological Carbon Ion Beam Line." Physics in Medicine and Biology 59 (12): 2863–82. https://doi.org/10.1088/0031-9155/59/12/2863.
9. Cortés-Giraldo, Miguel A., and Alejandro Carabe. 2015. "A Critical Study of Different Monte Carlo Scoring Methods of Dose Average Linear-Energy-Transfer Maps Calculated in Voxelized Geometries Irradiated with Clinical Proton Beams." Physics in Medicine and Biology 60 (7): 2645–69. https://doi.org/10.1088/0031-9155/60/7/2645.
10. Granville, Dal A., and Gabriel O. Sawakuchi. 2015. "Comparison of Linear Energy Transfer Scoring Techniques in Monte Carlo Simulations of Proton Beams." Physics in Medicine and Biology 60 (14): N283–91. https://doi.org/10.1088/0031-9155/60/14/N283.
11. Agostinelli, S., J. Allison, K. Amako, J. Apostolakis, H. Araujo, P. Arce, M. Asai, et al. 2003. "Geant4—a Simulation Toolkit." Nuclear Instruments and Methods in Physics Research Section A: Accelerators, Spectrometers, Detectors and Associated Equipment 506 (3): 250–303. https://doi.org/10.1016/S0168-9002(3)01368-8.
12. Allison, J., K. Amako, J. Apostolakis, H. Araujo, P. Arce Dubois, M. Asai, G. Barrand, et al. 2006. "Geant4 Developments and Applications." IEEE Transactions on Nuclear Science 53 (1): 270–78. https://doi.org/10.1109/TNS.2006.869826.
13. Allison, J., K. Amako, J. Apostolakis, P. Arce, M. Asai, T. Aso, E. Bagli, et al. 2016. "Recent Developments in Geant4." Nuclear Instruments and Methods in Physics Research Section A: Accelerators, Spectrometers, Detectors and Associated Equipment 835 (November): 186–225. https://doi.org/10.1016/j.nima.2016.06.125.

14. ———. 2016. "ICRU Report 90: Key Data for Ionizing-Radiation Dosimetry: Measurements Standards and Applications." Journal of the ICRU. Vol. 14. https://doi.org/10.1093/jicru/ndw043.

15. Souris, Kevin, John Aldo Lee, and Edmond Sterpin. 2016. "Fast Multipurpose Monte Carlo Simulation for Proton Therapy Using Multi- and Many-Core CPU Architectures." Medical Physics 43 (4): 1700–1712. https://doi.org/10.1118/1.4943377.

16. Grzanka, Leszek, Oscar Ardenfors, and Niels Bassler. 2018. "MONTE CARLO SIMULATIONS OF SPATIAL LET DISTRIBUTIONS IN CLINICAL PROTON BEAMS." Radiation Protection Dosimetry 180 (1–4): 296–99. https://doi.org/10.1093/rpd/ncx272.

17. Parisi, Alessio, Sabina Chiriotti, Marijke De Saint-Hubert, Olivier Van Hoey, Charlot Vandevoorde, Philip Beukes, Evan Alexander De Kock, et al. 2019. "A Novel Methodology to Assess Linear Energy Transfer and Relative Biological Effectiveness in Proton Therapy Using Pairs of Differently Doped Thermoluminescent Detectors." Physics in Medicine and Biology 64 (8): 085005. https://doi.org/10.1088/1361-6560/aaff20.

18. Petringa, G., L. Pandola, S. Agosteo, R. Catalano, P. Colautti, V. Conte, G. Cuttone, et al. 2020. "Monte Carlo Implementation of New Algorithms for the Evaluation of Averaged-Dose and -Track Linear Energy Transfers in 62 MeV Clinical Proton Beams." Physics in Medicine and Biology 65 (23): 235043. https://doi.org/10.1088/1361-6560/abaeb9.

19. McNamara, Aimee L., Jan Schuemann, and Harald Paganetti. 2015. "A Phenomenological Relative Biological Effectiveness (RBE) Model for Proton Therapy Based on All Published in Vitro Cell Survival Data." Physics in Medicine and Biology 60 (21): 8399–8416. https://doi.org/10.1088/0031-9155/60/21/8399.

20. Mairani, A., I. Dokic, G. Magro, T. Tessonnier, J. Bauer, T. T. Böhlen, M. Ciocca, et al. 2017. "A Phenomenological Relative Biological Effectiveness Approach for Proton Therapy Based on an Improved Description of the Mixed Radiation Field." Physics in Medicine and Biology 62 (4): 1378–95. https://doi.org/10.1088/1361-6560/aa51f7.

21. Rørvik, Eivind, Sara Thörnqvist, Camilla H. Stokkevåg, Tordis J. Dahle, Lars Fredrik Fjaera, and Kristian S. Ytre-Hauge. 2017. "A Phenomenological Biological Dose Model for Proton Therapy Based on Linear Energy Transfer Spectra." Medical Physics 44 (6): 2586–94. https://doi.org/10.1002/mp.12216.

22. Bertolet, A., A. Baratto-Roldán, S. Barbieri, G. Baiocco, A. Carabe, and M.A. Cortés-Giraldo. 2019. "Dose-Averaged LET Calculation for Proton Track Segments Using Microdosimetric Monte Carlo Simulations." Medical Physics 46 (9). https://doi.org/10.1002/mp.13643.

23. Grzanka, Leszek, Michael P R Waligórski, and Niels Bassler. 2019. "THE ROLE OF PARTICLE SPECTRA IN MODELING THE RELATIVE BIOLOGICAL EFFECTIVENESS OF PROTON RADIOTHERAPY BEAMS." Radiation Protection Dosimetry 183 (1–2): 251–54. https://doi.org/10.1093/rpd/ncy268.

24. Kalholm, Fredrik, Leszek Grzanka, Erik Traneus, and Niels Bassler. 2021. "A Systematic Review on the Usage of Averaged LET in Radiation Biology for Particle Therapy." Radiotherapy and Oncology 161 (August): 211–21. https://doi.org/10.1016/j.radonc.2021.04.007.

25. Grün, Rebecca, Thomas Friedrich, Erik Traneus, and Michael Scholz. 2019. "Is the Dose-averaged <scp>LET</scp> a Reliable Predictor for the Relative Biological Effectiveness?" Medical Physics 46 (2): 1064–74. https://doi.org/10.1002/mp.13347.

26. Furusawa, Y., K. Fukutsu, M. Aoki, H. Itsukaichi, K. Eguchi-Kasai, H. Ohara, F. Yatagai, T. Kanai, and K. Ando. 2000. "Inactivation of Aerobic and Hypoxic Cells from Three Different Cell Lines by Accelerated (3)He-, (12)C- and (20)Ne-Ion Beams." Radiation Research 154 (5): 485–96. https://doi.org/10.1667/0033-7587(2000)154[0485:ioaahc]2.0.co;2.

27. Baratto-Roldán A, Bertolet A, Baiocco G, Carabe A, Cortés-Giraldo MA (2021). "Microdosimetry and Dose-Averaged LET Calculations of Protons in Liquid Water: A Novel Geant4-DNA Application." Frontiers in Physics 9: 726787. doi: 10.3389/fphy.2021.726787

28. Bertolet, Alejandro, Miguel A. Cortés-Giraldo, and Alejandro Carabe-Fernandez. 2020. "On the Concepts of Dose-Mean Lineal Energy, Unrestricted and Restricted Dose-Averaged LET in Proton Therapy." Physics in Medicine and Biology 65 (7): ab730a. https://doi.org/10.1088/1361-6560/ab730a.

29. Wagenaar, Dirk, Linh T Tran, Arturs Meijers, Gabriel Guterres Marmitt, Kevin Souris, David Bolst, Benjamin James, et al. 2020. "Validation of Linear Energy Transfer Computed in a Monte Carlo Dose Engine of a Commercial Treatment Planning System Validation of Linear Energy Transfer Computed in a Monte Carlo Dose Engine of a Commercial Treatment Planning System." Physics in Medicine and Biology 65: 025006.

30. Lin, Liyong, Sheng Huang, Minglei Kang, Petri Hiltunen, Reynald Vanderstraeten, Jari Lindberg, Sami Siljamaki, et al. 2017. "A Benchmarking Method to Evaluate the Accuracy of a Commercial Proton Monte Carlo Pencil Beam Scanning Treatment Planning System." Journal of Applied Clinical Medical Physics 18 (2): 44–49. https://doi.org/10.1002/acm2.12043.

31. Lin, Liyong, Kevin Souris, Minglei Kang, Adam Glick, Haibo Lin, Sheng Huang, Kristin Stützer, et al. 2017. "Evaluation of Motion Mitigation Using Abdominal Compression in the Clinical Implementation of Pencil Beam Scanning Proton Therapy of Liver Tumors:" Medical Physics 44 (2): 703–12. https://doi.org/10.1002/mp.12040.

32. Deng, Wei, James E. Younkin, Kevin Souris, Sheng Huang, Kurt Augustine, Mirek Fatyga, Xiaoning Ding, et al. 2020. "Technical Note: Integrating an Open Source Monte Carlo Code 'MCsquare' for Clinical Use in Intensity-Modulated Proton Therapy." Medical Physics 47 (6): 2558–74. https://doi.org/10.1002/mp.14125.

33. Jia, Xun, Jan Schümann, Harald Paganetti, and Steve B. Jiang. 2012. "GPU-Based Fast Monte Carlo Dose Calculation for Proton Therapy." Physics in Medicine and Biology 57 (23): 7783–97. https://doi.org/10.1088/0031-9155/57/23/7783.

34. Giantsoudi, Drosoula, Jan Schuemann, Xun Jia, Stephen Dowdell, Steve Jiang, and Harald Paganetti. 2015. "Validation of a GPU-Based Monte Carlo Code (GPMC) for Proton Radiation Therapy: Clinical Cases Study." Physics in Medicine and Biology 60 (6): 2257–69. https://doi.org/10.1088/0031-9155/60/6/2257.

35. Schiavi, A., M. Senzacqua, S. Pioli, A. Mairani, G. Magro, S. Molinelli, M. Ciocca, G. Battistoni, and V. Patera. 2017. "Fred: A GPU-Accelerated Fast-Monte Carlo Code for Rapid Treatment Plan Recalculation in Ion Beam Therapy." Physics in Medicine and Biology 62 (18): 7482–7504. https://doi.org/10.1088/1361-6560/aa8134.

36. Wan Chan Tseung, H., J. Ma, and C. Beltran. 2015. "A Fast GPU-Based Monte Carlo Simulation of Proton Transport with Detailed Modeling of Nonelastic Interactions." Medical Physics 42 (6): 2967–78. https://doi.org/10.1118/1.4921046.

37. Pepin, Mark D., Erik Tryggestad, Hok Seum Wan Chan Tseung, Jedediah E. Johnson, Michael G. Herman, and Chris Beltran. 2018. "A Monte-Carlo-Based and GPU-Accelerated 4D-Dose Calculator for a Pencil Beam Scanning Proton Therapy System." Medical Physics 45 (11): 5293–5304. https://doi.org/10.1002/mp.13182.

38. Paganetti, Harald. 2012. "Range Uncertainties in Proton Therapy and the Role of Monte Carlo Simulations." Physics in Medicine and Biology 57 (11). https://doi.org/10.1088/0031-9155/57/11/R99.

39. Wilkens, Jan J., and Uwe Oelfke. 2003. "Analytical Linear Energy Transfer Calculations for Proton Therapy." Medical Physics 30 (5). https://doi.org/10.1118/1.1567852.

40. Sánchez-Parcerisa, D., M. Kondrla, A. Shaindlin, and A. Carabe. 2014. "FoCa: A Modular Treatment Planning System for Proton Radiotherapy with Research and Educational Purposes." Physics in Medicine and Biology 59 (23): 7341–60. https://doi.org/10.1088/0031-9155/59/23/7341.

41. Sanchez-Parcerisa, D., M A Cortés-Giraldo, D. Dolney, M. Kondrla, M. Fager, and A. Carabe. 2016. "Analytical Calculation of Proton Linear Energy Transfer in Voxelized

Geometries Including Secondary Protons." Physics in Medicine and Biology 61 (4): 1705–21. https://doi.org/10.1088/0031-9155/61/4/1705.

42. Marsolat, F, L De Marzi, F Pouzoulet, and A Mazal. 2016. "Analytical Linear Energy Transfer Model Including Secondary Particles: Calculations along the Central Axis of the Proton Pencil Beam." Physics in Medicine and Biology 61 (2). https://doi.org/10.1088/0031-9155/61/2/740.

43. Hirayama, Shusuke, Taeko Matsuura, Hideaki Ueda, Yusuke Fujii, Takaaki Fujii, Seishin Takao, Naoki Miyamoto, et al. 2018. "An Analytical Dose-Averaged LET Calculation Algorithm Considering the off-Axis LET Enhancement by Secondary Protons for Spot-Scanning Proton Therapy." Medical Physics 45 (7): 3404–16. https://doi.org/10.1002/mp.12991.

44. Deng, Wei, Xiaoning Ding, James E. Younkin, Jiajian Shen, Martin Bues, Steven E. Schild, Samir H. Patel, and Wei Liu. 2020. "Hybrid 3D Analytical Linear Energy Transfer Calculation Algorithm Based on Precalculated Data from Monte Carlo Simulations." Medical Physics 47 (2). https://doi.org/10.1002/mp.13934.

45. Bertolet, Alejandro, M. A. Cortés-Giraldo, Kevin Souris, and Alejandro Carabe. 2020. "A Kernel-based Algorithm for the Spectral Fluence of Clinical Proton Beams to Calculate Dose-averaged LET and Other Dosimetric Quantities of Interest." Medical Physics 47 (6): 2495–2505. https://doi.org/10.1002/mp.14108.

46. Bertolet, Alejandro, Miguel Antonio Cortés-Giraldo, Kevin Souris, Marie Cohilis, and Alejandro Carabe-Fernandez. 2019. "Calculation of Clinical Dose Distributions in Proton Therapy from Microdosimetry." Medical Physics 46 (12): 5816–23. https://doi.org/10.1002/mp.13861.

47. Carabe, Alejandro, Samuel España, Clemens Grassberger, and Harald Paganetti. 2013. "Clinical Consequences of Relative Biological Effectiveness Variations in Proton Radiotherapy of the Prostate, Brain and Liver." Physics in Medicine & Biology 58 (7): 2103. https://doi.org/10.1088/0031-9155/58/7/2103.

48. Kellerer, Albrecht M. 1985. "Fundamentals of Microdosimetry." In The Dosimetry of Ionizing Radiation, edited by Kenneth R. Kase, Bengt E. Bjärngard, and Frank H. Attix, I:77–162. Academic Press, Inc.

49. Papiez, L., and J. J. Battista. 1994. "Radiance and Particle Fluence." Physics in Medicine and Biology 39 (6): 1053–62. https://doi.org/10.1088/0031-9155/39/6/011.

# 5 Low energy hadronic processes in hadrontherapy

*Manuel Quesada*
Universidad de Sevilla, Seville, Spain

*Francesco Cerutti and Francesc Salvat Pujol*
CERN, European Organization for Nuclear Research, Geneva, Switzerland

*Maria Colonna*
Istituto Nazionale di Fisica Nucleare (INFN) Laboratori Nazionali del Sud (LNS), Catania, Italy

## CONTENTS

This chapter reviews the hadron beam interactions playing a role in medical applications, as implemented in the Geant4 and FLUKA codes or being modeled for further inclusion.

*Geant4*

Geant4 is a software tookit for the simulation of the passage of particles through matter. Hadronic physics in Geant4 spans the full energy range of interest and covers any reaction which can produce hadrons in its final state. As such, it covers purely hadronic interactions, lepton- and gamma-induced nuclear reactions, and radioactive decay. The interaction is represented as a Geant4 process which consists of a cross section to determine when the interaction will occur, and a model which determines the final state, i.e. produced secondary particles, of the interaction.

Models and cross sections are provided over the full energy range. As a characteristic Geant4 feature, for a given process within a certain energy range, more than one cross section and model

DOI: 10.1201/9781003023920-5

are usually offered in order to provide alternative approaches for different applications. Therefore several options exist which can be combined at user's choice or packed in a physics list (see below). In the following we are going to concentrate on particles, cross sections and models relevant for medical applications whose energy region of interest lies below 1 GeV.

Additional details and references can be found in the Physics Reference Manual [1] and the latest general review [2]. Recently, the main aspects and performance of the hadronic physics of Geant4 have been reported in a comprehensive benchmark for medical applications [3].

*FLUKA*

Likewise, FLUKA [4, 5, 6, 7], as a general purpose Monte Carlo code for calculations of particle transport and interactions with matter, deals with several ten particle types and, as far as hadrons are concerned, describes their reactions from threshold (or thermal energies in case of neutrons) up to collider energies (thanks to its interface with the DPMJET code [8, 9, 10], which takes over above 10 TeV in case of single hadron projectiles and 5 GeV/n in case of A>1 nucleus projectiles).

On the other hand, FLUKA was not conceived as a toolkit, rather with the aim to offer the users a fully integrated physics description, relying whenever possible on microscopic models deemed by the developers to be the most accurate ones and preserving correlations within interactions and among shower components, including photons and electrons from 100 eV and 1 keV, respectively. Only few specific processes are not activated by default but upon user's request as relevant to certain applications, mainly to optimize the simulation time for more general cases. Among those, such as photonuclear interactions or emission of heavy fragments in the evaporation stage of a reaction, there is the radionuclide decay calculation, which can be perfomed on-line.

Low energy (<1 GeV) hadronic processes of interest in hadrontherapy are handled with the same scheme earlier introduced, coupling interaction probabilities given by integral cross section evaluations and reaction models returning the final products. In the present scope, the most relevant models used in FLUKA (see section 5.2.2.1) are PEANUT, dealing with single hadron reactions on nuclei, and BME and RQMD, applied to nucleus-nucleus reactions for complementary energy ranges, namely up to 150 MeV/n and above 100 MeV/n, respectively (with an overlap in the 100 to 150 MeV/n interval). Moreover, the three of them, as any other nuclear reaction model of the code, are completed by a common module accounting for evaporation, fission, fragmentation, and gamma de-excitation, as discussed in the following.

An illustration of FLUKA's reliability for particle therapy can be found in [11] and references therein.

## 5.1 HADRONIC CROSS SECTIONS

### 5.1.1 ELASTIC CROSS SECTIONS

#### 5.1.1.1 Geant4

Neutron elastic cross sections are extracted by default from the evaluated G4PARTICLEXSDATA data set, whereas at higher energies they use the Barashenkov parameterization [12] and the Glauber-Gribov extension to high energies [13], being the first one the only relevant in medical applications since the threshold for transition to the high energy regime (91 GeV) is well above their energy range. Below 20 MeV, in order to preserve most of the resonant structure, they include (although simplified and smoothed in order to reduce CPU time) the detailed cross section data from the Geant4 Neutron Data Library (G4NDL) used by the *high precision* G4NeutronHP package, which in turn is based on the ENDF/B-VII.1 evaluated library [14].

Proton, $\pi^+$ and $\pi^-$ use the Barashenkov-Glauber-Gribov cross sections [12, 13].

Light clusters (deuterons, tritons and alphas) use the modified Glauber-Gribov cross sections [15]

When the G4ParticleHP physics package is activated (suffix *AllHP* in the physics lists), it encompasses the G4NeutronHP physics for neutrons (up to 20 MeV) whereas for protons it uses evaluated cross sections from ENDF/B-VII-1 database [14] (up to 150 MeV) when available, otherwise it uses TENDL database [16] (with data up to 200 MeV).

Elastic nucleus-nucleus process for projectiles with A>4 can be ignored in a first approximation since the screening of the atomic electrons leads to a small-angle scattering.

### 5.1.1.2 FLUKA

In FLUKA, nuclear elastic scattering of protons (above 10 MeV) and neutrons (see below on their particularities) is accounted for in the kinetic energy range of relevance for hadron therapy (up to a few hundred MeV). Nuclear elastic scattering cross sections for nucleons are derived from the Angeli-Csikai [17] and the Shen [18] parameterizations, with an ad-hoc Coulomb correction.

As further detailed in section 5.2.2.4, the transport of neutrons below 20 MeV is instead performed within FLUKA's multigroup approach, in which nuclear elastic scattering is treated in an aggregate manner along with inelastic and non-elastic channels via group-to-group transfer probabilities generated from evaluated nuclear data libraries (mainly ENDF).

Although dedicated nuclear elastic scattering of nuclear projectiles with $A > 1$ is presently not included, an extension based on the distorted wave Born approximation may be envisaged, considering the availability of optical potential models for deuterons, tritons, and alpha particles.

Finally, parameterized nucleon-nucleon elastic cross sections are employed in the cascade stage of a nucleon-nucleus interaction, accounting for in-medium effects (see section 5.2.2.1).

### 5.1.2 INELASTIC CROSS SECTIONS

#### 5.1.2.1 Geant4

As in the elastic case, neutron cross sections are extracted by default from the G4PARTICLEXSDATA data set and the Barashenkov-Glauber-Gribov parameterization [12, 13] is used for protons and pions.

For light clusters (deuterons up to alphas), the modified Glauber-Gribov cross section [15] is used for all energies.

When the G4ParticleHP physics package is activated, the same as in the elastic case holds for the inelastic cross sections.

For nucleus-nucleus cross sections, in Geant4 a variety of prescriptions are available for the energy range of interest (below 1 GeV): "Sihver," "Kox," "Tripathi," "Tripathi Light," and "Shen" [19]. The last one was previously recommended [2], but, after recent developments [15], the modified Glauber-Gribov cross section is used in the hadronic physics list recommended for medical applications (QGSP_BIC, see below) [3].

Neutron capture cross sections are extracted from the evaluated G4PARTICLEXSDATA data set for energies below 20 MeV and are set to zero above this limit.

When the G4ParticleHP physics package is activated, neutron capture cross sections are extracted from G4NDL data library (up to 20 MeV).

#### 5.1.2.2 FLUKA

In FLUKA, hadron–nucleus reaction cross sections are obtained by means of embedded tabulations, interpolations and parameterizations, covering the enormous energy range required by the variety of the code applications from gigantic colliders and cosmic ray physics down to MeV linear accelerators and radioisotope production by low-energy particle reinteractions.

For neutrons below 20 MeV, as already indicated, a special treatment is reserved, to better cope with their peculiar interaction properties that are strongly material dependent. Based on evaluated data, a dedicated library allows at the same time to transport them and account for the effects of their interactions, without invoking any interaction model, contrary to the regular scheme relying independently on the integral reaction cross section and the reaction description.

In the case of nucleus–nucleus reactions, a readjusted version [20] of the NASA cross section parameterization [21] is adopted on the low-energy side, with specific corrections for alpha projectiles as suggested by available measurements, and blent with DPMJET derived fits applicable from 3 GeV/n upwards.

## 5.2  HADRONIC MODELS

### 5.2.1  ELASTIC SCATTERING MODELS

#### 5.2.1.1  Geant4

The elastic scattering of neutrons and protons is modeled by default by the G4ChipsElasticModel (Chiral Phase Space Invariant Phase Space) [22] in the full energy range.

Light clusters (from deuteron to alpha), $\pi^+$ and $\pi^-$ use upto 1 GeV the G4HadronElastic model, which is a two-exponential momentum transfer model updated from Geant3 (*Gheisha*).

When the G4ParticleHP physics package is activated, evaluated elastic angular distributions are used with the same library provenance and energy ranges as for the cross sections.

#### 5.2.1.2  FLUKA

Exploiting the fact that the angular distribution of nucleons undergoing nuclear elastic scattering at intermediate energies generally consists of an intense forward-emission peak and a typically less accentuated tail, FLUKA employs a compact two-Gaussian parameterization effectively capturing both of these features [23].

Although not relevant in the present scope, pion-proton, kaon-proton, and kaonbar-proton elastic scattering relies on partial-wave analyzes and fits to experimental data, merging to the eikonal approximation at higher energies [24].

Recoiling target nuclei can be transported upon user request down to several 100 eV/n.

### 5.2.2  INELASTIC MODELS

#### 5.2.2.1  Intranuclear cascade models

##### 5.2.2.1.1  Geant4

The intranuclear cascade model makes a description of interactions in terms of particle-particle collisions on the basis that the deBroglie wavelength of the incident particle in nuclear collisions is, above a given threshold, comparable (or shorter) than the average intra- nucleon distance. The cascade begins when an incident particle strikes a nucleon in the target nucleus and produces secondaries. The secondaries may in turn escape, be absorbed or interact with other nucleons abiding by the Pauli blocking. The exciton number is updated at each step. At the end of the cascade the remnant is trasferred as an excited nuclear fragment to the pre-equilibrium model or directly to de-excitation. At that point energy conservation is checked. Relativistic kinematics is applied throughout the cascade.

Geant4 includes four intranuclear cascade models: Bertini, Binary, Liege intranuclear and Quantum Molecular Dynamics .

The extended Bertini cascade (BERT) [25] is valid for p, n, $\pi$, and strange particles as projectiles with incident energies between 0 and 15 GeV. It solves the Boltzmann equation on average and models the target nucleus as up to six concentric shells of constant density as an approximation to the continuously changing density distribution of nuclear matter within nuclei. The cascade ends when all particles, which are kinematically able to do so, escape the nucleus. Although this model has its own precompound and deexcitation code, an option exists for using the native Geant4 precompound and deexcitation modules discussed thereafter.

The Geant4 native Binary cascade (BIC) [26] simulates p and n-induced cascades below 10 GeV, and $\pi$-induced cascades below 1.3 GeV. Each participating nucleon is treated as a gaussian wave packet and the total wave function of the nucleus is assumed to be direct product of these (without anti-symmetrization). The centroids of these wave packets follow the classical Hamilton equations, which are solved numerically. The Hamiltonian includes a time independent nuclear optical potential. A 3-dimensional model of the nucleus is constructed, positioning the nucleons according to the local density approximation using the Fermi gas model. The nuclear density distributions are of the Wood-Saxon form for A>16 and harmonic-oscillator for A<17. Nucleon momenta are sampled in a correlated way from 0 to the Fermi momentum, with the local phase-space densities abiding by the Pauli's Exclusion Principle and the sum of these momenta being constrained to 0. The model accounts for the formation and decay of strong resonances. Cross section data (experimental when available) are used to select collisions. The cascade terminates when the average and maximum energy of secondaries is below threshold. The remaining fragment is then treated by the post-cascade native precompound and de-excitation models as described below. For nucleus-nucleus collisions, the G4BinaryLightIonReaction extension of the model is used.

The Liege intranuclear cascade (INCL) has been completely redesigned since its introduction in Geant4. The current version of the model is known as INCL++ [27] and is physics-wise equivalent to the legacy version as far as nucleon- and $\pi$-induced reactions are concerned. In addition, INCL++ has been extended to handle reactions induced by light ions (up to $A = 18$). At present by default, INCL++ uses the Geant4 native de-excitation model directly after the cascade stage; it does not include an intermediate pre-equilibrium step. Coupling to the ABLA de-excitation model [28] (as in its original version) is also possible.

The Quantum Molecular Dynamics cascade (QMD) is also a native Geant model based on an extension of the classical molecular dynamics model [29]. As in BIC, each nucleon in the target and projectile nuclei is treated as a Gaussian wave packet which propagates with scattering through the nuclear medium, taking Pauli exclusion into account. The nuclear potential is that of two merging nuclei and its shape is re-calculated at each time step of the collision. Participant-participant scattering is also taken into account. These last two facts combine to make the model rather slow for collisions of heavy nuclei, but the production of nuclear fragments versus energy is well reproduced. The model, which is Lorentz covariant, is valid for all projectile-target combinations and for projectile energies between 100 MeV/nucleon and 10 GeV/nucleon.

### 5.2.2.1.2 FLUKA

The IntraNuclear Cascade (INC) framework is adopted also in FLUKA, through the PEANUT (Pre-Equilibrium Approach to NUclear Thermalization) implementation [30]. The target nucleus is described as a nucleon gas volume divided into several radial zones of different proton and neutron densities. Additional sets of zones beyond the nucleus radius account for the nuclear and Coulomb potentials. The corresponding fields curve the trajectory of the incoming hadron and secondary particles, which in the present scope are practically limited to nucleons. In fact, new particle creation applies to higher energies, where the Dual Parton Model model, based on quark string treatment, takes over from the resonance model above a few GeV [31]. Here the nucleon–nucleon scattering probability takes into account the density dependent Fermi motion, incorporating also significant quantum ingredients such as Pauli blocking and antisymmetrization effects, which hinder a further interaction with a nucleon of the same kind as the one just hit in the vicinity. Energy, momentum and all additive quantum numbers are exactly conserved on an event-by-event basis, including the nuclear recoil and binding energies. Emission of light fragments by nucleon coalescence is also simulated, if requested by the user. In PEANUT the cascade stage proceeds until all not yet emitted nucleons have an energy less than 50 MeV in the continuum. Nevertheless, if they are above a lower threshold, they are still transported through the nucleus as far as they are emitted or shall reinteract. In the latter case, no interaction is actually performed but the exciton configuration is updated for the subsequent pre-equilibrium stage. This way, a smooth transition to the latter is assured.

As for nucleus–nucleus reactions in the range between 0.1 and 5 GeV/n, FLUKA is interfaced to a Relativistic Quantum Molecular Dynamics (RQMD) code [32], which for computation time reasons is used in the so-called "fast cascade" option. Contrary to the much more time-consuming full QMD mode, this default option makes the nucleons propagate in a mean field, similarly to the INC way. However, the original RQMD final state did not identify any nuclear fragment and was affected by a not rigorous energy conservation. Therefore, its FLUKA interface [20] exploits the available information on spectactor nucleons to reconstruct projectile- and target-like residuals and calculates their excitation energies from the actual hole depth of hit nucleons, taking into account the respective binding energies. More recently, analogously to the recipe above indicated, it also gathers inside the excited residuals nucleons below 50 MeV, preventing their reinteractions, such as to properly allow for the nucleus de-excitation by the PEANUT pre-equilibrium stage and so yield a better accuracy [11].

Finally, lower energy nucleus–nucleus reactions (from threshold up to 150 MeV/n) are dealt with thanks to the Boltzmann Master Equations (BME) built-in event generator [33]. Strictly speaking, the BME treatment refers to the pre-equilibrium stage of the composite system generated by the complete or incomplete fusion of the two interacting ions, as exposed in more detail in the following subsection. Prior to that, or to the alternative PEANUT pre-equilibrium stage that is applied to systems not covered by the pre-computed BME database [34], the code calculates the complete fusion probability as the ratio between the respective parameterized cross section and the reaction cross section. In case a more peripheral collision mechanism is then sampled, the impact parameter $b$ is chosen according to the differential expression of the reaction cross section $d\sigma_R/db$, as resulting from the development [35] of a model originally elaborated by P.J. Karol [36]. As a funtion of $b$, the integration of the nucleon densities over the projectile and target overlapping volume gives the mass of a so-called "middle source" preferentially excited, in the context of a three body picture featuring also projectile-like and target-like fragments, whose probabilities of exclusively fusing with the intermediate object is considered as well. For the largest impact parameters, the reaction mechanism naturally becomes a one-nucleon transfer or direct emission. As already mentioned, the excited residuals, whose number goes from one (in case of complete fusion) to three, pass to the pre-equilibrium stage.

### 5.2.2.2  Pre-equilibrium models

#### 5.2.2.2.1  Geant4

The pre-equilibrium stage is introduced since the equilibrium de-excitation models by themselves are not able to describe the high-energy tails of particle emission spectra; therefore it describes the post-cascade evolution until the nuclear system reaches equilibrium. Geant4 native pre-equilibrium model is based on the Cascade Exciton Model [37], which is a version of the semi-classical exciton model [38]. During this stage, transitions to states with different number of excitons compete with particle emissions, including emission of light compound fragments (up to alphas). The transition probabilities are calculated semimicroscopically, whereas the emission probabilities make use of the inverse reaction cross sections, which, via the reciprocity theorem, are expressed in terms of the Kalbach's parameterization of reaction cross sections from optical model calculations [39].

The transition to the state of statistical equilibrium is roughly characterized by an equilibrium number of excitons, which is determined consistently when all types of transitions (both increasing and decreasing the exciton number) are equiprobable.

At the end of the pre-equilibrium stage, the residual nucleus is assumed to be in a statistical equilibrium state in which the excitation energy is shared among by the entire nuclear system. Such an equilibrated compound nucleus, which has lost memory of all previous steps which led to its formation, is caracterizad by its mass, charge and excitation energy.

### 5.2.2.2.2   FLUKA

The PEANUT pre-equilibrium [30] is based on the exciton formalism of the Geometry Dependent Hybrid model [40] and proceeds through steps featuring either the emission of a nucleon in the continuum or a nucleon–nucleon collision that increases by two units the exciton number, namely by one both the number of holes below the Fermi surface and the number of nucleons above the Fermi surface (particle-type excitons). The respective probabilities are calculated as a function of local quantities, such as nuclear density and Fermi energy, taking into account that the position of the two-body elastic reinteraction is not known and so those local quantities converge to nucleus averaged values as the number of steps increases and the nucleus volume involved in the process becomes larger. Reinteraction cross sections are corrected according to the Pauli principle and nucleon correlations. Analogously to the intranuclear-cascade stage discussed above, a nucleon coalescence mechanism responsible for the emission of light fragments is included. The pre-equilibrium termination is not determined by an abrupt threshold corresponding to a predefined number of excitons, rather by a smoother probability law [41], preventing to spend an excessive amount of excitation energy in particle emissions that the subsequent evaporation stage can better deal with.

On the other hand, the BME theory [42] describes the time evolution of the momentum distribution of the nucleons of an excited nucleus created in the interaction of two low-energy ($<100$ MeV/n) ions. For this purpose, the nucleon momentum space is divided in bins and the time variation of the occupation probability of the states of each bin is evaluated by the integration of a set of coupled differential equations (the BME) that take into account nucleon–nucleon elastic collisions and emission into the continuum of single nucleons and nucleons bound in clusters. The bin occupation probabilities at the initial time depend on the previous dynamics of the two ion interaction. This procedure allows to obtain the double differential spectra of pre-equilibrium particles, but is not compatible with the computation time requirements of a Monte Carlo simulation of an irradiation problem. Thereby, it has been applied off-line to a representative set of ion pairs for different bombarding energies, in order to parameterize the calculated ejectile multiplicities and double differential spectra and create a database of the obtained parameters. Thanks to the interpolation of these parameters over the domain covered by the BME database, the pre-equilibrium stage of complete or incomplete fusion systems generated in low-energy nucleus–nucleus reactions can be reproduced on an event-by-event basis [33]. For cases outside the database domain, the PEANUT pre-equilibrium is invoked instead, as anticipated above.

### 5.2.2.3   Nuclear de-excitation models

### 5.2.2.3.1   Geant4

The Geant4 native de-excitation model includes in turn several alternative/competitor semi-classical models which are managed by the G4ExcitationHandler class, in which they are be invoked (in order of precedence):

- Fermi break-up for nuclei with $Z < 9$ and $A < 17$ [43]. It takes into account the Pauli blocking and all possible decay channels in stable and long lived fragments.
- statistical multifragmentation, for excitation energies $E_x > 3$ MeV [43]. It's not relevant for medical applications.
- evaporation of:
  - nucleons and light fragments up to $\alpha$, by the standard Weisskopf-Ewing model [44] with Kalbach's reaction cross sections [39]

- heavier nuclei with $Z \leq 12$ and $A \leq 28$, by the Generalized Evaporation Model [45].
- evaporation of photons:
  - discrete gammas according to tabulated E1, M1 and E2 transition probabilities taken from the Evaluated Nuclear Structure Data File (ENSDF) and
  - continuous, according to E1 Giant Dipole Resonance (GDR) strenght distribution,
- fission, based on Bohr-Wheeler semi-classical model [46]

For proton and ion beam therapy applications, the photon evaporation model, which is critical for the tracking of the Bragg peak from emitted prompt gammas, has been improved in recent years.

### 5.2.2.3.2   FLUKA

In FLUKA the module describing the final stage of all nuclear reactions (apart from those induced by neutrons below 20 MeV, handled by a specific multigroup treatment based on a dedicated data library) applies to any excited residual nucleus. With no additional memory of the previous reaction stages, this is fully characterized by its atomic and mass numbers, its excitation energy, which is supposed to be shared among many nucleons, as well as its spin and parity, as more recently implemented [47].

For light systems, possibly produced even in the course of this last de-excitation stage, the fundamental assumptions of the evaporation model no longer hold and therefore Fermi break-up is adopted if $A<18$, implying a one-step fragmentation into two or more pieces [48, 49]. The sampling of the final state is based on a total of almost 50,000 combinations, including up to 6 products and their relevant unstable levels (such as for $^8$Be or in case of important gamma decay). The available kinetic energy to be shared at disassembling is computed by subtracting the Coulomb repulsion among the charged products, which is then distributed to the latter ones. Angular momentum barriers are taken into account as a $L = 0$ fragmentation is forbidden by spin conservation, with the effect of suppressing the respective channels and significantly improving the predictions of nuclear residue yields from photonuclear reactions in the GDR range, for instance $^{11}$C from $(\gamma, n)$ on $^{12}$C [7].

More massive systems undergo evaporation, whose implementation is founded also in FLUKA on the Weisskopf-Ewing formalism and extended to the emission of "particles" with A up to 24 [44, 49]. For heavy nuclei, the fission channel becomes competitive with the evaporation ones. Fission barriers are calculated according to the Myers and Swiatecki recipe and the level density enhancement at the saddle point washes out as a function of the excitation energy [50]. The fission fragments, reflecting a mass distribution that for high Z has both a symmetric and an asymmetric component, can be subject to evaporation in turn.

Photon emission dissipates the remaining excitation energy, with a gamma cascade proceeding through a continuous nuclear level density and eventually discrete levels. For the first part an evaporation-like statistical model allows to determine the multipole type and order (among E1, M1, and E2) and consequently the energy of the emitted photon, which in the second part results instead from a rotational level structure or the tabulated values of excited levels [51].

### 5.2.2.4   Dedicated low-energy treatments

#### 5.2.2.4.1   Geant4

Originally a physics package named G4NeutronHP (*High Precision*) was provided for incident neutrons with energies below 20 MeV. It used nuclear data from evaluated ENDF-6 formatted nuclear data files. Recently the new package G4ParticleHP, which encompasses the former, has been developed for incident nucleons and light clusters up to alphas. It uses also the nuclear data from ENDF-6 evaluations, which includes the elastic and reaction channels. For protons the ENDF/B-VII.1 database is used wherever data are available, otherwise the TENDL database, which includes the full range of target isotopes with lifetime >1 sec, is used. In either case evaluated proton data extends up to 200 MeV. For incident light ions there are only a few evaluated data available in reduced energy ranges, but they do not include carbon and therefore are not relevant for present medical applications.

Neutron capture is modeled by default by the Photon Evaporation model of Geant4, which uses Evaluated Nuclear Structure Data File (ENSDF) [52] to create final state products including Internal Conversion electrons.

When the G4ParticleHP physics package is activated the final state of radiative capture is described by either photon multiplicities, or photon production cross sections, and the discrete and continuous contributions to the photon energy spectra, along with the angular distributions of the emitted photons. The photon energies are associated to the multiplicities or the cross sections for all discrete photon emissions. For the continuum contribution, the normalized emission probability is broken down into a weighted sum of normalized distributions. All these data are extracted from G4NDL data library (up to 20 MeV).

### 5.2.2.4.2   FLUKA

In FLUKA the neutron energy range from 20 MeV down to 0.01 meV is divided into 260 intervals (energy "groups") of approximately equal logarithmic width, 31 of which lie in the thermal and epithermal region. A corresponding library, covering a rich list of elements at room and cryogenic (87 K) temperatures and mostly derived from ENDF/B (but also from JENDL, JEFF, TENDL, ...), gives the group-to-group transfer probabilities reflecting in an inclusive way the neutron elastic and inelastic interactions in the concerned material. Multigroup cross sections, neutron angular distributions, kerma factors accounting for the energy deposition by all secondary charged particles that are not generated explicitly, production rates of residual nuclei (also not generated explicitly), and photon generation probabilities as a function of a respective energy group structure, are also included in the FLUKA library [6]. Thereby only neutrons and photons are tracked as a result of a low-energy neutron interaction, with the notable exception of recoil protons in hydrogen (where pointwise treatment is available above 10 eV, apart from $^2$H) and protons from the (n,p) reaction on $^{14}$N, as well as the charged products of the (n,$\alpha$) reaction on $^6$Li and $^{10}$B. This approach proves to be reliable for several purposes and faster than any other using continuous cross sections[1].

### 5.2.3   RADIOACTIVE DECAY MODEL

#### 5.2.3.1   Geant4

The G4RadioactiveDecay model handles $\alpha$, $\beta^+$, $\beta^-$, isomeric transition (IT) and electron capture (EC) decays, and can be applied to generic ions both in flight and at rest. Details for each decay or level transition, such as nuclear level energies, branching ratios and reaction Q values, come from the Geant4 RadioactiveDecay database, which currently contains entries for 2798 nuclides. Details of specific gamma levels used for IT decays are taken from the Geant4 PhotonEvaporation database. Both the PhotonEvaporation and RadioactiveDecay databases take their data from the Evaluated Nuclear Structure Data File (ENSDF) [52] and their common nuclear levels have identical values.

#### 5.2.3.2   FLUKA

As earlier mentioned, FLUKA can calculate in the same run both prompt and decay quantities, being the latter ones derived from the decay of the radionuclides produced in the prompt phase. Decay quantities are provided for a requested set of cooling times, by means of the analytical computation of the Bateman's coefficients accounting for buildup and decay as a function of an input irradiation

---

[1]Pointwise treatment has been recently implemented, after the completion of this chapter

profile [53]. FLUKA can also simulate a radioactive source in the so-called "semi-analog" mode, where the decay time is sampled according to the nuclide lifetime and the full decay chain is followed until a stable nucleus is reached. The description of the radioactive decay process is based on a database collecting in total more than 100,000 gamma, conversion electron, and alpha lines and beta (plus and minus) end points, down to 0.1% and 0.01% branching ratios for light and heavy radionuclides, respectively, and mostly from ENSDF [52], with corrections and additions.

### 5.2.4  PHOTON AND LEPTO-NUCLEAR MODELS

#### 5.2.4.1  Geant4

The photonuclear process is modeled with a Bertini style cascade model, which treats the incident gamma as if it were a hadron interacting with a nucleon within the nuclear medium.

The electro-nuclear process is also modeled factorizing the interaction into separate hadronic and electromagnetic parts and treating the exchanged virtual photon as if it were a hadron with a Bertini style cascade.

#### 5.2.4.2  Fluka

FLUKA performs photonuclear reactions either by real photons or virtual photons that mediate nuclear interactions by electrons, positrons, muons as well as electromagnetic dissociation of nuclei [54]. In the second case, the virtual photon spectrum, including more recently also the E2 component, is folded with the photon–nucleus cross section. The latter, as introduced for real photon interactions [55], covers the whole energy range by dividing it into four different regimes, namely (from threshold up) GDR, Quasi-Deuteron, Delta resonance, and high energy, where the vector meson dominance model applies. The reaction course is consistently described through PEANUT, which handles the photon absorption in the nucleus leading eventually to the de-excitation stage returning the final state.

### 5.3  PHYSICS LISTS

#### 5.3.1  GEANT4

In Geant4, physics lists refer to classes which provide the means to collect and organize the particle types, physics models and cross sections required for a particular simulation application. These classes allow physics processes to be registered to the run manager which in turn attaches them to tracks so that they may interact properly with the simulation geometry.

The reference physics lists are specialized to provide standard behavior in various application domains. In particular QGSP_BIC_AllHP provides a good overall description for medical applications [3]. It uses Binary Cascade, which embeds native pre-equilirium and de-excitation models as final stages (at higher incident energies, above the range of medical applications, it uses QGS string model followed by pre-equilibrium, for which the "P" is meant). For high precision neutron propagation the package G4NeutronHP is included in the physics list by appending the letters HP to its name, for example QGSP_BIC_HP. The generalization to any incident projectile, protons or light ions (when available), is made in the same way, by appending the letters AllHP, for example QGSP_BIC_AllHP.

### 5.4  OTHER MODELS

#### 5.4.1  NEW TRANSPORT MODELS FOR N-N COLLISIONS BELOW 100 MEV/U

In this energy regime, the reaction dynamics is governed by the nuclear mean-field potential and the residual nucleon-nucleon (n-n) short-range interaction (hard two-body scattering), on about equal footing. For the latter, a careful check of Pauli blocking effects is of crucial importance, to preserve the fermionic character of the nuclear system. As far as dynamical fragmentation models are concerned, stochastic extensions of transport theories, describing the time evolution of the nucleon one-body distribution function in phase space, $f(\mathbf{r}, \mathbf{p}, t)$, are among the most advanced approaches, together with improved molecular dynamics models (see [56] for a review).

### 5.4.1.1 Fluctuations in full phase space and the BLOB model

The Boltzmann-Langevin-One-Body (BLOB) model solves the semi-classical Boltzmann-Langevin (BL) equation for the distribution function $f(\mathbf{r}, \mathbf{p}, t)$. In particular, BLOB accounts for the stochastic character of n-n two-body collisions extending the standard Boltzmann-Uehling-Uhlenbeck (BUU) collision integral, $I_{BUU}$, towards the inclusion of explicit correlations at the nucleon-nucleon level. Namely, the following (BLOB) equation is solved [57, 58]:

$$\frac{\partial f}{\partial t} + \{f, H\} = I_{BUU} + \delta I, \qquad (5.1)$$

where $H$ denotes the mean-field Hamiltonian, including the nuclear effective interaction, and the term $\delta I$ accounts for n-n correlations. The strength of the collision integral is governed by the differential nucleon-nucleon cross section.

From the practical point of view, Eq.(5.1) is solved numerically, sampling the density distribution in phase space with $N_{test}$ test particles per nucleon. $N_{test}$ typically ranges from tens to hundreds, depending on the size of the colliding nuclei. The r.h.s. of Eq.(5.1) corresponds to the implementation of n-n collision processes. Within the BLOB treatment, a single n-n collision involves four phase-space portions $A$, $B$, $C$ and $D$, which are agglomerates of $N_{test}$ test-particles of the same type (neutrons or protons) each. $A$ and $B$ simulate the colliding nucleon wave packets, and Pauli-blocking factors act on the corresponding final states $C$, $D$, also treated as extended phase-space regions. The choice of defining each phase-space portion $A$, $B$, $C$ and $D$ so that the isospin number is either 1 or $-1$ is necessary to preserve the Fermi statistics for both neutrons and protons, and it imposes that blocking factors are defined accordingly in phase-space cells for the given isospin species. The method is schematically illustrated in Figure 5.1.

An approximated (and less time-consuming) way to solve the BL equation is represented by the Stochastic Mean Field (SMF) model. Both SMF and BLOB include an identical treatment of the mean-field propagation, on the basis of the same effective interaction, but they differ in the way effects beyond the mean-field description, such as correlations and related fluctuations, are included. In particular, SMF considers only fluctuations of the spatial density distribution, i.e., only in coordinate space.

SMF and BLOB were designed and developed to simulate heavy ion interactions in the Fermi-energy regime (below 100 MeV/u). The improved treatment of the fluctuation dynamics in BLOB leads to a better description of multi-fragmentation reactions [57, 59]. Moreover BLOB has been recently applied also to fragment production in spallation reactions [60]. We stress that the inclusion of fluctuations is essential to tackle the description of multi-fragment production. In this respect, stochastic models, such as SMF and BLOB, represent an important improvement over standard BUU-like models.

Within the same category of approaches, a further framework to treat the dissipation and fluctuation dynamics associated with n-n scattering in heavy-ion collisions has been recently introduced in [61]. Two-body collisions are effectively described in terms of the diffusion of nucleons in the viscous nuclear medium, according to a set of Langevin equations in momentum space. The new framework, combined with the usual mean-field dynamics, has been shown to be suited to simulate heavy-ion collisions at intermediate energies. Applications of the method, as well as the comparison with other transport models, are presently in progress.

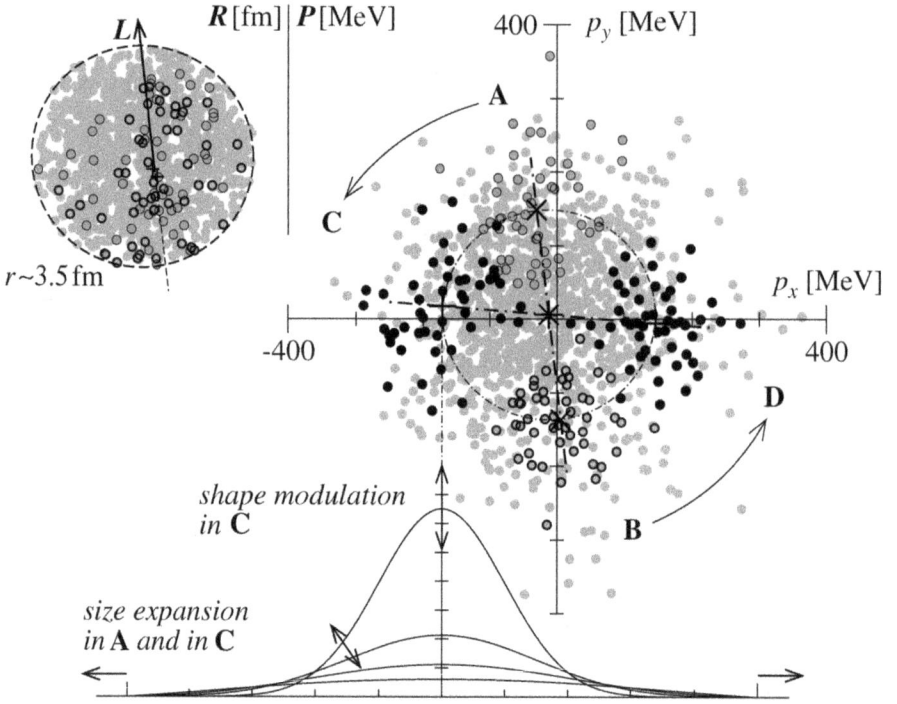

**Figure 5.1** Example of one collision event in BLOB. Two nucleons are represented by two agglomerates of test particles A and B which share the same volume in coordinate space $R$. In the momentum space $P$ the collision process induces a rotation, according to a given set of scattering angles $(\theta, \phi)$, to the destination sites C and D, where the test particles are distributed according to Pauli-blocking and energy conservation constraints. The latter are enforced by modulating the shape and the size of the nucleon packet (see the bottom part of the figure) [58].

### 5.4.1.2 Antisymmetrized Molecular Dynamics

Within the framework of molecular dynamics models, an important step forward in the direction of fully taking into account Pauli blocking effects is represented by the antisymmetrized molecular dynamics (AMD) approach. In AMD, a system of $A$-nucleon is represented by a Slater determinant of Gaussian wave packets,

$$|\Phi_{AMD}(Z)\rangle = \hat{A} \prod_{K=1}^{A} \varphi_K \tag{5.2}$$

where $\hat{A}$ is the full antisymmetrization operator. Each single-particle state $\varphi_k$ is a product of a Gaussian function and a spin-isospin state

$$\langle \mathbf{r} | \varphi_k \rangle = \exp\left[-\nu\left(\mathbf{r} - \frac{\mathbf{Z}_k}{\sqrt{\nu}}\right)^2\right] \otimes \chi_{\alpha_k}. \tag{5.3}$$

The spin and isospin of each nucleon are kept fixed, $\alpha_k = p\uparrow, p\downarrow, n\uparrow$ or $n\downarrow$. The width parameter $\nu$ of the Gaussian function is chosen to be $\nu = 1/(2.5\ fm)^2$ in almost all applications. It should be noticed that the single-particle states $\varphi_k$ are not orthogonal to each other, however, as long as they are linearly independent, the Slater determinant (5.2) is a proper fermionic many-body state. The latter results parametrized in terms of the Gaussian centroids $Z = \{\mathbf{Z}_1, \mathbf{Z}_2, \dots, \mathbf{Z}_A\}$, which are complex vectors. The time-dependent variational principle allows to determine the equations of motion for these quantities, according to the Hamiltonian of the system [62, 63, 64]. Similarly to the transport approaches discussed above, an effective interaction is employed in AMD to represent the mean-field potential, such as the Gogny force or the Skyrme force.

A stochastic collision integral, describing hard two-body scattering between nucleon packets and preserving the antisymmetrization is explicitly included in the description.

As in QMD models, in AMD the width parameter $v$ is always kept fixed. This is well suitable to describe fragmentation events, thanks to the localization of the nucleon wave packet, as shown already by the very first applications of the AMD approach to the simulation of heavy ion collisions [66, 67]. However, further extensions of AMD also include the possibility to consider deformation of the wave packects, which actually can be represented as a superposition of many Gaussian wave functions, see Ref. [68] for a review.

A recent upgrade of the AMD model considers the possibility to include explicit light cluster production, as an extension of the nucleon correlations induced by the collision integral [69].

### 5.4.2 POSSIBILITIES OF IMPLEMENTATION IN GEANT4

Some attempts to couple SMF and BLOB with Geant4 already exist [65], in view of their possible porting. To this purpose, two "dummy" models in Geant4, *G4SMF* and *G4BLOB*, were developed; the Geant4 guidelines for developing models were followed, by inheriting from the Geant4 pure virtual class *G4VIntraNuclearTransportModel*. *G4SMF* and *G4BLOB* load the output from SMF and BLOB, respectively, and sample one of their final states, in terms of the test particle distrubution. The reaction products are reconstructed by applying a clustering procedure to the corresponding one-body density distribution function $f$. This allows one to evaluate their mass, charge, kinematical properties and excitation energy [70]. The large fragments were then passed to the de-excitation model of Geant4, *G4ExcitationHandler*, for their statistical de-excitation. The 10.5.p1 version of Geant4 was used.

An extended benchmark with the data-set of De Napoli et al. [71], i.e. experimentally measured double differential cross sections of fragment production in $^{12}C + ^{12}C$ reactions at 62 MeV/u, is discussed in [65].

Results obtained for the double differential cross sections, scaled by the total experimental inelastic cross section, are shown in Figure 5.2, in the case of alpha particles (see [65] for a more extended analysis). The figure also shows the results corresponding to models already available in Geant4 (BIC and INCL), to be taken as a reference. From these studies, there emerge indications towards a better performance of SMF, and BLOB in particular, to reproduce the data set considered, with respect the other models. More systematic analyzes would be in order. Moreover, it would be worthwhile to consider employing also the AMD model, and its latest version in particular, which is expected to optimally describe light particle emission in the energy regime considered.

The main problems affecting the porting of BLOB to Geant4 are related to its computation time, which is too large for the usage in medical applications. Similar considerations would apply to the AMD model. In the case of BLOB, one possibility would be porting it to the GPU, profiting from the fact that BLOB uses the test particle method. Thus, according to its computing scheme, BLOB could take advantage of the "single instruction on multiple data" approach of the GPU programming with a low thread divergency. A speed up in the code by some orders of magnitude is expected in this case. Moreover, the possibility of training a Deep Learning algorithm, specifically a Variational Auto-Encoder (VAE), to emulate BLOB was investigated in Ref.[72]. It was shown that, once trained, the VAE could produce a BLOB final state in a negligible time. The interface of the generation part in Geant4 is foreseen.

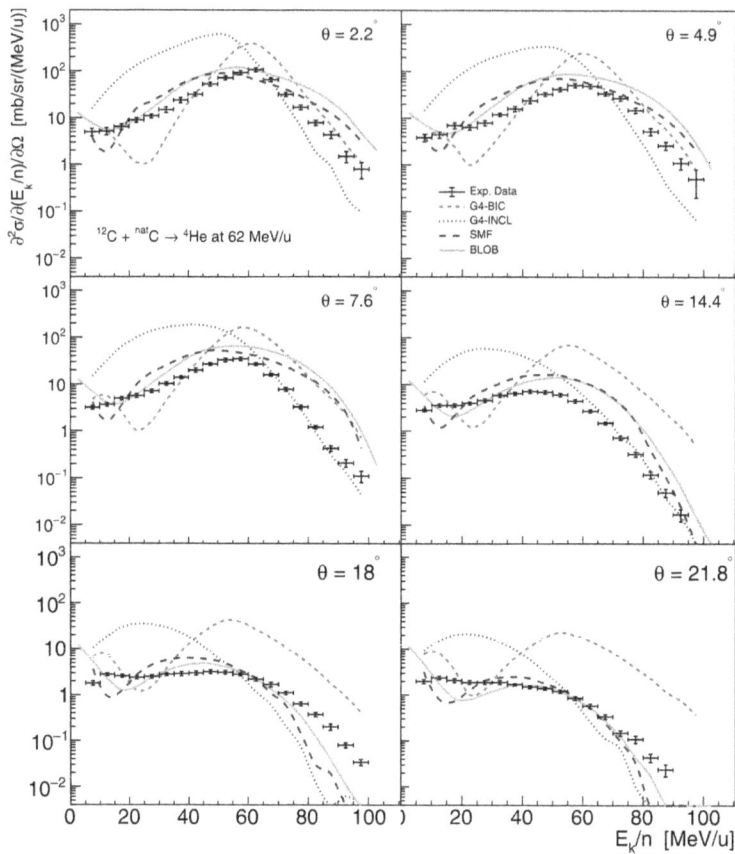

**Figure 5.2** Double differential cross sections of alpha particle production as a function of the kinetic energy, for different angles. The experimental data are compared to the results of different models: Binary Intranuclear Cascade (BIC) (short-dashed line), INCL++ (dotted line), SMF (dashed line) and BLOB (full line). From [65] (Fig.3).

## REFERENCES

1. "Geant4 Physics Reference Manual." `https://geant4-userdoc.web.cern.ch/UsersGuides/PhysicsReferenceManual/html/index.html`.
2. J. Allison and others (Geant4 Collaboration), "Recent developments in GEANT4," *Nuclear Instruments and Methods in Physics Research A*, vol. 835, pp. 186–225, 2016.
3. P. Arce *et al.*, "Report on G4-Med, a Geant4 benchmarking system for medical physics applications developed by the Geant4 Medical Simulation Benchmarking Group," *Medical Physics*, vol. 1, no. 48, pp. 19–56, 2021.
4. `https://fluka.cern`.
5. C. Ahdida, D. Bozzato, D. Calzolari, F. Cerutti, N. Charitonidis, A. Cimmino, A. Coronetti, G. D'Alessandro, A. Donadon Servelle, L. Esposito, R. Froeschl, R. Garcia Alia, A. Gerbershagen, S. Gilardoni, D. Horvath, G. Hugo, A. Infantino, V. Kouskoura, A. Lechner, B. Lefebvre, G. Lerner, M. Magistris, A. Manousos, G. Moryc, F. Ogallar Ruiz, F. Pozzi, D. Prelipcean, S. Roesler, R. Rossi, M. Sabate Gilarte, F. Salvat Pujol, P. Schoofs, V. Stransky,

C. Theis, A. Tsinganis, R. Versaci, V. Vlachoudis, A. Waets, and M. Widorski, "New Capabilities of the FLUKA Multi-Purpose Code," *Frontiers in Physics*, vol. 9:788253, 2022. `doi.org/10.3389/fphy.2021.788253`.

6. G. Battistoni, T. Boehlen, F. Cerutti, P. Chin, L. Esposito, A. Fasso, A. Ferrari, A. Lechner, A. Empl, A. Mairani, A. Mereghetti, P. G. Ortega, J. Ranft, S. Roesler, P. Sala, V. Vlachoudis, and G. Smirnov, "Overview of the FLUKA code," *Ann. Nucl. Energy*, vol. 82, pp. 10–18, 2015.

7. T. Boehlen, F. Cerutti, M. Chin, A. Fasso, A. Ferrari, P. Ortega, A. Mairani, P. Sala, G. Smirnov, and V. Vlachoudis, "The FLUKA Code: Developments and Challenges for High Energy and Medical Applications," *Nucl. Data Sheets*, vol. 120, pp. 211–214, 2014.

8. `https://github.com/afedynitch/DPMJET`.

9. S. Roesler, R. Engel, and J. Ranft, "The Monte Carlo Event Generator DPMJET-III," in *Proceedings of the Monte Carlo 2000 Conference*, pp. 1033–1038, Springer-Verlag Berlin, 2001.

10. A. Fedynitch, *Cascade equations and hadronic interactions at very high energies*. PhD thesis, `https://cds.cern.ch/record/2231593/files/CERN-THESIS-2015-371.pdf`, 2015.

11. G. Battistoni, J. Bauer, T. Boehlen, F. Cerutti, M. Chin, R. D. S. Augusto, A. Ferrari, P. G. Ortega, W. Kozlowska, G. Magro, A. Mairani, K. Parodi, P. Sala, P. Schoofs, T. Tessonnier, and V. Vlachoudis, "The FLUKA Code: An Accurate Simulation Tool for Particle Therapy," *Front. Oncol.*, vol. 6:116, 2016. `doi.org/10.3389/fonc.2016.00116`.

12. "Nea: Barashenkov cross sections from nuclear energy agency." `http://www.nea.fr/html/dbdata/bara.html`.

13. V. M. Grichine, "A simple model for integral hadron–nucleus and nucleus–nucleus cross-sections," *Nuclear Instruments and Methods in Physics Research B*, vol. 267, pp. 2460–2462, 2009.

14. *https://t2.lanl.gov/nis/data/endf/index.html*.

15. V. M. Grichine, "Integral cross-sections of light nuclei in the Glauber-Gribov representation," *Nuclear Instruments and Methods in Physics Research B*, vol. 427, pp. 60–62, 2018.

16. *https://tendl.web.psi.ch/tendl_2019/tendl2019.html*.

17. J. Wilson, L. Townsend, W. Buck, S. Chun, B. Hong, and B. Lamkin, "Nucleon-nucleus Interaction Data Base: Total Nuclear and Absorption Cross Sections," *NASA Technical Memorandum*, vol. 4053, pp. 349–356, 1988.

18. Q. Shen, "Systematics of intermediate energy proton nonelastic and neutron total cross section," *IAEA International Nuclear Data Committee*, no. 020, 1991.

19. Shen, Wen-qing, Wang, Bing, Feng, Jun, Zhan, Wen-long, Zhu, Yong-tai, Feng, and En-pu, "Total reaction cross section for heavy-ion collisions and its relation to the neutron excess degree of freedom," *Nuclear Physics A*, vol. 491, no. 1, pp. 130–146, 1989.

20. V. Andersen, F. Ballarini, G. Battistoni, M. Campanella, M. Carboni, F. Cerutti, A. Empl, A. Fasso, A. Ferrari, E. Gadioli, M. Garzelli, K. Lee, A. Ottolenghi, M. Pelliccioni, L. Pinsky, J. Ranft, S. Roesler, P. Sala, and T. Wilson, "The FLUKA code for space applications: recent developments," *Adv. Space Res.*, vol. 34, pp. 1302–1310, 2004.

21. R. Tripathi, F. Cucinotta, and J. Wilson, "Accurate universal parameterization of absorption cross-sections III – light systems," *Nucl. Instr. Meth. B*, vol. 155, pp. 349–356, 1999.

22. M. Kossov, "Chiral Invariant Phase Space model," *European Physical Journal*, vol. 36, no. 3, pp. 289–293, 2008.

23. J. Ranft, "Estimation of radiation problems around high energy accelerators using calculations of the hadronic cascade in matter," *Particle Accelerators*, vol. 3, pp. 129–161, 1972.

24. A. Fasso, A. Ferrari, S. Roesler, P. R. Sala, F. Ballarini, A. Ottolenghi, G. Battistoni, F. Cerutti, E. Gadioli, M. V. Garzelli, A. Empl, and J. Ranft, "The physics models of FLUKA: status and recent developments," in *Computing in High Energy and Nuclear Physics*, p. MOMT005, 2003.

25. D. H. Wright and M. H. Kelsey, "The Geant4 Bertini Cascade," *Nucl. Instr. Meth. A*, vol. 804, pp. 175–188, 2015.

26. G. Folger, V. Ivanchenko, and J. Wellisch, "The Binary Cascade," *The European Phisical Journal A*, vol. 21, pp. 407–417, 2004.

27. D. Mancusi, A. Boudard, J. Cugnon, J. David, P. Kaitaniemi, and S. Leray, "Extension of the Liege intranuclear-cascade model to reactions induced by light nuclei," *Physical Review C*, vol. 90, pp. 054602-1–054602-30, 2014.

28. J. Benlliure, A. Grewe, M. de Jong, K. Schmidt, and S. Zhdanov, "Calculated Nuclide Production Yields in Relativistic Collisions of Fissile Nuclei," *Nuclear Physics A*, vol. 628, pp. 458–478, 1998.

29. T. Koi, M. Asai, and D. H. Wright, "Interfacing the JQMD and JAM nuclear reaction codes to GEANT4," in *Computing in High Energy and Nuclear Physics SLAC-PUB-9978*, pp. 1–4, SLAC, 2003.

30. A. Ferrari and P. Sala, "The Physics of High Energy Reactions," in *Proc. Workshop on Nuclear Reaction Data and Nuclear Reactors Physics, Design and Safety*, p. 424, World Scientific, 1998.

31. A. Ferrari and P. Sala, "Nuclear reactions in Monte Carlo codes," *Radiat. Prot. Dosimetry*, vol. 99, no. 1-4, pp. 29–38, 2002.

32. H. Sorge, H. Stoecker, and W. Greiner, "Poincare invariant Hamiltonian dynamics: Modelling multi-hadronic interactions in a phase space approach," *Ann. Phys.*, vol. 192, p. 266, 1989.

33. F. Cerutti, G. Battistoni, G. Capezzali, P. Colleoni, A. Ferrari, E. Gadioli, A. Mairani, and A. Pepe, "Low energy nucleus–nucleus reactions: the BME approach and its interface with FLUKA," in *Proc. 11th International Conference on Nuclear Reaction Mechanisms*, p. 507, Ricerca Scientifica ed Educazione Permanente N. 126, 2006.

34. F. Cerutti, A. Ferrari, A. Mairani, and P. Sala, "New developments in FLUKA," in *Proc. 13th International Conference on Nuclear Reaction Mechanisms*, p. 469, CERN, 2012. http://cds.cern.ch/record/1537387?ln=en.

35. F. Cerutti, A. Clivio, and E. Gadioli, "A semiclassical formula for the reaction cross-section of heavy ions," *Eur. Phys. J. A*, vol. 25, p. 413, 2005.

36. P. Karol, "Nucleus–nucleus reaction cross sections at high energies: Soft-spheres model," *Phys. Rev. C*, vol. 11, p. 1203, 1975.

37. K. Gudima, S. G. Mashnik, and V. D. Toneev, "Cascade-exciton model of nuclear reactions," *Nuclear Physics A*, vol. 401, pp. 329–361, 1983.

38. J. J. Griffin, "Statistical Model of Intermediate Structure," *Physical Review Letters*, vol. 17, pp. 478–481, 1966.

39. C. Kalbach, *PRECO-2000 Exciton Model Preequilibrium Code with Direct Reactions*. Nuclear Energy Agency, 2002.

40. M. Blann and H. K. Vonach, "Global test of modified precompound decay models," *Phys. Rev. C*, vol. 28, p. 1475, 1983.

41. M. Veselsky, "Production mechanism of hot nuclei in violent collisions in the Fermi energy domain," *Nucl. Phys. A*, vol. 705, pp. 193–222, 2002.

42. M. Cavinato, E. Fabrici, E. Gadioli, E. Gadioli Erba, and E. Risi, "Boltzmann master equation theory of angular distributions in heavy-ion reactions," *Nucl. Phys. A*, vol. 643, pp. 15–29, 1998. And references therein.

43. J. Bondorf, A. Botvina, A. Iljinov, I. Mishustin, and K. Sneppen, "Statistical Multifragmentation Of Nuclei," *Physics Reports*, vol. 257, pp. 133–221, 1995.

44. V. E. Weisskopf and D. H. Ewing, "On the Yield of Nuclear Reactions with Heavy Elements," *Physical Review*, vol. 57, pp. 472–485, 1940.

45. S. Furihata, K. Niita, S. Meigo, Y. Ikeda, and F. Maekawa, *GEM code - a simulation program for the evaporation and the fission process of an excited nucleus, JAERI Data/Code 2001-015*. Japan Atomic Energy Research Institute (JAERI), 2001.

46. N. Bohr and J. A. Wheeler, "The Mechanism of Nuclear Fission," *Physical Review*, vol. 56, pp. 426–450, 1939.

47. A. Fontana, "Nuclear interaction model developments in FLUKA," in *Proc. 14th International Conference on Nuclear Reaction Mechanisms*, p. 283, CERN, 2015. https://cds.cern.ch/record/2115392?ln=en.

48. E. Fermi, "High Energy Nuclear Events," *Progress of Theoretical Physics*, vol. 5, no. 4, p. 570, 1950.

49. A. Ferrari, J. Ranft, S. Roesler, and P. Sala, "Cascade particles, nuclear evaporation, and residual nuclei in high energy hadron–nucleus interactions," *Z. Phys. C*, vol. 70, pp. 413–426, 1996.

50. G. Battistoni, F. Cerutti, A. Fasso, A. Ferrari, S. Muraro, J. Ranft, S. Roesler, and P. Sala, "The FLUKA code: description and benchmarking," in *AIP Conference Proceedings 896*, pp. 31–49, 2007. doi.org/10.1063/1.2720455.

51. A. Ferrari, J. Ranft, S. Roesler, and P. Sala, "The production of residual nuclei in peripheral high energy nucleus–nucleus interactions," *Z. Phys. C*, vol. 71, pp. 75–86, 1996.

52. https://www.nndc.bnl.gov/ensdf/.

53. M. Brugger, H. Khater, S. Mayer, A. Prinz, S. Roesler, L. Ulrici, and H. Vincke, "Benchmark studies of induced radioactivity produced in LHC materials, part II: Remanent dose rates," *Radiat. Prot. Dosimetry*, vol. 116, no. 1-4, pp. 12–15, 2005. doi.org/10.1093/rpd/nci052.

54. H. Braun, A. Fasso, A. Ferrari, J. Jowett, P. Sala, and G. Smirnov, "Hadronic and electromagnetic fragmentation of ultrarelativistic heavy ions at LHC," *Phys. Rev. ST - AB*, vol. 17, p. 021006, 2014.

55. A. Fasso, A. Ferrari, and P. Sala, "Photonuclear Reactions in FLUKA: Cross Sections and Interaction Models," in *AIP Conference Proceedings 769*, p. 1303, 2005. doi.org/10.1063/1.1945245.

56. M. Colonna, "Collision dynamics at medium and relativistic energies," *Progress in Particle and Nuclear Physics*, vol. 113, p. 103775, 2020.

57. P. Napolitani and M. Colonna, "Bifurcations in Boltzmann-Langevin one body dynamics for fermionic systems," *Physics Letters B*, vol. 726, p. 382, 2013.

58. P. Napolitani and M. Colonna, "Boltzmann-Langevin one-body dynamics for fermionic systems," *EPJ Web of Conferences*, vol. 31, p. 00027, 2012.

59. P. Napolitani and M. Colonna, "Nuclear jets in heavy-ion collisions," *Physics Letters B*, vol. 797, p. 313483, 2019.

60. P. Napolitani and M. Colonna, "Frustrated fragmentation and re-aggregation in nuclei: a non-equilibrium description in spallation," *Physical Review C*, vol. 92, p. 034607, 2015.

61. H. Lin and P. Danielewicz, "One-body Langevin dynamics in heavy-ion collisions at intermediate energies," *Physical Review C*, vol. 99, p. 024612, 2019.

62. A. Ono, S. Hudan, A. Chbihi, and J. Frankland, "Compatibility of localized wave packets and unrestricted single particle dynamics for cluster formation in nuclear collisions," *Physical Review C*, vol. 66, p. 014603, 2002.

63. A. Ono and H. Horiuchi, "Antisymmetrized molecular dynamics for heavy ion collision," *Progress in Particle and Nuclear Physics*, vol. 53, no. 2, p. 501, 2004.

64. A. Ono, "Dynamics of clusters and fragments in heavy-ion collisions," *Progress in Particle and Nuclear Physics*, vol. 105, p. 139, 2019.

65. C. Mancini-Terracciano *et al.*, "Preliminary results coupling "Stochastic Mean Field" and "Boltzmann-Langevin One Body" models with Geant4," *Physica Medica*, vol. 67, pp. 116–122, 2019.

66. A. Ono, H. Horiuchi, T. Maruyama, and A. Ohnishi, "Fragment formation studied with antisymmetrized version of molecular dynamics with two-nucleon collisions," *Progress of theoretical physics*, vol. 87, no. 5, p. 1185, 1992.

67. A. Ono, H. Horiuchi, T. Maruyama, and A. Ohnishi, "Fragment formation studied with antisymmetrized version of molecular dynamics with two-nucleon collisions," *Physical Review Letters*, vol. 68, no. 19, p. 2898, 1992.

68. Y. Kanada-En'yo, M. Kimura, and A. Ono, "Antisymmetrized molecular dynamics and its applications to cluster phenomena," *Progress of Theoretical and Experimental Physics*, p. 01A202, 2012.

69. A. Ono, "Dynamics of light clusters in fragmentation reactions," *Il Nuovo Cimento C*, vol. 39, p. 390, 2016.

70. A. Guarnera, M. Colonna, and P. Chomaz, "3D stochastic mean-field simulations of the spinodal fragmentation of dilute nuclei," *Physics Letters B*, vol. 373, no. 4, pp. 267–74, 1996.

71. M. D. Napoli *et al.*, "Carbon fragmentation measurements and validation of the Geant4 nuclear reaction models for hadrontherapy," *Phys. Med. Biol.*, vol. 57, no. 22, pp. 7651–71, 2012.

72. A. Cardiello *et al.*, "Preliminary results in using Deep Learning to emulate BLOB, a nuclear interaction model," *Physica Medica*, vol. 73, pp. 65–72, 2020.

# 6 Experimental data of nuclear fragmentation for validating Monte Carlo codes: Present availability and lacks

*Giuseppe Battistoni, Silvia Muraro, and Aafke C. Kraan*
Istituto Nazionale di Fisica Nucleare (INFN) Section of Milan,
Milan, Italy

## CONTENTS

Reliable nuclear fragmentation models in Monte Carlo codes are important for accurate 3D dose evaluation in patients treated with particle therapy, especially in complex cases where standard treatment planning systems may have limits. The ability of Monte Carlo codes to reproduce experimental data of cross sections and yields of secondary fragments plays hereby a fundamental role. In this chapter, we discuss the experimental data that can be used for building and validating nuclear fragmentation models.

## 6.1  INTRODUCTION

Charged hadrons of energies relevant in particle therapy (up to a few hundred MeV/nucleon) interact in tissue by electromagnetic and nuclear interactions [88]. The quality of Monte Carlo codes depends on the degree of accuracy in the modelling of both type of interactions. The theory of electromagnetic interactions is well established. Although modelling their implementation with sufficient details is still highly complicated in MC codes, it is generally considered a satisfactory and consolidated task.

This is not the case for nuclear interactions. Both elastic and inelastic nuclear reactions are relevant in particle therapy. In elastic nuclear collisions the kinetic energy is conserved. Elastic interactions contribute to the lateral broadening of the dose distribution and to lower of the height of the Bragg peak (similarly to the effect of Multiple Coulomb Scattering). In inelastic collisions more violent reactions between projectile and target occur. The projectile may knock out secondary particles (protons, neutrons, deuterons, alpha's, etc.) from the nucleus and break into fragments if the

DOI: 10.1201/9781003023920-6

incoming projectile is an ion. Inelastic nuclear interactions have a strong impact on dose distribution (see also Chapters 5 and 6 for a more extensive description), due to the build up of secondary particles [23, 12]. First of all, inelastic reactions cause beam attenuation, because the primary particles disappear with penetration depth. Furthermore, the secondary particles produced in inelastic reactions modify the buildup region of the Bragg curve (mostly due to target fragmentation). Also, in case of heavy ion projectiles there is dose deposition beyond the Bragg peak (from projectile fragmentation). Finally, the production of low energetic secondary particles including neutrons, which are typically emitted at larger angles cause a relatively large low dose region (low dose envelope). Thus, the production of neutrons should be included in dose calculations [71]. Since the inelastic reaction cross section grows as $A^{2/3}$, the impact of inelastic nuclear interactions is growing with increasing mass of the projectile. Secondary particles are responsible for the deterioration of the physical selectivity, especially around the Bragg peak region, and therefore their presence is considered as undesired. In fact, no projectiles heavier than oxygen are used in particle therapy. However, the production of secondaries also opens up the possibility to detect them, as is done in non-invasive range monitoring.

Contrary to electromagnetic interactions, no rigorous calculable models exist to describe nuclear interactions. The commonly used general purpose modern MC codes make use of phenomenological models, where the treatment of nuclear environment and all phases following the primary fast interaction (pre-equilibrium, evaporation, fission, de-excitation) is to be fully taken into account. Although a lot of progress has been achieved in the last years, none of the available hadronic physics models is considered as completely satisfactory [52, 23]. Among the difficulties are the fact that there are different models for different energy ranges and the presence of free parameters that must be tuned by means of experimental data at the single interaction level. In the next paragraphs a review of some of the most useful available data is presented. Generally speaking, the scientific community considers these data still far from being a complete set, not only in terms of available projectiles, targets, energies, and angles, but also in terms of reliability and precision. In addition is has to be remarked that MC models require a continuous work of upgrade and development and therefore the production of new and more precise experimental data is of great interest in this context.

## 6.2   THE NEED FOR VALIDATION AND BENCHMARK MEASUREMENTS

The accuracy of the predictions of nuclear interaction models ultimately relies on the ability to correctly model the relevant production cross sections. To do so, they should be built upon reliable physical bases to have full predictive capability. In practice, this means that these models have to be built according to a "microscopic" approach, *i.e.* starting from the fundamental properties of the nucleus and of its constituents. All relevant conservation laws have to be fulfilled and correlations within each single interaction must be preserved. However, due to their intrinsic phenomenological nature, even in the most advanced nuclear interaction models there exists a certain number of free parameters (depending on the specific model) which has to be determined, possibly minimizing the dependence on projectile, target and energy. Experimental data are fundamental and necessary to allow benchmarking and to drive further model development.

Typically, model benchmarking requires the measurement of total and differential nuclear cross sections. In addition, measurements related to secondary particle production can be used, including primary beam attenuation, multiplicity, angle and energy distributions. A collection of measured cross sections in the energy range from 100 MeV/u up to 10 GeV/u can be found in reviews by Norbury [55], Sihver [73], Bauhoff [11], focusing mostly on radiation protection in space. The handbook by Heilbronn and Nakamura [53] contains also lots of data for neutron production, mostly from design studies of heavy ion accelerator facilities and radiation protection in space. Finally, a work by Braunn et al. [15] contains a large number of references of total proton-nucleus cross section measurements as a function of energy in the range up to 250 MeV with tissue like targets. In

**Table 6.1**

*Cross section measurements on thin targets for tissue-like targets in the energy range up to 400 MeV/u.*

| Incident beam | Energy [MeV/u] | Target | Measurement | Reference |
|---|---|---|---|---|
| $^4$He | 70-220 | H, C, O, Si | Charge and mass changing cross sections | Horst et al. [36, 35] |
| $^4$He, C | 135, 290, 400 | C, Li | Double differential cross section measurements of neutron production | Handbook [53], Chapter 3 |
| $^{12}$C, $^{20}$Ne | 83, 200, 250, 300 | C, Al, Ca, Fe, Zn, Y, Ag | Total cross section | Kox et al. [38, 39] |
| $^{12}$C | 30 to 400 | Be, C, Al | Total reaction cross section as function of projectile energy | Takechi et al. [76] |
| $^{12}$C | 200 to 400 | Water, polycarbonate | Total and partial charge changing cross sections for production of fragments up to $Z = 4$ at various energies | Toshito et al. [81] |
| $^{12}$C | 62 | C | Double differential cross sections and angular distributions of secondary charged fragments up to $25^o$ | De Napoli et al. [16] |
| $^{12}$C | 95 | C, CH$_2$, Al, Al$_2$O$_3$, Ti | Double differential cross section for secondary charged fragment production ranging from protons to carbon isotopes | Dudouet et al. [22] |
| $^{12}$C | 50 | C, CH$_2$, Al, Al$_2$O$_3$, Ti, PMMA | Double differential cross section for secondary charged fragment production ranging from protons to carbon isotopes | Divay et al. [20] |
| $^{12}$C | 115, 153, 221, 281, 353 | C, Plastic Scintillator, PMMA | Energy differential cross section at $60^o$ and $90^o$ of fragments with $Z = 1$ | Mattei et al. [49] |

the context of radiotherapy, much effort has been done in the last decades to improve the accuracy of MC codes in the projectile energy range up to 400 MeV/u for tissue-like targets. In the following, we summarize some of the most relevant measurement that have to be considered, and identify the gaps. The data can be divided in two categories: i) measurements on thin targets; ii) measurements on thick targets.

## 6.3  EXPERIMENTAL DATA BASED ON THIN TARGETS

Measurements performed with thin targets are the most appropriate for tuning MC models, because the energy of the beam doesn't decrease, and the model parameters can be isolated from transport issues. Such measurements are particularly appropriate for determining the total cross sections, partial cross sections, and single and double differential cross sections of specific processes. While total cross sections are valuable to predict primary beam attenuation, partial cross sections, single and double differential cross sections are important to predict yields, angles and energies of secondary particles.

A non exhaustive selection of cross section measurements, that have frequently been used for tuning nuclear models in MC simulations in the particle therapy energy range, is reported in Table 6.1. The majority of the cross section measurements in Table 6.1 is for carbon projectiles, however the growing amount of interest in particle therapy with other projectiles has led to new initiatives.

Many of the measurements in Table 6.1 were used for the tuning of the hadronic models in several MC codes. A study by Böhlen et al. [12] aimed at the tuning of the hadronic models in FLUKA and GEANT4 revealed several shortcomings in both codes, in particular at lower energies. In GEANT4, several improvements in the nuclear models were introduced afterwards [16, 14, 21, 41]. In the

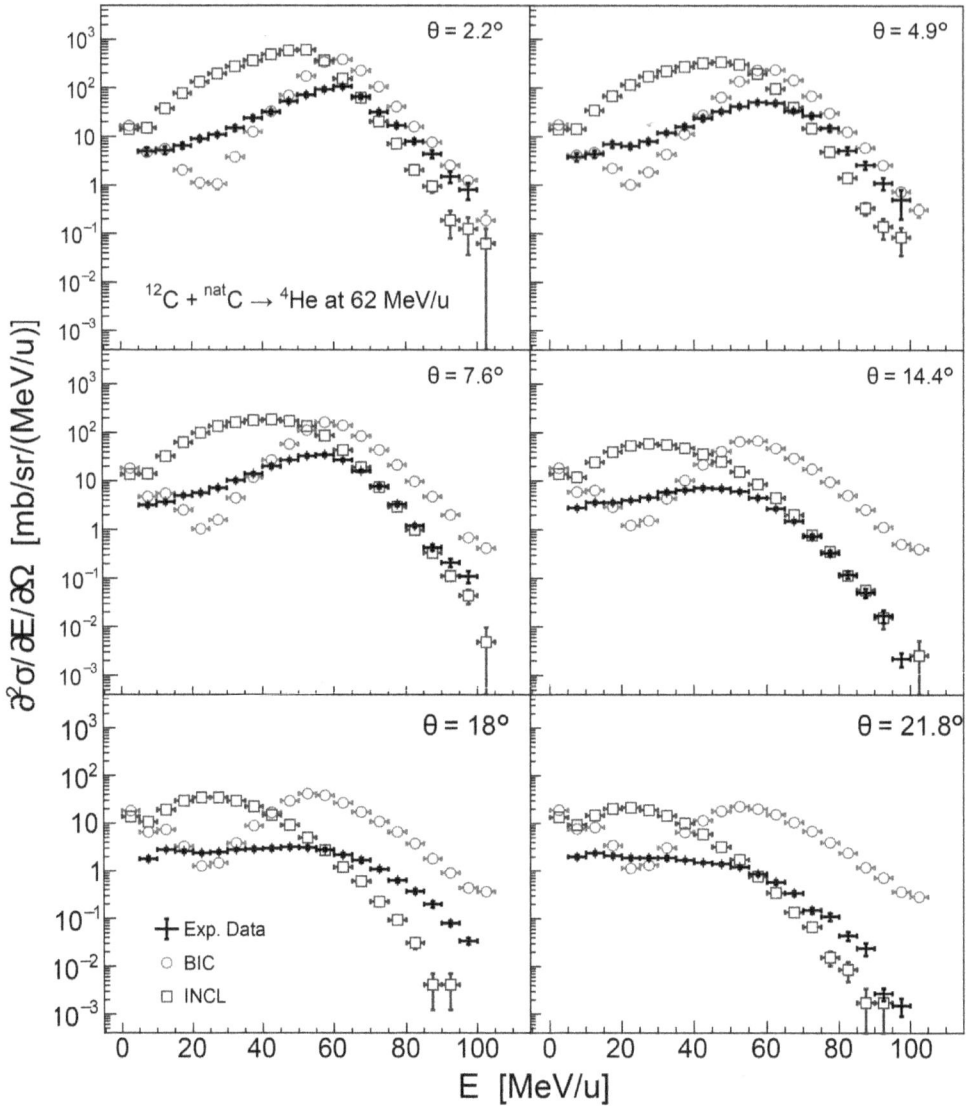

**Figure 6.1** The double-differential cross sections measured at different angles of $\alpha$-particle production in the interaction of a 62 MeV/u $^{12}$C beam with a thin C target, as a function of the $\alpha$-particle kinetic energy. Comparison between experimental data (filled dots) from De Napoli et al. [16] and the GEANT nuclear models BIC (open circles) and INCL (open squares). Taken from [6], with permission.

context of medical physics, a dedicated testing system was recently developed, denominated G4-Med [6], in order to respond to the need of benchmarking the code against reference data. An example of a GEANT4 benchmark is shown in Figure 6.1, where experimental data from De Napoli et al. [16] (in black) are compared with the two models available in Geant4 for ion interactions at particle therapy energies, namely INCL (in blue) and BIC (in red). Moreover, PHITS, FLUKA and MCNP6 were recently benchmarked with experimental data for neutron production cross sections [83]. An example for FLUKA is given in Figure 6.2, showing the FLUKA-RQMD predictions

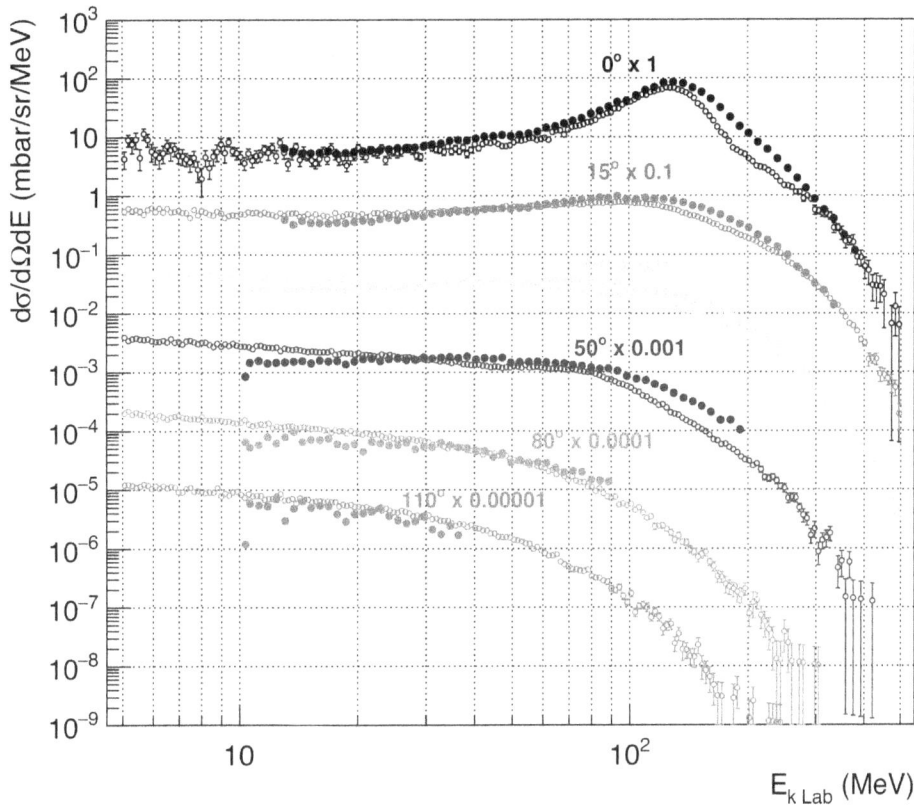

**Figure 6.2** The FLUKA–RQMD predictions of the double differential cross section for neutron production for 135 MeV/n $^{12}$C interactions in a thin carbon target as a function of neutron energy at several detection angles (empty circles in different grey scales) compared with experimental data (solid circles) from Sato et al. [68].

of the double differential cross section for neutron production in a thin carbon target compared to experimental data from Sato et al. [68].

Despite the progress made over the years, Table 6.1 shows that double differential cross section measurements for charged fragment production are still scarce, while such measurements are the most essential for tuning nuclear reaction models. Measurements that are specifically aimed at improving the knowledge for particle therapy are planned in the future by the FOOT collaboration [75].

## 6.4 EXPERIMENTAL DATA BASED ON THICK TARGETS

Measurements on thick targets comprehend primary beam attenuation studies, Faraday cup measurements, fragmentation yields, emission angles, and so on. Especially in the last two decades, a large amount of measurements were done with the purpose of range monitoring in particle therapy. Of all the measurements on thick targets, only a handful are actually useful for MC benchmarking. First, they should include a clear description of the experimental setup. Second, the physical quantities should be reported in absolute units. In some cases, measurements on thick targets allow to extract cross sections and are thus useful for the tuning of nuclear interaction models. In other cases, they cannot be directly used for the tuning of nuclear models, but they can still give the possibility to assess the overall accuracy of MC codes in terms of transport, nuclear and electromagnetic interaction models together.

In Table 6.2 a selection of valuable measurements is presented. Of these measurements, the cross section measurements by Schall [69], Haettner [30, 29] and Golvschenko [26, 25] are most suitable for benchmarking MC codes at particle therapy energies, and these data were used for benchmarking FLUKA [12], GEANT4 [12], PHITS [61], and SHIELD-HIT [32, 9]. An example of an attenuation measurement by Haettner at al for a $^{12}$C projectile in a thick water target is given in Figure 6.3. Measurements of emission angles and fragment yields were performed for the validation of PHITS [28], FLUKA [8] and GEANT4 [17], allowing for additional improvements in these codes. Figure 6.4 shows the yield of secondary particles with $Z = 1$ as a function of energy at forward angles ($\leq 30^o$) compared with PHITS predictions. In a recent work by Aricò et al. [7],

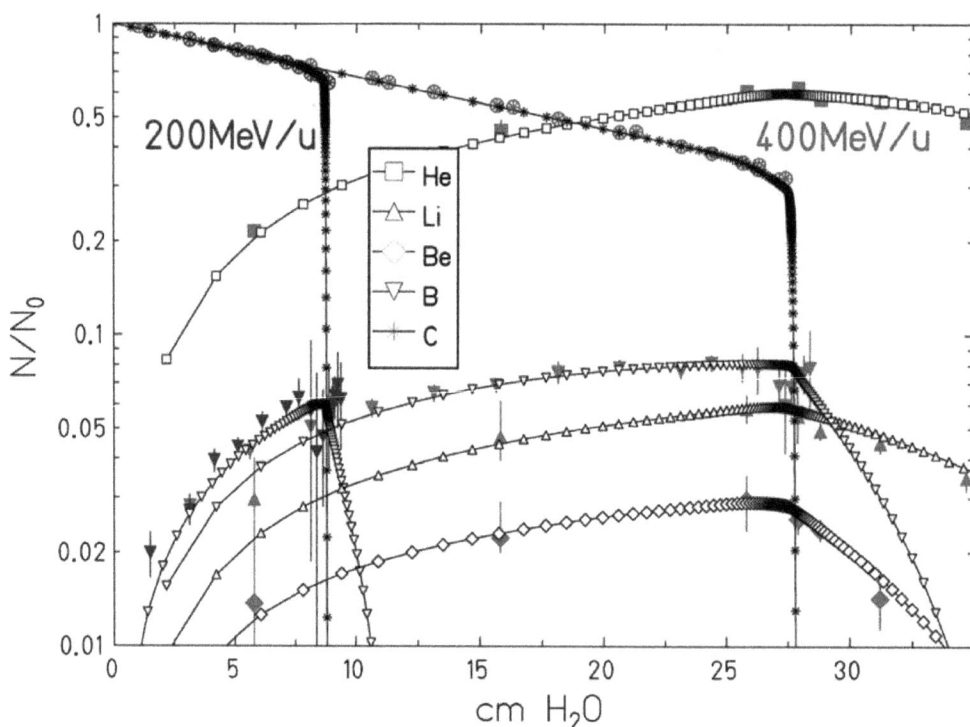

**Figure 6.3**   Primary beam attenuation and secondary buildup as a function of depth for 200 MeV/u and 400 MeV/u carbon beams. Data are compared with MC simulations. Reproduced from Haettner et al. [29].

where the amount of secondary fragments produced in water and PMMA targets with a $^{12}$C beam was measured, the authors found differences between the FLUKA code and the measurements, calling for improvements in the nuclear models.

A different approach is represented by charge measurements performed by means of a multi-layer Faraday Cup. Although such measurements cannot provide any specific check of a particular reaction channel, they can be used as integral test which allows to estimate the accuracy of MC models in reproducing the overall range of nuclear secondaries produced in target fragmentation. For example, in the work of Rinaldi et al. [62], a FLUKA simulation of protons at 160 MeV was compared to existing experimental data. Besides FLUKA, also other MC codes have been previously compared to the same kind of measurements, including SHIELD-HIT is considered in Henkner et al. [33], MCNPX in Mascia et al. [43], and GEANT4 in Zacharatou et al. [87] and in Hall et al. [31].

A distinct group of measurements with thick targets are the ones that are motivated by range monitoring, a topic where the reliability of nuclear models in MC is of particular relevance. These

## Table 6.2

*A non exhaustive selection of measurements on thick targets relevant to particle therapy: projectile, energy, target material, measurement, literature with MC-data comparisons, and reference with first author.*

| Incident beam | Energy [MeV/u] | Target | Measurement | Reference |
|---|---|---|---|---|
| $^4$He | 120, 200 | Water, PMMA | Attenuation of primary beam and build-up of secondary charged fragments in depths | Rovituso et al. [64] |
| $^4$He | 220 | Water, PMMA | Attenuation of primary beam, and build-up of secondary hydrogen ions due to fragmentation. | Aricò et al. [8] |
| $^4$He | 102, 125, 145 | PMMA | Flux of fragments behind Bragg peak at 5 angles between 0 and $30^o$ from beam-line | Marafini et al. [42] |
| $^{12}$C | 110 to 250 | C, paraffin, water | Total charge changing cross section and partial cross sections for B and Be fragment production | Golovschenko et al. [26, 25] |
| $^{11}$B, $^{12}$C, $^{14}$N, $^{16}$O, $^{26}$F, $^{20}$Ne | 200 to 670 | water, carbon, lucite, polyethylene, aluminum | Total and partial charge changing cross sections through primary beam attenuation measurements, buildup of nuclear fragments | Schall et al. [69] |
| $^4$He, $^{12}$C | 100 to 400 | C | Double differential cross section measurements for neutron production | Handbook [53], Chapter 2 |
| $^{12}$C, $^{16}$O | 57, 93, 95 | graphite, plexiglas, polyethylene | Fragment emission angle distributions | Sihver et al. [72]. |
| $^{12}$C | 56 | thick muscle, cortical bone | Production yields of produced fragments and energy spectra of most abundant fragments ($Z \leq 5$ isotopes) at $0^o$ | De Napoli et al. [17] |
| $^{12}$C | 150, 290, 400, 490 | PMMA | Fluence and LET of various fragments | Matsufuji et al. [44] |
| $^{12}$C | 200 | thick Water | Detect all fragments and present energy spectra at various angles ($0^o$, $5^o$, $10^o$, $20^o$, $30^o$) with respect to the beam axis for charged fragments ($Z \leq 2$ isotopes) and neutrons. | Gunzert-Marx et al. [28] |
| $^{12}$C | 200, 400 | thick Water | Energy and angular distributions of fragment isotopes from $Z = 1$ to $Z = 5$ at 6 depths before and behind Bragg peak, build-up curves of secondary fragments, attenuation of primary carbon beams | Haettner et al. [30, 29] |
| $^{12}$C | 213, 226, 250 | thick PMMA | Show back-projection of distributions on the beam-axis of secondary charged particle tracks detected at $30^o$ from the beam-axis, as well as lateral projections (HIT) | Gwosch et al. [27] |
| $^{12}$C | 290 | thick Water | Investigate spatial fragment distribution: primary beam angular distributions and projectile fragments ($Z \leq 5$) angular distributions. Also multiplicity distributions. They focus on the MCS model. | Matsufuji et al. [45] |
| $^{12}$C, $^{14}$N, $^{16}$O | 200, 270, 300 | thick water | Z distributions of beam fragments, total and charge-changing cross sections, Bragg peak measurements (10B etc. were produced as secondary beams from primary beams. | Schardt et al. [70] |
| $^{12}$C | 430 | water, PMMA | $^{12}$C attenuation and yield of different fragments | Aricò et al. [7] |

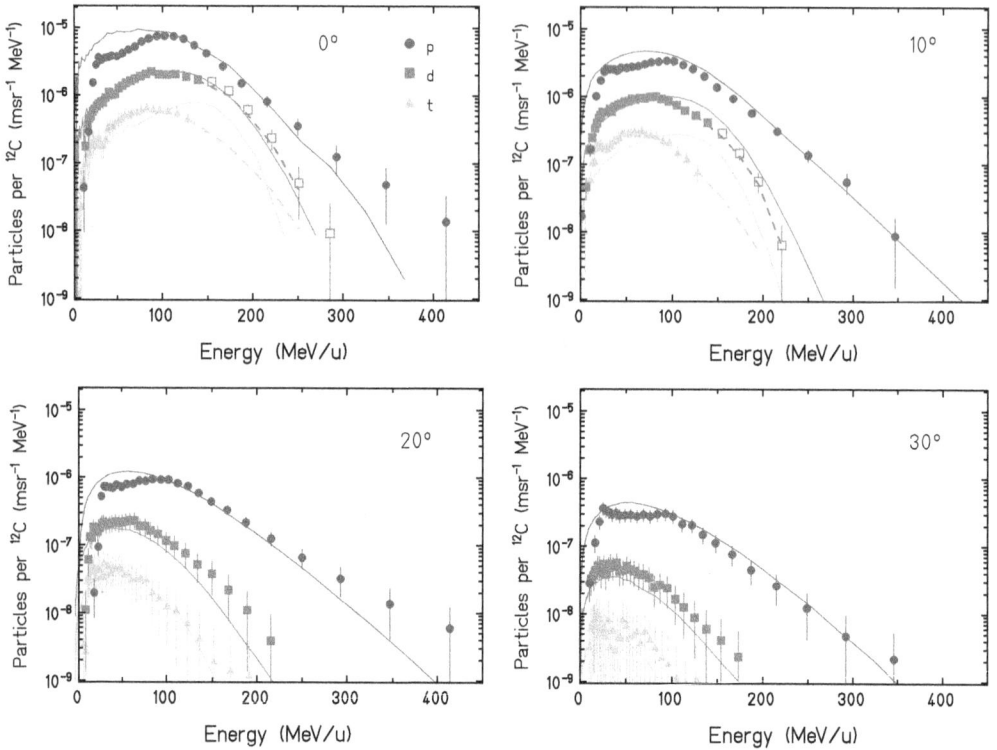

**Figure 6.4** Yield of $Z = 1$ secondary particles as a function of energy at forward angles ($\leq 30^o$) compared with PHITS predictions. Reproduced from Gunzert-Marx et al. [28]

secondaries include $\beta^+$ emitting nuclei, prompt gammas and energetic secondary charged fragments. We summarize a selection of these measurements in Table 6.3. Again such a list is non-exhaustive, and we selected only those measurements that were reported in absolute physics quantities on homogeneous targets.

As far as $\beta^+$ emitting nuclei are concerned, a large amount of measurements is available for offline, in-room, and online monitoring. Most of the measurements in Table 6.3 are dedicated to the detection of the activity spatial distribution. However, the data which are particularly useful for MC model tuning are cross section measurements. At presence, most data are available for the production of the most abundant isotopes $^{11}C$ and $^{15}O$. The work by Matsushida et al. contains valuable data for the production cross section of $^{11}C$ in carbon projectiles, up to 70 MeV [46]. New measurements in a wide energy range are available for $^{10}C$, $^{11}C$, and $^{15}O$, both for carbon and proton projectiles and for carbon ion projectiles are also available, as described in a recent work by Horst et al. [34]. More data for short lived isotope produced in carbon ion collisions with light targets including $^{10}C$, $^{13}N$, $^{14}O$, and $^{15}O$ are since recently available [67, 19]. Some of these available data has been used for benchmarking MC codes. Most validation and benchmarking work concerned the most abundant isotopes $^{11}C$ and $^{15}O$, including GEANT, PHITS and HIBRAC [63], as well as FLUKA [10], all showing satisfactory results. More recently, new efforts were made to compare GEANT4 with data for short-lived $\beta^+$ emitting nuclei [19], revealing the need for improvements [13].

Regarding prompt gammas, soon after the first proposal to use prompt gamma detection for particle therapy [50], it was realized that existing MC models were not reliable, see for instance [40]. Valuable new measurements were reported afterwards by Smeets et al. [74] and Pinto et al. [57], as

**Table 6.3**

*Summary of measurements in the context of range monitoring studies*

| Incident beam | Energy [MeV/u] | Target | Technique | Measurement | Reference |
|---|---|---|---|---|---|
| p | 160 | PMMA | Prompt $\gamma$ | Energy spectra and yields at $90^o$ | Smeets et al. [74] |
| p | 230 | water | Prompt $\gamma$ | Energy spectra and yields at $90^o$ | Verburg et al. [86, 85] |
| p | 48 | 4 samples with varying amount of O, C, H | Prompt $\gamma$ | Energy spectra and yields at $90^o$ | Polf et al. [59] |
| $^{12}$C | 73, 95, 305 | PMMA, water | Prompt $\gamma$ | Time-of-flight and energy spectra at $90^o$ | Testa et al. [78, 77, 79] |
| $^{12}$C | 220 | polymethyl methacrylate | Prompt $\gamma$ | Energy spectra and yields at $90^o$ | Vanstalle et al. [84] |
| $^{12}$C | 95, 310 | PMMA, water | Prompt $\gamma$ | Energy spectra and yields at $90^o$ | Pinto et al. [57] |
| $^{12}$C | 80 | PMMA | Prompt $\gamma$ | Energy spectra and yields at $90^o$ | Agodi et al. [2] |
| $^4$He, $^{12}$C, $^{16}$O | 100 to 300 | PMMA | Prompt $\gamma$ | Yields at $60^o$, $90^o$, and $120^o$ | Mattei et al. [48] |
| $^{12}$C | 80 | PMMA | Fast Charged Hadrons | Proton yields at $60^o$ and $90^o$ | Agodi et al. [1] |
| $^{12}$C | 220 | PMMA | Fast Charged Hadrons | Fragments with Z=1 at $90^o$ | Piersanti et al. [56], Mattei et al. [47] |
| $^4$He, $^{12}$C | 120-220 | PMMA | Fast Charged Hadrons | Secondary protons at $90^o$ | Rucinski et al. [65] |
| $^{16}$O | | PMMA | Fast Charged Hadrons | Yields of fragments with $Z = 1$ as function of energy and production position at $60^o$ and $90^o$ | Rucinski et al. [23] |
| $^{12}$C | 400 | composite target | Fast Charged Hadrons | Secondary fragments for angles $34^o$ to $81^o$ | Alexandrov et al. [4, 5] |
| p, $^{12}$C | 40-220(p), 65-430(C) | graphite, beryllium oxide | $\beta+$ | Cross section measurements of $^{10}$C, $^{11}$C, $^{15}$O | Horst et al. [34] |
| p, $^{12}$C | 110, 140, 175 (p), 212, 260, 343 (C) | PMMA | $\beta+$ | Absolute activity distributions and total production cross sections of $^{10}$C, $^{11}$C, $^{15}$O | Pshenichnov et al. [60] |
| p | 55 | water, carbon, phosphorus, calcium | $\beta+$ | Number of short lived $\beta+$ emitters | Dendooven et al. [19] |
| p | 10 to 70 | polyethylene, water | $\beta+$ | Cross sections of 4 specific reaction channels for production of $^{11}$C, $^{15}$O, $^{13}$N, | Akagi et al. [3] |
| p | 10 to 70 | polyethylene | $\beta+$ | Cross sections for specific reaction channels for production of $^{11}$C and $^{10}$C | Matsushita et al. [46] |

well as several studies aimed at improving the accuracy of MC codes like FLUKA [10], MCNPX [74], Geant4 [18, 58] and TOPAS [80].

Finally, charged fast hadrons were considered more recently for range monitoring purposes in the context of ion therapy [51, 82, 24] . Table 6.3 summarizes various measurements that are useful for MC benchmarking. A main goal remains achieving a higher spatial precision [82], which requires the use of fragments emitted at large angles (mostly protons). Simulating such processes is challenging, because only a few of the total number of charged hadron secondaries produced are emitted at large angles and not all standard available biasing techniques can be applied. In addition there is lack of data at large production angles to benchmark production models. A recent attempt to perform this kind of measurements for $^{12}$C interactions on different elements is reported in [49].

## 6.5  FUTURE DEVELOPMENTS

In the last decade the increasing importance of MC application in the context of particle therapy has stimulated the development of the available codes. Among the most relevant sources of uncertainties is the modelling of nuclear interactions. Generally speaking it turns out that most of the available hadronic models appear to be adequate for physical dose calculations. However it is also clear that none of such models is capable, alone, to provide reliable predictions for every clinical and research application. This situation drives the efforts of developers to constant search for improvements. Due to the intrinsic phenomenological nature of the calculation models, experimental data are necessary for benchmarking, so to allow such improvements. Efforts are also continuously ongoing to develop models and provide codes that require a more limited computing times, so that the application in clinical practise becomes more feasible.

It has to be noticed that the uncertainty of the predictions of MC models can be, at best, of the same order as the experimental uncertainty. Whether the level of accuracy of a certain model is high enough is a personal judgment that strongly depends on the scope of its use. The capability of correctly reproducing in detail the cross sections may not be necessary in all cases. For instance, a model can be accurate in reproducing the physical dose but not enough to give reliable predictions for range verification techniques.

Summarizing, in this chapter an attempt has been made to present examples of the available experimental data which have been used so far for the benchmarking of nuclear models. For this purpose, single and double differential cross sections, measured on thin target experiments, are probably the most useful data for the characterization of the MC models. There is however a general consensus that the set of available data is still far from being sufficiently complete, especially when nucleus-nucleus interactions are concerned, in terms of available projectile species, target, energies, secondary particles, angles, etc. So far, the attention has been mainly focused on the interactions of proton and $^{12}$C beams. More recently, the attention is focusing on new ions, such as $^{4}$He and $^{12}$O interactions. The case of helium is considered particularly promising for future clinical applications [54, 37].

## REFERENCES

1. C. Agodi, G. Battistoni, F. Bellini, G. A. P. Cirrone, F. Collamati, G. Cuttone, et al. Charged particle's flux measurement from PMMA irradiated by 80 MeV/u carbon ion beam. *Phys. Med. Biol.*, 57:5667, 2012.
2. C Agodi, F Bellini, GAP Cirrone, et al. Precise measurement of prompt photon emission for carbon ion therapy. *Journal of Instrumentation*, 7, 2012.
3. T Akagi, M Yagi, T Yamashita, et al. Experimental study for the production cross section of positron emitters induced from $^{12}$C and $^{16}$O nuclei by low-energy proton beams. *Radiation Measurements*, 59:262, 2013.

4. A Aleksandrov, L Consiglio, G De Lellis, A Di Crescenzo, A Lauria, MC Montesi, V Patera, C Sirignano, and v Tioukov. Measurement of large angle fragments induced by 400 MeV/u carbon ion beams. *Meas. Sci. Technol*, 26:094001, 2015.

5. A Alexandrov, G De Lellis, A Di Crescenzo, A Lauria, MC Montesi, A Pastore, V Patera, A Sarti, and V Tioukov. Measurements of $^{12}$C ions beam fragmentation at large angle with an emulsion cloud chamber. *Journal of Instrumentation*, 12:P08013, 2017.

6. P. Arce, D. Bolst, D. Cutajar, S. Guatelli, A. Le, A.B. Rosenfeld, D. Sakata, M-C. Bordage, J.M.C. Brown, P. Cirrone, G. Cuttone, L. Pandola, G. Petringa, M.A. Cortés-Giraldo, J.M. Quesada, L. Desorgher, P. Dondero, A. Mantero, A. Dotti, D.H. Wright, B. Faddegon, J. Ramos-Méndez, C. Fedon, S. Incerti, V. Ivanchenko, D. Konstantinov, G. Latyshev, I. Kyriakou, C. Mancini-Terracciano, M. Maire, M. Novak, C. Omachi, T. Toshito, A. Perales, Y. Perrot, F. Romano, L.G. Sarmiento, T. Sasaki, I. Sechopoulos, and E.C. Simpson. Report on G4-Med, a Geant4 benchmarking system for medical physics applications developed by the Geant4 Medical Simulation Benchmarking Group. *Medical Physics*, 48(1):19, 2021.

7. G. Aricò, T. Gehrke, R. Gallas, A. Mairani, O. Jäkel, and M. Martišíková. Investigation of single carbon ion fragmentation in water and PMMA for hadron therapy. *Phys. Med. Biol.*, 64(5):055018, 2019.

8. G. Aricó, T. Gehrke, J. Jakubek, R. Gallas, S. Berke, O. Jäkel, A. Mairani, A. Ferrari, and M. Martišíková. Investigation of mixed ion fields in the forward direction for 220.5 MeV/u helium ion beams: comparison between water and PMMA targets. *Phys. Med. Biol.*, 62(20):8003–8024, 2017.

9. N Bassler, DC Hansen, A Lühr, B Thomsen, JB Petersen, and N. Sobolevsky. SHIELD-HIT12A - a Monte Carlo particle transport program for ion therapy research. *J. Phys.: Conf. Ser.*, 489:012004, 2014.

10. G Battistoni, J Bauer, TT Böhlen, F Cerutti, MPW Chin, et al. The FLUKA code: an accurate simulation tool for particle therapy. *Fron. Oncol.*, 6:116, 2016.

11. W. Bauhoff. Tables of reaction and total cross sections for proton-nucleus scattering below 1 GeV. *Atomic Data and Nuclear Data Tables*, 35(3):429–447, 1986.

12. T. T. Böhlen, F. Cerutti, M. Dosanjh, A. Ferrari, I. Gudowska, A. Mairani, et al. Benchmarking nuclear models of FLUKA and GEANT4 for hadron therapy. *Phys Med Biol*, 55(19):5833–47, 2010.

13. A Bongrand, E Busato, P Force, et al. Use of short-lived positron emitters for in-beam and real-time beta+ range monitoring in proton therapy. *Physica Medica*, 69:248–255, 2020.

14. B Braunn, A Boudard, J Colin, J Cugnon, D Cussol, JC David, P Kaitaniemi, M Labalme, S Leray, and D Mancusi. Comparisons of hadrontherapy-relevant data to nuclear interaction codes in the GEANT4 toolkit. *Journal of Physics: Conference Series*, 420:1, 2013.

15. B Braunn, A Boudard, and J David. Assessment of nuclear-reaction codes for proton induced reactions on light nuclei below 250 MeV. *Eur. Phys. J. Plus*, 130:153, 2015.

16. M. De Napoli, C. Agodi, G. Battistoni, A.A. Blancato, G.A.P. Cirrone, G. Cuttone, et al. Carbon fragmentation measurements and validation of the GEANT4 nuclear reaction models for hadron therapy. *Phys. Med. Biol.*, 57(22):7651, 2012.

17. M De Napoli, F Romano, D D'Urso, et al. Nuclear reaction measurements on tissue-equivalent materials and GEANT4 Monte Carlo simulations for hadrontherapy. *Phys. Med. Biol.*, 59:7643, 2014.

18. G. Dedes, M. Pinto, D. Dauvergne, N. Freud, J. Krimmer, J. M. Létang, et al. Assessment and improvements of GEANT4 hadronic models in the context of prompt-gamma hadrontherapy monitoring. *Phys. Med. Biol.*, 59(7):1747, 2014.

19. P Dendooven, HJT Buitenhuis, F Diblen, et al. Short-lived positron emitters in beam-on PET imaging during proton therapy. *Phys. Med. Biol.*, 60:8923–8947, 2015.

20. C Divay, J Colin, D Cussol, Ch Finck, Y Karakaya, M. Labalme, M. Rousseau, S Salvador, and M Vanstalle. Differential cross section measurements for hadron therapy: 50 MeV/nucleon [12]C reactions on H, C, O, Al, and Ti targets. *Phys. Rev. C*, 95:044602, 2017.

21. J. Dudouet, D. Cussol, D. Durand, and M. Labalme. Benchmarking GEANT4 nuclear models for hadron therapy with 95 MeV/nucleon carbon ions. *Phys. Rev. C*, 89(5):054616, 2014.

22. J Dudouet, D Juliani, M Labalme, D Cussol, JC Angélique, B Braunn, J Colin, Ch Finck, JM Fontbonne, H Guérin, P Henriquet, J Krimmer, M Rousseau, MG Saint-Laurent, and S Salvador. Double-differential fragmentation cross-section measurements of 95 MeV/nucleon [12]C beams on thin targets for hadron therapy. *Phys. Rev. C*, 88:024606, 2013.

23. M. Durante and H. Paganetti. Nuclear physics in particle therapy: a review. *Reports on Progress in Physics*, 79(9):096702, 2016.

24. R. Félix-Bautista, T Gehrke, L Ghesquière-Diérickx, M Reimold, C Amato, D Turecek, J Jakubek, M Ellerbrock, and M. Martisíková. Experimental verification of a non-invasive method to monitor the lateral pencil beam position in an anthropomorphic phantom for carbon-ion radiotherapy. *Phys. Med. Biol.*, 64:175019, 2019.

25. AN Golovchenko, J Skvarc, N Yasuda, et al. Erratum: Total charge-changing and partial cross-section measurements in the reactions of 110-250 MeV/nucleon [12]C in carbon, paraffin and water. *Physical Review C*, 66:039901, 2002.

26. AN Golovchenko, J Skvarc, N Yasuda, et al. Total charge-changing and partial cross-section measurements in the reactions of 110-250 MeV/nucleon [12]C in carbon, paraffin and water. *Physical Review C*, 66(1):014609, 2002.

27. K. Gowsch, B. Hartmann, J. Jakubek, C. Granja, P. Soukup, O. Jäkel, et al. Non-invasive monotoring of therapeutic carbon ion beams in a homogeneous phantom by tracking of secondary ions. *Phys. Med. Biol.*, 58(11):3755, 2013.

28. K Gunzert-Marx, H Iwase, D Schardt, and RS Simon. Secondary beam fragments produced by 200 MeV u[−1] [12]C ions in water and their dose contributions in carbon ion radiotherapy. *New Journal of Physics*, 10:075003, 2008.

29. E. Haettner, H. Iwase, M. Krämer, G. Kraft, and D. Schardt. Experimental study of nuclear fragmentation of 200 and 400 Mev/u [12]C ions in water for applications in particle therapy. *Phys. Med. Biol.*, 58(23):8265–8279, 2013.

30. E. Haettner, H. Iwase, and D. Schardt. Experimental fragmentation studies with [12]C therapy beams. *Radiat. Prot. Dosim.*, 122(1-4):485, 2006.

31. D.C. Hall, A. Makarova, H Paganetti, and B Gottschalk. Validation of nuclear models in Geant4 using the dose distribution of a 177 MeV proton pencil beam. *Phys. Med. Biol.*, 61(1):N1–N10, 2016.

32. DC Hansen, A Lühr, N Sobolevsky, and N. Bassler. Optimizing SHIELD-HIT for carbon ion treatment. *Phys. Med. Biol.*, 57(8):2393, 2012.

33. K Henkner, N Sobolevsky, O Jäkel, and H Paganetti. Test of the nuclear interaction model in SHIELD-HIT and comparison to energy distributions from GEANT4. *Phys. Med. Biol.*, 54(22):N509–N517, 2009.

34. F Horst, W. Adi, G Aricò, K Brinkmann, M Durante, MC Reidel, M Rovituso, U Weber, HG Zaunick, K Zink, and C. Schuy. Measurement of PET isotope production cross sections for protons and carbon ions on carbon and oxygen targets for applications in particle therapy range verification. *Phys. Med. Biol.*, 64:205012, 2019.

35. F Horst, G Aricò, K Brinkman, et al. Measurements of [4]He charge and mass changing cross sections on H,C, O, and Si targets in the energy range 70-220 MeV/u for radiation transport calculations in ion-beam therapy. *Phys. Rev. C*, 99:014603, 2019.

36. F Horst, C Schuy, and U Weber. Measurements of [4]He charge and mass changing cross sections for [4]He+[12]C collisions in the energy range 80-220 MeV/u for applications in ion beam therapy. *Phys. Rev. C*, 96:024624, 2017.

37. B. Kopp, S. Mein, T. Tessonnier, J. Besuglow, S. Harrabi, E. Heim, A. Abdollahi, T. Haberer, J. Debus, and A. Mairani. Rapid effective dose calculation for raster-scanning 4he ion therapy with the modified microdosimetric kinetic model (mmkm). *Physica Medica*, 81:273–284, 2021.

38. S Kox, A. Gamp, R Cherkaoui, et al. Direct measurements of heavy ion total reaction cross section at 30 and 83 MeV/nucleon. *Nuclear Physics A*, 420:162–172, 1984.

39. S Kox, A Gamp, C Perrin, et al. Trends of total reaction cross sections for heavy ion collisions in the intermediate energy range. *Physical Review C*, 35(5):1678–1691, 1987.

40. F. Le Foulher, M. Bajard, M. Chevallier, D. Dauvergne, N. Freud, P. Henriquet, S. Karkar, J.M. Létang, L. Lestand, R. Plescak, C. Ray, D. Schardt, E. Testa, and M. Testa. Monte Carlo simulations of prompt-gamma emission during carbon ion irradiation. *IEEE Transactions on Nuclear Science*, 57(5):2768–2772, 2010. http://hal.in2p3.fr/in2p3-00480024.

41. C Mancini-Terracciano, M Asai, B Caccia, GAP Cirrone, A Dotti, R Faccini, P Napolitani, L Pandola, DH Wright, and M Colonna. Preliminary results coupling stochastic mean field and Boltzmann-Langevin One Body models with GEANT. *Physica Medica*, 67:116–122, 2019.

42. M. Marafini et al. Secondary radiation measurements for particle therapy applications: nuclear fragmentation produced by $^4$He ion beams in a PMMA target. *Phys. Med. Biol.*, 62:1291–1309, 2017.

43. A Mascia, J De Marco, P Chow, and T Solberg. Benchmarking of the MCNPX nuclear interaction models for use in the proton therapy energy range. In *Proc. 14th ICCR, Seoul, South Korea 2004*, pages 478–481, 2004.

44. N. Matsufuji, A. Fukumura, M. Komori, T. Kanai, and T. Kohno. Influence of fragment reaction of relativistic heavy charged particles on heavy-ion radiotherapy. *Phys. Med. Biol.*, 48(11), 2003.

45. N. Matsufuji, M Komori, et al. Spatial fragment distribution from a therapeutic pencil-like carbon beam in water. *Phys. Med. Biol.*, 50:3393, 2005.

46. K Matsushita, T Nishio, S Takana, et al. Measurement of proton induced target fragmentation cross sections in carbon. *Nuclear Physics A*, 946:104, 2016.

47. I. Mattei, G. Battistoni, F. Collini, E. De Lucia, M. Durante, S. Fiore, C. La Tessa, C. Mancini-Terracciano, M. Marafini, R. Mirabelli, S. Muraro, R. Paramatti, L. Piersanti, A. Rucinski, A. Russomando, A. Sarti, C. Schuy, A. Sciubba, E. Solfaroli Camillocci, M. Toppi, G. Traini, S. M. Valle, M. Vanstalle, and V. Patera. Addendum: Measurement of charged particle yields from PMMA irradiated by a 220 MeV/u $^{12}$C beam. *Phys. Med. Biol.*, 62(21):8483, 2017.

48. I Mattei, F Bini, F Collamati, E De Lucia, PM Frallicciardi, E Iarocci, C Mancini-Terracciano, M Marafini, S Muraro, R Paramatti, et al. Secondary radiation measurements for particle therapy applications: prompt photons produced by $^4$He, $^{12}$C and $^{16}$O ion beams in a PMMA target. *Phys. Med. Biol.*, 62(4):1438, 2017.

49. I. Mattei et al. Measurement of $^{12}$C fragmentation cross sections on C, O, and H in the energy range of interest for particle therapy applications. *IEEE TRANSACTIONS ON RADIATION AND PLASMA MEDICAL SCIENCES*, 4(2):269, 2020.

50. CH Min and CH. Kim. Prompt gamma measurements for locating the dose falloff region in the proton therapy. *Appl. Phys. Lett.*, 89(18):183517, 2006.

51. S. Muraro, G. Battistoni, F. Collamati, E. De Lucia, R. Faccini, F. Ferroni, S. Fiore, P. Frallicciardi, M. Marafini, I. Mattei, S. Morganti, R. Paramatti, L. Piersanti, D. Pinci, A. Rucinski, A. Russomando, A. Sarti, A. Sciubba, E. Solfaroli-Camillocci, M. Toppi, G. Traini, C. Voena, and V. Patera. Monitoring of hadrontherapy treatments by means of charged particle detection. *Front. Oncol.*, 6:177, 2016.

52. S. Muraro, G. Battistoni, and A. C. Kraan. Challenges in monte carlo simulations as clinical and research tool in particle therapy: A review. *Frontiers in Physics*, 8:567800, 2020.

53. T. Nakamura and L. Heilbronn. *Handbook On Secondary Particle Production And Transport*. World Scientific, 2006.

54. John W. Norbury, Giuseppe Battistoni, Judith Besuglow, Luca Bocchini, Daria Boscolo, Alexander Botvina, Martha Clowdsley, Wouter de Wet, Marco Durante, Martina Giraudo, Thomas Haberer, Lawrence Heilbronn, Felix Horst, Michael Krämer, Chiara La Tessa, Francesca Luoni, Andrea Mairani, Silvia Muraro, Ryan B. Norman, Vincenzo Patera, Giovanni Santin, Christoph Schuy, Lembit Sihver, Tony C. Slaba, Nikolai Sobolevsky, Albana Topi, Uli Weber, Charles M. Werneth, and Cary Zeitlin. Are further cross section measurements necessary for space radiation protection or ion therapy applications? helium projectiles. *Frontiers in Physics*, 8:409, 2020.

55. JW Norbury, J Miller, AM Adamczyk, LH Heilbronn, LW Townsend, SR Blattnig, RB Norman, SB Guetersloh, and CJ. Zeitlinet. Nuclear data for space radiation. *Radiation. Meas*, 12:315–363, 2012.

56. L. Piersanti, F. Bellini, F. Bini, F. Collamati, E. De Lucia, M. Durante, et al. Measurement of charged particle yields from PMMA irradiated by a 220 MeV/u $^{12}$C beam. *Phys. Med. Biol.*, 59(7):1857, 2012.

57. M. Pinto, M. Bajard, S. Brons, M. Chevallier, D. Dauvergne, Dedes G., et al. Absolute prompt-gamma yield measurements for ion beam therapy monitoring. *Phys. Med. Biol.*, 60(2):565, 2015.

58. M Pinto, D Dauvergne, N Freud, et al. Assessment of GEANT4 prompt-gamma emission yields in the context of proton therapy monitoring. *Front. Oncol.*, 28, 2016.

59. JC Polf, R Panthi, DS Mackin, M McCleskey, A Saastamoinen, BT Roeder, et al. Measurement of characteristic prompt gamma rays emitted from oxygen and carbon in tissue- equivalent samples during proton beam irradiation. *Phys. Med. Biol.*, 58(17):5821, 2013.

60. I. Pshenichnov, I. Mishustin, and W. Greiner. Distributions of positron-emitting nuclei in proton and carbon-ion therapy studied with GEANT4. *Phys. Med. Biol.*, 51(23):6099, 2006.

61. X Puchalska et al. Benchmarking of PHITS for carbon ion therapy. *International Journal of Particle Therapy*, 4(3):48, 2018.

62. I Rinaldi, A Ferrari, A Mairani, H Paganetti, K Parodi, and P Sala. An integral test of FLUKA nuclear models with 160 MeV proton beams in multi-layer Faraday cups. *Phys. Med. Biol.*, 56:4001–4011, 2011.

63. Heide Rohling, Lembit Sihver, Marlen Priegnitz, Wolfgang Enghardt, and Fine Fiedler. Comparison of PHITS, GEANT4, and hibrac simulations of depth-dependent yields of beta+-emitting nuclei during therapeutic particle irradiation to measured data. *Physics in Medicine and Biology*, 58(18):6355–6368, sep 2013.

64. M Rovituso, C Schuy, U Weber, S Brons, MA Cortés-Giraldo, C La Tessa, E Piasetzky, D Izraeli, D Schardt, and M Toppi. Fragmentation of 120 and 200 MeV/u $^4$He ions in water and PMMA targets. *Phys. Med. Biol.*, 62(4):1310, 2017.

65. A. Rucinski, G. Battistoni, F. Collamati, E. De Lucia, R. Faccini, P. M. Frallicciardi, C. Mancini-Terracciano, M. Marafini, I. Mattei, S. Muraro, R. Paramatti, L. Piersanti, D. Pinci, A. Russomando, A. Sarti, A. Sciubba, E. Solfaroli Camillocci, M. Toppi, G. Traini, C. Voena, and V. Patera. Secondary radiation measurements for particle therapy applications: charged particles produced by $^4$He and $^{12}$C ion beams in a PMMA target at large angle. *Phys. Med. Biol.*, 63(5):055018, 2018.

66. A. Rucinski, G. Traini, A. Baratto Roldan, G. Battistoni, M. De Simoni, Y. Dong, M. Fischetti, P. M. Frallicciardi, E. Gioscio, C. Mancini-Terracciano, M. Marafini, I. Mattei, R. Mirabelli, S. Muraro, A. Sarti, A. Schiavi, A. Sciubba, E. Solfaroli Camillocci, S.M. Valle, and V Patera. Secondary radiation measurements for particle therapy applications: Charged secondaries produced by $^{16}$O ion beams in a PMMA target at large angles. *Physica Medica*, 64:45–53, 2019.

67. S Salvador, J Colin, D Cussol, C Divay, JM Fontbonne, and M Labalme. Cross section measurements for production of positron emitters for pet imaging in carbon therapy. *Physical Review C*, 95:044607, 2017.

68. H Sato, T Kurosawa, H Iwase, T Nakamura, Y Uwamino, and N Nakao. Measurements of double differential neutron production cross sections by 135 mev/nucleon he, c, ne and 95 mev/nucleon ar ions. *Phys. Rev. C.*, 64:034607, 2001.

69. I Schall, D Schardt, H Geissel, et al. Charge-changing nuclear reactions of relativistic light-ion beams ($5 \leq Z \leq 10$) passing through thick absorbers. *Nucl. Instr. Meth. B*, 117:221–234, 1996.

70. D Schardt, I Schall, H Geissel, H Irnich, G Kraft, A Magel, MF Mohar, G Münzenberg, F Nickel, C Scheidenberger, W Schwab, and L Sihver. Nuclear fragmentation of high-energy heavy-ion beams in water. *Advances in Space Research*, 17(2):87–94, 1996.

71. Uwe Schneider and Roger Hälg. The impact of neutrons in clinical proton therapy. *Frontiers in Oncology*, 5:235, 2015.

72. L Sihver, M Giacomelli, S Ota, et al. Projectile fragment emission angles in fragmentation reactions of light ions in the energy region $< 200$ MeV/nucleon: Experimental study. *Radiation Measurements*, 48:73–81, 2013.

73. L. Sihver, M. Lantz, M. Takechi, A. Kohama, A. Ferrari, F. Cerutti, and T. Sato. A comparison of total reaction cross section models used in particle and heavy ion transport codes. *Adv. in Space Research*, 49:812–819, 2012.

74. J. Smeets, F. Roellinghoff, D. Prieels, F. Stichelbaut, A. Benilov, P. Busca, et al. Prompt gamma imaging with a slit camera for real time range control in proton therapy. *Phys. Med. Biol.*, 57(11):3371, 2012.

75. R. Spighi et al. Foot: Fragmentation of target experiment. *Nuovo Cim. C*, 42(2-3-3):134, 2019.

76. M Takechi, M Fukuda, M Mihara, et al. Reaction cross sections at intermediate energies and Fermi-motion effects. *Physical Review C*, 79:061601, 2009.

77. E Testa, M Bajard, M Chevallier, D Dauvergne, F Le Foulher, N Freud, et al. Dose profile monitoring with carbon ions by means of prompt-gamma measurements. *Nucl. Instr. Meth. B*, 267(6):993, 2009.

78. E Testa, M Bajard, M Chevallier, D Dauvergne, F Le Foulher, JC Poizat, et al. Monitoring the Bragg peak location of 73 MeV/u carbon ion beams by means of prompt gamma-ray measurements. *Appl. Phys. Lett.*, 93(9):093506, 2008.

79. M Testa, M Bajard, M Chevallier, D Dauvergne, N Freud, P Henriquet, et al. Real-time monitoring of the Bragg peak position in ion therapy by means of single photon detection. *Radiat. Environ. Biophys.*, 49(3):337, 2010.

80. M. Testa, C. H. Min, J. M. Verburg, J. Schümann, H.M. Lu, and H. Paganetti. Range verification of passively scattered proton beams based on prompt gamma time patterns. *Phys. Med. Biol.*, 59(15):4181, 2014.

81. T Toshito, K Kodama, L Sihver, et al. measurements of total and partial change-changing cross sections for 200 and 400 MeV/nucleon $^{12}$C on water and polycarbonate. *Physical Review C*, 75:054606, 2007.

82. G. Traini et al. Review and performance of the dose profiler, a particle therapy treatments online monitor. *Physica Medica*, 65:84, 2019.

83. P Tsai, B Lai, LH Heilbronn, and R Sheu. Benchmark of neutron production cross sections with Monte Carlo codes. *Nucl. Inst. Meth. in Phys Research B*, 416:16–29, 2018.

84. M. Vanstalle, I. Mattei, A. Sarti, F. Bellini, F. Bini, F. Collamati, E. De Lucia, M. Durante, R. Faccini, F. Ferroni, C. Finck, S. Fiore, M. Marafini, V. Patera, L. Piersanti, M. Rovituso, C. Schuy, A. Sciubba, G. Traini, C. Voena, and C. La Tessa. Benchmarking GEANT4 hadronic models for prompt-$\gamma$ monitoring in carbon ion therapy. *Med. Phys.*, 44(8):4276–4286, 2017.

85. J.M. Verburg and J. Seco. Proton range verification through prompt gamma-ray spectroscopy. *Phys. Med. Biol.*, 59(23):7089, 2014.

86. M. J. Verburg, K. Riley, T. Bortfeld, and J. Seco. Energy and time resolved detection of prompt gamma rays for proton range verification. *Phys. Med. Biol.*, 58(20):L37–49, 2013.
87. C Zacharatou Jarlskog and H Paganetti. Physics setting for using GEANT4 toolkit in proton therapy. *IEEE Trans. Nucl. Sci.*, 55:1018–25, 2008.
88. P.A. Zyla, R.M. Barnett, J. Beringer, et al. The Review of Particle Physics (2020). *Prog. Theor. Exp. Phys.*, page 083C01, 2020.

# 7 Quality assurance in particle therapy with PET

*Maria Giuseppina Bisogni*
Pisa University, Pisa, Italy
Istituto Nazionale di Fisica Nucleare (INFN) Section of Pisa, Pisa,
Italy

## CONTENTS

## 7.1 PHYSICAL BASIS OF POSITRON EMISSION TOMOGRAPHY

Particle therapy make use of ions (mainly protons and carbon ions) to treat solid and radioresistant tumors ([1]). The depth dose curve of charged particles in the matter with the characteristic peak at the end of their range (dubbed Bragg Peak) was suggested for cancer therapy of deep seated tumors by Robert Wilson in 1946 ([11]). The integral dose (meaning, the total energy released in the crossed tissues) for a given target dose is always lower than the one delivered by photons in conventional radiotherapy due the lower entrance and minimal exit dose. Furthermore, the steep dose gradients allow a more precise definition of the target volume suitable for treating tumors located in proximity of critical organs (for instance, chondrosarcomas of the skull base located close to the spinal cord)([12]).

Nevertheless, particle therapy is more sensitive to uncertainties than conventional radiotherapy and the impact of an improper quantification can be more severe. Uncertainties arise from treatment planning (approximations in the dose calculation, calibration errors, imaging artifacts) and from treatment delivery (organ motion, anatomical/morphological changes, patient set-up)([13]). As a clinical good practice, conservative safety margins are considered in the treatment plan to take into account range uncertainties. For instance, in proton treatments an uncertainty in proton range of 3.5% of the range plus additional 1–3 mm is assumed ([14]). To fully exploit the potential of particle therapy and, potentially, reduce the safety margins, prediction of the particles range in patient must be as accurate as possible in the planning and delivery of the treatment. Several imaging tools can be used to improve the quality of the treatments. Range uncertainties can be reduced with pre-treatment imaging, like dual energy Computed Tomography (CT) ([15]) and proton radiography ([16]) [71]. *In vivo* range verification systems offer instead the possibility to check the accuracy of beam delivery providing an in-vivo confirmation of the planned treatment. In addition *in vivo* verification could also provide a feedback on a possible disagreement between the planned and actual delivered dose thus enabling an adaptation of the plan before the next treatment fraction ([17]).

DOI: 10.1201/9781003023920-7

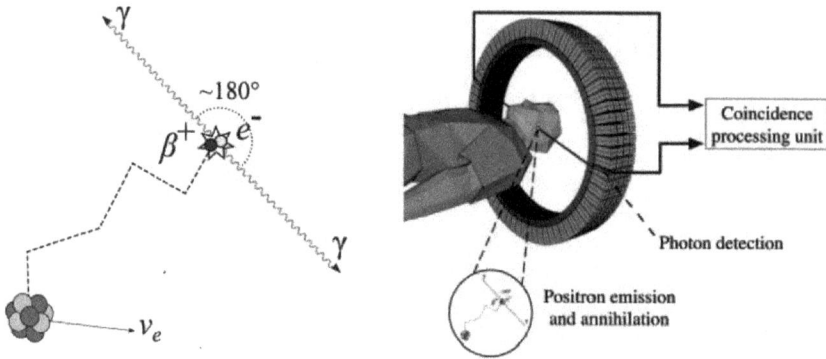

**Figure 7.1**   PET principle of operation. Left: A positron (β+) is emitted by a radioisotope together with an electron neutrino (νe). The positron slows down in tissue until it reaches thermal equilibrium and annihilates with an electron. Right: Detection of the photons in time coincidence by two opposing detectors. Reprinted with permission from ([18]).

Most of the *in vivo* verification systems rely on the detection of the secondary radiation exiting the patient after nuclear reactions occurring along the beam path. Indeed, nuclear reactions may occur all along the projectile path, until close to the Bragg peak region when the kinetic energy falls below the Coulomb barrier. Therefore, secondary radiation emission is correlated to the primary ion range, although the underlying hadronic interaction processes differ from the electromagnetic interaction ruling dose deposition.

Positron Emission Tomography (PET) is the most consolidated and clinically investigated *in vivo* verification technique ([2]). As in conventional nuclear medicine, it exploits the coincidence detection of the gamma rays coming from the annihilation of a positron with an atomic electron. The difference here is that the positron is emitted in the decay of a radioisotope created by the interaction of the primary beam with the tissue while in standard PET the radioisotope is chemically bonded to a radiochemical injected in the patient body.

The scheme of the PET principle is represented in Figure 7.1. The annihilation photons detected in time coincidence by opposite pairs of detectors are used to reconstruct the volumetric activity distribution $r(x,y,z)$ of the $b^+$ radioisotope that is correlated with the beam range in tissue, the degree of correlation depending on the primary ion species. Thanks to the nearly collinear emission of the gamma rays from the annihilation it is possible to define the line L along which the annihilation occurred. L is called line-of-flight (LOF). The activity distribution is measured in terms of projections along the LOF by using the line integral operator. Thus, for an ideal model and for a pair of detectors i and j, the line integral operator is defined as:

$$N_{ij} = k \int_{LOR_{ij}} \rho\,(x,y,z)\,dL \tag{7.1}$$

where $LOR_{ij}$ is the line of response connecting the two detectors.

The positron emitting radioisotopes are atoms whose nuclei have an excess of protons with respect to neutrons and decay to a stable configuration through $b^+$ decay:

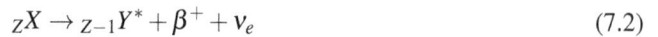

$$_Z X \rightarrow\, _{Z-1}Y^* + \beta^+ + \nu_e \tag{7.2}$$

The daughter nucleus $_{Z-1}Y^*$ can be produced in an excited state that decays to the ground state $_{Z-1}Y$ through gamma emission. The $\beta^+$ decays is a three-particle process. Given the mass of the recoil nucleus, its kinetic energy can be neglected so the released energy is shared between the $\beta^+$

e the $v_e$ and the energy spectrum of the $\beta^+$ is continuous with the maximum kinetic energy called endpoint.

Positron sources have to be artificially produced via nuclear reactions where positively charged particles bombard stable isotopes. In particle therapy the beam itself interacts with the target nuclei in the body to produce $\beta^+$-emitting isotopes or the projectile breaks down to an unstable $\beta^+$-emitting nucleus (see section 2). In nuclear medicine cyclotrons with typical energy of 10–20 MeV to overcome the Coulomb barrier are used to accelerate protons on targets.

Positrons lose their energy mostly through anelastic Coulomb interactions with the atomic electrons of the biological tissue. Finally the positron reaches thermal equilibrium with the medium and annihilation with an electron occurs. The range of the positron in water (i.e. the distance in water between the emission point and the position where thermal equilibrium takes place) for most of the PET radionuclides is about 1–2 mm. When the positron annihilates with an electron it is assumed in first approximation that both particles are at rest and for energy and momentum conservation the annihilation can only generate two gamma rays back-to-back. However, due to the bounding energy of the electron, the annihilation does not happen at rest and it results in a non-collinearity of the two gammas that shows a Gaussian dispersion around $180^o$ of about $0.5^o$ FWHM. Extensive reviews of the physics and technology of PET can be found in ([18, 19, 20, 21]).

## 7.2   PET MONITORING IN PARTICLE THERAPY

PET monitoring relies on the physical process of $\beta^+$-activation that includes target and projectile nuclear fragmentation with production of positron-emitting nuclei ([22]).

Nuclear interactions relevant for range monitoring are inelastic collisions, that are reactions between projectile and target where total kinetic energy is not conserved ([3, 4]). The projectile may knock out secondary particles (protons, deuterons, alphas, etc.) from the target nucleus and breaks into fragments if it is an ion. For primary protons, the secondary particles emission is entirely due to the target nuclei. In the so-called "dynamical" phase of the reaction (time scale of $10^{-22}$ s) protons, neutron and light fragments (through coalescence) are emitted and the residual nucleus is left in an excited state. De-excitation happens mostly through Fermi-breakup where the excited nucleus dissociates in one step into smaller fragments. This last step is "slow" (time scale $10^{-18}$–$10^{-16}$ s) and can be accompanied with gamma emissions. For primary ions, the nucleus-nucleus interaction can be described with the "abrasion-ablation" model. In the fast stage (abrasion, time scale $10^{-22}$ s), projectile and target nuclei overlap in a hot reaction zone. An excited quasi-projectile with much of the initial velocity, a quasi-target fragment at rest and several excited light fragments are formed. During the slow step (ablation, time scale $10^{-18}$–$10^{-16}$ s), the reactions products de-excite evaporating light nuclei and gammas. Differently to proton irradiation, in this case both projectile and target can fragment. In addition, projectile fragments travel further in the forward direction having the same velocities and directions as the primaries but longer ranges (charged particles range scales with $A/Z^2$) leading to the characteristic tail beyond the Bragg peak ([22]).

Protons and light ions (Z<= 4) produce positron-emitting target nuclei such as $^{11}$C, $^{15}$O, $^{13}$N with half-lives of about 20, 2, and 10 minutes respectively. The activation occurs as long as the beam energy is above the nuclear reaction threshold that typically corresponds to 1–4 mm of residual range of the primaries in tissue. Figure 7.2 shows an activation profile in a homogeneous plastic target (dotted line) produced by 95 MeV protons showing a slow rise followed by an abrupt distal fall-off a few mm's before the Bragg peak.

On top of the $\beta^+$-activated target nuclei, heavier ions (Z>= 5) can also yield positron emitting projectile fragments when they stop, near the end of their range. The peak in the activation profile just before the Bragg peak is due to nuclear reaction kinematics and different stopping power of the produced radioactive fragments with respect to the stable primary. For instance, for primary $^{12}$C beams, the activity is mainly due to $^{11}$C and, to a lesser extent, to the short lived $^{10}$C ($T_{1/2}$= 20 s).

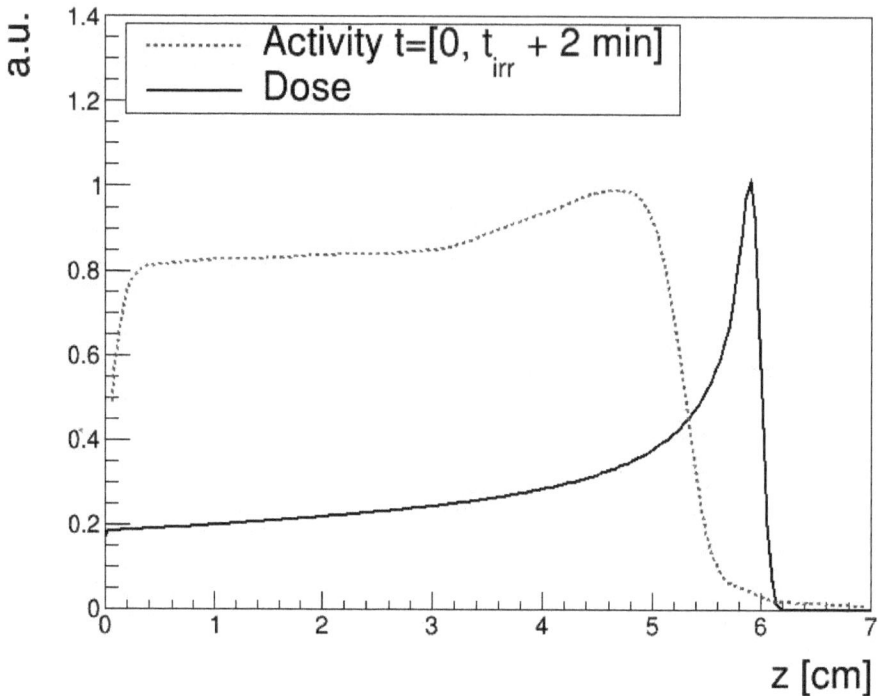

**Figure 7.2** Calculated depth dose distribution (solid line) and corresponding measured activity profiles (dotted line) for a homogeneous polymethyl methacrylate (PMMA) target irradiated with a 95 MeV proton beam.

Both those radionuclides accumulate shortly before the $^{12}$C Bragg peak. The tail after the activity peak is due to non $\beta^+$-emitting projectile fragments that in turn induce secondary fragmentation in the target.

The positron emitted after $\beta^+$ decay annihilates with an atomic electron of the tissue, most likely when coming to a rest, yielding a pair of 511keV gammas traveling in almost opposite directions. These energetic photons have an high probability to escape from the patient and be detected by detector pairs operated in time coincidence as in conventional nuclear medicine PET applications. PET imaging in particle therapy monitoring is mostly used to infer the range of the primary particles crossing the tissues. There is in fact no direct correlation between $\beta^+$ induced activity and the dose since induced activity and dose deposition rely on different physical processes. Nevertheless, comparing the measured PET data with a reference distribution it is still possible to assess the compliance between the planned and the actual dose delivered to the patient. The reference PET data can be obtained mostly by MC simulations or by analytical models and in that case the accuracy of the plan is tested. Otherwise, the treatment verification is done comparing the measured PET distributions with first day measurement to test the reproducibility among different fractions of the same treatment. PET in particle therapy has been widely studied for about 20 years and it is now an established although not widely used technique. Main problems preventing its widespread use is in clinics are the low induced signal levels and the physiological washout. In fact, the b+ activity formed in nuclear interactions (a few kBq/ml/Gy) is almost two orders of magnitude below the typical activity concentrations in diagnostic nuclear medicine (order of 50 kBq/ml in hot spots). In addition, the induced activity is rapidly lost due to physical decay of the sources (the main isotopes produced, $^{15}$O and $^{11}$C, have half-lives of 2 min and 20 min respectively) and physiological washout, with isotopes produced binding to different molecules and undergoing functional pathways such as perfusion and diffusion ([2]).

PET imaging for *in-vivo* range verification of ion beams is performed with commercial scanners placed in an room close to the treatment site (off-line PET) ([23, 24]). This solution is economically advantageous however the delay between the dose delivery and the PET verification greatly limits the quality of the results due to the physical and biological signal decay. Alternatively, *ad-hoc* systemslocated in close proximity to the patient (in-room PET) ([24]) can be used. In this case the delay is minimized and the physical decay and washout impact is greatly reduced. However, the longer treatment room occupancy and the difficulties in co-registering PET and planning CT prevents this method to be widely applied. PET scanners integrated in the treatment gantry or nozzle and operating during the delivery of the beam (in-beam PET) allows achieving higher sensitivities in the measurement of the low induced activity levels([25]) since $^{15}$O and other short-lived isotopes can be detected and the biological washout effect is greatly mitigated. Moreover, the patient repositioning is avoided. On the other hand, in-beam PET implies high cost for development and integration. Moreover, restrictions from the patient couch and the beam directions implies the adoption of dual-head PET geometries with associated image artifacts due to uncompleted angular coverage. In addition, the in-beam PET systems operation greatly depends on the beam time structure. Cyclotron machines (the vast majority for proton therapy) produce continuous beams. Due to the high background during the continuous beam delivery, the PET signal is usually acquired after the end of the irradiation ([5]), although data-taking during beam extraction was demonstrated to be feasible with the DOPET system, a PET scanner with high count rate capability ([26]). Synchrotron machines are used to accelerate both protons and light ions, with a beam delivery time structure characterized by an extraction phase (spill) and a pause between two spills when the beam acceleration phase takes place (inter-spill). In such facilities, in-beam PET systems have been previously developed and operated in the clinic during the pause of the spills or immediately after the irradiation ([6]), but their functioning was hampered during the actual beam delivery due to the high background radiation consisting of high energy prompt photons and neutrons ([27, 28]).

The ultimate clinical exploitation of PET monitoring should provide the actual dose delivered to the patient starting from the measured activity. Owing to the different beta+ activity formation process (due to nuclear interactions ) and the dose deposition process (due to Coulomb inelastic interactions), the inverse solution of the dose retrieval starting from the induced activity is an ill-posed problem. Practical approximate solutions ([29]), more rigorous mathematical approaches ([30, 31, 32]) and, recently, machine learning based methods ([33]) were proposed but they were never really extensively applied in clinics. In practice *in vivo* PET verification was mostly used to infer beam range information from the position of the distal activity fall-off. To this aim, different methods have been studied starting from point-like analysis to more sophisticated automated approaches that make use of activity iso-surfaces definition, distal fall-off shift in beam-eye view or correlation coefficient in selected distal 3D regions of interest ([34, 35, 36]).

## 7.3   THE ROLE OF MONTE CARLO METHODS IN PET MONITORING

Monte Carlo (MC) simulations are an essential tool in PET monitoring. First of all, they can accurately describe particle transport and interaction of radiation with patients whose anatomical description can be derived from CT scans, making them a powerful tool for system design studies ([3, 4]). Nonetheless, the main use of MC simulations is in the treatment quality assurance. PET and other *in-vivo* range monitoring techniques are generally based on direct comparisons between measured and MC predictions. By comparing the measured PET data with a reference distribution, it is possible to infer whether the dose was imparted as planned. Large discrepancies between expected and measured PET images can be related to problems in beam delivery, set-up or morphological changes in the patient anatomy. Reference distributions are generally calculated with

MC simulations based on the treatment plan, time-course of irradiations and PET scanner geometry and acquisition modality. In this respect, MC simulations were essential in the analysis and interpretation of the data obtained in the clinical studies reported in the next section ([37, 38, 7, 8]).

However, those studies highlighted important limitation in MC simulations that must be addressed in order to unleash the full potential of PET in range monitoring. The capability of MC codes to provide a reliable prediction of the production of the $b^+$ emitting isotopes formed during the irradiation is strongly correlated to the physical models of nuclear fragmentation processes and all the other stages following the fast interaction.

The most important general-purpose codes (FLUKA, GEANT4, MCNP6/X, to cite the most used) can predict the production of the most abundant nuclides (like $^{11}C$ and $^{15}O$) with sufficient accuracy. However, the prediction of other nuclides (for instance, those with short lifetime as $^{12}N$, $^{14}O$, $^8B$) remains a challenge due to the scarcity of experimental cross section data.

Other sources of inaccuracies come from the modeling of biological washout and of moving targets. These are largely uncovered by MC simulations and their correct implementation in the codes is complex but fundamental to extend the use of PET as range monitoring tool to a larger pool of clinical cases.

Finally, speed and complexity of the current frameworks are inadequate to the application in clinical practice. Recently, fast simulation techniques have been developed ([4]), exploiting new technologies in computing hardware and dedicated algorithms or simplifying the structure of the code to speed up the dose calculation. Research work is ongoing to extend those codes to model *in vivo* range monitoring techniques.

## 7.4   CLINICAL IMPLEMENTATION

After the first pioneering experience with He beams 50 years ago at the Lawrence Berkeley National Laboratory ([39]), a more extensive clinical study was performed at the horizontal beamline of the GSI Helmholtzzentrum für Schwerionen forschung in Darmstadt, Germany. Here a commercial PET scanner based on BGO crystals was modified in a dual head camera to be adapted at the beam port ([29]). Over 400 patients treated for head and neck and pelvis tumors with Carbon ions were successfully monitored with the PET scanner between 1997 and 2008. To avoid contamination from prompt radiation background, the data collection was performed during the pauses between two consecutive beam extractions and in the 40 sec after the treatment end.

At the National Cancer Center Hospital East in Kashiwa, Japan, a beam on-line planar PET system ([5]) was mounted on a rotating gantry port for dose–volume delivery-guided proton therapy. Activity measurements were performed in patients with head and neck tumors, liver, lungs, prostate, and brain. The position and intensity of the activity were measured during the 200 s immediately after the proton irradiation. Differences between a reference activity image (taken at the first treatment) and the daily activity-images indicated changes in the proton-irradiated volume. More recently the in-beam PET INSIDE system started a clinical trial at the National Center of Oncological Hadrontherapy (CNAO) in Pavia, Italy. The PET system is a dual head systems based on LFS crystals and SiPMs ([6]). The system can operate both in-spill and inter-spill but data with patients were only collected during beam extraction pauses to avoid any contamination from background radiation . Specific head-and neck and brain pathologies treated with both protons and Carbon ions were included in the trial and 20 patients were monitored so far. A reliable approach for range accuracy and reproducibility assessment was developed and tested on simulated and measured patients. The activity images acquired during irradiation were analyzed with a robust approach based on a multi-threshold procedure in order to detect possible particle range deviations ([37]). A color map overlaid on the patient CT was designed to highlight the critical regions where a difference between the reference and the actual range was found (see Figure 7.3). The developed map help clinicians to foresee a possible dose discrepancy in the treatment so as to better plan for a control CT and look

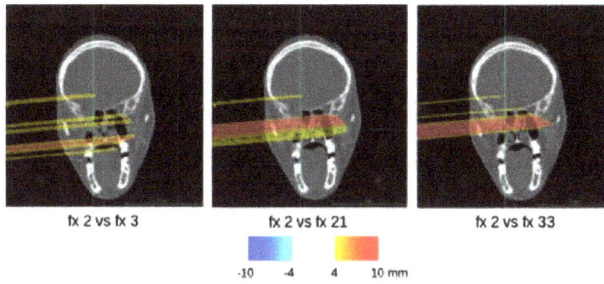

**Figure 7.3**   Color maps referring to activity image analysis of different fractions of a patient treated with protons at CNAO and monitored with the INSIDE in-beam PET showing a morphological variation during the course of the therapy. The maps are overlaid on the planning CT and the LUT of the range difference is shown in the lower part. Reprinted with permission from ([37]).

for possible morphological changes with a patient-tailored schedule. Reproducibility test showed that a sensitivity of 4 mm was achieved in patients treated with protons.

In room solutions have been clinically explored for passive scattering proton therapy at the Massachusetts General Hospital ([38]), where a prototype PET scanner was positioned next to the treatment head after treatment. The MC method was used to reproduce PET activities for each patient. To assess the proton beam range uncertainty, the measured PET activity surface distal to the target at the end of range was compared with MC predictions. The measured PET images show overall good spatial correlations with MC predictions. Some discrepancies could be attributed to uncertainties in the local elemental composition and biological washout and co-registration errors between PET and CT.

Offline PET/CT-based treatment verification was clinically explored at the Heidelberg Ion Beam Therapy Centre (HIT) with actively scanned proton and Carbon ion beams ([7, 8]). A commercial full-ring PET/CT scanner installed in close vicinity to the treatment rooms was used to image the patients after selected irradiation fractions. The expected activity distribution is obtained from the production of $\beta^+$-active isotopes simulated by a MC code on the basis of the patient-specific treatment plan, post-processed considering the time course of the respective treatment fraction, the estimated biological washout of the induced activity and a simplified model of the imaging process. Reproducibility tests were also performed comparing different fractions of the same patient. Head, head/neck, liver and pelvic tumors were monitored. Quantitative range analysis showed that the reproducibility was better than 1 mm while accuracy was limited to 1–5 mm for most examined cases due to the limitations of the physical prediction and washout model.

Clinical studies with off-line PET/CT were also reported by Hyogo facility ([40]) and Florida Proton Therapy Institute ([41]). In particular, in the latter one systematic analyzes of proton activated positron emitter distributions provided patient specific information on intra-fractional prostate motion and patient position variability during proton beam delivery. Such data were useful in establishing patient-specific planning target volume (PTV) margins.

## 7.5   ACTUAL TRENDS AND FUTURE DEVELOPMENTS

Despite the inherent limitations related to the delay of decay signals and to the suboptimal instrumentation, PET is still the most used technique for range monitoring and to date the most tested in the clinic. Latest generation in-beam dual-head PET prototypes were recently proposed with improved performances. In particular ultra-fast time-of-flight detectors with time resolution below 10 ps ([42]) would allow the direct localization of the annihilation events and the reconstruction of the 3D activity distribution with minimal degradation of the image due to the limited angle geometry.

On the other hand, recent advances in photosensors, front-end electronics and data acquisition, also combined with artificial intelligence techniques, allowed to develop smart PET detectors with improved spatial and time resolution ([43]). Suitable combinations of those sensors read-out by means of parallel data read-out architectures could actually perform range monitoring during beam-on. In fact, it has recently been shown that using fast integrated electronics and appropriate signal processing algorithms that analyze the temporal structure of events from PET data, it is possible to suppress most of the noise due to the background radiation and increase the noise signal ratio of the PET images acquired beam-on ([44]). Other interesting approaches rely on the possibility to detect short-lived positron emitters like $^{12}$N ($T_{1/2} = 11$ ms) with dual head PET systems stand-alone ([45, 46, 47]) or in combination with prompt-gamma detection to furtherly suppress the background noise ([48]).

Completely different approaches undertaken to overcome the limitations of the dual head geometry are those based on special full-rings featuring both a dual ring and a slanted or axially-shifted single ring configuration leaving an opening for the beam path. This option has been made viable by the depth-of-interaction capability of the PET detectors, enabling the exploitation of obliques line of response ([49]). This system has been used at HIMAC in Chiba Japan to visualize the full path of a $^{11}$C in the body ([50]) renewing the interest of PET range verification with radioactive beams now that facilities with high intensity beams are in construction ([9]).

An innovative approach on range monitoring relies on hybrid detection schemes that offers the combination of complementary information from different modalities. Multimodal systems based on the combination of in-beam PET and a charged particle tracking system ([10]) or a gamma detector ([51]) would make it possible to increase the global sensitivity, for example with the detection of $b^+$-g simultaneous emissions by $b^+$ isotopes such as $^{14}$O or $^{10}$C ([51]). Furthermore, complementing the 1D information produced by the tracking systems with the volumetric information offered by the PET system would open to the possibility of performing biological studies (for example, tumor sub-regions investigation), dynamic studies (tumor time-resolved analysis) and tests on radiobiological models.

## REFERENCES

1. Durante, M., R. Orecchia, and J. S. Loeffler. 2017. "Charged-particle therapy in cancer: clinical uses and future perspectives." Nat Rev Clin Oncol 14 (8): 483–495. https://doi.org/10.1038/nrclinonc.2017.30. https://www.ncbi.nlm.nih.gov/pubmed/28290489.
2. Parodi, K. 2015. "Vision 20/20: Positron emission tomography in radiation therapy planning, delivery, and monitoring." Med Phys 42 (12): 7153–68. https://doi.org/10.1118/1.4935869. https://www.ncbi.nlm.nih.gov/pubmed/26632070.
3. Kraan, A. C. 2015. "Range verification methods in particle therapy: Underlying physics and Monte Carlo modelling." Frontiers in Oncology 5 (JUN). https://doi.org/10.3389/fonc.2015. 00150. https://www.scopus.com/inward/record.uri?eid=2-s2.0-84934279767&doi=10.3389% 2ffonc.2015.00150&partnerID=40&md5=778f2f14ff07420ecdf477e99663c283.
4. Muraro, S., G. Battistoni, and A. C. Kraan. 2020. "Challenges in Monte Carlo Simulations as Clinical and Research Tool in Particle Therapy: A Review." Frontiers in Physics 8. https://doi.org/10.3389/fphy.2020.567800. https://www.scopus.com/inward/record.uri?eid=2-s2.0-85097364123&doi=10.3389%2ffphy.2020.567800&partnerID=40&md5=224073e3f76cb34338 e077cacd64d836.
5. Nishio, T., A. Miyatake, T. Ogino, K. Nakagawa, N. Saijo, and H. Esumi. 2010. "The Development and Clinical Use of a Beam ON-LINE PET System Mounted on a Rotating Gantry Port in Proton Therapy." International Journal of Radiation Oncology Biology Physics 76 (1): 277–286. https://doi.org/10.1016/j.ijrobp.2009.05.065. https://www.scopus.com/inward/record.uri?eid=2-s2.0-72049110976&doi=10.1016%2fj.ijrobp.2009.05.065& partnerID=40&md5=e655e3b76f225d6b545c329722689cda.

6. Bisogni, M. G., A. Attili, G. Battistoni, N. Belcari, N. Camarlinghi, P. Cerello, S. Coli, A. Del Guerra, A. Ferrari, V. Ferrero, E. Fiorina, G. Giraudo, E. Kostara, M. Morrocchi, F. Pennazio, C. Peroni, M. A. Piliero, G. Pirrone, A. Rivetti, M. D. Rolo, V. Rosso, P. Sala, G. Sportelli, and R. Wheadon. 2017. "INSIDE in-beam positron emission tomography system for particle range monitoring in hadrontherapy." Journal of Medical Imaging 4 (1). https://doi.org/10.1117/1.JMI. 4.1.011005. https://www.scopus.com/inward/record.uri?eid=2-s2.0-85000504286&doi= 10.1117%2f1.JMI.4.1.011005&partnerID=40&md5=3c4dd4c7e2512dd0fd71a75c13dba308.

7. Nischwitz, S. P., J. Bauer, T. Welzel, H. Rief, O. Jäkel, T. Haberer, K. Frey, J. Debus, K. Parodi, S. E. Combs, and S. Rieken. 2015. "Clinical implementation and range evaluation of in vivo PET dosimetry for particle irradiation in patients with primary glioma." Radiotherapy and Oncology 115 (2): 179–185. https://doi.org/10.1016/j.radonc.2015.03.022. https://www. scopus.com/inward/record.uri?eid=2-s2.0-84931572746&doi=10.1016%2fj.radonc.2015. 03.022&partnerID=40&md5=cf4d20be4dedc5dde35a58448d3ae97b.

8. Handrack, J., T. Tessonnier, W. Chen, J. Liebl, J. Debus, J. Bauer, and K. Parodi. 2017. "Sensitivity of post treatment positron emission tomography/computed tomography to detect interfractional range variations in scanned ion beam therapy." Acta Oncologica 56 (11): 1451–1458. https://doi.org/10.1080/0284186X.2017.1348628. https://www.scopus.com/inward/record. uri?eid=2-s2.0-85029580843&doi=10.1080%2f0284186X.2017.1348628&partnerID=40&md5= 136937a87b5b88ce21231162a2ad17a5.

9. Durante, M., A. Golubev, W. Y. Park, and C. Trautmann. 2019. "Applied nuclear physics at the new high-energy particle accelerator facilities." Physics Reports 800: 1–37. https://doi.org/ 10.1016/j.physrep.2019.01.004. https://www.scopus.com/inward/record.uri?eid=2-s2.0-85064323596&doi=10.1016%2fj.physrep.2019.01.004&partnerID=40&md5=fc683446a2eba 84654bb86f001e5869f.

10. Fischetti, M., G. Baroni, G. Battistoni, G. Bisogni, P. Cerello, M. Ciocca, P. De Maria, M. De Simoni, B. Di Lullo, M. Donetti, Y. Dong, A. Embriaco, V. Ferrero, E. Fiorina, G. Franciosini, F. Galante, A. Kraan, C. Luongo, M. Magi, C. Mancini-Terracciano, M. Marafini, E. Malekzadeh, I. Mattei, E. Mazzoni, R. Mirabelli, A. Mirandola, M. Morrocchi, S. Muraro, V. Patera, F. Pennazio, A. Schiavi, A. Sciubba, E. Solfaroli Camillocci, G. Sportelli, S. Tampellini, M. Toppi, G. Traini, S. M. Valle, B. Vischioni, V. Vitolo, and A. Sarti. 2020. "Inter-fractional monitoring of 12 C ions treatments: results from a clinical trial at the CNAO facility." Scientific Reports 10 (1). https://doi.org/10.1038/s41598-020-77843-z. https://www.scopus.com/ inward/record.uri?eid=2-s2.0-85096713822&doi=10.1038%2fs41598-020-77843-z&partnerID=40&md5=37257bd1df1d08e248aec93f43461d41.

11. Wilson, R. R. 1946. "Radiological use of fast protons." Radiology 47 (5): 487–91. https://doi.org/10.1148/47.5.487. https://www.ncbi.nlm.nih.gov/pubmed/20274616.

12. Durante, M., and H. Paganetti. 2016. "Nuclear physics in particle therapy: a review." Rep Prog Phys 79 (9): 096702. https://doi.org/10.1088/0034-4885/79/9/096702. https://www.ncbi.nlm.nih.gov/pubmed/27540827.

13. Knopf, A. C., and A. Lomax. 2013. "In vivo proton range verification: a review." Phys Med Biol 58 (15): R131–60. https://doi.org/10.1088/0031-9155/58/15/R131. https://www.ncbi.nlm.nih.gov/pubmed/23863203.

14. Paganetti, H. 2012. "Range uncertainties in proton therapy and the role of Monte Carlo simulations." Phys Med Biol 57 (11): R99–117. https://doi.org/10.1088/0031-9155/57/11/R99. https://www.ncbi.nlm.nih.gov/pubmed/22571913.

15. Bär, Esther, Arthur Lalonde, Gary Royle, Hsiao-Ming Lu, and Hugo Bouchard. 2017. "The potential of dual-energy CT to reduce proton beam range uncertainties." Medical Physics 44 (6): 2332–2344. https://doi.org/10.1002/mp.12215.

16. Johnson, Robert P. 2017. "Review of medical radiography and tomography with proton beams." Reports on Progress in Physics 81 (1): 016701. https://doi.org/10.1088/1361-6633/aa8b1d. http://dx.doi.org/10.1088/1361-6633/aa8b1d.

17. —. 2016. "On- and off-line monitoring of ion beam treatment." Nuclear Instruments and Methods in Physics Research, Section A: Accelerators, Spectrometers, Detectors and Associated Equipment 809: 113–119. https://doi.org/10.1016/j.nima.2015.06.056. https://www.scopus.com/inward/record.uri?eid=2-s2.0-84959335919&doi=10.1016%2fj.nima.2015.06.056&partnerID=40&md5=89cbef05ef54cedd42dba29f2d41fa1b.

18. Del Guerra, A., N. Belcari, and M. Bisogni. 2016. "Positron emission tomography: Its 65 years." Rivista del Nuovo Cimento 39 (4): 155–223. https://doi.org/10.1393/ncr/i2016-10122-6. https://www.scopus.com/inward/record.uri?eid=2-s2.0-84964053167&doi=10.1393%2fncr%2fi2016-10122-6&partnerID=40&md5=8dfc6f748a5495e3397953c69d2f0fd1.

19. Morrocchi, M., and A. Del Guerra. 2020. "Positron Emission Tomography: Alive and kicking after more than 65 years on stage." Journal of Instrumentation 15 (3). https://doi.org/10.1088/1748-0221/15/03/C03050. https://www.scopus.com/inward/record.uri?eid=2-s2.0-85084182757&doi=10.1088%2f1748-0221%2f15%2f03%2fC03050&partnerID=40&md5=ff87d398f9f05b01118b643a0a296e88.

20. Jonesa, T., and D. Townsend. 2017. "History and future technical innovation in positron emission tomography." Journal of Medical Imaging 4 (1). https://doi.org/10.1117/1.JMI.4.1.011013. https://www.scopus.com/inward/record.uri?eid=2-s2.0-85016630051&doi=10.1117%2f1.JMI.4.1.011013&partnerID=40&md5=dc0ce65d1b904310578cea12822d36c7.

21. Vaquero, J. J., and P. Kinahan. 2015. Positron Emission Tomography: Current Challenges and Opportunities for Technological Advances in Clinical and Preclinical Imaging Systems. In Annual Review of Biomedical Engineering.

22. —. 2021. "Ion range and dose monitoring with Positron Emission Tomography." In Radiation Therapy Dosimetry: a practical handbook, edited by Arash Darafsheh, 413–426. Boca Raton: CRC Press, Taylor&Francis Group.

23. Zhu, X., and G. El Fakhri. 2013. "Proton therapy verification with PET imaging." Theranostics 3 (10): 731–40. https://doi.org/10.7150/thno.5162. https://www.ncbi.nlm.nih.gov/pubmed/24312147.

24. Zhu, X., S. Espana, J. Daartz, N. Liebsch, J. Ouyang, H. Paganetti, T. R. Bortfeld, and G. El Fakhri. 2011. "Monitoring proton radiation therapy with in-room PET imaging." Phys Med Biol 56 (13): 4041–57. https://doi.org/10.1088/0031-9155/56/13/019. https://www.ncbi.nlm.nih.gov/pubmed/21677366.

25. Shakirin, G., H. Braess, F. Fiedler, D. Kunath, K. Laube, K. Parodi, M. Priegnitz, and W. Enghardt. 2011. "Implementation and workflow for PET monitoring of therapeutic ion irradiation: A comparison of in-beam, in-room, and off-line techniques." Physics in Medicine and Biology 56 (5): 1281–1298. https://doi.org/10.1088/0031-9155/56/5/004. https://www.scopus.com/inward/record.uri?eid=2-s2.0-79951877696&doi=10.1088%2f0031-9155%2f56%2f5%2f004&partnerID=40&md5=6e33ec3c6530d3cde2315fbd97bf12c6.

26. Sportelli, G., N. Belcari, N. Camarlinghi, G. A. P. Cirrone, G. Cuttone, S. Ferretti, A. Kraan, J. E. Ortuño, F. Romano, A. Santos, K. Straub, A. Tramontana, A. D. Guerra, and V. Rosso. 2014. "First full-beam PET acquisitions in proton therapy with a modular dual-head dedicated system." Physics in Medicine and Biology 59 (1): 43–60. https://doi.org/10.1088/0031-9155/59/1/43. https://www.scopus.com/inward/record.uri?eid=2-s2.0-84890692894&doi=10.1088%2f0031-9155%2f59%2f1%2f43&partnerID=40&md5=3e619d26bf418317bf4e9e66d620c1e3.

27. Testa, M., M. Bajard, M. Chevallier, D. Dauvergne, N. Freud, P. Henriquet, S. Karkar, F. Le Foulher, J. M. Létang, R. Plescak, C. Ray, M. H. Richard, D. Schardt, and E. Testa. 2010. "Real-time monitoring of the Bragg-peak position in ion therapy by means of single photon detection."

Radiation and Environmental Biophysics 49 (3): 337–343. https://doi.org/10.1007/s00411-010-0276-2. https://www.scopus.com/inward/record.uri?eid=2-s2.0-77955467857&doi=10.1007%2fs00411-010-0276-2&partnerID=40&md5=633d2fa3c501bde4788e8cde2bad8180.

28. Biegun, A. K., E. Seravalli, P. C. Lopes, I. Rinaldi, M. Pinto, D. C. Oxley, P. Dendooven, F. Verhaegen, K. Parodi, P. Crespo, and D. R. Schaart. 2012. "Time-of-flight neutron rejection to improve prompt gamma imaging for proton range verification: A simulation study." Physics in Medicine and Biology 57 (20): 6429–6444. https://doi.org/10.1088/0031-9155/57/20/6429. https://www.scopus.com/inward/record.uri?eid=2-s2.0-84867280532&doi=10.1088%2f0031-9155%2f57%2f20%2f6429&partnerID=40&md5=f270951034fcf2de31f31e10f3742eb8.

29. Enghardt, W., K. Parodi, P. Crespo, F. Fiedler, J. Pawelke, and F. Pönisch. 2004. "Dose quantification from in-beam positron emission tomography." Radiotherapy and Oncology 73 (SUPPL. 2): S96–S98. https://doi.org/10.1016/S0167-8140(04)80024-0. https://www.scopus.com/inward/record.uri?eid=2-s2.0-21444447195&doi=10.1016%2fS0167-8140%2804%2980024-0&partnerID=40&md5=be95b85674dc5064b3178a412a6f3373.

30. Fourkal, E., J. Fan, and I. Veltchev. 2009. "Absolute dose reconstruction in proton therapy using PET imaging modality: Feasibility study." Physics in Medicine and Biology 54 (11): N217–N228. https://doi.org/10.1088/0031-9155/54/11/N02. https://www.scopus.com/inward/record.uri?eid=2-s2.0-69249206907&doi=10.1088%2f0031-9155%2f54%2f11%2fN02&partnerID=40&md5=2e1f7486106e404208dbc549e640f86d.

31. Parodi, K., and T. Bortfeld. 2006. "A filtering approach based on Gaussian-powerlaw convolutions for local PET verification of proton radiotherapy." Physics in Medicine and Biology 51 (8): 1991–2009. https://doi.org/10.1088/0031-9155/51/8/003. https://www.scopus.com/inward/record.uri?eid=2-s2.0-33645541395&doi=10.1088%2f0031-9155%2f51%2f8%2f003&partnerID=40&md5=1a5578e4b5bbd808e11d165743553ba2.

32. Rutherford, H., A. Chacon, A. Mohammadi, S. Takyu, H. Tashima, E. Yoshida, F. Nishikido, T. Hofmann, M. Pinto, D. R. Franklin, T. Yamaya, K. Parodi, A. B. Rosenfeld, S. Guatelli, and M. Safavi-Naeini. 2020. "Dose quantification in carbon ion therapy using in-beam positron emission tomography." Physics in Medicine and Biology 65 (23). https://doi.org/10.1088/1361-6560/abaa23. https://www.scopus.com/inward/record.uri?eid=2-s2.0-85097958686&doi=10.1088%2f1361-6560%2fabaa23&partnerID=40&md5=4c98e3abf80880ef554893b06cd8ee01.

33. Liu, C., Z. Li, W. Hu, L. Xing, and H. Peng. 2019. "Range and dose verification in proton therapy using proton-induced positron emitters and recurrent neural networks (RNNs)." Phys Med Biol 64 (17): 175009. https://doi.org/10.1088/1361-6560/ab3564. https://www.ncbi.nlm.nih.gov/pubmed/31342940.

34. Frey, K., D. Unholtz, J. Bauer, J. Debus, C. H. Min, T. Bortfeld, H. Paganetti, and K. Parodi. 2014. "Automation and uncertainty analysis of a method for in-vivo range verification in particle therapy." Physics in Medicine and Biology 59 (19): 5903–5919. https://doi.org/10.1088/0031-9155/59/19/5903. https://www.scopus.com/inward/record.uri?eid=2-s2.0-84907212847&doi=10.1088%2f0031-9155%2f59%2f19%2f5903&partnerID=40&md5=d70c07c6e0add70e14ebad11ab64884c.

35. Ferrero, V., E. Fiorina, M. Morrocchi, F. Pennazio, G. Baroni, G. Battistoni, N. Belcari, N. Camarlinghi, M. Ciocca, A. Del Guerra, M. Donetti, S. Giordanengo, G. Giraudo, V. Patera, C. Peroni, A. Rivetti, M. D. D. R. Rolo, S. Rossi, V. Rosso, G. Sportelli, S. Tampellini, F. Valvo, R. Wheadon, P. Cerello, and M. G. Bisogni. 2018. "Online proton therapy monitoring: Clinical test of a Silicon-photodetector-based in-beam PET." Scientific Reports 8 (1). https://doi.org/10.1038/s41598-018-22325-6. https://www.scopus.com/inward/record.uri?eid=2-s2.0-85043263471&doi=10.1038%2fs41598-018-22325-6&partnerID=40&md5=721685fe472a731dccf67362ad7f2682.

36. Min, C. H., X. Zhu, K. Grogg, G. El Fakhri, B. Winey, and H. Paganetti. 2015. "A Recommendation on How to Analyze In-Room PET for In Vivo Proton Range Verification

Using a Distal PET Surface Method." Technology in Cancer Research and Treatment 14 (3): 320–325. https://doi.org/10.1177/1533034614547457. https://www.scopus.com/inward/record.uri?eid=2-s2.0-84954533234&doi=10.1177%2f1533034614547457&partnerID=40&md5=bebddbe4491b965f7f1375bd4fbc53b0.

37. Fiorina, E., V. Ferrero, G. Baroni, G. Battistoni, N. Belcari, N. Camarlinghi, P. Cerello, M. Ciocca, M. De Simoni, M. Donetti, Y. Dong, A. Embriaco, M. Fischetti, G. Franciosini, G. Giraudo, A. Kraan, F. Laruina, C. Luongo, D. Maestri, M. Magi, G. Magro, E. Malekzadeh, C. Mancini Terracciano, M. Marafini, I. Mattei, E. Mazzoni, P. Mereu, R. Mirabelli, A. Mirandola, M. Morrocchi, S. Muraro, A. Patera, V. Patera, F. Pennazio, A. Retico, A. Rivetti, M. D. Da Rocha Rolo, V. Rosso, A. Sarti, A. Schiavi, A. Sciubba, E. Solfaroli Camillocci, G. Sportelli, S. Tampellini, M. Toppi, G. Traini, S. M. Valle, F. Valvo, B. Vischioni, V. Vitolo, R. Wheadon, and M. G. Bisogni. 2021. "Detection of Interfractional Morphological Changes in Proton Therapy: A Simulation and In Vivo Study With the INSIDE In-Beam PET." Frontiers in Physics 8. https://doi.org/10.3389/fphy.2020.578388. https://www.scopus.com/inward/record.uri?eid=2-s2.0-85100777341&doi=10.3389%2ffphy.2020.578388&partnerID=40&md5=7c0d688a5df127ced0058bd4bf1fd6e9.

38. Zhu, X., S. España, J. Daartz, N. Liebsch, J. Ouyang, H. Paganetti, T. R. Bortfeld, and G. El Fakhri. 2011. "Monitoring proton radiation therapy with in-room PET imaging." Physics in Medicine and Biology 56 (13): 4041–4057. https://doi.org/10.1088/0031-9155/56/13/019. https://www.scopus.com/inward/record.uri?eid=2-s2.0-79960382081&doi=10.1088%2f0031-9155%2f56%2f13%2f019&partnerID=40&md5=85e77648026ac93dd5bdd70d7a2b35cf.

39. MacCabee, H. D., U. Madhvanath, and M. R. Raju. 1969. "Tissue activation studies with alpha-particle beams." Physics in Medicine and Biology 14 (2): 213–224. https://doi.org/10.1088/0031-9155/14/2/304. https://www.scopus.com/inward/record.uri?eid=2-s2.0-0014493044&doi=10.1088%2f0031-9155%2f14%2f2%2f304&partnerID=40&md5=bd20535ee993025202e65e26335ae82f.

40. Abe, M. 2007. "Charged particle radiotherapy at the Hyogo Ion Beam Medical Center: Characteristics, technology and clinical results." Proceedings of the Japan Academy Series B: Physical and Biological Sciences 83 (6): 151–163. https://doi.org/10.2183/pjab.83.151. https://www.scopus.com/inward/record.uri?eid=2-s2.0-34548575233&doi=10.2183%2fpjab.83.151&partnerID=40&md5=7a14c0c4ec0fe10c19bfd2ef9ae6ba06.

41. Hsi, W. C., D. J. Indelicato, C. Vargas, S. Duvvuri, Z. Li, and J. Palta. 2009. "In vivo verification of proton beam path by using post-treatment PET/CT imaging." Medical Physics 36 (9): 4136–4146. https://doi.org/10.1118/1.3193677. https://www.scopus.com/inward/record.uri?eid=2-s2.0-69549095923&doi=10.1118%2f1.3193677&partnerID=40&md5=90413c060cb25a228c8bdece3809e54e.

42. Lecoq, P., C. Morel, J. O. Prior, D. Visvikis, S. Gundacker, E. Auffray, P. Križan, R. M. Turtos, D. Thers, E. Charbon, J. Varela, C. De La Taille, A. Rivetti, D. Breton, J. F. Pratte, J. Nuyts, S. Surti, S. Vandenberghe, P. Marsden, K. Parodi, J. M. Benlloch, and M. Benoit. 2020. "Roadmap toward the 10 ps time-of-flight PET challenge." Physics in Medicine and Biology 65 (21). https://doi.org/10.1088/1361-6560/ab9500. https://www.scopus.com/inward/record.uri?eid=2-s2.0-85094971199&doi=10.1088%2f1361-6560%2fab9500&partnerID=40&md5=fff58f5b7d3442a252a73253fb2a7f4a.

43. N. Belcari, M. G. Bisogni, N. Camarlinghi, P. Carra, E. Ciarrocchi, G. Sportelli, M. Morrocchi, V. Rosso, M. D'Inzeo, G. Franchi, L. Perillo, A. Puccini, C. Bruschini, E. Charbon, F. Gramuglia, E. Venialgo, K. Deprez, C. Thyssen, R. Van Holen, M. Stockhoff, E. Vansteenkiste, S. Vandenberghe. 2019. "UTOFPET: a highly scalable TOF-PET detector concept." IEEE NSS-MIC, Manchester, UK.

44. Kostara, E., G. Sportelli, N. Belcari, N. Camarlinghi, P. Cerello, A. Del Guerra, V. Ferrero, E. Fiorina, G. Giraudo, M. Morrocchi, F. Pennazio, M. Pullia, A. Rivetti, M. D.

Rolo, V. Rosso, R. Wheadon, and M. G. Bisogni. 2019. "Particle beam microstructure reconstruction and coincidence discrimination in PET monitoring for hadron therapy." Physics in Medicine and Biology 64 (3). https://doi.org/10.1088/1361-6560/aafa28. https://www.scopus.com/inward/record.uri?eid=2-s2.0-85060145294&doi=10.1088%2f1361-6560%2faafa28&partnerID=40&md5=b53ca713dc1860868e646d46bae278d9.

45. Dendooven, P., H. J. Buitenhuis, F. Diblen, P. N. Heeres, A. K. Biegun, F. Fiedler, M. J. van Goethem, E. R. van der Graaf, and S. Brandenburg. 2015. "Short-lived positron emitters in beam-on PET imaging during proton therapy." Phys Med Biol 60 (23): 8923–47. https://doi.org/10.1088/0031-9155/60/23/8923. https://www.ncbi.nlm.nih.gov/pubmed/26539812.

46. Ozoemelam, I., E. van der Graaf, M. J. van Goethem, M. Kapusta, N. Zhang, S. Brandenburg, and P. Dendooven. 2020a. "Feasibility of quasi-prompt PET-based range verification in proton therapy." Phys Med Biol 65 (24): 245013. https://doi.org/10.1088/1361-6560/aba504. https://www.ncbi.nlm.nih.gov/pubmed/32650323.

47. —. 2020b. "Real-Time PET Imaging for Range Verification of Helium Radiotherapy." Frontiers in Physics 8. https://doi.org/10.3389/fphy.2020.565422. https://www.scopus.com/inward/record.uri?eid=2-s2.0-85093537317&doi=10.3389%2ffphy.2020.565422&partnerID=40&md5=cf9882fff53ba3c5c8de1ba01128b000.

48. Ferrero, V., P. Cerello, E. Fiorina, V. Monaco, M. Rafecas, R. Wheadon, and F. Pennazio. 2019. "Innovation in online hadrontherapy monitoring: An in-beam PET and prompt-gamma-timing combined device." Nuclear Instruments and Methods in Physics Research, Section A: Accelerators, Spectrometers, Detectors and Associated Equipment 936: 48–49. https://doi.org/10.1016/j.nima.2018.08.065. https://www.scopus.com/inward/record.uri?eid=2-s2.0-85053010985&doi=10.1016%2fj.nima.2018.08.065&partnerID=40&md5=0c6e60c9c5fe102e5f20e1ae7008b44f.

49. Tashima, H., E. Yoshida, N. Inadama, F. Nishikido, Y. Nakajima, H. Wakizaka, T. Shinaji, M. Nitta, S. Kinouchi, M. Suga, H. Haneishi, T. Inaniwa, and T. Yamaya. 2016. "Development of a small single-ring OpenPET prototype with a novel transformable architecture." Physics in Medicine and Biology 61 (4): 1795–1809. https://doi.org/10.1088/0031-9155/61/4/1795. https://www.scopus.com/inward/record.uri?eid=2-s2.0-84959125466&doi=10.1088%2f0031-9155%2f61%2f4%2f1795&partnerID=40&md5=63e6f161794376734000c6aa3998dc13.

50. Hirano, Yoshiyuki, Hiroyuki Takuwa, Eiji Yoshida, Fumihiko Nishikido, Yasunori Nakajima, Hidekatsu Wakizaka, and Taiga Yamaya. 2016. "Washout rate in rat brain irradiated by a11C beam after acetazolamide loading using a small single-ring OpenPET prototype." Physics in Medicine and Biology 61 (5): 1875–1887. https://doi.org/10.1088/0031-9155/61/5/1875. http://dx.doi.org/10.1088/0031-9155/61/5/1875.

51. Lang, C., D. Habs, K. Parodi, and P. G. Thirolf. 2014. "Sub-millimeter nuclear medical imaging with high sensitivity in positron emission tomography using $\beta+\gamma$ coincidences." Journal of Instrumentation 9 (01): P01008–P01008. https://doi.org/10.1088/1748-0221/9/01/p01008. http://dx.doi.org/10.1088/1748-0221/9/01/P01008.

52. Parodi, K., F. Pönisch, and W. Enghardt. 2005. "Experimental study on the feasibility of in-beam PET for accurate monitoring of proton therapy." IEEE Transactions on Nuclear Science 52 (3 II): 778–786. https://doi.org/10.1109/TNS.2005.850950. https://www.scopus.com/inward/record.uri?eid=2-s2.0-23844461860&doi=10.1109%2fTNS.2005.850950&partnerID=40&md5=d1fa6c95c3f787d6ce59a0a9734ddf4chttps://ieeexplore.ieee.org/document/1487723/.

# 8 Radioactive beams for ion therapy: Monte Carlo simulations and experimental verifications

*Mitra Safavi-Naeini and Andrew Chacon*
Australian Nuclear Science and Technology Organisation (ANSTO),
Lucas Heights, Australia

*Susanna Guatelli*
University of Wollongong, Wollongong, NSW, Australia

*Akram Mohammadi and Taiga Yamaya*
National Institute for Quantum and Radiological Science and
Technology, Chiba, Japan

*Anatoly Rosenfeld*
University of Wollongong, Wollongong, Australia

*Marco Durante*
GSI Helmholtzzentrum für Schwerionenforchung, Darmstadt,
Germany and Technische Universität Darmstadt, Darmstadt,
Germany

## CONTENTS

DOI: 10.1201/9781003023920-8

## 8.1 INTRODUCTION

Cancer is a leading cause of death worldwide with over 19 million new cases and 10 million deaths expected in 2020 [Hyuna et al.]. The precision of heavy ion therapy makes it particularly useful for treating deeply situated tumors while minimising damage to adjacent healthy tissue. However, due to the steep dose gradients, any deviation between the treatment plan and the delivered dose distribution can result in significant adverse effects on normal tissue, particularly if the treatment region is in the proximity of an organ at risk (OAR). Accurate and, ideally, real-time measurement of spatial dose distribution during irradiation would provide a mechanism for closed-loop control over the treatment process, minimising errors between the treatment plan and the actual delivered dose.

During heavy ion therapy, a fraction of the ions in the beam will undergo nuclear inelastic collisions. Fragmentation of nuclei in either the primary beam or the target results in the production of a range of stable and radioactive isotopes. Some of these fragments are positron-emitting radionuclides, which continue to travel some distance[1] in target before stopping, where they eventually decay. Measuring the distribution of these secondary positron-emitting fragments offers a unique opportunity for non-invasive, quasi real-time and / or offline quality assurance (QA) in heavy ion therapy via positron emission tomography (PET).

Many annihilation photons must be detected to obtain a PET image of sufficient quality for useful treatment QA. The cross sections for inelastic ion collisions depend on several parameters, including incident ion species and energy, and the density and composition of the target. These factors determine the mix of fragments produced, which, in turn, determines the number and distribution of positron-emitting radionuclides produced during irradiation. To improve image quality, a number of authors have proposed the use of positron-emitting radioactive nuclei (such as $^{11}$C, $^{15}$O or $^{10}$C) as the primary particle in the heavy ion beam. In such radioactive ion beams (RIBs), most primary particles will survive intact to decay via positron emission at their stopping point, corresponding to the location of the Bragg peak. Therefore, for radioactive beams, the spatial distribution of the stopping points of primary particles is the dominant component of the PET image, while positron-emitting fragments of the target and beam nuclei make up a secondary component. This approach was first explored during the charged particle therapy pilot program at the Lawrence Berkeley Laboratory (LBL), where radioactive neon ions were used range verification. Following the LBL pilot program, The Heavy Ion Medical Accelerator in Chiba (HIMAC) clinical facility demonstrated the combined use of $^{11}$C and $^{10}$C ions together with the spot scanning method. In 2001, Urakabe et al. demonstrated that a positron-emitting $^{11}$C scanned spot beam could be directly used as the therapeutic agent, while using the previously acquired relative biological effectiveness factors derived for $^{12}$C in water. A variation to this approach was explored by Iseki et al. at NIRS, where a low-intensity monoenergetic $^{10}$C probe beam was used to estimate the depth of the therapeutic $^{12}$C beam's Bragg peak with an uncertainty of $\pm 0.3$ mm, while keeping the dose received during the range measurement under 100 mGyE (a few percent of the therapeutic dose). After the treatment configuration was confirmed with a small number exploratory beams, the $^{12}$C beam was used to deliver the full therapeutic dose. The European Light Ion Accelerator framework (EULIMA EU) has also explored the inclusion of radioactive isotopes of carbon and oxygen for therapeutic dose delivery, as well the GSI therapy trial in Germany and experiments at the MEDICIS facility at CERN.

While a number of different positron-emitting radionuclei have been proposed for therapeutic use in particle therapy, including $^{9}$C, $^{10}$C, $^{11}$C, $^{15}$O, $^{17}$F, and $^{19}$Ne (see Table 8.1) , in order for radioactive beams to be used for treatment and QA, their precise radiobiological properties need to be fully characterized. Specifically, the following questions need to be answered:

1. How does the relative biological effectiveness (RBE) of polyenergetic radioactive ion beams vary as a function of depth within a spread out Bragg peak, and how does this compare to the corresponding stable ion species?

---

[1]The distance depends on the positron-emitting nuclei's provenance; if it is produced via target fragmentation, then the range is negligible whereas the range of projectile ion species is determined by their mass (i.e., the low-Z fragments travel farther than the high-Z fragments).

**Table 8.1**

**Positron emitting nuclei which has been proposed for use in RIB therapy**

| Isotope | Half-life |
|---------|-----------|
| $^{9}C$ | 126.5 ms |
| $^{10}C$ | 19.3 s |
| $^{11}C$ | 20.33 min |
| $^{15}O$ | 2.04 min |
| $^{17}F$ | 1.83 h |
| $^{19}Ne$ | 17.26 s |

2. What quantitative differences are expected between the distributions of positron annihilations resulting from treatment with stable and positron-emitting radioactive ion beams, and how will these impact the use of PET images as an intra-treatment or post-treatment QA mechanism? Finally,

3. What additional dose will be received by the patient if a positron-emitting radioactive beam is used instead of a stable beam?

## 8.2  PHYSICAL, BIOLOGICAL AND TECHNICAL ASPECTS OF RADIOACTIVE BEAMS

### 8.2.1  PHYSICAL ASPECTS

#### 8.2.1.1  Energy deposition, scatter, range straggling

Radioactive ion beams undergo the same electromagnetic interactions as their respective stable counterparts, since they have the same number of protons, and hence overall electrostatic charge. However, as positron-emitting radioisotopes are neutron-deficient, they have a lower mass compared to stable isotopes of the same element. Therefore, there will be a small increase in the scattering and range straggling of a beam of positron-emitting radioactive ions compared to its stable counterpart. Nuclei in both the primary beam and the target will fragment via the same processes as for stable ion beams, with the specific cross sections depending on the nuclei present in the primary beam and target. However, a key difference is that as the range of the radioactive primary beams increases, the abundance of positron emitting nuclei of interest decreases since a portion of the particles in the primary beam undergo fragmentation (with only some fragments being positron emitters). This characteristic contrasts with stable ion beams, where, as the range increases, there is an *increase* in positron yield as more of the stable beam undergoes fragmentation, resulting in more positron emitting nuclei.

#### 8.2.1.2  LET

Several researchers have experimentally measured the linear energy transfer (LET) of different RIBs. Using a water column and LET counter, Li et al. measured the LET of $^{11}C$ and $^{9}C$ beams, finding that the dose-averaged LET of $^{9}C$ and $^{11}C$ was 15 keV/mm and 20 keV/mm in the entrance region [1]. In the peak region, the dose-averaged LET of $^{9}C$ was found to be 80 keV/mm, while it was measured at 110 keV/mm for $^{11}C$. Further measurements made by Chacon et al. obtained estimates of the dose-averaged LET of $^{11}C$ and $^{15}O$ ion beams using silicon-on-insulator microdosimeters and compared them to the corresponding stable ion beams [2]. The dose-averaged LETs of the radioactive beams were found to be very similar to those of the stable beams in most cases, despite the radioactive and stable beams having different beam energies, energy spreads and beam sizes.

## 8.2.2 BIOLOGICAL ASPECTS (MONOENERGETIC AND POLYENERGETIC BEAM SPECTRA)

### 8.2.2.1 RBE

The relative biological effectiveness (RBE) of ion beams is very different to that of photon or electron radiation due to the specific energy deposition and electron track structure induced by the passage of energetic ions through matter (see Chapter 3). Before RIBs can translate to clinical use, the RBE of these beams needs to be characterized and compared to the corresponding stable ion beams so any differences can be accounted for by the treatment planning system.

As introduced in Chapter 4, the relative biological effectiveness of a radiation field can be predicted by measuring the microdosimetric spectrum of the radiation field and then applying the modified microdosimetric kinetic model (MKM). The microdosimetric spectrum can either be theoretically predicted using Monte Carlo simulations, or measured using microdosimeters. Using Geant4 Monte Carlo simulations, the $RBE_{10}$ of three RIBs – $^{11}C$, $^{10}C$, and $^{15}O$ – was found to be within one standard deviation of the corresponding non-radioactive ion beams for all evaluated energies, indicating that the therapeutic efficacy of such beams should be very similar to beams of the corresponding non-radioactive ion [3]. Experimentally, the microdosimetric spectra of $^{11}C$ and $^{15}O$ have been measured using silicon-on-insulator microdosimeters. It was found that the predicted $RBE_{10}$ of $^{11}C$ and $^{12}C$ are in close agreement, with the mean value for each isotope being within the 95% confidence interval of the other in the entrance, Bragg peak and tail regions. Similarly, for $^{15}O$ and $^{16}O$, the $RBE_{10}$ values are within mutual 95% confidence intervals in the entrance and build-up/Bragg peak regions [2].

To date, there have been limited experimental biological studies using RIBs due to the low dose rates currently achievable with ion sources capable of generating RIBs. At a dose rates of 0.5 Gy/h, the $RBE_{50}$ of $^{9}C$ at the distal end of the Bragg peak (in HSG cells) was found to be greater than that of $^{12}C$ by a factor of 1.87 [4]. This increase in $RBE_{50}$, which was not observed experimentally with pure positron emitter $^{11}C$, was attributed to the decay modes of $^{9}C$, which result in the production of high-LET alpha particles and protons as well as positrons. Since these initial studies, there has been little research into the therapeutic use of $^{9}C$ as a therapeutic beam due to the difficulty in producing high intensity beams of $^{9}C$ ions.

Substantial further in-vitro and in-vivo research is needed to experimentally characterize the RBE of RIBs prior to clinical use. This work requires development of new beamlines which can provide higher and more clinically relevant beam intensities and purities.

### 8.2.2.2 Washout

One of the challenges in PET-based quality assurance for particle therapy with stable ion beams is that tissue- and isotope-dependent metabolic washout of the produced activity can degrade the quality of PET images [5, 6, 7, 8, 9].

The impact of washout on PET image quality can be mitigated by minimising the delay between irradiation and image acquisition, with in-beam PET the most effective method. To minimize the effect of post-acquisition metabolic washout, a correction factor can be applied to the PET image based on the estimated washout rates of tissues in the treatment region [10]. Several studies have attempted to quantify the rate and impact of biological washout on distributions of positron annihilations obtained following the delivery of stable and RIB beams, specifically in rat brains and rabbits, by fitting the observed PET signal in different tissues to a multi-exponential model with fast, medium and slow decay constants, or interpretation of the image based on radiochemistry [12, 11, 13, 14, 15]. However, metabolic washout of positron-emitting isotopes created through fragmentation is a complex process and is dependent on many factors such as the specific treatment region, physiological state of the tumor, and the species of positron-emitting fragments present [12, 15, 16].

A possible approach to minimising metabolic washout of positron-emitting nuclei is to use RIBs with relatively short half-lives, and then perform inter-spill image acquisition (i.e., during the beam-off interval). Several positron-emitting RIBs, such as $^9$C, $^{10}$C and $^{15}$O satisfy this criterion. For such short-lived radioisotopes, the point of decay will be very close to the stopping point of the particle. In this case, the appropriate dose rate would need to be carefully selected to ensure that the PET image signal would be dominated by true coincidences rather than randoms (the latter of which may become excessive if the induced activity rate is too high). This remains an open area for future research and optimization.

### 8.2.2.3   Additional radiation dose

An important consideration in the potential use of RIBs for particle therapy is the question as to whether the use of such beams would result in any additional impacts on the patient relative to the corresponding stable ion beam. From this perspective, the main difference for the patient is that an additional radiation dose will result from the use of a radioactive beam. The dose resulting from the decay of a positron-emitting radionuclide includes the kinetic energy of the positrons together with the 511 keV gamma photons resulting from their eventual annihilation; for a $^{11}$C beam, a 70 Gy(RBE) dose delivered to a 100 mm cubic treatment volume would require approximately $2.3 \times 10^{11}$ particles, distributed throughout the treatment volume. This corresponds to an initial activity concentration of 1.3 MBq/cc, which is comparable to tissue concentrations of radiotracer which would be used in diagnostic $^{11}$C clinical PET imaging and would deliver a biological dose within the treatment volume of the order of 3-10 mSv. The high energy of the annihilation photons means that a relatively small proportion of these photons would deposit energy in the patient, with the additional dose rapidly falls off outside the treatment volume. Therefore, for irradiation with purely positron-emitting radioactive ion beams, the contribution of positron annihilation photons to normal tissue dose outside of the treatment volume is insignificant compared to the dose due to lateral scattering of particles. This is not the case for other positron-emitting radionuclides such as $^9$C, which also produce high-LET alpha particles and protons; these may contribute significantly to the delivered radiation dose to both the target and surrounding tissues, and are the reason for the relatively high RBE of $^9$C.

## 8.3   TECHNICAL ASPECTS

### 8.3.1   BEAM PRODUCTION

The biggest challenge which needs to be overcome for RIBs is the low beam intensities that are currently available relative to stable ion beams. Currently, achievable intensities of RIBs are of the order of $10^5$–$10^6$ pps, which makes them several orders of magnitude too small to be of clinical interest. There are currently two methods of producing RIBs: isotope-on-line (ISOL) and in-flight (see Figure 8.1).

In ISOL production, there is a light-ion fission of *thick targets* (e.g. H on Ta) which produces radioactive fragments ($^{11}$C, $^{15}$O, etc.). The radioactive fragments are then selectively extracted from the target and used as the ion source for acceleration in a synchrotron.

The in-flight method uses fragmentation of an accelerated stable beam with a *thin* target (typically C or Be). The stable beam is then stripped of one (or more) neutrons as it passes through the target and retains a momentum almost the same as the original beam. Generally, when the in-flight method is used to generate RIBs, for every neutron removed from the primary atom, there is a reduction in beam intensity by an order of magnitude compared to the original beam.

### 8.3.2   YIELD VERSUS FLUX

The distribution of positron-emitting radionuclides within a phantom is different for RIBs and stable beams. For RIBs, positron annihilations principally occur in the vicinity of the stopping point of the primary particle. The intensity of the decay radiation observed in a PET image is therefore

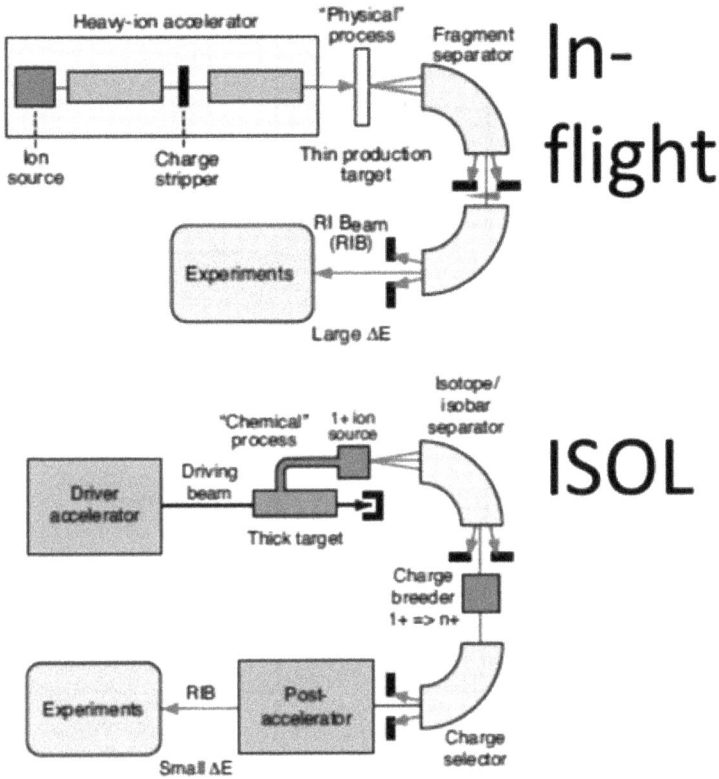

**Figure 8.1**    Current methods for the production of RIBs.

proportional to the number of primary particles which have arrived at that particular depth. The energy weightings required to achieve a flat biological dose have a bias towards higher energies (since more deeply penetrating high-energy particles also deposit an entrance dose which is added to the dose deposited by lower energy beams). By contrast, the contribution of primary or target fragmentation, which is relatively minor for RIBs, is the only source of positrons in the case of stable ion beams, and positron-emitting fragmentation products are produced to a varying extent along the entire length of the beam path. Therefore, the stable beams exhibit a flatter (although not completely flat) activity distribution in the SOBP, and weaker contrast between the SOBP and the entrance region.

Monte Carlo simulations have played an important role in the prediction of positron distributions when using radioactive primary beams. Augusto et al. used the FLUKA Monte Carlo toolkit to investigate the use of $^{11}$C and $^{15}$O beams, either alone or in conjunction with $^{12}$C and $^{16}$O, respectively [17]. It was found that for beams with equivalent energy per nucleon incident on the same water phantom, $^{11}$C and $^{15}$O beams produce very similar fragmentation products when compared with their stable counterparts, with the main differences being the relative yield of helium ions and several boron isotopes (see Figure 8.2 and Figure 8.3). Subsequent studies using Geant4 by Chacon et al. found that positron-emitting primary beams offered a factor of ten increase in the signal to background ratio (SBR) of PET images compared to using stable ion beams [3]. These results have since been confirmed experimentally by the authors; PET images of a range of targets irradiated with $^{11}$C and $^{15}$O RIBs and their stable counterparts were compared, and the SBRs in images obtained with $^{11}$C were better than those obtained with $^{12}$C by a factor of 10 and 11 after 5 and 20 minutes of image acquisition, respectively, and for $^{15}$O, improvement factors of 5.18 and 5.15 were obtained over $^{16}$O for 5 and 20-minute acquisitions, respectively [2].

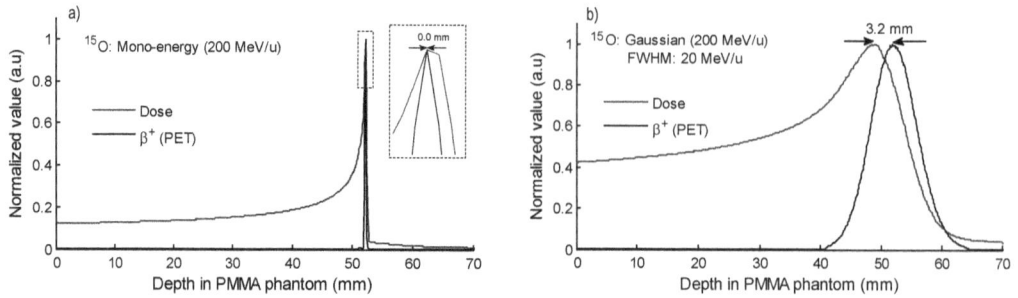

**Figure 8.2**  Comparison of the positron-emitting fragment distribution and dose profile in a PMMA phantom irradiated with a 200 MeV/u $^{15}$O beam (a) without an energy spread (perfectly mono-energetic) and (b) with an energy spread of 20 MeV/u FWHM (Gaussian distribution).

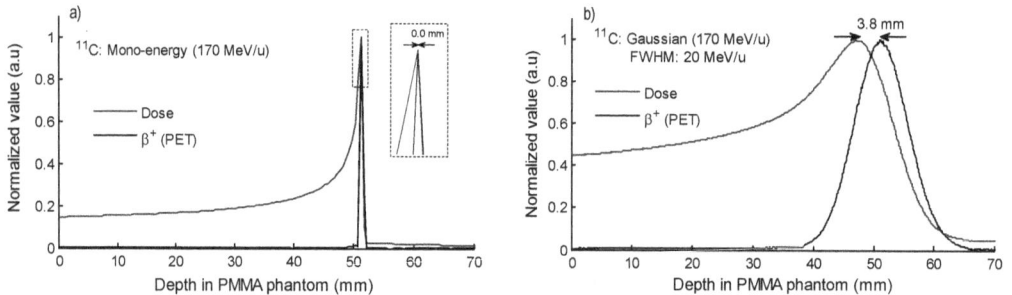

**Figure 8.3**  Comparison of the positron-emitting fragments distribution and the dose in the PMMA phantom irradiated with the $^{11}$C beam of 170 MeV/u (a) without an energy spread (mono-energetic) and (b) with an energy spread (Gaussian distribution).

One of the key differences between RIBs and stable ion beams is that for RIBs, positron emission predominantly occurs at the end of a particles range rather than through fragmentation. This makes RIBs useful for range verification, since there is a direct relationship between the positron emission distribution and particle range. Recently, this relationship has been explored by Mohammadi et al., where both in simulations and experiments it was observed that the difference in position between the Bragg peak and the positron emission peak depends on the momentum spread of the of the monoenergetic RIB [18, 2]. For 200 MeV/u $^{15}$O RIBs, the difference between the positron emission peak and Bragg peak was found to be 1.8 mm and 0.3 mm for momentum acceptances of 5% and 0.5%, respectively. For 170 MeV/u $^{11}$C RIBs, differences of 2.1 mm and 0.1 mm were observed for 5% and 0.5% momentum acceptances, respectively. The results of these studies demonstrate that small energy acceptances are required to ensure that the target volume is adequately treated if RIBs are to be used for range verification, particularly if RIBs are to be used as a probing beam.

### 8.3.3   REVIEW OF PRODUCTION METHODS AND CHALLENGES

#### LAWRENCE BERKELEY LABORATORY (LBL)

At LBL, physicists used $^{19}$Ne produced from a beam of $^{20}$Ne striking a beryllium target, followed by a magnetic separator [19]. This positron-emitting radioactive beam was used both in phantom studies (including with Lexan and water targets) and in vivo experiments on dogs, with the aim of improved range verification compared with non-radioactive ion beams [20, 21]. In-beam PET detectors, PEBA and PEBA-II, consisting of 64 NaI and later BiGe scintillators, were used to detect the annihilation photons from the beam with each detector placed ~1 m away from the phantom. From PET imaging of the RIB, the range of the beam was able to be determined with an accuracy of ~1 mm. Unfortunately, with the shutdown of the Bevalac accelerator in 1992 (due to the deterioration of the detector performance), this work has been discontinued; additionally, neutron irradiation from the passive-scattering range shifter caused problematic activation of the BiGe detectors, generating a large background signal.

## GSI

The GSI Helmholtz Centre for Heavy Ion Research in Darmstadt, Germany was the first facility in the world to use PET imaging for dose quality assurance. Using the GSI fragment separator (FRS), the beam was able to produce $^{15}O$, $^{17}F$, and $^{19}Ne$ beams for the testing of their dual-headed PET scanner. The first application of radioactive ion beams was for treatment plan verification prior to irradiation with stable $^{12}C$ ions [22, 5]. GSI is now running the Biomedical Applications of Radioactive Ion Beams (BARB) project, funded in 2020 with an ERC Advanced Grant (www.gsi.de/BARB) [23]. The project aims at pre-clinical validation of radioactive ion beams in therapy (i.e. both for dose delivery and online imaging), with a transfer line from the projectile fragment separator to Cave M where mice can be irradiated in a dedicated small animal in-beam PET scanner [24] built by the Ludwig Universität Munich in the framework of another ERC project SIRMIO ([25], www.lmu.de/SIRMIO).

## HEAVY ION MEDICAL ACCELERATOR IN CHIBA (HIMAC)

Japan's HIMAC has had the longest history in the production and evaluation of RIBs for cancer therapy. Following LBL, HIMAC was the first center to routinely treat patients with ions heavier than protons. The facility uses the inflight method to strip neutrons from stable nuclei beam to produce a positron-emitting RIB. Currently, the facility is only able to produce low intensity beams which can be used as a probing beam prior to treatment with a higher intensity stable beam. The facility is currently able to produce $^{11}C$, $^{10}C$, $^{9}C$ and $^{15}O$ for scientific studies (including phantom, in vitro and small-animal irradiation and washout studies), however to date only stable ion beams have been used clinically.

## 8.4    DISCUSSIONS AND FUTURE DIRECTIONS

One of the challenges related to the development of RIBs is the need for validated hadronic physics models for accurate Monte Carlo simulation of particle therapy. To date, there has only been limited development in the hadronic physics models for stable ion beams in terms of fragmentation and positron yields (for example,[26]). This work needs to be extended to RIBs so that next generation of beamlines, treatment planning systems and imaging systems can be optimized for use with these beams using Monte Carlo simulations. Additionally, improved physics models for complex hadronic interactions can be used as input to biophysical models to better predict biological outcomes when irradiating living cells and tissues with RIBs.

Another critical area for development prior to potential clinical translation of RIBs is in-vitro and in-vivo experimental measurements of each radioactive ion's RBE and how it compares to its respective stable counterpart. Current simulations and biophysical models predict that purely positron-emitting RIBs (such as $^{11}C$ and $^{15}O$) will have essentially the same RBE as the respective stable isotopes, while RIBs with more complex decay pathways (such as $^{9}C$, which is doubly neutron-deficient) can exhibit an RBE which is considerably higher. However, due to the low intensities which are currently achievable with radioactive ion beams (especially the more highly neutron-deficient isotopes), these predictions have yet to be experimentally measured.

### 8.4.1    CONCLUSION

In summary, experimental evidence indicates that purely positron-emitting RIBs are approximately equivalent to the corresponding stable isotope with respect to expected therapeutic properties in heavy ion radiotherapy, while being greatly superior to non-radioactive beams in terms of the potential for accurately imaging the treatment volume during and after treatment. In contrast, RIBs with more complex decay paths are clearly not biologically equivalent to their stable counterparts due to the presence of additional decay products other than positrons, and the therapeutic use of such Ribs would require modifications to the design of treatment planning systems.

In simulations, the $RBE_{10}$ of the pure positron-emitting RIBs was found to be within one standard deviation of the corresponding non-radioactive ion beams for all evaluated energies, indicating that the therapeutic efficacy of such beams should be very similar to beams of the corresponding non-radioactive ion. Monte Carlo simulations and experimental studies have demonstrated the substantial increase in positron yield offered by positron-emitting radioactive beams for the same biological effective dose, with the result that the boundaries of the spread-out Bragg peak in a PET image could be unambiguously identified. Moreover, in-situ mapping of the implanted isotopes and their different washout rates might provide new knowledge related to the biological effects of irradiation, making RIB act as in-vivo tracers [23].

Therefore, with the potential for a large increase in statistics and hence PET image quality for radiotherapy quality assurance and biological imaging applications, without requiring significant changes to treatment planning procedures, positron emitting primary beams are an enticing choice for heavy ion therapy. While production of RIBs with a sufficient intensity for clinical use remains a challenge, further preclinical programs, including in vivo evaluation with dedicated in-beam PET instrumentation, will be necessary to pave the way for their ultimate clinical translation. Several such studies are currently underway or being planned, including those in small animals at NIRS/QST with low-intensity beams and upcoming experiments at GSI/FAIR with RIBs at therapeutic intensities.

## REFERENCES

1. Q. Li *et al.*, 'The LET spectra at different penetration depths along secondary $^9$ C and $^{11}$ C beams', *Phys. Med. Biol.*, vol. 49, no. 22, pp. 5119–5133, Nov. 2004, doi: 10.1088/0031-9155/49/22/007

2. A. Chacon *et al.*, 'Experimental investigation of the characteristics of radioactive beams for heavy ion therapy', *Med. Phys.*, vol. 47, no. 7, pp. 3123–3132, Jul. 2020, doi: 10.1002/mp.14177.

3. A. Chacon *et al.*, 'Monte Carlo investigation of the characteristics of radioactive beams for heavy ion therapy'. Sci Rep 9, 6537 (2019). doi: 10.1038/s41598-019-43073-1

4. Q. Li *et al.*, 'Enhanced efficiency in cell killing at the penetration depths around the Bragg peak of a radioactive 9C-ion beam', *International Journal of Radiation Oncology\*Biology\*Physics*, vol. 63, no. 4, pp. 1237–1244, Nov. 2005, doi: 10.1016/j.ijrobp.2005.08.006.

5. W. Enghardt, K. Parodi, P. Crespo, F. Fiedler, J. Pawelke, and F. Pönisch, 'Dose quantification from in-beam positron emission tomography', *Radiotherapy and Oncology*, vol. 73, pp. S96–S98, Dec. 2004, doi: 10.1016/S0167-8140(4)80024-0.

6. C. Ammar *et al.*, 'Comparing the biological washout of $\beta^+$ -activity induced in mice brain after $^{12}$ C-ion and proton irradiation', *Phys. Med. Biol.*, vol. 59, no. 23, pp. 7229–7244, Dec. 2014, doi: 10.1088/0031-9155/59/23/7229.

7. M. Priegnitz, D. Möckel, K. Parodi, F. Sommerer, F. Fiedler, and W. Enghardt, 'In-beam PET measurement of $^7$ Li $^{3+}$ irradiation induced $\beta^+$ -activity', *Phys. Med. Biol.*, vol. 53, no. 16, pp. 4443–4453, Aug. 2008, doi: 10.1088/0031-9155/53/16/015

8. T. Tomitani *et al.*, 'Washout studies of $^{11}$ C in rabbit thigh muscle implanted by secondary beams of HIMAC', *Phys. Med. Biol.*, vol. 48, no. 7, pp. 875–889, Apr. 2003, doi: 10.1088/0031-9155/48/7/305.

9. C. Toramatsu *et al.*, 'Biological washout modelling for in-beam PET: rabbit brain irradiation by $^{11}$C and $^{15}$O ion beams'. *Phys. Med. Biol.* 2020 May 28; 65(10):105011. doi: 10.1088/1361-6560/ab8532

10. Parodi, K., Paganetti, H., Shih, H.A., Michaud, S., Loeffler, J.S., DeLaney, T.F., Liebsch, N.J., Munzenrider, J.E., Fischman, A.J., Knopf, A., Bortfeld, T., 2007b. Patient study of in

vivo verification of beam delivery and range, using positron emission tomography and computed tomography imaging after proton therapy. *Int. J. Radiat. Oncol. Biol. Phys.* 68, 920–934. https://doi.org/10.1016/j.ijrobp.2007.01.063

11. H. Mizuno *et al.* 2003 *Phys. Med. Biol.* 48 2269 DOI 10.1088/0031-9155/48/15/302.

12. I. Martínez-Rovira, C. Jouvie, and S. Jan. Technical note: Implementation of biological washout processes within GATE/GEANT4–a Monte Carlo study in the case of carbon therapy treatments. *Med. Phys.* 2015 Apr; 42(4):1773-8. doi: 10.1118/1.4914449. PMID: 25832067.

13. Y. Hirano *et al.* Compartmental analysis of washout effect in rat brain: in-beam OpenPET measurement using a 11C beam. *Phys. Med. Biol.* 58 8281 DOI 10.1088/0031-9155/58/23/8281 (2013).

14. Y. Hirano *et al.* Washout rate in rat brain irradiated by a (11)c beam afer acetazolamide loading using a small single-ring openpet prototype. *Phys. Med. Biol.* 61, 1875–87, https://doi.org/10.1088/0031-9155/61/5/1875 (2016).

15. C. Toramatsu *et al.* Washout effect in rabbit brain: in-beam PET measurements using (10)C, (11)C and (15)O ion beams. Biomed. *Phys. Eng.* Express 4 035001 DOI 10.1088/2057-1976/aaade7 (2018).

16. A. C. Knopf *et al. Int. J. Radiat. Oncol. Biol. Phys.* 79(1), 297–304. DOI 10.1016/j.ijrobp. 2010.02.017 (2011).

17. R. S. Augusto, 'New developments in 11C post-accelerated beams for hadron therapy and imaging'. *Nucl. Instrum. Meth. B.* 2016 Jun 1; 376. doi: 10.1016/j.nimb.2016.02.045

18. A. Mohammadi *et al.*, 'Influence of momentum acceptance on range monitoring of [11] C and [15] O ion beams using in-beam PET', *Phys. Med. Biol.*, vol. 65, no. 12, p. 125006, Jun. 2020, doi: 10.1088/1361-6560/ab8059.

19. J. Alonso *et al.*, 'Radioactive Beam Production at the Bevalac'. Lawrence Berkeley National Laboratory. LBNL Report #: LBL-28114 1989. Retrieved from https://escholarship. org/uc/item/2jx4p9jc

20. J. Llacer *et al.*, 'An Imaging Instrument for Positron Emitting Heavy Ion Beam Injection', *IEEE Trans. Nucl. Sci.*, vol. 26, no. 1, pp. 634-647, Feb. 1979, doi: 10.1109/TNS.1979.4329701.

21. A. Chatterjee. 'PHYSICAL MEASUREMENTS WITH HIGH ENERGY RADIOACTIVE BEAMS'. Lawrence Berkeley National Laboratory. LBNL Report #: LBL-13606 1981. Retrieved from https://escholarship.org/uc/item/33z0t1j7

22. J. Pawelke *et al.*, 'The investigation of different cameras for in-beam PET imaging'. *Phys. Med. Biol.* 1996 Feb;41(2):279-96. doi: 10.1088/0031-9155/41/2/006.

23. D. Boscolo *et al.*, 'Radioactive Beams for Image-Guided Particle Therapy: The BARB Experiment at GSI'. *Front. Oncol.* 2021 Aug 19;11:737050. doi: 10.3389/fonc.2021.737050

24. S. Gerlach *et al.*, 'Beam characterization and feasibility study for a small animal irradiation platform at clinical proton therapy facilities'. *Phys. Med. Biol.* 2020 Dec 22;65(24):245045. doi: 10.1088/1361-6560/abc832

25. K. Parodi *et al.*, 'Towards a novel small animal proton irradiation platform: the SIRMIO project'. *Acta Oncol.* 2019 Oct; 58(10):1470-1475. doi: 10.1080/0284186X.2019.1630752.

26. A. Chacon *et al.*, 'Comparative study of alternative Geant4 hadronic ion inelastic physics models for prediction of positron-emitting radionuclide production in carbon and oxygen ion therapy', *Phys. Med. Biol.*, vol. 47, no. 7, pp. 3123–3132, Jul. 2020, doi: 10.1002/mp.14177.

27. M. Durante and K. Parodi, 'Radioactive Beams in Particle Therapy: Past, Present, and Future', *Front. Phys.*, vol. 8, p. 326, Aug. 2020, doi: 10.3389/fphy.2020.00326.

28. A. Mohammadi *et al.*, 'Range verification of radioactive ion beams of [11] C and [15] O using in-beam PET imaging', *Phys. Med. Biol.*, vol. 64, no. 14, p. 145014, Jul. 2019, doi: 10.1088/1361-6560/ab25ce.

29. H. Sung *et al.*, 'Global Cancer Statistics 2020: GLOBOCAN Estimates of Incidence and Mortality Worldwide for 36 Cancers in 185 Countries', *CA A Cancer J Clin*, vol. 71, no. 3, pp. 209–249, May 2021, doi: 10.3322/caac.21660.

# 9 Monte Carlo and microdosimetry in particle radiotherapy

*Stefano Agosteo*
Politecnico di Milano, Milan, Italy

*Valeria Conte*
Istituto Nazionale di Fisica Nucleare (INFN) Laboratori Nazionali
di Legnaro (LNL), Legnaro, Italy

*Susanna Guatelli and Anatoly Rosenfeld*
University of Wollongong, Wollongong, Australia

*Giulio Magrin*
EBG MedAustron, Wiener Neustadt, Austria

*Giada Petringa*
Istituto Nazionale di Fisica Nucleare (INFN) Laboratori Nazionali
del Sud (LNS) Catania, Italy

## CONTENTS

## 9.1 INTRODUCTION

The nature and the relative yield of ionizations and excitations produced by ionizing particles in subcellular structures depend only to a small extent on the average energy deposited by the particles on larger scales. Differences in the relative biological effectiveness (RBE) between various radiations must be due to differences in the microscopic patterns of energy deposition within the irradiated objects, rather than on average quantities. Treatment Planning systems (TPS) are commercially available that include the variation of LET or RBE along the penetration depth, however, while the dose prescriptions calculated by the TPS are routinely verified with certified ionization chambers as part of the quality assurance (QA) program in any radiotherapy department, there is not a defined procedure for the quality assurance of LET or biological effectiveness calculations.

Microdosimetry measures the random processes of energy deposition in small volumes that mimic sub-cellular sizes, therefore it may be used to perform routine verification of the LET or RBE distributions calculated by the TPS. The standard detector for microdosimetry is the tissue equivalent proportional counter (TEPC). Alternatively, solid-state microdosimeters have been developed that offer practical advantages over TEPCs: they do not require high voltage for operation, the size of the active cross-sectional area can be reduced to a few tens of nanometers to cope with the high intensities of therapeutic particle beams, they can be arranged in an array of matrices to perform two-dimensional microdosimetric characterization with high spatial resolution, e.g. ([1]). The drawback is the lower sensitivity of these detectors, which is limited to an energy deposition of a few keV. In contrast, TEPCs take advantage of the gas avalanche that amplifies the number of initial electrons produced by an individual ionizing radiation event, therefore augmenting the detector sensitivity.

## 9.2 DEFINITION OF MICRODOSIMETRIC QUANTITIES

Microdosimetry measures the energy deposited in a microscopic volume as a stochastic process, and results are presented both as single and as multiple-event spectra. However, the measurement of the energy deposited locally in individual events gives more information on the radiation quality, and it is therefore generally preferred. Microdosimetric quantities, and the way to represent them, are defined and discussed extensively in ICRU Rep36 [2]. The two main quantities are the specific energy $z$ and the lineal energy, $y$, that are defined by the following equations (1):

$$z = \frac{\varepsilon}{m} \quad and \quad y = \frac{\varepsilon_1}{\bar{l}} \tag{9.1}$$

where $\varepsilon$ is the energy imparted to a microscopic volume, $m$ is the mass of the volume and $\bar{l}$ is its mean chord length. $z$ is commonly expressed in units of Gy and $y$ in units of keV/μm.

The specific energy can be defined both for single events, in which case it is indicated as $z_1$, and for multiple events, while the lineal energy is defined for single events only. $z$ and $y$ are the stochastic equivalents of the Dose and the *LET*, respectively. They both can be either experimentally determined or computed. The probability density functions of the specific, $f(z)$, and of the lineal energy, $f(y)$, obey to the normalization rule:

$$\int_0^\infty f(z)dz = 1 \quad and \quad \int_0^\infty f(y)dy = 1 \tag{9.2}$$

The dose probability density of $z$ and $y$ are also defined, representing the fraction of dose delivered within a unit interval of $z$ or $y$ respectively. The following relations apply:

$$d(z) = \frac{zf(z)}{\int_0^\infty zf(z)\,d(z)} \quad and \quad d(y) = \frac{yf(y)}{\int_0^\infty yf(y)\,d(y)} \tag{9.3}$$

The expectation values of the distributions $f(y)$ and $d(y)$ are called mean lineal energy, $\bar{y}_F$, and dose-mean lineal energy, $\bar{y}_D$:

$$\bar{y}_F, = \int_0^\infty yf(y)dy \quad ; \quad \bar{y}_D = \int_0^\infty yd(y)dy \tag{9.4}$$

Similar definitions hold for $\bar{z}_F$ and $\bar{z}_D$. The two quantities $\bar{y}_F$ and $\bar{y}_D$ are analogous, but not equal, to the macroscopic quantities track-averaged $\overline{LET}_T$ and dose-averaged $\overline{LET}$, respectively. The microdosimetric distributions are usually represented in a semilogarithmic plot of $yf(y)$ and $yd(y)$ versus $y$, as shown in Figure 9.1. In this representation, equal areas under the curve correspond to equal

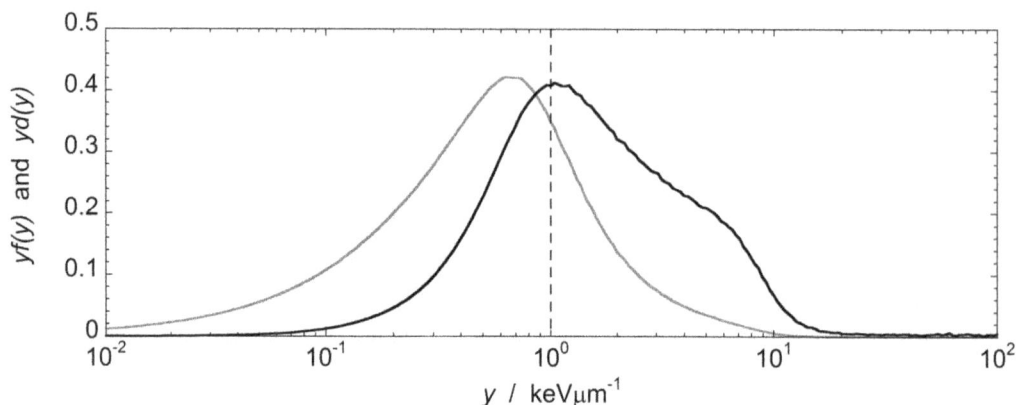

**Figure 9.1**  Example of frequency (grey line) and dose (black line) distributions measured at the 62 MeV modulated proton beam of Catana with a mini-TEPC placed at the entrance position.

contributions to the total number of events or to the total dose, respectively. For instance, from Figure 9.1 the fraction of events with lineal energy below 1 keV/μm is about Ÿ of the total, while the correspondent contribution to the dose is less than 40%.

## 9.3  ROLE OF MONTE CARLO SIMULATIONS IN MICRODOSIMETRY

The Monte Carlo method has been extensively recognized as a well-established theoretical approach to perform microdosimetric calculations, thanks to its capability to describe the stochastic nature of particle interactions and energy depositions ([3, 4]).

General purpose Monte Carlo codes, including FLUKA ([5]), PENELOPE ([6]), Geant4 ([7]), MCNP ([8]) and PHITS ([9, 10]), have been extensively used to perform microdosimetric calculations, for different hadrontherapy treatments, such as proton and carbon ion therapy, Boron Neutron Capture Therapy and Targeted Alpha Therapy (e.g. [11, 12]).

An aim of microdosimetric simulation studies is to investigate the Radiobiological Effectiveness (RBE) of radiation as it has been extensively recognized that the RBE of HZE particles can't be uniquely determined from the *LET*, as it depends on the track structure and the stochastic nature of the energy deposition ([3]). In addition, MC simulations are extensively used to characterize novel detectors aimed to perform experimental microdosimetry.

Monte Carlo simulation set-ups as the ones described in ([4]) and ([13]) may be adopted to calculate microdosimetric quantities. In ([4]), an incident particle and its secondaries are tracked in a semi-infinite water medium and the microdosimetric spectra are calculated positioning a spherical sensitive volume SV randomly multiple times in the water medium. This set-up is implemented in the Geant4 Advanced Example *microdosimetry*. In ([13]), the incident radiation field is modeled as a pencil beam travelling towards the center of the SV, set ideally in a semi-infinite volume, called in the following *Container*, made of the same material (water). However, to track the radiation field in a semi-infinite medium may be computationally demanding. To limit this problem, the sizes of the *Container* could be carefully limited to achieve a satisfactory compromise between particle equilibrium and computational times. In this second simulation set-up, depending on the specific goal of the simulation study, it could be useful to adopt a broader particle beam as incident radiation. Monte Carlo simulation set-up of interest for experimental microdosimetry, involving the modelling of realistic microdosimetric devices, are described in Section 3.2.

### 9.3.1    TRACK STRUCTURE VS CONDENSED HISTORY APPROACH FOR MICRODOSIMETRY

General purpose MC codes adopt the condensed history (CH) approach to describe particle inter-actions. In summary, several physical interactions are "condensed" into a single simulated "step" ([14, 15]), thus speeding up the simulation at the cost of accuracy in the description of the physical interactions. CH models rely upon the restricted linear energy transfer $L_\Delta$ of the particle to deter-mine the continuous energy loss $dE_\Delta$ due to electronic collisions. In particular, $dE_\Delta = L_\Delta \cdot dx$, where $dx$ is the step length. $dE_\Delta$ does not include the contribution of secondary electrons, which would be generated in the simulation with kinetic energy larger than $\Delta$. In CH Monte Carlo codes, $\Delta$ is often called *cut*, and can be expressed either in kinetic energy or range of the secondary electron in the specific medium considered; if an electron is generated with a kinetic energy above $\Delta$, it is explicitly tracked in the simulation. A multiple scattering theory of elastic collisions describes the change in direction after each simulated step ([16]).

While this approach is adequate to calculate the dose in macroscopic volumes, it fails when reducing the sizes of the sensitive volume *SV* as it can't describe the local energy deposition dis-tribution. In other words, the stochastic nature of the particle interactions can't be neglected when reducing the dimensions of the *SV*. These dimension limits depend strictly on the radiation field and on the *SV* considered. In addition, multiple scattering theories are valid for electrons with energy above approximately 1 keV ([4]).

Track Structure (TS) codes such as KURBUC ([17]), PARTRAC ([18]), Geant4-DNA ([19]), among others, describe particle interactions down to low energy (down to few eV) and event-by-event, without adopting any multiple scattering theory. The TS approach provides a more accurate description of the stochastic nature of energy deposition, however, it is available for only few tar-get materials (water vapour, liquid water and some solid-state materials, depending on the specific Monte Carlo code considered) and is very computationally intensive. In addition, depending on the radiation field considered and the size of the *SV*, this approach may not be necessary, and a CH Monte Carlo simulation code could be adequate for microdosimetric calculations (see section 3.2). Therefore, it is important to define the simulation study conditions for which a TS code is deemed to be necessary for microdosimetry. Lazarakis et al. 2018 [16] studied the case of incident monochro-matic electrons with energy below 10 keV (major part of the energy is deposited via electrons with energy below 10 keV in a clinical Spread Out Bragg Peak), in liquid water *SV*s with diameters ranging from 1 nm to 10 μm.

As an example, Figure 9.2 shows the frequency of energy deposition in the *SV*, which is then used to calculate microdosimetric spectra, obtained with a TS approach (Geant4-DNA) and a CH approach (Geant4 Livermore Physics List e) with Geant4 10.02.p02, for a 10 keV electron beam incident on a 10 nm diameter *SV*.

It is possible to see that the TS and CH approaches provide different energy deposition distri-butions. In addition, the distribution obtained with a CH approach shows an unphysical peak at an energy corresponding to the cut. Figure 9.3 shows the ratio of the energy deposition calculated in the *SV* by means of Geant4 CH physics models and Geant4-DNA. *R* is the ratio of the variable *SV* diameter and the average track length of incident 10 keV electrons. It is possible to notice that the agreement between CH and TS approach is obtained for $R > 1$. For lower $R$ values, the CH ap-proach overestimates the mean energy deposition. In summary, the study showed that for electrons a TS approach is more adequate when the SV is small. In this situation, if using a CH Monte Carlo code, the maximum step size and cut should be set carefully. These results agree with [4].

As mentioned before, one of the problems of a TS approach is that it is computationally intensive. A strategy to overcome this problem is to activate CH physics models in the macroscopic volume and the TS in specific *SV*s in positions of interest. This strategy is for example adopted in Geant4, where the TS Geant4-DNA models are activated in specific regions of interest. Another approach has been developed by Sato and co-authors and available in PHITS ([3]). In this case the probability

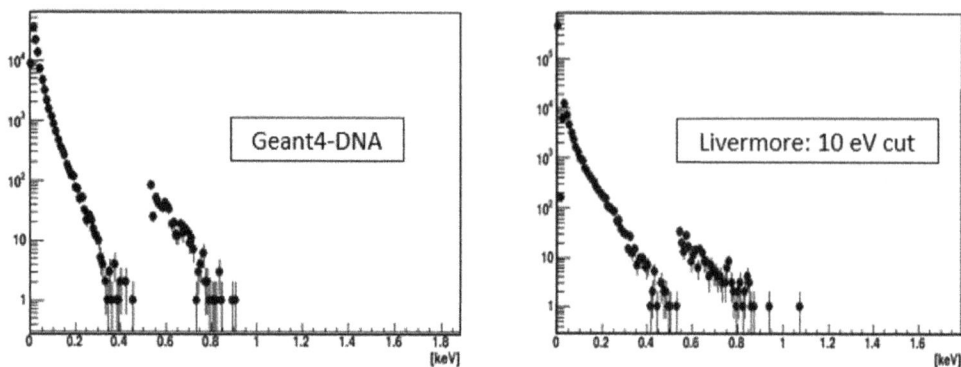

**Figure 9.2** Frequency of the energy deposition (on the x-axis), per incident particle, given by 10 keV electrons in a 10 nm diameter SV, calculated using a TS approach (Geant4-DNA) and a CH approach (Geant4 Livermore). The peak at about 530 eV is due to the ionization of tightly bound electrons. The secondary peak observed when using the Livermore models results from the application of a production cut. Figure from [16].

densities (PDs) of microdosimetric quantities were calculated with the TS code TRACION ([20]), around the trajectories of protons and $^4$He, $^{12}$C, and $^{56}$Fe ions with energies from 1 MeV/n up to 100 GeV/n in water. Then the PDs were fitted with a mathematical function based on Olko's model ([21]). The PHITS simulations in macroscopic geometries can then use these analytical expressions of the PDs to calculate physical quantities of interest, e.g. RBE$_{10}$ (Sato T. 2009).

In conclusion, depending on the physical size and density of the *SV* and of the incident radiation field considered, a TS approach may be more adequate for microdosimetry. This should be evaluated case by case, also considering that a TS approach is currently applicable for a limited set of materials, e.g. liquid and water vapor, silicon, gold and propane, among others.

### 9.3.2 DETECTOR MODELING

Microdosimeters can be characterized by comparing the experimental microdosimetric spectra acquired in controlled conditions to the ones simulated by reproducing the experiment as strictly as possible. In many cases, as discussed in section 3.1, the CH approach is sufficient for providing satisfactory agreement with the experimental data. This has been demonstrated for the characterization of some detectors irradiated with high-*LET* hadron beams. In particular, the CH approach can be used with some cautions for ion beams when the secondary electron equilibrium holds. It is recommended to set the minimum energy cut-off in the detector sensitive regions (e.g. for a TEPC in the filling gas and in the tissue-equivalent walls). Moreover, the step length for multiple scattering should be set to reasonable small values (e.g., to a few percent of the kinetic energy of the particle facing each step). If the secondary electron equilibrium holds in a TEPC, the energy lower than the cut-off which is deposited locally in the detector walls (but which would have been deposited in the filling gas with no cut-off) is compensated by that energy lower than the cut-off deposited in the filling gas and vice versa.

Monte Carlo simulations performed with FLUKA ([22, 23]) showed that FLUKA can predict with a reasonably good agreement microdosimetric spectra in correspondence of a simulated site size of 1 µm for photon fields and proton beams. Böhlen et al. (2011) [24], comparing simulations and experimental data, showed that FLUKA can predict with sufficient accuracy the spatial

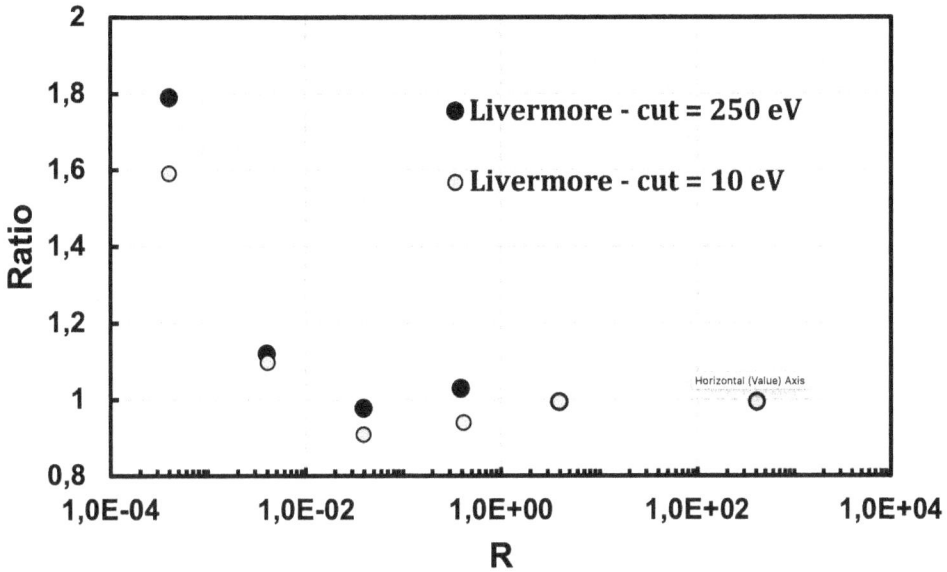

**Figure 9.3** Ratio of the energy deposition calculated with Geant4 CH and TS approach in a liquid water SV, for an incident 10 keV electron beam. R is the ratio of the target diameter and the mean track length of the incident electrons. In the case of the CH approach, the Geant4 Livermore physics moles have been used with a cut of 250 eV and, alternatively, 10 eV. Figure from [16].

energy deposition patterns around ion tracks down to sub-micron scale. Rollet et al. (2012) [25] showed a fair agreement between FLUKA numerical simulation and 5-$\mu$m thick synthetic diamond microdosimeters for $^{241}$Am alpha source.

Mazzucconi et al. (2019) [26] simulated the response of an avalanche-confinement TEPC at different depths inside a PMMA phantom irradiated with the 62 MeV per nucleon carbon ion beam from the superconductive cyclotron of the INFN Laboratori Nazionali del Sud (LNS, Catania, Italy). This TEPC is capable of simulating microdosimetric sites from 0.3 $\mu$m down to 25 nm. The FLUKA code was used for this purpose. The whole geometry of the TEPC was reproduced strictly together with that of the beam delivery system (i.e., vacuum window, ripple filters, etc.). In order to achieve the best accuracy in the simulation (i.e. influence of wall effects) and avoid unnecessary long computation times, the generation and transport thresholds were set by subdividing the detector regions into shells. In particular, the electron production and transport thresholds were set to 1 keV in the sensitive region and in all the surrounding regions (e.g. cathode wall, anode, helix) and to 10 keV in the other detector regions that are not directly adjacent to the sensitive zone (e.g. aluminum case and surrounding air). Considering the very low density of the gas-filled regions, the simulation would require the activation of the Single Scattering option for hadrons and electrons. Spectra obtained by enabling this option did not show noticeable differences with those derived with the Multiple Coulomb Scattering option. Therefore, this option was used and optimized through EMFFIX and FLUKAFIX cards which allow reducing the step size of particle transport: a step size of 1% in total energy for both hadrons and electrons was set for DME gas and graphite, and a step size of 5% was used in the remaining surrounding materials. Simulations and irradiations were performed by placing the TEPC at different depths inside the PMMA phantom (i.e. across the Bragg peak) and at various gas pressures for simulating different sites, showing a good agreement. Figure 9.4, left side, shows the (FLUKA) simulated and the experimental microdosimetric spectra at 5.63 mm in

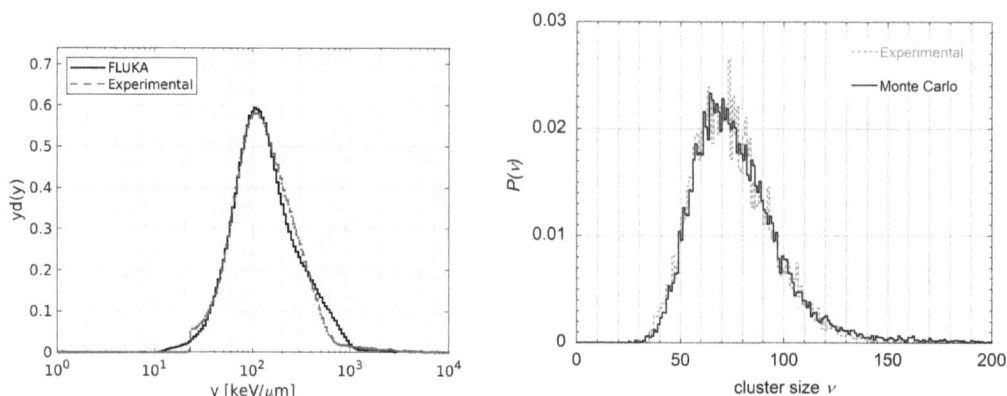

**Figure 9.4** Left: comparison between simulated and experimental microdosimetric spectra for 62 MeV/u carbon ions in a 25 nm site at depth = 5.63 mm. Right: comparison between simulated (MC-Startrack) and experimental microdosimetric spectra for $^{244}$Cm alpha-particles in a 25 nm site.

depth (shallower part of the distal Bragg peak fall-off) for a 25 nm site size. Figure 9.4, right side, shows the probability of a cluster of n ionizations produced in a 25 nm site size from a $^{244}$Cm alpha particle, measured and simulated by means of a TS code ([27, 28]). The agreement between the experimental and the simulated spectra is very satisfactory.

Monte Carlo simulation codes have been also extensively used to describe the microdosimetric response of solid state microdosimeters, including Silicon-On-Insulator microdosimeters developed at the Center For Medical and Radiation Physics, University of Wollongong, fabricated with both planar and Micro-Electro-Mechanical Systems (MEMS) 3D detector technology at SINTEF Mi-NaLab, Norway, and described in ([29]).

In this simulation domain Geant4 has been extensively validated for microdosimetry against experimental measurements performed by means of SOI microdosimeters at the Massachusetts General Hospital, US, ([30]) and at the CATANA facility, Italy ([31]) for proton therapy, at the Biological beamline in HIMAC, Chiba, Japan, for heavy ion therapy ([32, 1]), and at the iThemba LABS in South Africa for a fast neutron therapeutic beam ([33]). The Geant4 advanced example *Radiopro-tection* (https://geant4.web.cern.ch/collaboration/working_groups/advanced_examples) is provided to show how to perform microdosimetric calculations in solid state microdosimeters. Research of the past decade shows that Geant4, and more in general, general purpose Monte Carlo simulations describing particle transport in matter, can be used to characterize the response of microdosimeters in radiation fields of interest, supporting experimental activities (e.g. [30, 31, 33]). In addition, Monte Carlo codes can help to solve problems, as to improve the design of the detector and of its packaging (e.g. [33]), and to fill some methodological gaps. For example, Geant4 was used to develop a methodology to convert microdosimetric measurements in a solid state material to those in biological targets such as water or soft tissue (e.g. [34, 35]) and to optimize the design of microdosimetric devices (e.g. Vohradky et al. 2021).

## 9.4 COMPUTATIONAL AND EXPERIMENTAL MICRODOSIMETRY IN CLINICAL PRACTICE

### 9.4.1 QUALITY ASSURANCE OF RADIATION QUALITY: TPS – MC – EXPERIMENTAL MICRODOSIMETRY

When discussing microdosimetry in clinical practice, the clinical feasibility cannot be ignored. Any experimental characterization of the radiation quality should undergo the severe scrutiny of the clinical feasibility and the need to have limited impact on beam time and workflow of treatment procedures. Those are not discussed here, however, they are the strategic factors which, finally, determine if any clinical implementations of microdosimetry will be successful.

Several scientific papers discuss the implementation of microdosimetric measurements in clinical routines. These can be separated in two categories according to their final purpose within the clinical process: (i) planning the tumor treatments with specific reference to the biological effectiveness of the radiation, or (ii) quality assurance as verification of the radiation quality considered as pure physical parameters. At present, there is no standard use of microdosimetry in ion-beam therapy and the scientific publications should be considered as preparatory steps in the two topics.

### 9.4.1.1   Biological effectiveness and Treatment Planning System (TPS).

TPS are based on three-dimensional images of the location of the tumor volume and the surrounding tissue. Using different tools which combine simulations and analytical computations, TPSs allow delineating the target and calculate the optimized beam directions and intensities. In current clinical practice, this is the element of the treatment workflow where the radiation-quality parameters are taken into consideration. The radiation-qualities parameters calculated on the base of TPSs are the three-dimensional maps of $\overline{LET}_T$ and $\overline{LET}_D$. Although these mean values are evaluated from the $LET$ distributions, the explicit access to those estimations is challenging since TPSs are commercial products. Independent MC simulations play, in this respect, an instrumental role as they are the essential "missing link" in between the $LET$ maps of the TPSs and the microdosimetric spectra [REF]. Inevitably, the focus should also be on how $LET$ distributions could be related to microdosimetric spectra.

The impact of the different radiation qualities on the tissue target is evaluated through computations which refer to the models of radiation effectiveness. In a plan created by TPSs for actively scanned radiation, the irradiation is the results of the overlapping of beams with different directions and energies; in many voxels (i.e. the sub volumes of few squared millimeters in which the total volume is subdivided), the total dose is the sum of contributions from hundreds of beams and, consequently, of hundreds of different beam qualities. Monte Carlo simulations are used in TPS both for the definition of the beam model, and for the implementation of the biological effective models. In current TPSs for actively scanned irradiation, the biological effectiveness is computed independently for each of the thousands of voxels irradiated. In proton therapy, the biological response is currently considered proportional to the absorbed dose and, consequently, no biological model is used. This assumption is a matter of discussion within the ion-beam therapy community.

The correlation between the microdosimetric measurement and the biological effectiveness has been studied for many years using radiobiological functions to weight the microdosimetric spectra at different depths in the SOBP ([36, 37]). Those investigations are not focusing on the direct implementation to TPS but provide the indication of the biological effectiveness based on the so-called microdosimetric relative biological effectiveness, $RBE_\mu$. Pioneering investigations started more than twenty years ago on clinical proton beams ([38, 39]) and carbon-ion beams ([40]). Recently, several experimental investigations were carried out using different classes of microdosimeters and the MC characterization of the entire clinical beam line including transport lines and passive elements. Recent investigations have been reported on the use of mini-TEPC, silicon MicroPlus-Bridge detectors ([41, 29]), other silicon microdosimeters developed at Milan Politecnico ([42]) and synthetic single-crystal diamond microdosimeters ([43]). For a clinical proton beam, Kase et al. calculated the RBE values (for human salivary gland cell death) based on experimental microdosimetric spectra collected with TEPC and the microdosimetric kinetic model (MKM) ([44]). The microdosimetric-calculated values showed to agree well with the experiments in cells. The MKM is the biological model that was developed originally by Hawkins ([45]) and was successively implemented in TPSs developed for carbon ions at the Heavy Ion Medical Accelerator in Chiba center in Japan ([46]). In the studies of Tran and colleagues, the results of microdosimetric experiments carried out with silicon microdosimeters in carbon-, nitrogen- and oxygen-ion beams are directly linked to the bio-logical outcomes assessed with the modified MKM ([47]).

-Microdosimetry and Radiobiological Efficiency in Heavy Ion Therapy

Microdosimetric kinetic model (MKM) was developed by [45, 48] based on the theory of dual radiation action ([49, 50]) in order to estimate cell survival after irradiation with a heavy ion beam. In the MKM, the surviving fraction of cells can be predicted from the specific energy, z, deposited to a subcellular structure referred to as a "domain" for any kind of radiation [Kase 2006]. Kase et al. 2006 [51] presented a modified MKM with revising the saturation correction for expressing the reduction of RBE due to overkill effect in very high specific energy z region, can predict the survival fraction of human salivary gland (HSG) cells from the microdosimetric quantities measured with the tissue equivalent proportional counter (TEPC) with a spherical sensitive volume [Kase 2006]. These predictions were performed for complex mixed radiation field of heavy ion beams from protons to silicon ions. Following successful results using modified MKM, several studies were carried out to evaluate the biological effects of the carbon ion irradiation field [Sato 2009, Nose 2009]. Therefore, MKM is a good approach for RBE prediction in treatment planning for heavy ion therapy (HIT).

In the modified MKM, the survival fraction, S, of certain cells is calculated with the biological model parameters ($\alpha_o$, $\beta$, $r_d$ and $y_0$) and is given by:

$$S = exp\left[-\alpha D - \beta D^2\right] \qquad (9.5)$$

$$\alpha = \alpha_o + \frac{\beta}{\rho \pi r_d^2} y^* \qquad (9.6)$$

Where $\alpha_0 = 0.13\ Gy^{-1}$ is a constant that represents the initial slope of the survival fraction curve in the limit of zero *LET*, $\beta = 0.05\ Gy^{-2}$ is a constant independent on *LET*, $\rho = 1 g/cm^3$ is the density of tissue, $r_d = 0.42\ \mu m$ is the radius of a sub-cellular domain in the MK model and y* is the restricted dose-mean lineal energy which is taking into account cell overkilling effect for $y > 150$ keV/μm and $y_o = 150$ keV/μm for HSG cells.

$$y^* = \frac{y_o^2 \int_0^\infty \left(1 - exp\left(-y^2/y_o^2\right)\right) f(y)\,dy}{\int_0^\infty y f(y) dy}$$

Then the biological RBE of the HSG cells is calculated by:

$$RBE_{10} = \frac{D_{10,R}}{D_{10}} = \frac{2\beta D_{10,R}}{\sqrt{\alpha^2 - 4\beta ln(0.1)} - \alpha} \qquad (9.7)$$

Where $D_{10}$ is 10% survival dose of in-vitro HSG cells for radiation of interest, and $D_{10,R}$= 5.0 Gy is the 10% survival dose obtained from the empirical survival curve of the HSG cells irradiated by 200 kVp X-rays.

-Example of application for TPS in HIT utilizing Monte Carlo simulations of microdosimetric parameters

As mentioned in Section 3.2, Geant4 was adopted to simulate the microdosimetric response of the Silicon on Insulator (SOI) microdosimeter described in ([29]), when exposed to a proton pencil beam at Massachusetts General Hospital (MGH) ([30]), and to mono energetic and Spread Out Bragg peak (SOBP) 290 MeV/u $^{12}$C ion beam, mono energetic 150 MeV/u $^4$He, 180 MeV/u $^{14}$N, 400 MeV/u $^{16}$O and 400 MeV/u $^{20}$Ne ions at the HIMAC biological beam line. The frequency mean lineal energy, $\bar{y}_F$, the dose mean lineal energy, $\bar{y}_D$, and the RBE$_{10}$, estimated using the modified MKM, were obtained by means of the experiments and compared to the Geant4 simulation results [1] [Bolst 2020].

Figure 9.5 shows the RBE$_{10}$ values obtained for a mono-energetic 290 MeV/u $^{12}$C ion beam at various depths, with the pinnacle of the BP occurring at approximately 149 mm. Good agreement

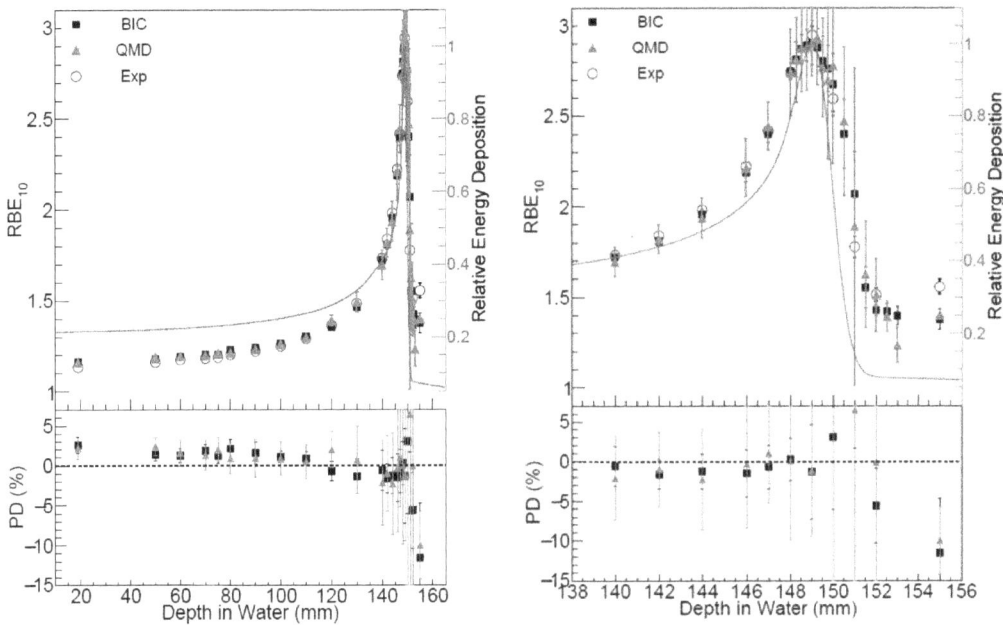

**Figure 9.5**   Left: Calculated $RBE_{10}$ values in the 290 MeV/u $^{12}$C ion beam using the experimental microdosimetric spectra measured with the SOI Mushroom microdosimeter in a water phantom and simulated with Geant 4 using different physics list. [Bolst, 2020], Right: Zoomed in view of the results at the BP region.

was observed between the experimental and simulation results, with the difference being $\sim 2\%$ before the distal part of the BP. At the entrance of the phantom the $RBE_{10}$ is $\sim 1.17$ and reaches a maximum at the pinnacle of the BP with a value of $\sim 2.9$. These results show that Geant4 and, more widely, general purpose Monte Carlo codes, are an appropriate in-silico instrument to link the *LET* maps of the TPSs to the microdosimetric spectra.

### 9.4.1.2   Quality assurance (QA) and verification of beam characteristics

The QA process guarantees with tests – which are repeated with regular frequencies, daily, weekly, monthly, or longer – that the characteristics of all aspects of the irradiation are maintained within the values assessed during the commissioning of the facility, in the limits of the predefined uncertainty. Currently, in proton and carbon-ion therapy centers, the beam characteristics as well as the dosimetric properties are part of the QA but no clinical program contemplates QA of radiation-quality parameters. A program in that sense should focus, at first, on the capability of microsimeters to provide detector independent results. In what can be considered as one of the first attempt in that sense, Colautti and colleagues performed an inter-comparison in carbon-ion beams of data calculated using Geant4 code and $\bar{y}_D$ microsimetric data collected experimentally ([52]). Four different types of microsimeters were used with a 62 MeV/u modulated carbon ion beam (Figure 9.6). The microdosimetric spectra were calibrated at water depth = 7.5 mm to represent the spectra in water and the experimental $\bar{y}_D$ values were compared with Geant4 simulations representing the $\overline{LET}_D$. The relative standard deviation of the four dose-mean lineal energy values measured with four different detectors is 6%, confirming the general agreement among different microsimeters.

A similar intercomparison of the response of different detectors was also performed at a 62 MeV modulated proton beam used to treat ocular melanoma. The results are shown in Figure 9.7. Larger differences are visible in the entrance and plateau regions, when the *LET* is less than 10 keV/mm and

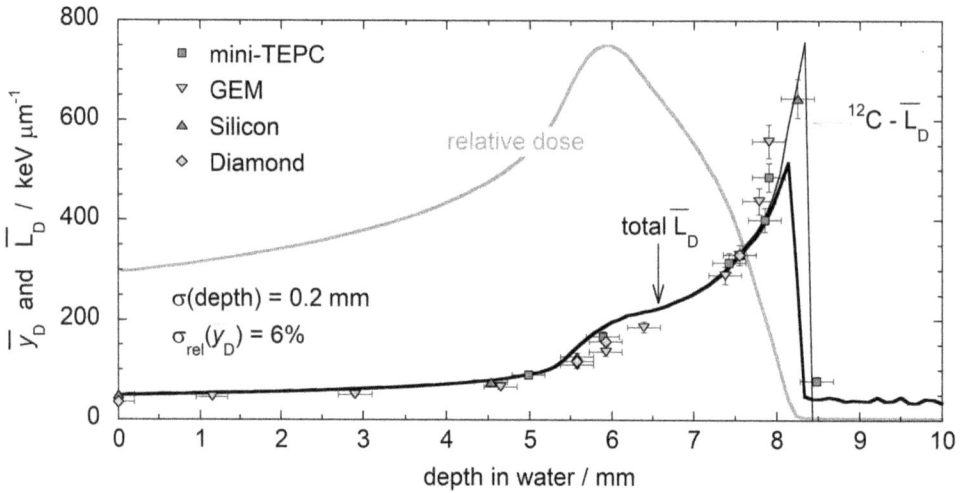

**Figure 9.6**  Intercomparison of mean dose lineal energy $\bar{y}_D$ measured with four different detectors at a 62 MeV/u spread out carbon ion beam. Data adapted from ([52]).

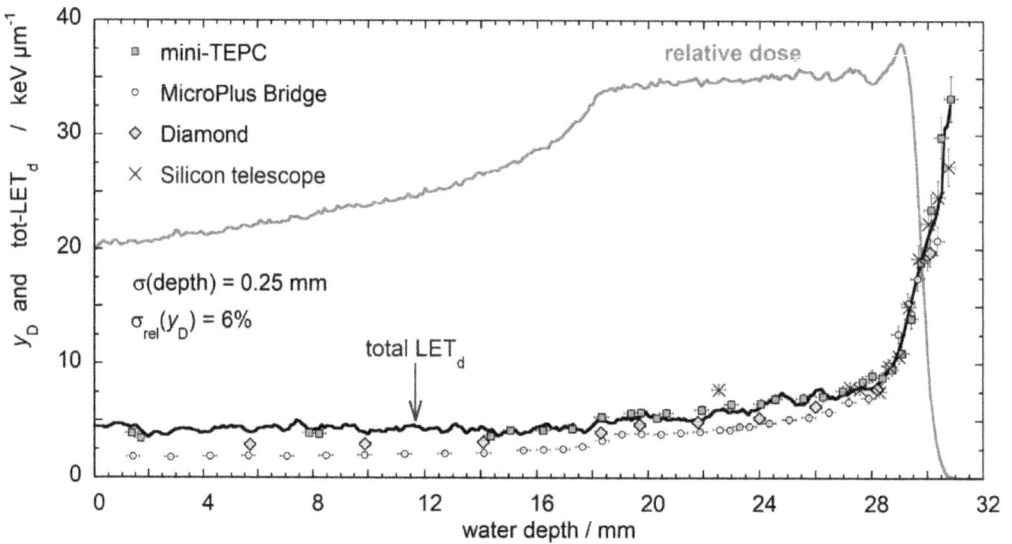

**Figure 9.7**  Intercomparison of mean dose lineal energy $\bar{y}_D$ measured with four different detectors at a 62 MeV spread out proton beam. Mini-TEPC and MicroPlus Bridge data adapted from ([41]), Silicon telescope data from ([42]) and Diamond results from ([43]).

energy loss straggling is a dominant factor in the stochastic distributions of the energy imparted. The agreement between different detectors is much better in the Bragg peak region, where the standard deviation of the four measurements is less than 5%.

Monte Carlo simulations play a key and complementary role for interpreting the response of two distinct detectors under the same radiation fields (see for instance [53]).

## 9.4.2 RETROSPECTIVE STUDIES.

A process which may have large clinical impact is collecting microdosimetric data for patients treated in a similar location and couple this information with the clinical outcomes evaluated in retrospective studies. These results are key for the assessment of the clinical-based biological effectiveness and potentially become part of the treatment planning described above. A novel approach used Monte-Carlo evaluated $\overline{LET}_D$ for characterizing the carbon-ion irradiation fields for patients in analogous conditions and compared the results in terms of tumor control probability at different periods after the treatments ([54]). A correlation between the doses delivered by $\overline{LET}_D$ above 50 KeV·μm$^{-1}$ and the tumor control at five years has been shown. These results, although only preliminary, are outstanding because for the first time a radiation quality concept (the $\overline{LET}_D$) is used outside treatment planning. This constitutes a completely new perspective in which microdosimetry studies may develop in the framework of ion beam therapy.

## 9.5  CONCLUSIONS

Computing instruments and techniques have become fast and powerful in recent years; and because codes are less expensive and faster to run than experiments, they are frequently preferred to study the stochastic processes of ionizing interactions. Simulations offer a high degree of flexibility; numerical experiments can be performed by turning specific terms on or off, isolating physical effects, or by varying input parameters, boundary or initial conditions. However, experiments are the real scenario where the simulated results are ultimately tested. On the other hand, measurements of reality are highly incomplete and imperfect. Parameters can be varied only over a limited range and particular physical effects are difficult to isolate. Theory and computation on the one hand and experiments on the other should be seen not as competitive activities but as complementary ones. The interaction of computation and experiments allows the mutual identification of interesting or important phenomena, the testing of basic physical models, the optimization of detector design and the validation of codes and calculations.

## REFERENCES

1. Tran T. L. et al. (2018) The relative biological effectiveness for carbon, nitrogen, and oxygen ion beams using passive and scanning techniques evaluated with fully 3D silicon microdosimeters. Med. Phys. 45 (5).
2. Booz J., L. Braby, J. Coyne, P. Kliauga, L. Lindborg, H-G. Menzel, N. Parmentier, ICRU Report 36: Microdosimetry, Journal of the International Commission on Radiation Units and Measurements, Volume os19, Issue 1, Bethesda (1983)
3. Sato T, Watanabe R, Sihver L, Niita K. Applications of the microdosimetric function implemented in the macroscopic particle transport simulation code PHITS. Int J Radiat Biol.; 88(1-2):143-50 (2012).
4. Kyriakou I. et al., Microdosimetry of electrons in liquid water using the low-energy models of Geant4, J. Appl. Phys. 122, 024303 (2017).
5. Ferrari A. et al., A Multi-Particle Transport Code (Program Version 2005) (CERN, Geneva, 2005).
6. Barò J., Sempau J., Fernàndez-Varea J. M., and Salvat F., Nucl. Instrum. Methods Phys. Res., Sect. B 100, 31 (1995).
7. Agostinelli S. et al. Nucl. Instrum. Methods Phys. Res., Sect. A 506, 250 (2003).
8. Briesmeister J. F., "MCNP-A general Monte Carlo Code for neutron and photon transport," Report No. LA-7396-M 3A, Los Alamos National Laboratory, Los Alamos, 1986.
9. Sato T. et al. Radiat. Prot. Dosim. 122, 41 (2006)

10. Sato T, Kase Y, Watanabe R, Niita K, Sihver L. Biological dose estimation for charged-particle therapy using an improved PHITS code coupled with a microdosimetric kinetic model. Radiat Res. (2009);171(1):107-17. doi: 10.1667/RR1510.1. PMID: 19138056.

11. Sato T. et al., Individual dosimetry system for targeted alpha therapy based on PHITS coupled with microdosimetric kinetic model, EJNMMI Physics; Heidelberg Vol. 8, Iss. 1, (2021). DOI:10.1186/s40658-020-00350-7

12. M. Elbast et al., Microdosimetry of alpha particles for simple and 3D voxelised geometries Radiation Protection Dosimetry, Volume 150(3) 2012, Pages 342–349.

13. Selva A. et al., Energy imparted and ionization yield in nanometre-sized volumes, Radiat. Phys. and Chem. 192 109910 (2022).

14. Nahum A.E., Radiat. Environ. Biophys. 38, 163 (1999).

15. H. Nikjoo, S. Uehara, D. Emfietzoglou, and F. A. Cucinotta, Radiat. Meas. 41, 1052 (2006).

16. Lazarakis, P. et al., "Investigation of track structure and condensed history physics models for applications in radiation dosimetry on a micro and nano scale in Geant4", Biomedical Physics and Engineering Express, 4 (2), 024001-1-024001-11 (2018).

17. Nikjoo, H., ONeill, P., Goodhead, D. T. & Terrissol, (1997) M. Computational modeling of low-energy electron-induced DNA damage by early physical and chemical events. Int. J. Radiat. Biol. 71, 467–483.

18. Friedland, W. et al. (1998) Monte Carlo simulation of the production of short DNA fragments by low-linear energy transfer radiation using higher-order DNA models. Radiat. Res. 150, 170–182.

19. Bernal, M. A. et al. (2015) Track structure modeling in liquid water: a review of the Geant4-DNA very low energy extension of the Geant4 Monte Carlo simulation toolkit. Phys. Med. 31, 157–178.

20. Watanabe R, et al., Monte Carlo simulation of radial distribution of DNA strand breaks along the C and Ne ion paths. Radiation Protection Dosimetry 143:186–190 (2010).

21. Olko P, Booz J., Energy deposition by protons and alpha particles in spherical sites of nanometer to micrometer diameter. Radiation and Environmental Biophysics 28:1–17 (1990).

22. Rollet S., Colautti P., Grosswendt B., Moro D., Gargioni E., Conte V., De Nardo L., Monte Carlo simulation of mini TEPC microdosimetric spectra: Influence of low energy electrons. Radiat. Meas. 45, 1330–1333 (2010).

23. Rollet S. et al., Microdosimetric assessment of the radiation quality of a therapeutic proton beam: comparison between numerical simulation and experimental measurements. Radiat. Prot. Dosim. 143 (2-4), 445-449 (2011).

24. Böhlen, T. T., Dosanjh, M., Ferrari, A., Gudowska, I., Mairani, A., 2011. FLUKA simulations of the response of tissue-equivalent proportional counters to ion beams for applications in hadron therapy and space. Phys. Med. Biol. 55, 6545-6561.

25. Rollet S. et al., A Novel Microdosimeter Based Upon Artificial Single Crystal Diamond, IEEE TRANSACTIONS ON NUCLEAR SCIENCE, VOL. 59, NO. 5, p 2409 (2012).

26. Mazzucconi D., Bortot D., Pola A. et al., Monte Carlo simulation of a new TEPC for microdosimetry at nanometric level: response against a carbon ion beam, Radiation Measurements 123 (2019) 26-33.

27. Grosswendt B, Conte V, Colautti P. An upgraded track structure model: experimental validation. Radiat Prot Dosimetry. 161(1-4): 464-468. doi: 10.1093/rpd/nct322. (2014).

28. Mazzucconi D. et al., A wall-less tissue equivalent proportional counter as connecting bridge from microdosimetry to nanodosimetry, Radiation Physics and Chemistry (2020) 108729.

29. Tran., T. L. et al. (2022) Silicon 3D Microdosimeters for Advanced Quality Assurance in Particle Therapy. Applied Sciences 12(1): 328. DOI:10.3390/app12010328

30. Tran T. L. et al. (2017), Characterization of proton pencil beam scanning and passive beam using a high spatial resolution solid-state microdosimeter. Med. Phys. 44 (11).

31. James B, et al. (2021) In-field and out-of-field microdosimetric characterisation of a 62 MeV proton beam at CATANA, Med. Phys. 48 (8).

32. Bolst D. et al. (2020) Validation of Geant4 for silicon microdosimetry in heavy ion therapy, Physics in Medicine and Biology, 2020, 65(4), 045014.

33. Vohradsky J. et al. (2021) Response of SOI microdosimeter in fast neutron beams: experiment and Monte Carlo simulations, Physica Medica, vol. 90:176-187.

34. Bolst D et al. (2017) Correction factors to convert microdosimetry measurements in silicon to tissue in 12 C ion therapy, Phys Med Biol, 62(6):2055–2069.

35. Davis, J. A, et al. (2019) Tissue equivalence of diamond for heavy charged particles, Radiation measurements, Vol.122:1–9.

36. Pihet P, Menzel HG, Schmidt R, Beauduin M, Wambersie A. Biological weighting function for rbe specification of neutron therapy beams. Intercomparison of 9 European centres. Radiat Prot Dosim. (1990) 31:1-4. doi: 10.1093/oxfordjournals.rpd.a080709.

37. Loncol T, Cosgrove V, Denis JM, Gueulette J, Mazal A, Menzel HG, et al. Radiobiological effectiveness of radiation beams with broad LET spectra: microdosimetric analysis using biological weighting functions. Radiat Prot Dosim. (1994) 52:347–52. doi: 10.1093/rpd/52.1-4.347

38. Gueulette J, Gregoire V, Octave-Prignot M, Wambersie A. Measurements of radiobiological effectiveness in the 85 MeV proton beam produced at the cyclotron CYCLONE of Louvain-la-Neuve. Belgium Radiat Res. (1996) 145:70–74. doi: 10.2307/3579197

39. De Nardo L, Cesari V, Iborra N, Conte V, Colautti P, Herault J, et al. Microdosimetric assessment of nice therapeutic proton beam biological quality. Phys Med. (2004) 20:71–77. doi: 10.1093/rpd/ncq483

40. Gerlach R, Roos H, Kellerer AM. Heavy Ion RBE and microdosimetric spectra. Radiat Prot Dosim. (2002) 99:413–8. doi: 10.1093/oxfordjournals.rpd.a006821

41. Conte V. et al., Microdosimetry of a therapeutic proton beam with a mini-TEPC and a MicroPlus-Bridge detector for RBE assessment. Phys Med Biol. 65 (2020): 245018. doi: 10.1088/1361-6560/abc368.

42. Bianchi A. et al., Microdosimetry with a sealed mini-TEPC and a silicon telescope at a clinical proton SOBP of CATANA, Radiation Physics and Chemistry, Volume 171, 2020.

43. Verona C. et al., Microdosimetric measurements of a monoenergetic and modulated Bragg Peaks of 62 MeV therapeutic proton beam with a synthetic single crystal diamond microdosimeter. Med. Phys., 47: 5791-5801 (2020). https://doi.org/10.1002/mp.14466

44. Kase Y. et al., Microdosimetric calculation of relative biological effectiveness for design of therapeutic proton beams, Journal of Radiation Research, 2013, 54, 485–493 doi: 10.1093/jrr/rrs110

45. Hawkins RB., Statistical Theory of Cell Killing by Radiation of Varying Linear Energy Transfer, Radiation Research 140, 360-374 (1994) 360-374 https://doi.org/10.2307/3579114

46. Inaniwa T. et al., Treatment planning for a scanned carbon beam with a modified microdosimetric kinetic model, Phys Med Biol. 2010 Nov 21;55(22):6721-37. 10.1088/0031-9155/55/22/008

47. Tran LT. et al., The relative biological effectiveness for carbon, nitrogen, and oxygen ion beams using passive and scanning techniques evaluated with fully 3D silicon microdosimeters, Med Phys. 45-5 (2018) p 2299-2308 doi: 10.1002/mp.12874

48. Hawkins R. B., A microdosimetric-kinetic model for the effect of non-Poisson distribution of lethal lesions on the variation of RBE with LET. Radiat. Res. 160, 61–69 (2003).

49. Kellerer M and Rossi H H 1978 A generalized formation of dual radiation action Radiat. Res. 75 471–88

50. Zaider M and Rossi H H 1980 The synergistic effects of different radiations Radiat. Res. 83 732–9

51. Kase Y, Kanai T,Matsumoto Y, Furusawa Y, Okamoto H, Asaba T, SakamaMand Shinoda H 2006 Microdosimetric measurements and estimation of human cell survival for heavy-ion beams Radiat. Res. 166 629–38

52. Colautti P, Conte V, Selva A, Chiriotti S, Pola A, Bortot D, et al. Miniaturized microdosimeters as LET monitors: first comparison of calculated and experimental data performed at the 62 MeV/u 12C beam of INFN-LNS with four different detectors. Phys Med. (2018) 52:113–21. doi: 10.1016/j.ejmp.2018.07.004

53. Magrin G, Verona C, Ciocca M, Marinelli M, Mastella E, Stock M, et al. Microdosimetric characterization of clinical carbon-ion beams using synthetic diamond detectors and spectral conversion methods. Med Phys. (2020) 47:713–21. doi: 10.1002/mp.13926

54. Hagiwara Y, Bhattacharyya T, Matsufuji N, Isozaki Y, Takiyama H, Nemoto K,et al. Influence of dose-averaged linear energy transfer on tumour control after carbon-ion radiation therapy for pancreatic cancer. Clin Transl Radiat Oncol. (2020) 21:19–24. doi: 10.1016/j.ctro.2019.11.002

55. Bolst D. (2019) "Silicon microdosimetry in hadron therapy using Geant4", Doctor of Philosophy thesis, School of Physics, University of Wollongong.

56. Kase Y, Kanai T., Sakama M. et al. (2011), "Microdosimetric approach to NIRS-defined biological dose measurement for carbon-ion treatment beam", J Radiat. Res. 52(1):59-68. doi: 10.1269/jrr.10062. Epub 2010 Dec 13.

57. Nose H, Kase Y, Matsufuji N and Kanai T 2009 Field size effect of radiation quality in carbon therapy using passive method Med. Phys. 36 870–875

58. Tran T. L., Bolst D., Guatelli S., Pogossov A., Petasecca M., Lerch M., Chartier L., Prokopovich D., Reinhard M., Povoli M., Kok A., Perevertaylo V., Matsufuji N., Kanai T., Jackson M. and Rosenfeld A. (2018), "The relative biological effectiveness for carbon, nitrogen and oxygen ion beams using passive and scanning techniques evaluated with fully 3D silicon microdosimeters" Med Phys.; 45(5): 2299-2308

# 10 Monte Carlo to link RBE with radiation quality quantities

*Andrea Attili*
INFN National Institute for Nuclear Physics, Rome, Italy

*Giuseppe Magro*
CNAO National Center for Oncological Hadrontherapy, Pavia,
Italy

*Marco Calvaruso*
Institute of Molecular Bioimaging and Physiology, National
Research Council, IBFM-CNR, Cefalù, Italy

## CONTENTS

## 10.1 INTRODUCTION – RELATIVE BIOLOGICAL EFFECTIVENESS (RBE), FROM GENERAL TO THE SPECIFIC: CAN CANCER HETEROGENEITY AFFECT CELL RESPONSE TO RADIATION?

By definition, the Relative Biological Effectiveness (RBE) represents the ratio between a radiation of reference and a specific type of radiation, with its proper physical characteristics and linear energy transfer (LET). RBE is often used in radiobiology to test the capability of a particular radiation in inducing a biological effect in comparison to the reference one. Mathematically RBE can be expressed by the following formula:

$$\text{RBE} = \frac{D}{D_{\text{ref}}} \tag{10.1}$$

where $D$ is adsorbed dose of given by a radiation and $D_{\text{ref}}$ is a reference absorbed dose of radiation of a standard type that gives the same amount of damage. The reference radiations considered are usually low-LET X-rays or $^{60}$Co $\gamma$-rays with an energy of 250 kVp In other words, RBE answers the question: "how much radiation of reference do we need to reach the same biological effect with the tested radiation?" [30].

Despite being considered as a "physical quantity," RBE is strictly linked to biology, especially when we evaluate the effect induced by radiotherapy (RT) in biological systems like the human body, nevertheless the RBE is fundamental to plan a therapeutic RT schedule. Moreover, while mathematical sciences are usually based on a linear bond between causes and effects, a "biological response" relies on a complex network of events which do not always lead to the same endpoint, even if the triggering factor remains the same.

Hence, from a biological point of view, if some expected endpoints may appear controversial in respect to what expected, on the other hand, they are just the alternative side of the same coin which depends on a specific biological *momentum/punctum temporis* or to specific and intrinsic features. On these basis, biologists and clinicians have overturned, in the last years, the approach known as "one-size fits all" and, especially for cancer research and cancer treatment, the common sense has changed toward the definition of a more targeted approach. That means, both at microscopic and macroscopic levels, to calibrate an experimental setting or a cure, considering the biological variability among patients, or more simply, among different biological samples. The application of ionizing radiation (IR) in medicine is nowadays widely diffuse. Together with chemotherapy and surgery, radiotherapy (RT) is one of the three clinical criteria aimed at the eradication of tumors. RT for cancer is used to hit the tumor bulk with a definite amount of energy using conventional IR such as X and g-rays or using high-LET protons and carbon ions (hadrons). The use of hadrons has proved to be more efficient in releasing the dose within the targets thanks to their physical properties and, while proton therapy is associated with an RBE value of 1.1, RBE for carbon ions has a range between 2-5 [12].

However, since radiation is *per se* a physical entity, in the past years improvements regarding RT were mainly finalized to ameliorate techniques for a more precise dose distribution, thus neglecting the influence of all those biological aspects that may interfere with an effective therapy. RT is currently used, in association to chemotherapy and surgery, to treat several types of neoplasms including: brain, breast, ocular, bone tumors, etc. Nevertheless, there is a wide heterogeneity in terms of RT response among cancers, such differences are even more astonishing if we consider that they may change also between tumors affecting the same organ [2].

The variability of effects induced by RT on tumors relies on a resilience capability of the latter which can counteract the first, in other words, each kind of neoplasm is characterized by a specific radioresistance. Radioresistance is multifaceted and its degree depends on many biological factors including the ones deriving from the tumor itself and from its surrounding microenvironment. The following biological and tumor-related aspects are responsible for radioresistance: tumor efficiency in repairing DNA damage induced by RT; cancer capability to arrest cell-cycle; change in the immunological milieu associated to the tumor bulk; the decrease of tumor oxygenation and the tumor-associated hypoxia; cancer metabolism; the overlap and coexistence of several genetic aberrations within the same cancer. Together, all these features, are referred as "Hallmarks of cancer" [58, 22]

Response to radiotherapy is usually predicted basing on tumor cell-survival following RT, one of the first mathematical models proposed to evaluate cell-survival is the so-called Linear Quadratic (LQ) model. Formulated in the 70s, the LQ model is still a valid and widely accepted method to analyze RT effects on cells, both *in-vitro* and *in-vivo*. The LQ is based on two parameters which directly influence the tumor response to IR: the $\alpha$, the $\beta$, and their ratio ($\alpha/\beta$). $\alpha$ and $\beta$ represent different kinds of damage: the $\alpha$ account for a lethal damage caused by a single incident particle that cannot be repaired, on the contrary, $\beta$ is not responsible for a direct cell-killing but it can be rather repaired [9, 45]. Since radioresistance measures the ability of cells to recover from IR-induced damage, both $\alpha$ and $\beta$ mirror the ability of cell targets to counteract IR effects.

RT-schedules in clinical practice are usually planned basing on the $\alpha/\beta$ ratio of the tumor to be treated, in other words, tumors affecting the same organ (e.g. breast cancers) are considered to exhibit the same $\alpha/\beta$ ratio. Thus, radiation treatment is not administered considering cancer heterogeneity but it's rather based on a mathematical assumption. On these bases, to predict and to carry out an effective tumor eradication, a thorough evaluation of many aspects should be undertaken to orient medical approaches towards more personalized rather than general criteria [55].

In conclusion, the above-mentioned considerations are not aimed by any means at the underestimation of new and innovative approaches to predict IR-induced damage. As a matter of fact, Monte Carlo (MC)-based simulations represent valuable and potent tools to foresee the impact of IR on the living matter. However, future simulation platforms will need to be implemented by integrating physics and mathematics with as much biological information as possible, thus to achieve more and more precise predictions.

## 10.2    GENERAL STATISTICAL ASPECTS

Usually, radiobiological simulations are performed in two main steps. In the first step, MC simulations are used to generate the phase space of primary and secondary particles interacting with a cell population. In a second step the particle phase space is used as an input of a radiobiological model to evaluate a biological effect for a specific biological endpoint, such as the RBE of the cell survival. It is important to remark that both steps of the evaluation try to simulate two stochastic processes. In a common irradiation configuration, the particle phase space that interact with the cell population fluctuates from cell to cell. These fluctuations are particularly relevant in the case of high-LET radiation. Furthermore, even considering cells irradiated with the same phase space, the biological response of the cell is not strictly deterministic. Two different cells irradiated with the same particle configuration could evolve in two different conditions.

In practice, the majority of the radiobiological evaluation implementation commonly used in ion beam therapy, including implementation based on mechanistic model such as the Local Effect Models (LEM) [56, 17, 20] or the Microdosimetric Kinetic Model (MKM) [23, 24, 25, 26] (see Section 10.6 for details), approximate the stochastic processes by using evaluations that try to reproduce the behavior of the expectation value of the radiobiological effect. From the physical point of view, these implementations often don't use the complete phase particle space space as input, but use quantities already averaged over the cell population, such as the dose averaged LET or, equivalently, the first and the second moment of the representative energy deposition spectrum (see section 10.4.1). General purpose condensed history MC codes, such as GEANT4 [1, 3], FLUKA [18, 6], PHITS [54, 53], and others, can be used to evaluate these physical quantities at a micrometric (cell) scale. By making use of Monte Carlo track structure (MCTS) simulations with radiochemistry models, such as PARTRAC [15], TRAX [37, 61] and GEANT4-DNA [29], or by using approximated track structure models [33, 16], the physical and chemical quantities could also be evaluated directly at a nanometric scale in order include relevant information for radiobiological evaluations.

Starting from these input physical quantities, the radiobiological evaluations are then carried out by assuming specific statistics, such as the Poisson statistics of lethal lesions to evaluate the probability of cell survival [45]. The stochastic nature of the processes manifests itself as a deviation from the Poisson assumption, observed experimentally in the high LET region, and it is usually accounted for by introducing *ad hoc* corrective factors in the model [38, 25, 34], although alternative attempts to directly account for the non-Poisson statistics have been made [52, 44, 13].

## 10.3    MIXED FIELD APPROACHES

Strategies to account for some biological effects in Monte Carlo (MC) dose calculations have recently been developed, to better understand the biological impact of a primary ion beam, which

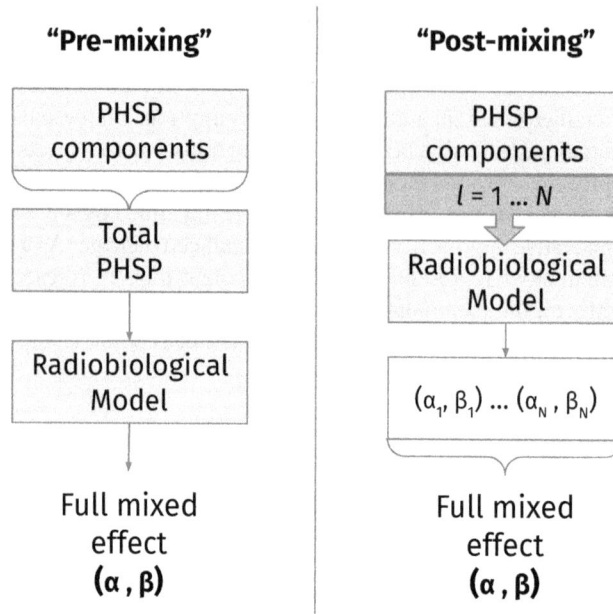

**Figure 10.1** Schematic representation of the "pre-mixing" and "post-mixing" for the evaluation of a mixed field radiobiological effect. Details are given in the text.

inevitably gives rise to a mixed radiation field, with particles and fragments having different charge, energy and linear energy transfer (LET), hence different ionization density along their track [47].

In a realistic treatment simulation, the particle phase space of the mixed-radiation field interacting with the cells in each voxel of the treated volume, can be thought as composed by different components. These components can be identified as the different intersecting beams that constitute the treatment field or, at a more microscopic level, as the different particle species and energies of the particle phase space seen by the cell. Each one of these component represents a different irradiation with different radiation quality and the global radiobiological effect depends in a complex and non linear way on the combination of these contributions. In practice two different main approaches to evaluate the net radiobiological effect of a mixed field can be identified, depending also on the specific radiobiological model. These approaches are schematically illustrated in Figure 10.1.

In a first approach, here identified as "pre-mixing" approach, the different physical quantities needed as physical inputs of the radiobiological evaluations, such as the dose average LET, or the micro- and nanodosimetric spectra, associated to the different components of the phase space are evaluated through independent MC simulations. These quantities are combined to evaluate the net values of the complete radiation field. Once the net physical values are available, they are used as input of the radiobiological model in a single evaluation step. In other words, the mixing is evaluated at the level of the physical quantities, before ("pre") the applications of the radiobiological model. The result is usually given in terms of the net LQ parameters $(\bar{\alpha}, \bar{\beta})$. This approach can be used in combination with dose averaged LET based models or with micro- and nano-dosimetric based models, such as the MKM. This approach will be discussed in Section 10.6.2.1

In a complementary approach, here identified as "post-mixing" approach, the radiobiological model is used to evaluate the biological effect of the single components of the phase space. In this step of the evaluation the effects are computed using as physical input of the model quantities associated to the separated phase space components, virtually considering these components as separated irradiation on different cell populations. The net radiobiological effect is then obtained by combining the the single component radiobiological effects with proper weights. In other words the mixing is evaluated at the level of the biological effects, after ("post") the applications of the radiobiological model. In the case of radiobiological models consistent with the LQ model, the net effect can be evaluated using the mixed field formalism in which the net LQ parameters $(\bar{\alpha}, \bar{\beta})$ are determined by dose-averaged mean values of the single component $\alpha_l$ and $\sqrt{\beta_l}$ [65]:

$$\bar{\alpha} = \frac{1}{D} \sum_l D_l \alpha_l \text{ and } \sqrt{\bar{\beta}} = \frac{1}{D} \sum_l D_l \sqrt{\beta_l}, \qquad (10.2)$$

where the subscript $l$ indicates the phase space component, $D_l$ is the dose contribution of the corresponding component, and $D = \sum_l D_l$ is the total dose. It is important to remark that the formalism expressed in Equations (10.2) approximate inherently the stochastic effects of the irradiation process (see section 10.2). This approach is commonly used in combination with the LEM. This approach will be discussed in Section 10.6.1.1.

In order to accelerate the MC evaluations, in both of these approaches the radiobiological evaluations usually can rely on a database of precomputed data as a function of energy per nucleon and particle species, that describe the phase space component. Each data has the fundamental characteristic that it can be approximated as being statistically independent. Hence, the net effect can be easily obtained via a linear combination accordingly to the weights associated to the different components as evinced in the case of Equations (10.2). In the case of the "pre-mixing" approach and the MKM based models, the precomputed data consists in the first and second moment of specific deposited energy distribution in the cell, obtained from the micro- and nanodosimetric evaluations for monoenergetic irradiations. This approach will be described in details in Section 10.6.2.1. In the case of the "post-mixing" approach, used in combination with the LEM, the data basically consists of the LQ coefficients $\alpha$ and $\sqrt{\beta}$ as evinced in Equations (10.2), or, equivalently, the $\text{RBE}_\alpha = \alpha/\alpha_X$ and $\text{RBE}_\beta = \sqrt{\beta/\beta_X}$, precomputed for each radiation component. A discussion of the latter approach will be given in Section 10.6.1.1.

## 10.4  DOSE-AVERAGED LET-BASED EVALUATIONS

### 10.4.1  LET AS A PREDICTOR OF THE RBE

Relative biological effectiveness (RBE) models, exploiting the linear-quadratic (LQ) parameterization of the cell survival, estimate RBE based on LET, dose per fraction and the cell-specific parameters $\alpha$ and $\beta$ for the reference radiation.

Starting from purely physical considerations, the LET is a non-stochastic one-dimensional macroscopic quantity, defined as the average energy locally transferred to the material by a charged particle per unit path-length [49]. It is, therefore, straightforward to identify LET as a descriptor of the radiation quality, and to correlate it with RBE: both of them, in fact, are known to increase along the treatment depth. Although neglecting the spatial envelope of the LET distribution, its dose-averaged value, $\text{LET}_D$, or track-averaged value, $\text{LET}_T$, have been suggested to be potentially used in biological treatment optimization even without knowing dose- and endpoint-specific RBE values accurately [49]. The need of averaging explains with the fact that the definition of LET is strictly valid only for a pure and mono-energetic beam of ions. Due to the build-up of a secondary spectrum and superposition of energies in a real treatment field, this definition is not adequate. In a MC environment, these quantities can be easily calculated even in complex voxelized patients' geometries. For instance, the $\text{LET}_D$ at depth $z$ is obtained as the absorbed dose delivered by a particle of type $i$ and energy $E$ multiplied by the corresponding particle energy loss per particle step (or stopping power, $S$) summed over all events relative to the total dose deposited [49], as shown in equation (10.3):

$$\text{LET}_D(z) = \frac{\sum_i \int dE \, S_i(E) \, D_i(E,z)}{\sum_i \int dE \, D_i(E,z)} \simeq \frac{\sum_i \int dE \, S_i^2(E) \, \Phi_i(E,z)}{\sum_i \int dE \, \Phi_i(E,z)} \quad . \qquad (10.3)$$

The term on the right approximates the absorbed dose as the product of fluence $\Phi$ and stopping power $S$ and is the form in which $\text{LET}_D$ is typically calculated numerically in a MC system. It has been shown that by considering spatial variations in $\text{LET}_D$ within treatment plan optimization, it might be possible to increase the therapeutic ratio in intensity-modulated proton therapy. There is, however, a need to understand whether or not differences in plans optimized using ($\text{LET}_D \times$ absorbed dose) vs (RBE $\times$ absorbed dose) for relevant molecular or cellular endpoint are large enough to be clinically relevant when viewed against the uncertainties and gaps in our understanding of the underlying clinical endpoint and patient-specific biology [49]. $\text{LET}_D$ is an average value of polyenergetic particle tracks and is thus combining different beam qualities contributing to cell kill in a single value. This raises the question if it can be used as a good predictor for RBE of any mixed radiation field, even for protons. Due to the higher complexity of the radiation fields, for treatment planning, for example, in carbon ion therapy more sophisticated (micro-dosimetric) approaches have to be adopted, which need to be discussed separately. Conversely, for biological optimization in proton or helium-ion therapy, phenomenological models have been proposed to estimate the RBE for the irradiated tissue. Commonly these models are based on a purely linear relationship between RBE and $\text{LET}_D$ or on $\text{LET}_D$-dependent analytical functions *ad hoc* defined to satisfy the empirical properties of RBE, as suggested by experimental findings.

In addition to the physical factors such as absorbed dose or LET, the RBE also depends on biological factors such as the cell or tissue type under consideration, which can be roughly summarized, to a first approximation, as the reference radiation fractionation sensitivity – $(\alpha_x/\beta_x)$.

Within the LQ framework, RBE, as a function of the absorbed dose per fraction $(D)$, can be rearranged in terms of the linear and quadratic parameters for both the reference photon radiation $(\alpha_x, \beta_x)$ and the ion of interest $(\alpha, \beta)$:

$$\text{RBE}(D;\alpha,\alpha_x,\beta,\beta_x) = \frac{1}{2D}\left(\sqrt{\left(\frac{\alpha_x}{\beta_x}\right)^2 + 4D\left(\frac{\alpha_x}{\beta_x}\right)\text{RBE}_\alpha + 4D^2\text{RBE}_\beta} - \left(\frac{\alpha_x}{\beta_x}\right)\right) \quad . \quad (10.4)$$

### 10.4.2  OVERVIEW OVER MODELS

Protons are currently the most frequently used particles in hadrontherapy. Despite the fact that RBE for protons depends on LET, dose level and tissue radiosensitivity, a constant factor of 1.1 is currently recommended and used for patient treatment. However, several phenomenological and biophysical models have been proposed for taking into account the main RBE dependencies and the potential effect of its variability [4, 64, 59, 11, 7, 62, 31, 46, 41, 51]. There are considerable variations between the estimations of RBE and RBE-weighted doses from the different models, which are a consequence of fundamental differences in experimental databases, model assumptions and regression techniques. The databases consist of multiple experiments, with both x-rays and $^{60}$Co $\gamma$-rays applied as reference radiation. As these rays have different radiation quality, there is a difference in the cellular response. Some models account for this effect, either by adjusting the $\text{LET}_D$ value ($\text{LET}_D^* = \text{LET}_D - \text{LET}_x + \text{LET}_\gamma$) or the RBE value of the data point (RBE$^* = $ RBE $\times D_\gamma/D_x$) [50].

$\text{LET}_D$ values above 20 keV/$\mu$m are rarely present in clinical proton therapy [48]. This restriction was acknowledged by the [59, 7, 46]'s models, while the [64, 62]'s models set the cut-off limit at 30 keV/$\mu$m. On the other hand, the [41]'s model is based on the [62]'s database, but with a higher cut-off value of around 40 keV/keV/$\mu$m. While the range of the scalar value $\text{LET}_D$ is limited, dose deposition from particles with very high LET values will still occur. The models developed with the LET spectrum of a mixed radiation field as a parameter for the radiation quality (see [41]) can therefore justify the inclusion of experiments with very high LET values in their database. There are also notable differences between the model databases in the low LET data. The [64, 7, 46]'s

2 Gy                                              8 Gy

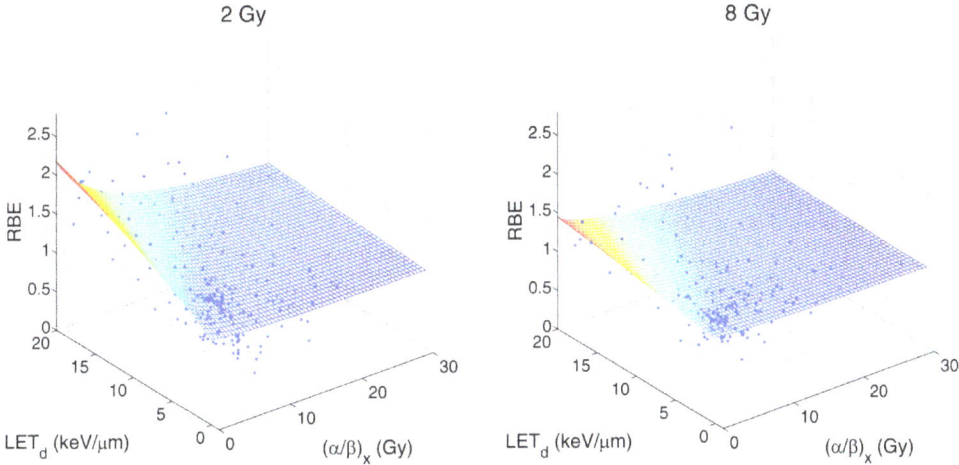

**Figure 10.2** The RBE for cell survival as a function of $\mathrm{LET}_D$ and $(\alpha_x/\beta_x)$ for a dose of 2 Gy (left panel) and 8 Gy (right panel) as predicted by a formulation of equation (10.5) [46]. The experimental data used in the fit is also plotted. The $\mathrm{LET}_D$ is given relative to the reference photon radiation. Figure taken from [46].

databases are dominated by data points below 5 keV/μm, while the [4, 59, 11, 62, 41]'s databases first start at 7.7 keV/μm [50].

For most models, the $\mathrm{RBE}_\alpha$ and $\mathrm{RBE}_\beta$ functions were found by regression to experimental databases, differing in size and selection of the *in vitro* data, with an explicit dependence of the proton $\alpha$ and $\beta$ parameters on LET and cell type, expressed in different variants for different models. At the same time, models exist, which are developed as an alternative to the phenomenological approach and are not directly based on cell experiments. They assume the RBE to be linearly dependent on $\mathrm{LET}_D$ [49]. Several empirical proton RBE models show a common dependence on physical and radiobiological quantities, for what concerns proton $\alpha$ and $\beta$, which can be summarized as follows:

$$\mathrm{RBE}_\alpha = \frac{\alpha}{\alpha_x} = p_0 + p_1 \frac{\mathrm{LET}_D}{(\alpha_x/\beta_x)} \quad , \quad \mathrm{RBE}_\beta = \sqrt{p_2 + p_3\, h\,(\mathrm{LET}_D)} \quad , \tag{10.5}$$

where $p_{[0\div3]}$ are model-specific fitted parameters and $h(\mathrm{LET}_D)$ is a LET-dependent function, weighting the $\mathrm{LET}_D$ either by $(\alpha_x/\beta_x)^{-1}$ or $(\alpha_x/\beta_x)^{1/2}$ according to [7] or [46], respectively. Models predict an increasing RBE with decreasing $(\alpha/\beta)$. One would also expect the slope to be greater for higher $\mathrm{LET}_D$ values. These trends are not statistically significant when analyzing all published *in vitro* cell survival data simultaneously. An increase in $\mathrm{RBE}_\beta$ as a function of $\mathrm{LET}_D$ is not significant and is visible only for $\mathrm{LET}_D \gtrsim 5\,\mathrm{keV}/\mu\mathrm{m}$. Others have indicated that the increasing RBE with decreasing $(\alpha/\beta)$ significant only at low $(\alpha/\beta)$ ($\lesssim 5$ Gy) [49]. The combined data are too noisy to confirm this. Hence, while maintaining a linear dependency for $\mathrm{RBE}_\alpha$ or rather doing efforts towards the use of strongly non-linear LET spectrum-dependent functions (see [51]'s weighted model), it is often assumed $\beta = \beta_x$ (i.e. $\mathrm{RBE}_\beta = 1$), as for [64, 59, 62, 41, 51]. An example of the behavior of $\mathrm{RBE}_\alpha$ and $\mathrm{RBE}_\beta$ as functions of $\mathrm{LET}_D$ and $(\alpha_x/\beta_x)$ is shown in Figure 10.2.

Most models assume specific dependencies *a priori* for $\mathrm{RBE}_\alpha$ and $\mathrm{RBE}_\beta$, by fitting a single function to the data set. However, the [62, 41, 51]'s models were made by fitting multiple functions with different dependencies and applying statistical testing to determine the best fitting function. When fitting the models to the databases, the majority of the models apply an unweighted regression technique.

Model selection should ideally be based on knowledge of the models and their suitability to the particular cases where the models are to be applied. The phenomenological models are limited by their empirical data and underlying assumptions. Hence, to minimize extrapolation of data in the modeling, the fits should be based on an experimental database similar to their usage [50].

### 10.4.3   DATABASE GENERATION: BEAM QUALITY AND MODELING ASSUMPTIONS

The procedure of building a self-consistent database is of crucial importance if a phenomenological, data-driven approach is thought to be used for implementing a radiobiological model. The works by [43, 41] can be taken as a figure of merit to extrapolate the main steps to link data available in literature to finally have an easy-to-use analytical function, which is able to predict the RBE in a clinically relevant range of doses, based on LET and the tissue specific LQ parameter $(\alpha_x/\beta_x)$ at least for light ions beams, like protons and helium ions, producing similar and relatively simple mixed radiation fields, phenomenological analytic expressions can be investigated to describe how the $RBE_\alpha$ varies with LET and then tested against statistical goodness-of-fit methods.

In order to study and determine the radiobiological properties of light ions beams, a predefined database can be taken as a reference (see the *Particle Irradiation Data Ensemble* – PIDE by [21], for example) and possibly reviewed. Data should be reanalyzed in order to fully handle the fitting results, taking into account the parameter uncertainties, if available. All the publications reported herein should be examined to eventually exclude the ones for which it is not possible to extract the LQ parameters of the response both to the ions and to the reference radiation, either in tables or retrievable by fitting data from the reported figures of survival curves. When photons and ion LQ parameters are reported as numbers, they may be directly taken. If not, whenever possible, they can be calculated from other related published quantities, e.g. from RBE and the reference radiation dose for a certain survival level. When only survival curves are provided, experimental points and their error bars may be acquired and digitized. Since all data reported in the published tables should be derived from the LQ model, those ones, for which the suggested best fit model is different, should be excluded, in order to build up a consistent analysis based on the LQ formalism only. Data from survival curves where the experimental points, mainly at low doses, are indistinguishable or difficult to determine should be also rejected.

It should be noticed that an intrinsic uncertainty affects the LET values usually reported in literature. In fact, LET is not always unequivocally calculated: some papers use the dose-average, others the track-average, but most of the time the method of LET calculation may be not even specified. LET renormalization could also be required, as discussed in the above, to make consistency among the photon reference radiations. Moreover, in some experiments, before hitting the cells, the ion beam is modulated by means of passive elements, thus degrading its energy and producing secondary particles. Including these data in the analysis, when the calculation approach is based on the dose-weighted averages quantities and the biological response is not linearly linked to the estimated LET, could influence the capability of the model in predicting the biological effect in case of a mixed radiation field.

Only data from experiments performed with asynchronous cells should be selected, excluding those that result from the irradiation of cells synchronized in a certain phase of the cell cycle. Asynchronous cells are indeed more representative of an *in vivo* scenario related to clinical practice.

Possible $RBE_\alpha$ parameterizations must be developed with the aim to capture basic features of the $RBE_\alpha$ using a minimum of assumptions supported by experimental data and published papers:

- experiments suggest that $RBE_\alpha$ usually increases with increasing LET ($L$) approximately up to a maximum value $L^*$ and then it starts decreasing;
- one can assume that $RBE_\alpha$ approaches the unity for decreasing LET values;
- one can assume that the initial slope might affect the cell line via the inverse of $(\alpha_x/\beta_x)$ so that $RBE_\alpha$ of cell lines with high $(\alpha_x/\beta_x)$ results to be less dependent on LET;

- as experimentally observed, $RBE_\alpha$ generally increases with decreasing $(\alpha_x/\beta_x)$ and with increasing LET, however, at high $(\alpha_x/\beta_x)$, the change in $RBE_\alpha$ due to different LET is very limited. For low LET, the $(\alpha_x/\beta_x)$-induced variation of $RBE_\alpha$ is also small.

All this can be turned into:

$$RBE_\alpha = 1 + \left[ p_0 + \left( \frac{\alpha_x}{\beta_x} \right)^{-1} \right] \cdot f(L) \quad , \tag{10.6}$$

where the multiplicative function $f(L)$ should act on $RBE_\alpha$ to possibly satisfy the empirical properties suggested by experimental findings, i.e. $RBE_\alpha(L) \geq 0, \forall L \lesssim L_{max}$ and $RBE_\alpha(L^*) \approx \max(RBE_\alpha)$, where $L_{max}$ is the maximum LET of the ion beam in water and $\max(RBE_\alpha)$ is the maximum $RBE_\alpha$ for a given cell line.

In order not to include any bias in the estimation of the fitting parameters, no *a priori* boundary limits for their variation may be specified and the requirements for the $RBE_\alpha$ function can be only verified *a posteriori*. The first free parameter $p_0$ may correct for null $\beta_x$ cell lines, with $RBE_\alpha \geq 1$. This further assumption is confirmed by experimental evidence.

Fitting functions $f(L)$ of increasing complexity and number of parameters can be chosen (see Figure 10.3), starting from purely polynomial expressions and then mixing polynomial and exponential terms. Combinations of polynomial and $\exp(-L^2)$ terms can be also tested for evaluating their capability in fitting $RBE_\alpha$ in the fall-off region after the maximum. The aim is improving the description of the experimental data until no relevant gain could be appreciated, for example, via an $F$-statistic analysis, which turns to be useful, among non-nested models, when quantifying whether the decrease of the sum of squared residuals (SSR) is worth the cost of the additional variables (loss of degrees of freedom).

To deal with the highly inhomogeneous and relatively poor data set, where the LQ parameters as well as LET are mixed up either having experimental uncertainties or not, Mairani proposed a data resampling technique coupled with a "leave-one-out" iterative data processing, to randomly work with equally weighted squared residuals when minimizing the SSR and to examine, at the same time, how one observation can influence the overall outcome.

With this phenomenological approach it is possible to model easily the RBE for proton and helium ion therapy, offering an improved description of the mixed radiation field. Absorbed dose in proton therapy is the sum of the dose deposited by the primary beam as well as by the secondary particles produced in nuclear interactions, mainly protons and helium ions ($Z = 1$ and $Z = 2$ particles). Both proton and helium ion beams have similar mixed radiation fields in terms of particle species. The major contributions are protons, deuterons, tritons ($Z = 1$) and $^3He$, $^4He$ ($Z = 2$) ions, produced in the target fragmentation in the case of proton beams or in both projectile and target fragmentation in the case of helium ion beams. According to [43, 41], the resulting $RBE_\alpha$ parameterization would therefore be:

$$RBE_\alpha = \frac{D_p}{D_p + D_{He}} RBE_\alpha^p + \frac{D_{He}}{D_p + D_{He}} RBE_\alpha^{He} \quad , \tag{10.7}$$

with

$$RBE_\alpha^p = 1 + \left( \frac{\alpha_x}{\beta_x} \right)^{-1} \cdot p_{1,p} L_p \tag{10.8}$$

and

$$RBE_\alpha^{He} = 1 + \left[ p_{0,He} + \left( \frac{\alpha_x}{\beta_x} \right)^{-1} \right] \cdot p_{1,He} L_{He} \exp\left(-p_{2,He} L_{He}^2\right) \quad , \tag{10.9}$$

where $L_{He,p}$ and $D_{He,p}$ are the $LET_D$ and the physical dose of protons and helium ions, respectively.

For these LET-based phenomenological models, the calculation framework coupled with the MC code essentially requires the LET to be estimated by the simulation program. For example, within

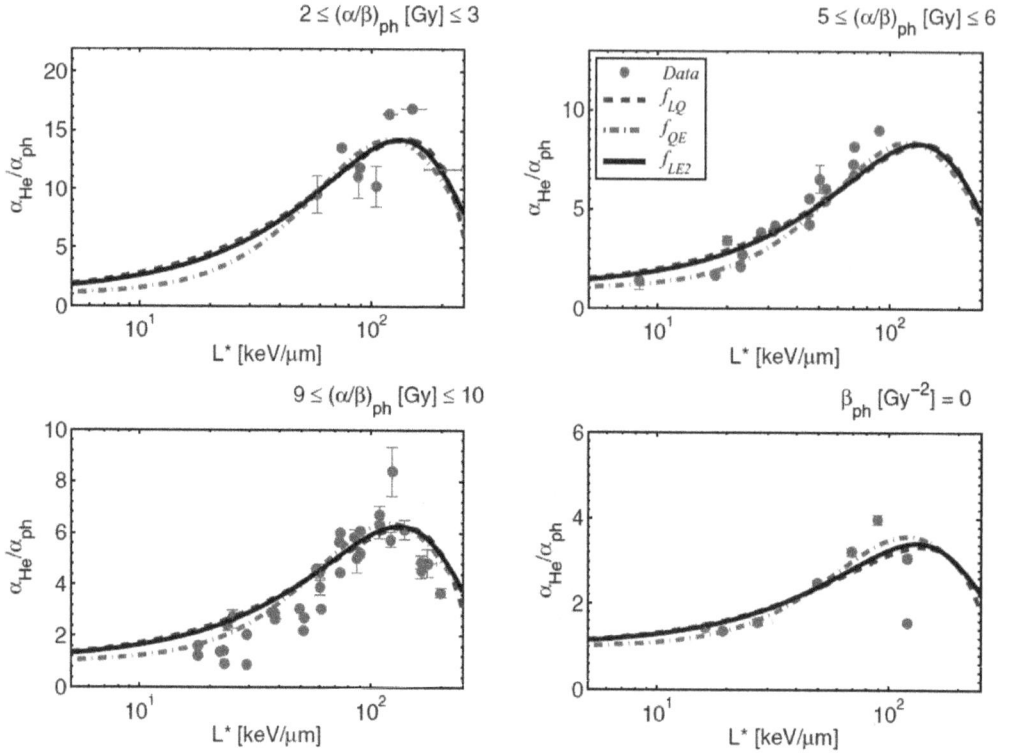

**Figure 10.3**  Comparison between experimental data (points with error bars) and fits (lines) for $RBE_\alpha$ as a function of corrected LET by applying three phenomenological parameterization as reported in the legend for four representative cell lines. Figure taken from [42].

the general purpose tool FLUKA, the user can call the built-in double precision function GETLET() depending on the particle type (FLUKA particle index), particle kinetic energy (GeV), particle momentum (GeV/$c$), maximum secondary electron energy (GeV, or $< 0$ for unrestricted LET) and material index for which LET is requested. The output would be the (un)restricted LET in keV/($\mu$m g/cm$^3$). When the user routine fluscw is activated by option USERWEIG, fluences $\Phi$ calculated, for example with USRBIN, are multiplied by a value returned by this function. Therefore, if this value matches the GETLET() output, the $LET_D$ for a given particle species in a water-equivalent geometry can be straightforwardly scored by an off-line element-wise division between the (absorbed dose $\times$ LET) matrix (i.e. $\Phi \times$ LET $\times$ LET) and the absorbed dose matrix ($\Phi \times$ LET). Then, summing up $RBE_\alpha$ as in equation (10.7) for the different ion species (p and He, for instance) allows the calculation of the RBE for the mixed radiation field.

## 10.5  OER-BASED EVALUATIONS

Besides physical factors such as ion energy and LET, environmental factors such as oxygen concentration will influence the RBE. There is strong evidence that the presence of hypoxic cells can limit the probability of tumor cure due to their largely reduced radiation sensitivity to photon radiation. This increased resistance is characterized by the oxygen enhancement ratio (OER), defined by the absorbed doses required to achieve a given effect under hypoxic and oxic conditions, respectively: OER $= D_h/D_o$. The OER is less pronounced for high-LET radiation. Whereas for photon radiation, typical OER values are close to 3, for high-LET radiation this value can drop down to approximately 1. In the latter case, the presence or absence of oxygen will not affect radiosensitivity. Consequently $RBE_h \simeq (3/OER_{ion}) \cdot RBE_o$, therefore the reduced oxygen effect for high-LET radiation corresponds to significantly higher RBE values for hypoxic conditions as compared to oxic conditions [27]. The reduced effect of oxygen thus represents one of the major rationales for application of high-LET beams in tumor therapy, because the cell killing probability is much less dependent on the oxygen status of the cells as compared to conventional radiation.

The FLUKA MC code can be prepared for inclusion of OER calculations specifically for (but nor limited to) proton therapy, in order to explore the impact of hypoxia [14]. The RBE-weighted dose is adapted for hypoxia by making RBE model parameters dependent on the OER, in addition to the LET. The OER depends on the partial oxygen pressure ($pO_2$) and LET. The oxygen levels, given as $pO_2$, can be estimated using positron emission tomography (PET) images with [$^{18}$F]-EF5 as hypoxia tracer.

The OER can be calculated, for example, by applying the model by [63]. This OER model calculates the survival fraction of cells, $S$, after ion irradiation according to the LQ model, with $\alpha$ and $\beta$ parametrized as follows:

$$\alpha(L,p) = \frac{(a_1 + a_2 L)\, p + (a_3 + a_4 L)\, K}{p + K} \quad , \quad \beta(p) = \frac{b_1\, p + b_2\, K}{p + K} \quad , \tag{10.10}$$

where $L$ is the dose-averaged LET, $p$ is the $pO_2$, and $K$ is set to 3 mmHg [63]. By non-linear least square curve fit of *in vitro* data the model parameters can be found. The OER can be calculated as:

$$\text{OER} = \frac{\sqrt{\alpha^2(L,p_h) - 4\beta(p_h)\ln S} - \alpha(L,p_h)}{\sqrt{\alpha^2(L,p_o) - 4\beta(p_o)\ln S} - \alpha(L,p_o)} \cdot \frac{\beta(p_o)}{\beta(p_h)} \quad , \tag{10.11}$$

where $p_h$ and $p_o$ are the oxygen pressure at the hypoxic and normoxic conditions, respectively. $p_h$ can be obtained from the PET image and $p_o$ usually is kept equal to 30 mmHg as this is a typical $pO_2$ value for tissues [63].

To account for hypoxia in the calculations of RBE and OER weighted dose, similar to [57] and [60], one can replace the normoxic response parameters in equation (10.4) (see the definition of $RBE_{max/min}$ therein) with hypoxic response parameters which vary with the OER:

$$\alpha_h = \frac{\alpha_o}{\text{OER}(L,p_h)} \quad , \quad \beta_h = \frac{\beta_o}{\text{OER}^2(L,p_h)} \quad . \tag{10.12}$$

This model allows to apply $\alpha$ and $\beta$ as defined in most of the existing RBE models derived from normoxic *in vitro* data and then estimate their hypoxic versions by applying equations above.

To score $pO_2$, a method for importing estimated $pO_2$ values in a patient geometry on a voxel-by-voxel basis in FLUKA using `fluscw` can be implemented, as shown in [14]. The subroutine may read the $pO_2$ values from a table, created from the PET images; the coordinate system of the PET image must be converted into FLUKA coordinates, and for each particle position, the corresponding $pO_2$ value from the PET image can be retrieved. Subsequently, $pO_2$ times dose-to-water ($pO_2 \times \Phi \times \text{LET}$) and dose-to-water ($\Phi \times \text{LET}$) can be scored in FLUKA, as previously described. Then, $pO_2$ is given by the quotient of the two scored quantities. To achieve the needed accuracy on the scored values without increasing the simulation time significantly, the fraction of the kinetic energy to be lost in a simulation step can be set to 0.0125, which is 25% of the default value when applying the FLUKA HADROTHErapy defaults [14].

## 10.6  MECHANISM-INSPIRED MODELS FOR RBE

There is general agreement that the microscopic, spatial energy deposition pattern of charged particles is a major determinant for their increased biological effectiveness. Since the physical properties

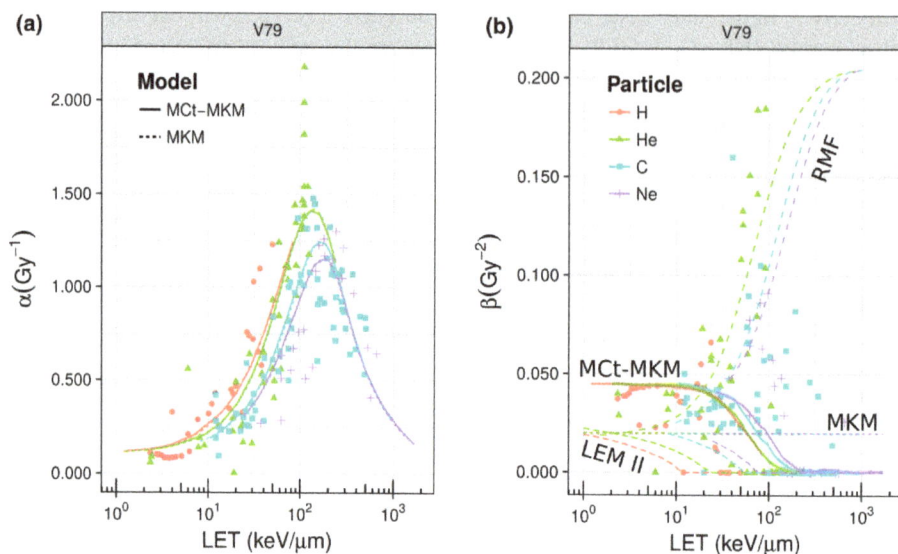

**Figure 10.4** Linear quadratic $\alpha$ (panel $a$) and $\beta$ (panel $b$) parameters as a function of LET for the irradiation of V79 cells with different ions. Points represent experimental data taken from PIDE [21] and different colors and shapes refer to H, He, C, and Ne ions. In panel $a$, dashed and solid lines represent the evaluations with the MKM and a Monte Carlo variant, named MCt-MKM [44]. In panel $b$, a comparison between different models is reported (namely MKM, MCt-MKM, LEM-II, and RMF). Figure taken from [44].

of the different radiation types can be described in great detail, different strategies have been developed as to how to translate the knowledge about the energy deposition pattern at different levels of detail into a prediction of the radiobiological effectiveness of particle beams in experimental and therapeutic situations [27].

The microdosimetric-kinetic model (MKM) [23, 24, 25, 26], recent versions of the local effect model (LEM) [17] and the repair-misrepair-fixation (RMF) model [8, 19, 32] are instead examples of mechanism-inspired models that explain the effects of particle characteristics such as LET on clonogenic cell survival in terms of putative mechanisms connecting the induction and biological processing of double strand breaks (DSB), for example, into more lethal forms of damage (e.g., chromosome aberrations). An example of monoenergetic evaluations performed using the LEM, MKM and RMF models compared to experimental data are reported in Figure 10.4. Differences in the models arise from the emphasized mechanisms of action as well as differences in the way proximity and domain-size effects (a domain is defined as a subcellular volume) are treated [49].

## 10.6.1 BIOLOGICAL EFFECT MIXING APPROACHES

### 10.6.1.1 MC codes coupled with the LEM

The LEM aims to derive the biological effects of ion radiation from the response of cells or tissues to photon radiation [49]. The LEM makes use of the concept of a local dose, which is defined as the expectation value of the energy deposition at any position in the radiation field for a given pattern of particle trajectories. The key assumption made in the LEM is that equal "local doses" produce equal local biological effects, independent of the radiation quality[1]. The relevant local

---

[1] In the latest version (LEM IV), it is assumed that the final biological response of a cell to radiation is directly linked to the initial spatial distribution and density of DSB within subnuclear targets, rather than the local dose distribution itself. In

dose is derived from an amorphous track structure representation of the energy deposition as a function of the radial distance to the particle trajectory. Particle effectiveness is calculated based on the microscopic local dose distribution pattern of ion traversals within the cell nucleus, assuming the nucleus is the sensitive target for the observed radiation effects. The LEM is used clinically to compute RBE-weighted dose distribution for carbon ion therapy.

In the LEM the biological effect in a cell nucleus (cn), defined in terms of the logarithm of the cell survival $-\ln S$ and obtained by summing up over the entire nucleus the biological damage calculated in small sub-volumes of the cell nucleus, can be expressed in terms of traversals of particles of a particular type and energy:

$$-\ln S(z_{cn}) = \alpha_z z_{cn} + \beta_z z_{cn}^2 \quad . \tag{10.13}$$

where $z_{cn}$ is the specific energy deposited by the particle in the cell nucleus, which is assumed to be the critical target in the model, while $\alpha_z$ and $\beta_z$ are the coefficients of the linear and quadratic terms, respectively. These parameters are calculated as described in detail in [56], and then stored in an external database for both primary beam and secondary fragments as a function of the particle energy, particle type and cell line. This database is the main input for performing biological calculations in the FLUKA MC framework [40].

To calculate the macroscopic biological effect, $-\ln S(D)$, for a given radiation field, the so-called low dose approximation approach may be implemented in FLUKA, as described in [38], which is valid for therapeutic dose levels up to the order of 10 GyE per fraction. This method links the LEM calculated intrinsic parameters, $\alpha_z$ and $\beta_z$ to the macroscopic dose ones, $\alpha_D$ and $\beta_D$. The initial slope $\alpha_D$, reported in [38], is obtained as $\alpha_D = (1 - S_1)/d_1$, where $d_1$ is the dose deposited by the particle in the cell nucleus and $S_1 = \exp(-\alpha_z d1$ is the surviving fraction due to a single traversal of a particle in the cell nucleus. For the determination of $\beta_D$, the following expression is adopted according to [38]: $\beta_D = \beta_Z (\alpha_D/\alpha_z)^2$, with $\beta_z \simeq (s_{max} - \alpha_z)/(2D_t)$. $D_t$ represents the transition dose at which the survival curve for the photon radiation is assumed to have an exponential shape with the maximum slope $s_{max} = \alpha_x + 2\beta_x D_t$. $\alpha_x$ and $\beta_x$ represent the coefficients of the linear and quadratic terms for the photon radiation.

The coupling of the FLUKA code with the LEM has been carried out following the theory of dual radiation action (TDRA) [35], which has been used in [38] for the low dose approximation approach. The authors of the TDRA stated that a biological system exposed to more than one radiation type shows synergism, implying that the total number of lesions is larger than the sum of the lesions produced by each particle, due to interactions between sub-lesions produced by different components.

Referring to the formalism introduced in the above, the number of lethal lesions after the exposure to a macroscopic dose $D$ can be expressed as:

$$N(D) = -\ln S(D) = \alpha_D D + \beta_D D^2 \quad , \tag{10.14}$$

while the sequential exposure to $n$ doses from different radiation types gives the following number of lesions:

$$N(D_1, \ldots, D_n) = \sum_{i=1}^{n} \alpha_{D,i} D_i + \left( \sum_{i=1}^{n} \sqrt{\beta_{D,i}} D_i \right)^2 \quad , \tag{10.15}$$

where $\alpha_{D,i}$ and $\beta_{D,i}$ are the parameters for the radiation type $i$.

Within this formalism the dose-averaged parameters for a mixed field can be calculated as:

$$\bar{\alpha}_D = \frac{\sum_i \alpha_{D,i} D_i}{\sum_i D_i} \quad , \sqrt{\bar{\beta}}_D = \frac{\sum_i \sqrt{\beta_{D,i}} D_i}{\sum_i D_i} \quad . \tag{10.16}$$

---

line with the general concepts of the LEM formalism, similar spatial patterns of DSB induction produce the same biological response, independent of the properties of the radiation creating the spatial pattern of initial damage.

At the initialization stage, the interface reads the LEM calculated initial RBE database tabulated in terms of particle type and energy per nucleon together with the LEM input parameters for a particular cell line. This initial RBE is defined as $\alpha_z/\alpha_x$, where $\alpha_z$ is the LEM calculated intrinsic parameter representing the initial slope of the ion–dose effect curve. $\alpha_D$ and $\beta_D$ are then calculated online using a dedicated `fluscw`-based routine, exploiting the `GETLET()` $\times \alpha_z$ (or $\sqrt{\beta_z}$) value as scoring weight. Through this routine it is possible to determine all ingredients useful for biological calculations, i.e. charge, mass, energy and unrestricted LET in water of the particles (primary carbon ions and secondary fragments) traversing the cell nucleus. The characterization of the charged particle traversal (charge, mass and energy per nucleon) allows to interpolate $\alpha_z$ from the correct table. Using the corresponding LET, one can calculate the dose deposited in the cell nucleus $d_1 = C \cdot \text{LET}/A_n$, where $A_n$ represents the cell nucleus area while $C$ is a constant as reported in [38]. The $\alpha_D$ and $\beta_D$ parameters are then determined according to the expressions mentioned in the above. Whenever an energy is deposited by a certain radiation type, the following two quantities, in addition to the dose $D$, are stored in different arrays: $\alpha_D \cdot D$ and $\sqrt{\beta_D} \cdot D$, using the FLUKA scoring capabilities. At the end of the simulation one obtains the dose-weighted averages $\alpha$ and $\beta$ for the mixed radiation field using equation (10.16). Finally the biological effect $-\ln S$, RBE-weighted dose $D_{\text{RBE}}$ and RBE are calculated using the same formalism introduced in [38]:

$$-\ln S = \begin{cases} \overline{\alpha}_D D + \overline{\beta}_D D^2 & \text{for } D \leq D_t \\ \overline{\alpha}_D D_t + \overline{\beta}_D D_t^2 + (D - D_t)\, s_{\max} & \text{for } D > D_t \end{cases} \quad , \tag{10.17}$$

$$D_{\text{RBE}} = \begin{cases} -\frac{\alpha_x}{2\beta_x} + \sqrt{\left(\frac{\alpha_x}{2\beta_x}\right)^2 - \frac{\ln S}{\beta_x}} & \text{for } -\ln S \leq -\ln S_t \\ D_t + (\ln S_t - \ln S)/s_{\max} & \text{for } -\ln S > -\ln S_t \end{cases} \quad , \quad \text{RBE} = \frac{D_{\text{RBE}}}{D} \quad , \tag{10.18}$$

where $D$ is the absorbed dose and $-\ln S_t = \alpha_x D_t + \beta_x D_t^2$. In the case of two or more irradiation fields, the FLUKA results ($D$, $\alpha_D \cdot D$ and $\sqrt{\beta_D} \cdot D$) for each beam port are summed up linearly and then equations (10.16), (10.17) and (10.18) are applied to obtain the total biological response.

## 10.6.2 MICRODOSIMETRIC QUANTITIES MIXING APPROACHES

### 10.6.2.1 MC codes coupled with the MKM

A review of different variants of MKM can be found in [5]. The main assumption of the modified and current clinically adopted version of the MKM developed in [34, 28] is that the cell nucleus is divided into many microscopic sub-volumes, called domains. The cell survival fraction is predicted from the energy deposited within these domains – the specific energy $z$, i.e. the ratio of the energy imparted and the mass – for any radiation quality. [28] introduced the saturation-corrected specific energy ($z_{\text{sat}}$) to account for the decrease of RBE due to the over-killing effect for high specific energy values.

In the MKM, the surviving fraction of cells, $S$, after ion irradiation delivering a physical dose $D$, is described as follows [34]:

$$-\ln S = (\alpha_0 + \beta\, z_{1D}^*)D + \beta D^2 \quad , \tag{10.19}$$

where $\alpha_0$ is the constant that represents the initial slope of the surviving fraction curve in the limit of LET = 0. $\beta$ is a constant quadratic term, independent on the radiation type, and $z_{1D}^*$ denotes the saturation-corrected dose-mean specific energy of the domain delivered in a single event, which depends on both $z$ and $z_{\text{sat}}$. It is derived by the following equation:

$$z_{1D}^* = \frac{\int_0^{X_{\max}} z(x)\, z_{\text{sat}}(x)\, 2\pi x \mathrm{d}x}{\int_0^{X_{\max}} z(x)\, 2\pi x \mathrm{d}x} \quad , \tag{10.20}$$

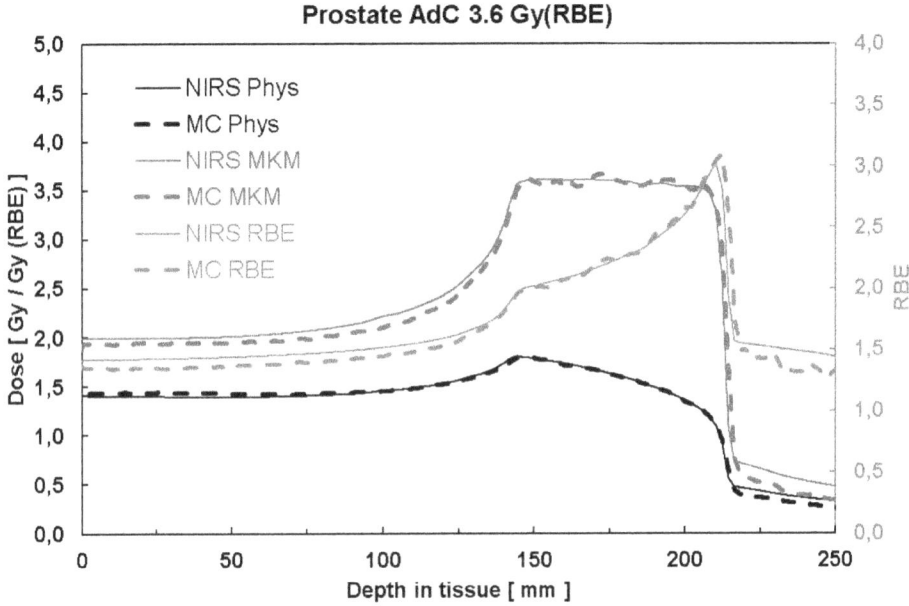

**Figure 10.5**   Comparison of depth physical (lowest line) or effective (flat line) dose (left y-axis) and RBE (right y-axis, middle line) profiles acquired in the target volume for a prostate cancer case. Solid and dashed lines represent original treatment planning curves and MC calculations, respectively. Figure taken from [39].

where $z(x)$ is the specific energy delivered to the domain as a function of the impact parameter $x$ (i.e. the distance between the center of the domain and the ion trajectory) and $X_{max}$ is the maximum impact parameter where the ions can still give an energy deposition to the domain. $z_{sat}$ represents the saturation-corrected specific energy and is given as follows:

$$z_{sat} = \frac{z_0^2}{z}\left[1 - \exp\left(-\frac{z^2}{z_0^2}\right)\right] \quad , \quad z_0 = \frac{(R_n/r_d)^2}{\sqrt{\beta\left[1 + (R_n/r_d)^2\right]}} \quad , \tag{10.21}$$

where $R_n$ is the nucleus radius, $r_d$ is the domain radius and $\beta$ is the quadratic parameter of the LQ model.

To calculate $z(x)$ in the MKM, the Kiefer-Chatterjee (KC) track structure model [10, 36] is applied. The KC-model gives the local dose (the core dose ($D_c$) and the penumbra dose ($D_p$)) as a function of the track radius, once the core radius ($R_c$) and the penumbra radius ($R_p$) for a particle with a given energy $E$, mass $A$, unrestricted linear energy transfer LET, effective charge $Z_{eff}$ (given by the Barkas expression) and velocity $\beta_{ion}$ (relative to the speed of light) are known.

When an ion has an impact parameter $x$, the specific energy delivered to the domain for this impact parameter results from the sum of the dose contributions to the domain from each given distance from the ion trajectory multiplied by the volume receiving this dose, divided by the total volume of the domain. The specific energy for a given impact parameter is, in other words, given by the average dose delivered to the domain with radius $r_d$.

For a proper coupling via the above described interface based on the LEM (see 10.6.1.1), one way to describe the biological effect with FLUKA is to provide an external radiobiological database, which meets the requirement of any LQ formalism [39]. Hence, for the MKM, a biological database can be prepared in terms of the linear variable $z_{1D}^*$, as a function of the kinetic energy per nucleon for each particle species (H, He, Li, Be, B, C). With this input table, FLUKA applies an approach based on the dose-weighted average $z_{1D}^*$ of the mixed radiation field, i.e.

$$\overline{z_{1DD}^*} = \frac{\sum_i z_{1D_{D,i}}^* D_i}{\sum_i D_i} \quad , \tag{10.22}$$

where $D_i$ is the dose from the $i^{\text{th}}$-charged particle of the mixed radiation field, with associated $z_{1D_{D,i}}^*$ and the summation is performed over all particles depositing dose. Finally, the $z_{1D}^* \cdot D$ quantity, in addition to the absorbed dose matrix $D$, is stored using the FLUKA scoring capabilities. Starting from equation (10.19), with the dose average of $z_{1D}^*$ in place of its original value, one can calculated the biological dose (i.e. the RBE-weighted) distribution $D_{\text{bio}}$ of a mixed-radiation field of a carbon ion beam irradiation, as:

$$D_{\text{bio}} = -\frac{\alpha_r}{2\beta} + \sqrt{\left(\frac{\alpha_r}{2\beta}\right)^2 + \frac{\alpha_0 D + \overline{z_{1DD}^*}D + \beta D^2}{\beta}} \quad , \tag{10.23}$$

where $\alpha_r$ is the linear coefficient of the LQ model for the reference radiation. When photons are used as reference radiation, $\alpha_r = \alpha_0 = \alpha_x$. An example of the application of the coupling formalism is given in Figure 10.5.

## REFERENCES

1. Sea Agostinelli, John Allison, K al Amako, John Apostolakis, H Araujo, P Arce, M Asai, D Axen, S Banerjee, G 2 Barrand, et al. Geant4—a simulation toolkit. *Nuclear instruments and methods in physics research section A: Accelerators, Spectrometers, Detectors and Associated Equipment*, 506(3):250–303, 2003.

2. JCL Alfonso and L Berk. Modeling the effect of intratumoral heterogeneity of radiosensitivity on tumor response over the course of fractionated radiation therapy. *Radiation Oncology*, 14(1):1–12, 2019.

3. John Allison, Katsuya Amako, JEA Apostolakis, HAAH Araujo, P Arce Dubois, MAAM Asai, GABG Barrand, RACR Capra, SACS Chauvie, RACR Chytracek, et al. Geant4 developments and applications. *IEEE Transactions on nuclear science*, 53(1):270–278, 2006.

4. M Belli, A Campa, and I Ermolli. A semi-empirical approach to the evaluation of the relative biological effectiveness of therapeutic proton beams: the methodological framework. *Radiation research*, 148(6):592–598, 1997.

5. V. E. Bellinzona, F. Cordoni, M. Missiaggia, F. Tommasino, E. Scifoni, C. La Tessa, and A. Attili. Linking Microdosimetric Measurements to Biological Effectiveness in Ion Beam Therapy: A Review of Theoretical Aspects of MKM and Other Models. *Frontiers in Physics*, 8(February):1–28, 2021.

6. TT Böhlen, F Cerutti, MPW Chin, Alberto Fassò, Alfredo Ferrari, P Garcia Ortega, Andrea Mairani, Paola R Sala, G Smirnov, and V Vlachoudis. The fluka code: developments and challenges for high energy and medical applications. *Nuclear data sheets*, 120:211–214, 2014.

7. Alejandro Carabe, Maryam Moteabbed, Nicolas Depauw, Jan Schuemann, and Harald Paganetti. Range uncertainty in proton therapy due to variable biological effectiveness. *Physics in Medicine & Biology*, 57(5):1159, 2012.

8. David J Carlson, Robert D Stewart, Vladimir A Semenenko, and George A Sandison. Combined use of monte carlo dna damage simulations and deterministic repair models to examine putative mechanisms of cell killing. *Radiation research*, 169(4):447–459, 2008.

9. KH Chadwick and HP Leenhouts. Molecular theory of cell survival. Technical report, Instituut voor Toepassing van Atoomenergie in de Landbouw, Wageningen ..., 1973.

10. A Chatterjee and HJ Schaefer. Microdosimetric structure of heavy ion tracks in tissue. *Radiation and environmental biophysics*, 13(3):215–227, 1976.

11. Y Chen and S Ahmad. Empirical model estimation of relative biological effectiveness for proton beam therapy. *Radiation protection dosimetry*, 149(2):116–123, 2012.

12. Jinhyun Choi and Jin Oh Kang. Basics of particle therapy ii: relative biological effectiveness. *Radiation oncology journal*, 30(1):1, 2012.

13. F Cordoni, M Missiaggia, A Attili, SM Welford, E Scifoni, and C La Tessa. Generalized stochastic microdosimetric model: The main formulation. *Physical Review E*, 103(1):012412, 2021.

14. Tordis Johnsen Dahle, Espen Rusten, Camilla Hanquist Stokkevåg, Antti Silvoniemi, Andrea Mairani, Lars Fredrik Fjæra, Eivind Rørvik, Helge Henjum, Pauliina Wright, Camilla Grindeland Boer, et al. The fluka monte carlo code coupled with an oer model for biologically weighted dose calculations in proton therapy of hypoxic tumors. *Physica Medica*, 76:166–172, 2020.

15. Michael Dingfelder, Detlev Hantke, Mitio Inokuti, and Herwig G Paretzke. Electron inelastic-scattering cross sections in liquid water. *Radiation physics and chemistry*, 53(1):1–18, 1998.

16. Thilo Elsässer and Michael Scholz. Cluster effects within the local effect model. *Radiation research*, 167(3):319–329, 2007.

17. Thilo Elsässer, Wilma K Weyrather, Thomas Friedrich, Marco Durante, Gheorghe Iancu, Michael Krämer, Gabriele Kragl, Stephan Brons, Marcus Winter, Klaus-Josef Weber, et al. Quantification of the relative biological effectiveness for ion beam radiotherapy: direct experimental comparison of proton and carbon ion beams and a novel approach for treatment planning. *International Journal of Radiation Oncology\* Biology\* Physics*, 78(4):1177–1183, 2010.

18. Alfredo Ferrari, Johannes Ranft, Paola R Sala, and A Fassò. *FLUKA: A multi-particle transport code (Program version 2005)*. Number CERN-2005-10. Cern, 2005.

19. Malte C Frese, K Yu Victor, Robert D Stewart, and David J Carlson. A mechanism-based approach to predict the relative biological effectiveness of protons and carbon ions in radiation therapy. *International Journal of Radiation Oncology\* Biology\* Physics*, 83(1):442–450, 2012.

20. Thomas Friedrich, Uwe Scholz, Thilo Elsässer, Marco Durante, and Michael Scholz. Calculation of the biological effects of ion beams based on the microscopic spatial damage distribution pattern. *International journal of radiation biology*, 88(1-2):103–107, 2012.

21. Thomas Friedrich, Uwe Scholz, Thilo ElsäSser, Marco Durante, and Michael Scholz. Systematic analysis of rbe and related quantities using a database of cell survival experiments with ion beam irradiation. *Journal of radiation research*, 54(3):494–514, 2013.

22. Douglas Hanahan and Robert A Weinberg. The hallmarks of cancer. *cell*, 100(1):57–70, 2000.

23. RB Hawkins. A microdosimetric-kinetic model of cell death from exposure to ionizing radiation of any let, with experimental and clinical applications. *International journal of radiation biology*, 69(6):739–755, 1996.

24. Roland B Hawkins. A microdosimetric-kinetic theory of the dependence of the rbe for cell death on let. *Medical physics*, 25(7):1157–1170, 1998.

25. Roland B Hawkins. A microdosimetric-kinetic model for the effect of non-poisson distribution of lethal lesions on the variation of rbe with let. *Radiation research*, 160(1):61–69, 2003.

26. Roland B Hawkins. The relationship between the sensitivity of cells to high-energy photons and the rbe of particle radiation used in radiotherapy. *Radiation research*, 172(6):761–776, 2009.

27. Icru. Prescribing, recording, and reporting photon beam therapy. *ICRU Report 93*, 2016.

28. Taku Inaniwa, Takuji Furukawa, Yuki Kase, Naruhiro Matsufuji, Toshiyuki Toshito, Yoshitaka Matsumoto, Yoshiya Furusawa, and Koji Noda. Treatment planning for a scanned carbon beam with a modified microdosimetric kinetic model. *Physics in Medicine & Biology*, 55(22):6721, 2010.

29. Sébastien Incerti, Gérard Baldacchino, M Bernal, Riccardo Capra, Christophe Champion, Ziad Francis, Paul Guèye, Alfonso Mantero, Barbara Mascialino, Philippe Moretto, et al. The

geant4-dna project. *International Journal of Modeling, Simulation, and Scientific Computing*, 1(02):157–178, 2010.

30. Michael C Joiner and Albert J van der Kogel. *Basic clinical radiobiology*. CRC press, 2018.

31. Bleddyn Jones. A simpler energy transfer efficiency model to predict relative biological effect for protons and heavier ions. *Frontiers in oncology*, 5:184, 2015.

32. Florian Kamp, Gonzalo Cabal, Andrea Mairani, Katia Parodi, Jan J Wilkens, and David J Carlson. Fast biological modeling for voxel-based heavy ion treatment planning using the mechanistic repair-misrepair-fixation model and nuclear fragment spectra. *International Journal of Radiation Oncology\* Biology\* Physics*, 93(3):557–568, 2015.

33. Yuki Kase, Tatsuaki Kanai, Naruhiro Matsufuji, Yoshiya Furusawa, Thilo Elsässer, and Michael Scholz. Biophysical calculation of cell survival probabilities using amorphous track structure models for heavy-ion irradiation. *Physics in Medicine & Biology*, 53(1):37, 2007.

34. Yuki Kase, Tatsuaki Kanai, Yoshitaka Matsumoto, Yoshiya Furusawa, Hiroyuki Okamoto, Toru Asaba, Makoto Sakama, and Hiroshi Shinoda. Microdosimetric measurements and estimation of human cell survival for heavy-ion beams. *Radiation research*, 166(4):629–638, 2006.

35. Albrecht M Kellerer and Harald H Rossi. A generalized formulation of dual radiation action. *Radiation research*, 75(3):471–488, 1978.

36. Jürgen Kiefer and Hermann Straaten. A model of ion track structure based on classical collision dynamics (radiobiology application). *Physics in Medicine & Biology*, 31(11):1201, 1986.

37. Michael Krämer and Gerhard Kraft. Calculations of heavy-ion track structure. *Radiation and environmental biophysics*, 33(2):91–109, 1994.

38. Michael Krämer and Michael Scholz. Rapid calculation of biological effects in ion radiotherapy. *Physics in Medicine & Biology*, 51(8):1959, 2006.

39. G Magro, TJ Dahle, S Molinelli, M Ciocca, P Fossati, A Ferrari, T Inaniwa, N Matsufuji, KS Ytre-Hauge, and A Mairani. The fluka monte carlo code coupled with the nirs approach for clinical dose calculations in carbon ion therapy. *Physics in Medicine & Biology*, 62(9):3814, 2017.

40. A Mairani, S Brons, F Cerutti, A Fasso, A Ferrari, M Krämer, K Parodi, M Scholz, and F Sommerer. The fluka monte carlo code coupled with the local effect model for biological calculations in carbon ion therapy. *Physics in Medicine & Biology*, 55(15):4273, 2010.

41. A Mairani, I Dokic, G Magro, T Tessonnier, J Bauer, TT Böhlen, M Ciocca, A Ferrari, PR Sala, O Jäkel, et al. A phenomenological relative biological effectiveness approach for proton therapy based on an improved description of the mixed radiation field. *Physics in Medicine & Biology*, 62(4):1378, 2017.

42. A Mairani, I Dokic, G Magro, T Tessonnier, F Kamp, DJ Carlson, M Ciocca, F Cerutti, PR Sala, A Ferrari, et al. Biologically optimized helium ion plans: calculation approach and its in vitro validation. *Physics in Medicine & Biology*, 61(11):4283, 2016.

43. A Mairani, G Magro, I Dokic, SM Valle, T Tessonnier, R Galm, M Ciocca, K Parodi, A Ferrari, O Jäkel, et al. Data-driven rbe parameterization for helium ion beams. *Physics in Medicine & Biology*, 61(2):888, 2016.

44. Lorenzo Manganaro, Germano Russo, Roberto Cirio, Federico Dalmasso, Simona Giordanengo, Vincenzo Monaco, Silvia Muraro, Roberto Sacchi, Anna Vignati, and Andrea Attili. A monte carlo approach to the microdosimetric kinetic model to account for dose rate time structure effects in ion beam therapy with application in treatment planning simulations. *Medical physics*, 44(4):1577–1589, 2017.

45. Stephen Joseph McMahon. The linear quadratic model: usage, interpretation and challenges. *Physics in Medicine & Biology*, 64(1):01TR01, 2018.

46. Aimee L McNamara, Jan Schuemann, and Harald Paganetti. A phenomenological relative biological effectiveness (rbe) model for proton therapy based on all published in vitro cell survival data. *Physics in Medicine & Biology*, 60(21):8399, 2015.

47. S Muraro, G Battistoni, and AC Kraan. Challenges in monte carlo simulations as clinical and research tool in particle therapy: a review. *Front. Phys. 8: 567800. doi: 10.3389/fphy*, 2020.

48. Harald Paganetti. Relative biological effectiveness (rbe) values for proton beam therapy. variations as a function of biological endpoint, dose, and linear energy transfer. *Physics in Medicine & Biology*, 59(22):R419, 2014.

49. Harald Paganetti, Eleanor Blakely, Alejandro Carabe-Fernandez, David J Carlson, Indra J Das, Lei Dong, David Grosshans, Kathryn D Held, Radhe Mohan, Vitali Moiseenko, et al. Report of the aapm tg-256 on the relative biological effectiveness of proton beams in radiation therapy. *Medical physics*, 46(3):e53–e78, 2019.

50. Eivind Rørvik, Lars Fredrik Fjæra, Tordis J Dahle, Jon Espen Dale, Grete May Engeseth, Camilla H Stokkevåg, Sara Thörnqvist, and Kristian S Ytre-Hauge. Exploration and application of phenomenological rbe models for proton therapy. *Physics in Medicine & Biology*, 63(18):185013, 2018.

51. Eivind Rørvik, Sara Thörnqvist, Camilla H Stokkevåg, Tordis J Dahle, Lars Fredrik Fjæra, and Kristian S Ytre-Hauge. A phenomenological biological dose model for proton therapy based on linear energy transfer spectra. *Medical physics*, 44(6):2586–2594, 2017.

52. Tatsuhiko Sato and Yoshiya Furusawa. Cell survival fraction estimation based on the probability densities of domain and cell nucleus specific energies using improved microdosimetric kinetic models. *Radiation research*, 178(4):341–356, 2012.

53. Tatsuhiko Sato, Yosuke Iwamoto, Shintaro Hashimoto, Tatsuhiko Ogawa, Takuya Furuta, Shinichiro Abe, Takeshi Kai, Pi-En Tsai, Norihiro Matsuda, Hiroshi Iwase, et al. Features of particle and heavy ion transport code system (phits) version 3.02. *Journal of Nuclear Science and Technology*, 55(6):684–690, 2018.

54. Tatsuhiko Sato, Koji Niita, Norihiro Matsuda, Shintaro Hashimoto, Yosuke Iwamoto, Shusaku Noda, Tatsuhiko Ogawa, Hiroshi Iwase, Hiroshi Nakashima, Tokio Fukahori, et al. Particle and heavy ion transport code system, phits, version 2.52. *Journal of Nuclear Science and Technology*, 50(9):913–923, 2013.

55. Gaetano Savoca, Marco Calvaruso, Luigi Minafra, Valentina Bravatà, Francesco Paolo Cammarata, Giuseppina Iacoviello, Boris Abbate, Giovanna Evangelista, Massimiliano Spada, Giusi Irma Forte, et al. Local disease-free survival rate (lsr) application to personalize radiation therapy treatments in breast cancer models. *Journal of personalized medicine*, 10(4):177, 2020.

56. M Scholz, AM Kellerer, W Kraft-Weyrather, and G Kraft. Computation of cell survival in heavy ion beams for therapy. *Radiation and environmental biophysics*, 36(1):59–66, 1997.

57. E Scifoni, W Tinganelli, WK Weyrather, M Durante, A Maier, and M Krämer. Including oxygen enhancement ratio in ion beam treatment planning: model implementation and experimental verification. *Physics in Medicine & Biology*, 58(11):3871, 2013.

58. Le Tang, Fang Wei, Yingfen Wu, Yi He, Lei Shi, Fang Xiong, Zhaojian Gong, Can Guo, Xiayu Li, Hao Deng, et al. Role of metabolism in cancer cell radioresistance and radiosensitization methods. *Journal of Experimental & Clinical Cancer Research*, 37(1):1–15, 2018.

59. Nina Tilly, Jonas Johansson, Ulf Isacsson, Joakim Medin, Erik Blomquist, Erik Grusell, and Bengt Glimelius. The influence of rbe variations in a clinical proton treatment plan for a hypopharynx cancer. *Physics in Medicine & Biology*, 50(12):2765, 2005.

60. Walter Tinganelli, Marco Durante, Ryoichi Hirayama, Michael Krämer, Andreas Maier, Wilma Kraft-Weyrather, Yoshiya Furusawa, Thomas Friedrich, and Emanuele Scifoni. Kill-painting of hypoxic tumours in charged particle therapy. *Scientific reports*, 5(1):1–13, 2015.

61. C Wälzlein, M Krämer, E Scifoni, and M Durante. Advancing the modeling in particle therapy: From track structure to treatment planning. *Applied Radiation and Isotopes*, 83:171–176, 2014.

62. Minna Wedenberg, Bengt K Lind, and Björn Hårdemark. A model for the relative biological effectiveness of protons: the tissue specific parameter $\alpha/\beta$ of photons is a predictor for the sensitivity to let changes. *Acta oncologica*, 52(3):580–588, 2013.

63. Tatiana Wenzl and Jan J Wilkens. Modelling of the oxygen enhancement ratio for ion beam radiation therapy. *Physics in Medicine & Biology*, 56(11):3251, 2011.

64. JJ Wilkens and U Oelfke. A phenomenological model for the relative biological effectiveness in therapeutic proton beams. *Physics in Medicine & Biology*, 49(13):2811, 2004.

65. M Zaider and HH Rossi. The synergistic effects of different radiations. *Radiation research*, pages 732–739, 1980.

# 11 Physical and biological impact of projectile and target fragmentation

*Elettra Bellinzona and Francesco Tommasino*
TIFPA-INFN Trento Institute for Fundamental Physics, Trento,
Italy
University of Trento, Trento, Italy

*Andrea Attili*
Roma Tre Section, INFN National Institute for Nuclear Physics,
Rome, Italy

*Emanuele Scifoni*
TIFPA-INFN Trento Institute for Fundamental Physics and
Applications, Trento, Italy

## CONTENTS

THE BIOPHYSICAL IMPACT of nuclear fragmentation of particle beams relevant for therapy, accounting for both processes arising from projectile and target nuclei, is here reviewed and summarized, emphasizing the role and relevance of nuclear fragmentation measurements and calculations in different media, for getting correct assessments of the biological weighted dose profile in particle therapy plans.

## 11.1 INTRODUCTION

Fragmentation processes are part of the interactions taking place when charged particles traverse matter. Such processes play a significant role in different scenarios of practical interest, as for instance charged particle therapy (CPT) and space radioprotection [13, 14]. Here, the focus will be on CPT related Monte Carlo applications. In this context, it is useful to mention that, despite several ions having been proposed for therapeutic applications, only protons and carbon ions are currently employed. It is however worth mentioning that extensive studies are ongoing to evaluate the clinical potential of helium and oxygen ions [65, 47, 62, 51] In this Section, the basics of charged particles' interactions with matter will be shortly described, with special emphasis on the aspects of interest for the radiobiological implications of fragmentation. Several excellent reviews exist on the topic, to which the reader is addressed for further details [14, 70].

When considering the use of accelerated ions for cancer therapy, it is appropriate to focus on the energy range that is sufficient to cover a deep-seated target (i.e. up to 25-30 cm depth). Depending on the particle, this corresponds to an energy up to about 450 MeV/n, which reflects into $\beta = v/c$ in the order of 0.6-0.7. In this context, the main mechanism of energy loss is the ionization of atomic shell electrons. This process can be well described by means of the Bethe equation, which provides the energy loss per travel path length:

$$\frac{dE}{dx} = \frac{4\pi e^4 Z_t Z_p^2}{m_e v^2} \left[ \ln \frac{2m_e v^2}{I} - \ln(1 - \beta^2) - \frac{C}{Z_t} - \frac{\delta}{2} \right] \tag{11.1}$$

where $\beta = v/c$, with $v$ speed of the particle and $c$ speed of the light, $Z_p$ and $Z_t$ indicate the projectile and target charge respectively, $m_e$ and $e$ refer to electron mass and charge, while $I$ is the mean ionization energy for a target atom or molecule. The last two terms between brackets are correction terms. The mean energy loss provided by Eq. 11.1 corresponds to the stopping power of the particle, which usually goes under the name of linear energy transfer (LET) in radiobiology and related applications. Summarizing, Eq. 11.1 indicates that the LET is directly proportional to the squared effective charge of the incoming particle and inversely proportional to its energy. Once the charged particle fluence is known, the LET can be used to estimate the dose received by a given cell (expressed in Gy, 1 Gy = 1 J/kg), taking into account the density of the medium:

$$D[Gy] = 1.6 \cdot 10^{-9} \frac{dE}{dx} \left[ \frac{keV}{\mu m} \right] F[cm^{-2}] \frac{1}{\rho} \left[ \frac{cm^3}{g} \right] \tag{11.2}$$

Eq. 11.2 shows that, at first approximation, the physical dose received by a cell is directly proportional to the particle LET. However, further considerations to translate this information in terms of expected biological effect are needed (see below).

According to the particle initial energy and to the related stopping power, the range of a particle in a given medium can be calculated, under the continuous slowing down approximation as:

$$R_{CSDA} = \int_0^L dx = \int_E^0 \frac{dE}{dE/dx} \tag{11.3}$$

Importantly, for different particles of the same energy traversing a given medium, the range can be scaled based on their mass and charge, according to:

$$\frac{R_2}{R_1} = \frac{M_2}{M_1} \frac{z_1^2}{z_2^2} \tag{11.4}$$

This indicates that, for instance, the lighter fragments produced by an incoming carbon ion in the patient tissues will travel more than the primary beam. This also leads us to a short reminder on fragmentation aspects of interest for CPT. In the case of proton therapy, only fragmentation of the target is possible, which results in the generation of neutrons, secondary protons and heavier recoils. The latter, due to the heavier mass compared to the primary proton beam and according to Eq. 11.4 are expected to have a much shorter range and higher LET, leading to peculiar radiobiological considerations. When carbon ions are considered, fragmentation of the primary beam takes place too. In a typical carbon ion treatment, this is responsible for about 50% of primary ions reaching the target, with the remaining fraction transformed into lighter fragments that distort the depth-dose profile. Remarkably, such lighter fragments are responsible for the dose tail observed distal from the carbon Bragg peak. As for target fragments, this also deserves a dedicated radiobiological analysis. In the energy range of interest, the fragmentation processes are reasonably well described by nucleus-nucleus collision models, which are based on the two-step process of abrasion-ablation. In this framework, the nucleus-nucleus reaction cross section is obtained by subtracting the elastic cross section from the total one:

$$\sigma_R = \sigma_{Tot} - \sigma_{el} \tag{11.5}$$

The reaction cross section can be described by means of the Bradt-Peters formula:

$$\sigma_R = \pi r_0^2 (A_p^{1/3} + A_t^{1/3} - b)^2 \tag{11.6}$$

where $r_0$ indicates the nucleus radius and $b$ is a correction factor for overlap. While Eq. 11.6 well describes high energy interactions, several parameterizations were obtained to extend its application to the energy range of interest in CPT [67, 66, 13].

What described so far indicates that, in a typical mixed field originating from fragmentation processes, we will have to deal with a spectrum of particles. For each of these particles, we expect a distribution of energies (and therefore of range) and LET values. This obviously has an impact on the biological effects associated with the irradiation [59]. The detailed description of methods suitable to take into account such effects is demanded in later Sections. We can anticipate that such methods will aim at an accurate description of the so-called RBE (relative biological effectiveness, i.e. the ratio of photon to charged particle dose needed to achieve the same biological effect) associated with a specific irradiation. In fact, the RBE parameter depends on a number of physical and biological quantities. Among the first, in a mixed irradiation field, the RBE will be influenced by the LET of different particle species, each of them contributing with a specific dose. The general trend will show an RBE increasing for increasing LET and decreasing physical dose. Track structure criteria and microdosimetry can be also employed to describe the effects of a mixed field.

In the effort to elucidate the biological effects of a mixed radiation field, a remarkable role is played by Monte Carlo codes. In fact, such codes are adopted to describe, at different levels of accuracy, the spectra of secondary particles arising from the interaction of the primary beam with target materials. As discussed above, this is the starting information for algorithms dedicated to radiobiological calculations. While for several years Monte Carlo was limited to research applications in CPT, with the advent of modern calculators and more efficient software it is now possible to find clinical applications of Monte Carlo codes. On the one hand, being associated with the distortion of the depth-dose profile, projectile fragmentation effects cannot be neglected in carbon ion treatment planning. On the other hand, target fragmentation is usually not explicitly taken into account, or at least strongly approximated, in proton therapy dose calculations. In both cases, an accurate description of fragmentation processes is needed in order to translate such effects first into a physical dose contribution, and finally into a biological effect.

From this point of view, one limitation is currently represented by the limited set of nuclear reaction cross sections on which Monte Carlo codes rely. In fact, the large investigations performed in the 60'–70's in nuclear physics left some gaps in the energy range and materials of interest for CPT [8]. Even though that represents an intrinsic obstacle, recent scientific initiatives could contribute to expanding the available nuclear cross section data. In this context, it is worth mentioning the FOOT (fragmentation of target) experiment [4], financed by the INFN (Italian national institute for nuclear physics). Based on a large scientific collaboration, FOOT will build a new experimental apparatus that will be dedicated to the systematic investigation of reaction cross section for particle species of interest for both CPT and space radioprotection (e.g. protons, carbon, helium, oxygen

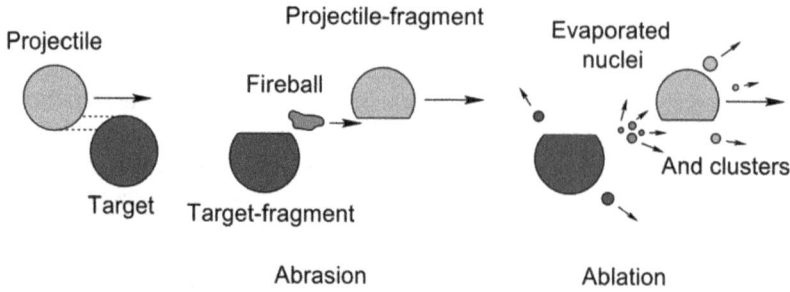

**Figure 11.1**   Illustration of the abrasion-ablation model of collisions at high energies according to Serber [61]. Figure taken from [25].

ions). By exploiting a direct and inverse kinematic approach, FOOT will provide new data for both projectile and target fragmentation, respectively.

## 11.2   PHYSICAL ASPECTS IN MC SIMULATIONS

Particles generated from ion fragmentation reactions are typically described as either "projectile" fragments or "target" fragments. The charge and mass of the primary particles are relevant to determine the specific contribution of fragments. In the case of an ion beam irradiation with high $Z$ ($Z \gtrsim 2$) the projectile fragments play the major role, while for proton beams a potentially non negligible dose enhancement can be observed due to the presence of target fragments.

Fragmentation reactions have been extensively studied in nuclear physics (see, e.g. [22, 32, 49] and experimental data are available for many projectile-target combinations and for a wide range of beam energies [20]. However, the production cross-section data of the target fragments and their energy spectra in the clinical energy ranges has still uncertainties, caused by the difficulty of the measurement of few events with low energy and range.

The nucleus-nucleus collision models used in therapy transport codes to evaluate the fragment generation processes, such as the intra-nuclear cascade, molecular dynamics, etc. (for a review see [42, 53]) are mainly variants of the abrasion-ablation model [61]. According to this model production of fragments is interpreted as a two-step process (see Figure 11.1). In the first step (abrasion, time scale $\sim 10^{-23} - 10^{-22}$s), nucleons are abraded in the overlapping reaction zone (the "fireball") while the outer spectator nucleons are only slightly affected. In the second step (ablation, time scale $\sim 10^{-18} - 10^{-16}$s), the residual projectile and target fragments de-excite by evaporation of nucleons or clusters.

While charged target fragments consist of short-ranged high-LET particles and deposit energy mainly along the path of the incident ion, the fragmentation of the projectile has more varied effects, significantly increasing the complexity of the treatment planning. Projectile fragmentations cause a loss of primary beam particles and a buildup of lighter lower-Z fragments. The target fragments (TF) are fewer than the projectile fragments and have low kinetic energies and/or high atomic numbers compared to the incident beam.

Although deterministic corrections to the dose profiles evaluations that accounts for the nuclear reaction and tissue material compositions have been proposed [33] (see also section 4), the most proper way to account for their effects is to explicitly track each one of them through MC simulations, since they can propagate significantly from the interaction vertex and can undergo further complex interactions through the heterogeneous medium.

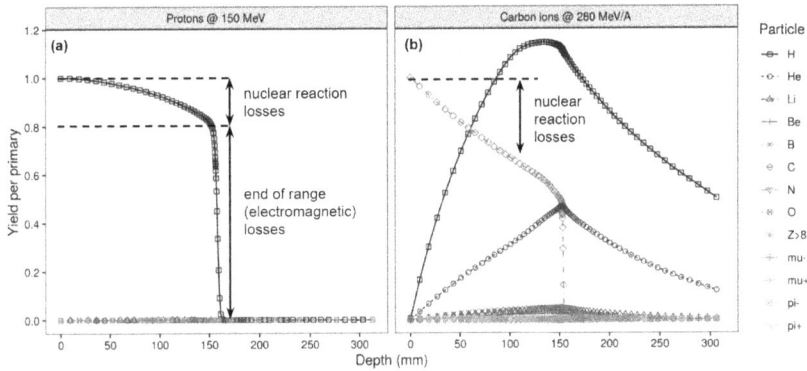

**Figure 11.2** Example of a simulation of particle yields (primary and fragments) versus depth in a water phantom for a monoenergetic 150 MeV proton beam (a) and 280 MeV/u carbon ion beam (b). The simulation has been performed with the FLUKA code.

### 11.2.1 EXPLOITING PROJECTILE AND TARGET FRAGMENTS

In some cases, projectile and target fragments can actually be profitably exploited. For instance, the production of $\beta\pm$ unstable fragments, such as $^{10}$C, $^{11}$C, $^{15}$O, and $^{13}$N, can be used for in vivo range monitoring applications in quality assurance of the beam delivery [17, 55]. The decay positrons from the $\beta+$ emitters are quickly stopped and annihilate, producing two characteristics back-to-back gamma rays that can be detected and traced to the annihilation vertex. This technique (positron-emission tomography, PET) can be applied during the beam delivery or after the irradiation. The $\beta+$ activity profiles exhibit two different components: a flat decreasing background resulting from target fragmentation and a pronounced peak structure caused by projectile fragments. For these applications, the most important general purpose codes such as Fluka and Geant4 are able to predict the production of the most abundant nuclides (like $^{11}$C, $^{15}$O,) with sufficient quality. The main challenge remains in the capability of predicting nuclides with short lifetimes, where also the available experimental measurements are scarce [53].

Fast fragments, mainly protons produced in the abrasion step, capable of escaping out of the patient can also be used for range monitoring applications [2]. The main issue in these kinds of simulations is that the most accurate measurement of a proton emission distribution correlates with the dose profiles achieved by detecting particles emitted at large angles with respect to the beam direction. From the modelling point of view, it is not a trivial task to reproduce with the same quality both fragmentation at small angles, the most important as far as the dose is concerned, and the emission at large angles [53].

### 11.2.2 PROJECTILE FRAGMENTS

Nuclear reactions involving the fragmentation of the primary projectiles play an important role in medical applications of radiation physics and space shielding. A relevant example of medical application is cancer therapy using ions beams [43]. In particular, in carbon ion beam therapy [44, 3], nuclear fragmentation of the carbon projectiles yields fast light nuclei which may deposit undesired energy in healthy tissues around and beyond the target, thereby degrading the conformity of the delivered dose distribution.

In a typical carbon ion therapy treatment, projectile fragmentation greatly reduces the fluence of primary ions. As an example, in the case of a 280 MeV/u only $\sim$50% of the ions actually reach the Bragg peak, the others undergoing fragmentation (see Figure 11.2).

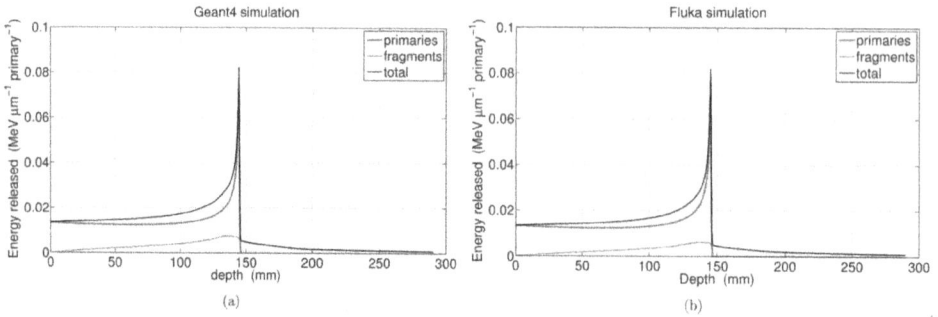

**Figure 11.3** Comparison of Geant4 (a) and Fluka (b) simulated Bragg peaks, generated by a 270 MeV/u carbon ion beam incident on a homogeneous water phantom. The decomposition of the two Bragg Peaks in the contributions of primaries and fragments is also shown.

The produced lighter and lower-LET particles usually have greater ranges than the primary beam ions and deposit energy well beyond the Bragg peak. This leads to the characteristic tail beyond the Bragg peak (see Figure 11.3). Furthermore, although projectile fragments approximately preserve the direction and velocity of the incident particle, a part of low-LET particles may also be produced at significant angles with respect to the incoming beam (see Figure 11.4) and are subjected to greater lateral straggling caused by multiple Coulomb scattering due to their smaller mass [52, 26]. Even though the dose contribution of a single pencil beam is small, when combining thousands of them, they could result in a significant lateral contribution of dose into healthy tissues.

The projectile fragmentation effects effectively limit the maximum ion charge that can be used in treatments. Current practice in Japan and Europe has largely been focused on carbon ions (Z=6) as representing a more optimal trade. Helium ions (Z=2, A=4) are also of considerable interest, and our analysis of recently obtained cross-sectional data suggests that they may provide a localization advantage. This arises from the fact that the nucleons in helium nuclei are especially tightly bound, making them relatively less likely to fragment [58].

### 11.2.3 TARGET FRAGMENTS

Similarly to projectile fragments, also TF produce a decrement in primary beam fluence alongside a higher penetration depth and a build-up effect [23, 64, 54, 56], although smaller than the case of projectile fragmentation. The build-up, mainly forward-emitted secondary protons and alpha particles, affects the entrance channel region [5] and therefore may also affect particularly healthy tissues. The Monte Carlo codes are widely used to distinguish the primary contribution with respect to the secondaries' one, where the fluence or the track-length fluence distribution are scored in the interested volumes. The second scoring method is usually preferred in the case of a proton irradiation where the short range of fragments implies high statistics, and therefore high calculation time, to score a significant amount of secondary particles. Various nuclear models are available that extrapolate the poor experimental data [4]. An example of a track-length fluence divided for species obtained with FLUKA MC is given in Figure 11.5.

The contribution of target fragments to the dose can be approximately evaluated considering the energy lost per unit depth in inelastic nuclear interactions for each depth $i$, as deposited locally at a depth $z_i$ and hence determined by the product of the proton energy, $E_i$, for the probability per unit path length of a non-elastic nuclear interaction, $\mu_{nuc}$, weighted by the fraction of energy converted into charged particles, $f_{cp}$, and by the length of the depth interval $\Delta z_i$[9]. The energy imparted in the layer $\Delta z_i$ due to inelastic nuclear interactions, $\varepsilon_n$, is then

$$\varepsilon_n[\Delta z_i] = \mu_{nuc}(E_i)f_{cp}(E_i)E_i\Delta z_i \qquad (11.7)$$

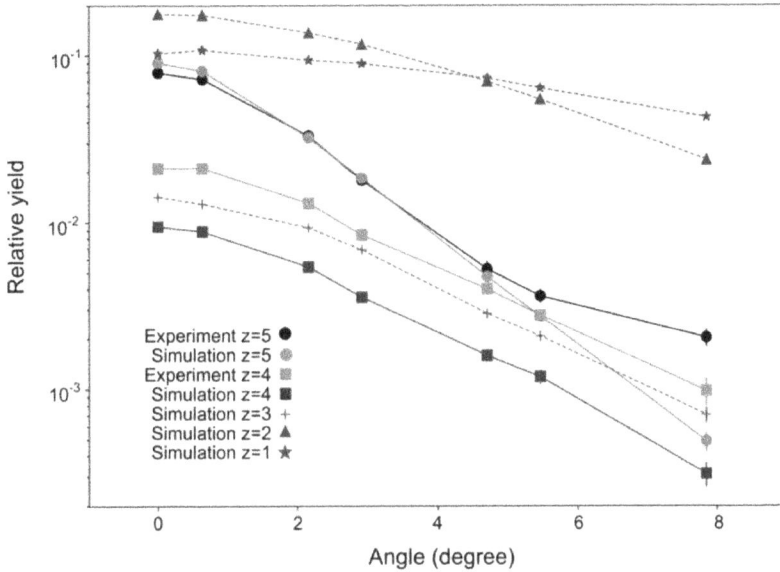

**Figure 11.4**   Angular distribution of the yield of fragments collected from a 380 MeV/u carbon ion beam interacting in a water thickness. $0°$ corresponds to the beam direction. The yield was normalized to the total number of $Z = 4$ and 5 at $0°$. For $Z = 4$ and 5, both simulations (performed using Geant4) and experimental results (measurements obtained using a CR39 plastic detector) were drawn. For $Z = 1, 2,$ and 3, only simulation results were drawn. Figure taken from [30].

Such quantity is then added to the energy from primary particles, $\varepsilon_{prim}$, to evaluate the total energy imparted in the step $z_i$, $\varepsilon_{tot}$ by weighting for the two contributions with the nuclear survival weight factor $W_n$, that considers the probability that a primary has not been lost from the beam in an inelastic interaction:

$$\varepsilon_{tot}\,[\Delta z_i] = W_n(E_i)(\varepsilon_{prim}[\Delta z_i] + \varepsilon_n[\Delta z_i]\mu_{nuc})\tag{11.8}$$

This approach evaluates the physical dose contribution of secondary particles, which results mainly in the build-up effect in the entrance region and a nuclear fragmentation tail after the BP particularly enhanced for projectile fragments.

## 11.3   RADIOBIOLOGICAL EVALUATIONS

A basic radiobiological parameter used in ion beam therapy is the relative biological effectiveness (RBE), defined as the ratio of doses of photons and charged particles inducing the same biological effect. Heavier particles irradiation exhibit potential advantages due to their increasing RBE toward the Bragg peak position. However, the RBE depends not only on depth, but in a complex way also on other parameters, such as ion charge and energy, dose level, and intrinsic tissue radiosensitivity. From a biological point of view, the biological effects of fragments cannot be neglected, because the charged fragments with high LET can be particularly damaging and are functional to the determination of the exact value of RBE, in particular in the healthy tissues surrounding the tumor volume.

   Among the various models to consider the biological effect of fragments, two categories can be depicted:

1. including secondary particles in LET calculation to predict RBE, used in particular in the case of proton beam and target fragments [50];

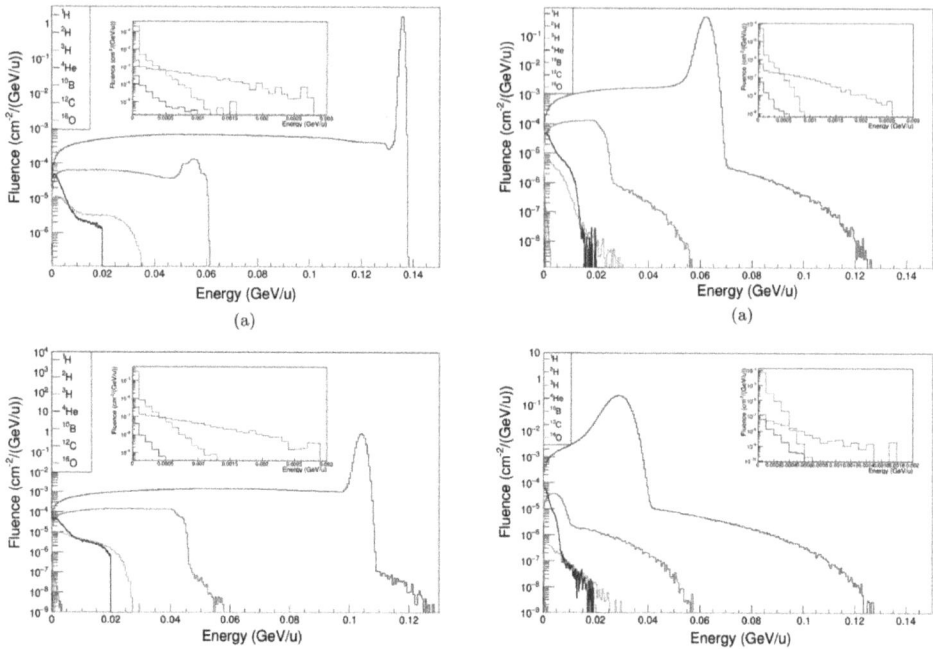

**Figure 11.5** Fluence of target fragments induced by 150 MeV protons in water, calculated with FLUKA MC code, at a depth of 2.5 (a) , 7.5 cm (b) 12.5 (a) and 15 cm (b) where the Bragg Peak position is 15.8 cm. Picture from [16].

  2. mechanistic RBE models in which the TF are considered in a more general mixed field
     approach.

The main mechanistic RBE models used in ion beam therapy are the local effect model (LEM) [60, 15, 21] the microdosimetric kinetic model (MKM) [28, 29, 41, 40] and the repair-misrepair-fixation (RMF) model [7, 19, 37]. The original version of LEM, referred to as LEM I, as well as the MKM are in routine clinical use for carbon ion treatment planning [46, 1]. For a review of RBE models see [39] and [63]. Further details are also given in Chapter 10 (Monte Carlo to link RBE with radiation quality quantities).

The generated fragments can be treated as secondary particles that contribute to create a mixed radiation field. The $LET_D$-based approaches, as the one described in [50] that includes also the effects of fragments with Z=1 and Z=2, approximate the mixed field effects and give reasonable predictions in the case of proton beams. Although an attempt to evaluate the RBE using a $LET_D$-based functional dependence has been made also for carbon ion beams, including the effects of the fragments [11], in general, the exclusive use of the $LET_D$ is not appropriate to describe the RBE of any mixed radiation field of protons and heavier ions [24]. In the case of complex mixed radiation fields that occur in clinical cases, where various energies, inhomogeneities and fragments are present causing an increase in the LET distribution width, significant deviations are found from $LET_D$-based evaluations with respect to the experimental data. These deviations are due in particular to the non-linear radiobiological effects, overkilling and/or saturation effects, observed and predicted by the mechanistic models for the high-LET beam components [24, 5]. A quantification of this deviation is reported in Figure 11.6.

A general method to account for a complex mixed field with different irradiations of different qualities is given by a formalism derived by [69]. This approach considers the radiobiological contribution of each single component separately, evaluating the average parameters $\alpha$ and $\beta$ to be used

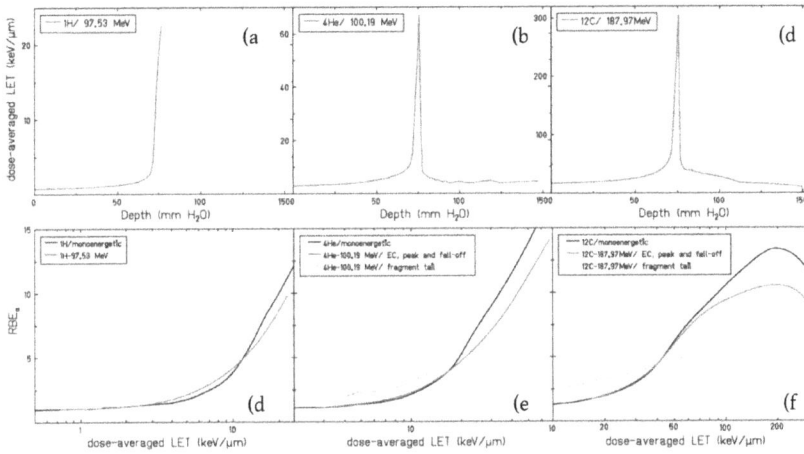

**Figure 11.6** (a-c) LET$_D$ vs. depth in water for proton (97.53 MeV), helium (100.19 MeV) and carbon ion (187.97 MeV) beams (the energies have been chosen in a way that the range in water is equivalent to 72 mm for protons). (d-f) (RBE$_\alpha$) vs LET$_D$ for the same beams. The RBE is based on the predictions of the LEM considering the complete LET spectra (primary and fragments) and refers to cell with linear quadratic ratio $\alpha/\beta = 2$ Gy. The black line in each subfigure is the corresponding RBE evaluated considering monoenergetic radiation as composed only by primary particles with LET = LET$_D$. Figure from [24].

in the linear-quadratic model of cell survival $S$ as a function of delivered dose $D$:

$$-\ln(S(D)) = \bar{\alpha}D + \bar{\beta}D^2 \tag{11.9}$$

where

$$\bar{\alpha} = \left( \sum_i w_i dE(i)/dx \right)^{-1} \sum_i w_i dE(i)/dx\,\alpha_i; \; \sqrt{\bar{\beta}} = \left( \sum_i w_i dE(i)/dx \right)^{-1} \sum_i w_i dE(i)/dx\sqrt{\beta_i}; \tag{11.10}$$

with $w_i$ that denotes the relative weight of the radiation component $i$ that comprise contributions from all particle types and energies from all pencil beams at a given voxel, $dE(i)/dx$ its energy loss (LET), and $\alpha_i$, $\beta_i$ are the radio-sensitivity coefficients of the $i$ component. Further details for mixed field approaches are given also in Chapter 10 (Monte Carlo to link RBE with radiation quality quantities)

The radiobiological effects of fragments also play an important role in comparative studies of dose distributions and cell survival fractions as functions of different primary ion types. These studies shows that the optimal normal tissue sparing was highly dependent on the $\alpha/\beta$ ratio of both the normal and the target tissue [57, 6]. However, this optimality is also very sensitive to the specific implementation of the simulations and the adopted nuclear and radiobiological models [18]. Different physical and radiobiological implementations could bring to different results and this could be obviously relevant when the simulations are used to support treatment choices among competitive modalities [68]. This sensitivity ultimately arises due to the delicate interplay between the conformity of the dose distribution and the RBE, and their complex dependence on both primary particles and projectile fragments contributions, found in the tumoral target volume and in the surrounding healthy tissues. For a thorough discussion see also Section 5.2. Towards Multiple Ion therapy in Particle therapy.

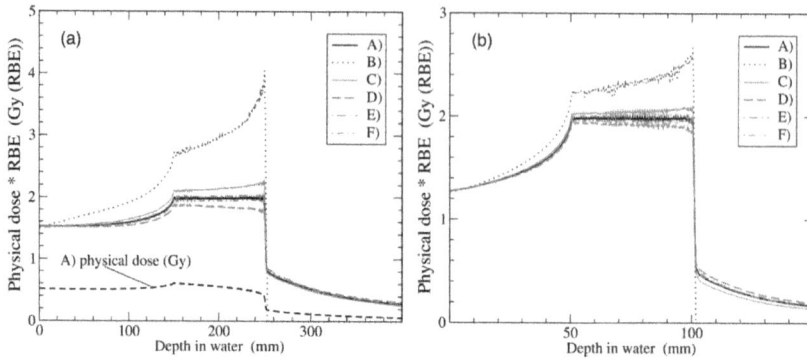

**Figure 11.7**   Dose distributions for carbon ions in water using the six different cases (A)–(F) of modelling nuclear interactions as specified in the following: (A) Reference: nuclear models as in SHIELD-HIT10A. (B) Turning off nuclear reactions entirely. (C) Decreasing all inelastic cross sections by 20%. (D) Increasing all inelastic cross sections by 20%. (E) Fermi-breakup model parameters: $V_{ft}/V_0 = 1$ and $V^C_{ft}/V_0 = 1$. (F) Fermi-breakup model parameters: $V_{ft}/V_0 = 30$ and $V^C_{ft}/V_0 = 30$. The free volume, $V_{ft}/V_0$, and the Coulomb volume, $V^C_{ft}/V_0$, are two adjustable parameters of SHIELD-HIT's Fermi-breakup model [27]. Figure taken from [48].

## 11.3.1   PROJECTILE FRAGMENTS

In order to determine the influence of modeling projectile nuclear fragmentation in the evaluation of the RBE weighted dose, a comparison between different evaluation modalities has been performed in [48] using the MC code SHIELD-HIT(10A) [27] in combination with the TPS TRiP98 [46]. An example of these comparisons for a longitudinal profile of a biologically optimized carbon ion SOBP are reported in Figure 11.7, together with a brief description of the different evaluation modalities. The RBE is obtained through an implementation of the LEM I [60]. These evaluations show the impact of nuclear fragmentation and how the uncertainties in nuclear model implementations could propagate on both the physical dose and the radiobiological assessments. The fragments, due to their Coulomb scattering, play a significant role in the assessment of the RBE in out-of-field conditions. An exemplary evaluation of RBE in the case of the lateral distribution is reported in Figure 11.8 for the case of a carbon ion beam crossing a water phantom, using a MKM implementation [41].

## 11.3.2   TARGET FRAGMENTS

The interest in considering secondary particles originated for the fragmentation of the target is mainly radio-biological; even if the TF constitute no more than 6% of the total fluence [5], they show a non negligible impact on the relative biological effectiveness (RBE) of a proton beam [12, 54, 5] due to an LET$_D$ that reaches a factor up to 10 higher than those of the primary protons at the same depth [23], as reported in Figure 11.9 for a 150 MeV pencil beam in a prostate patient.

An example of the non negligible radiobiological impact of target fragments is shown in Figure 11.10 where the survival curves are evaluated for a proton BP of initial energy of 160 MeV with a mixed field approach in TRiP98 TPS [45, 46] considering only primary protons or including also target fragments and compared with experimental survival values published in [31] for T98 cell line at different depths.

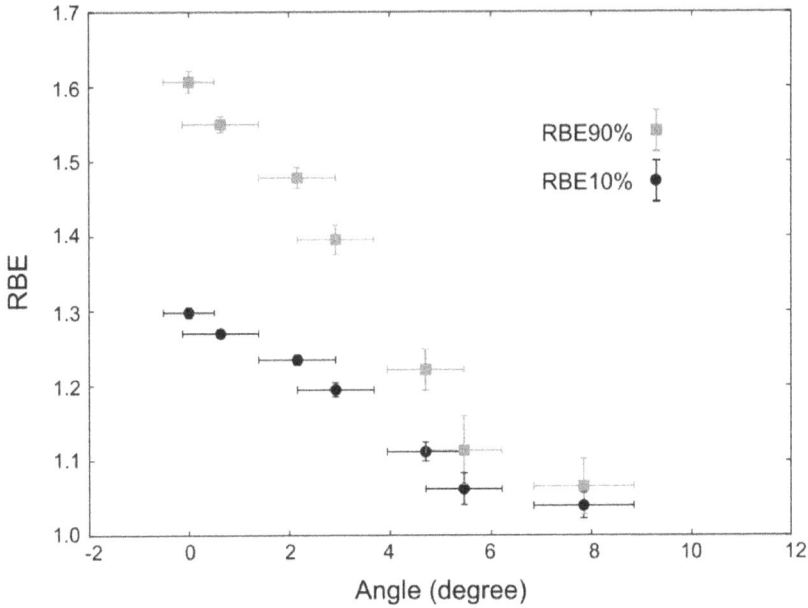

**Figure 11.8**   Angular RBE distributions (90% and 10% cell survival) derived from secondary fragments (reported in figure fragments-angle) produced from a 380 MeV/u carbon ion beam in a water phantom. The evaluation has been carried out using the MKM. Figure taken from [30].

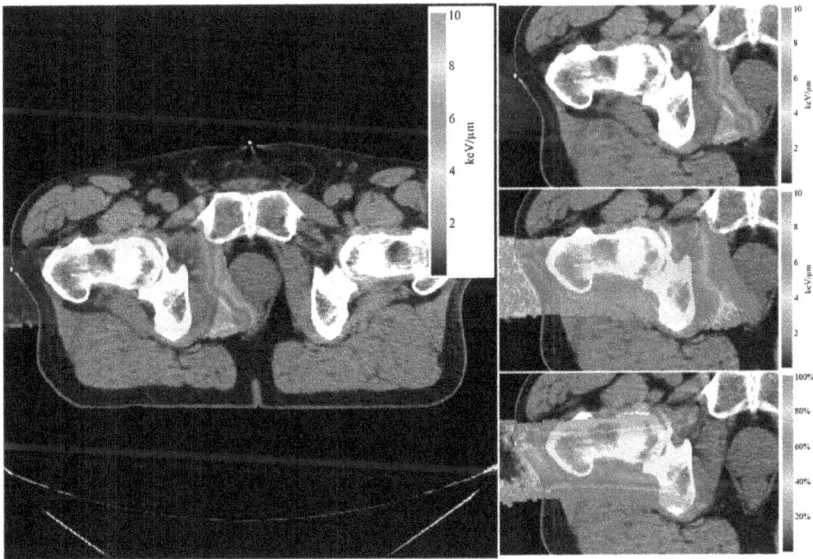

**Figure 11.9**   Prostate patient irradiated with a pristine proton beam (160 MeV): $\text{LET}_D$ of primary and secondary protons combined (a). $\text{LET}_D$ of primary protons only (b), secondary protons only (c) and the percentage difference between primary protons only and the combined dose-averaged $\text{LET}_D$ of primary and secondary protons (d). All $\text{LET}_D$ values are in $keV/\mu m$ in unit density tissue. The evaluations have been performed using GEANT4 Monte Carlo code. Figure from [23].

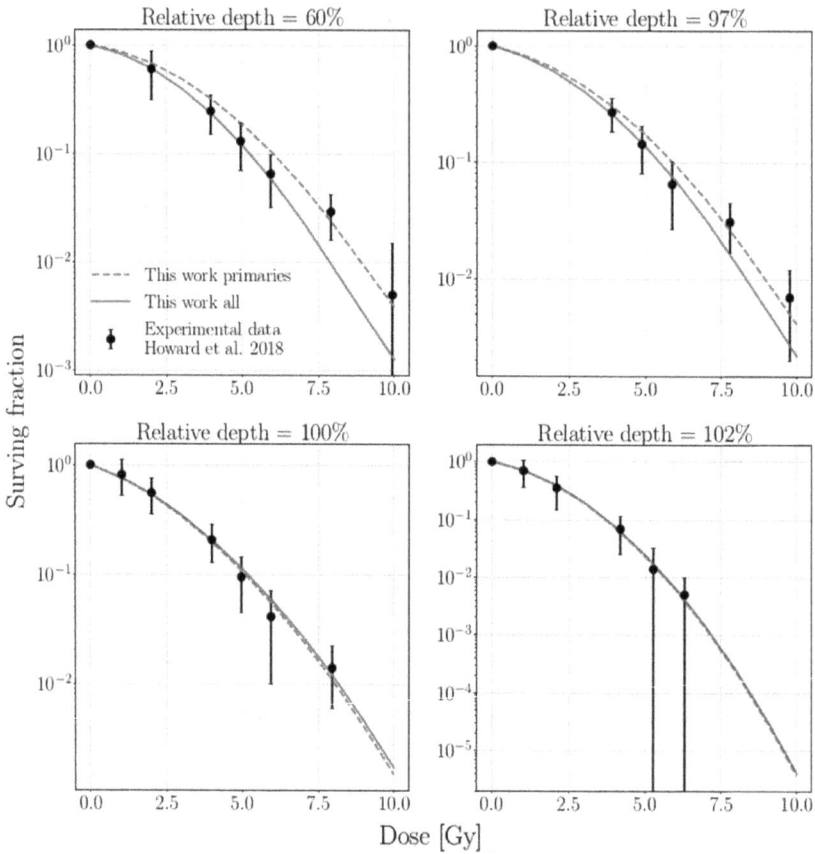

**Figure 11.10**  Surviving fraction for T98 cell line as a function of dose for an initial proton beam energy of 160 MeV. Solid lines represent linear interpolations for the surviving fraction evaluated with 1 MeV step considering the contribution of only primary protons (dashed) or all particles (solid). Figure from [5].

## 11.4  THE IMPORTANCE OF THE MATERIAL DEFINITIONS IN TREATMENT SIMULATIONS

Both in the case of projectile and target fragmentation, a major complication is arising from the need to describe different types of target media, in a physiologic environment, which can imply different nuclei interactions as the conventional assumption of the water molecule components, with the projectile particles ( p or C namely). Major advancements in this field in order to consider approximated methods have been realized by the NIRS group, while recent measurements performed at GSI open the way to consider explicitly experimentally characterized cross-sections and primary particle attenuation / secondary particle yields from the ion interaction with bone material. The elemental composition is in fact relevant information for defining the nuclear interaction at play in each voxel but is normally disregarded. Such composition can be ideally linked to the CT information (through the Hounsfield look-up table) as it is for example already provided in some advanced Monte Carlo Treatment Planning Systems like RayStation, in order to provide a voxel-by-voxel election of nuclear interactions, to be propagated in the beam transport algorithms and consequent dose calculations engine.

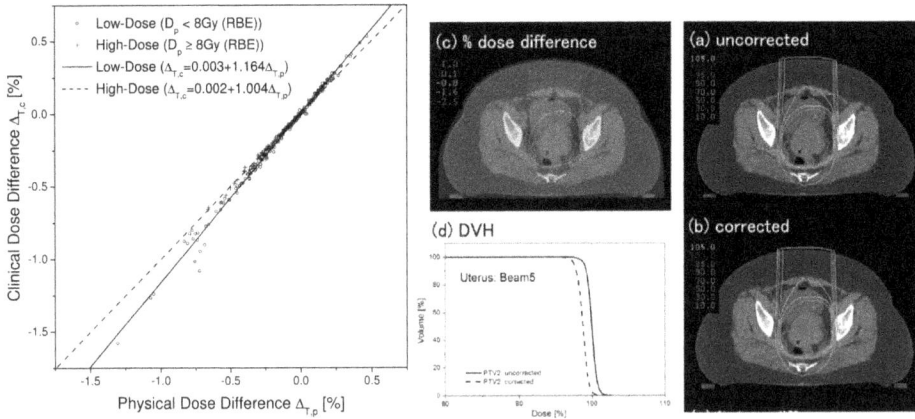

**Figure 11.11**    Approximated approach [35] for evaluating the impact of nuclear fragmentation of high dense target materials (bones,left) and its propagation to treatment plans (right).

## 11.4.1   BEYOND THE WATER APPROXIMATION

Predicting the effect of radiation for different materials was typically done only on the level of relative stopping power ratios and density scaling. However, such an approach neglects completely the effect of different nuclear fragmentation arising from the different constituent nuclei, producing different particle yields, and thus, not only a potentially different absorbed dose profile, but, especially in the case of heavier ions (C, O) an importantly different energetic spectrum of particles and thus, in a mixed field based calculation of the RBE weighted dose, as above mentioned, the final biological effects can be relevantly different, especially in the regions close to the major inhomogeneities (bones, entrance of the patient), cases which may a larger importance for example in a bone metastasis treatment or in a lung treatment close to the ribs, or in a prostate treatment, close to the femoral head. Besides the organic materials, indeed, other relevant compositions are those from dose delivery devices, such as the PMMA of range shifters, or the Graphite (Carbon) composing the beds often traversed, with irradiations from angles below the patient.

## 11.4.2   THE NIRS APPROACH

Recently the National Institute of Radiological Sciences (NIRS) group pioneered this field, introducing several approximated methods to keep into account the beam fragmentation in non-water like targets. These studies [38, 33, 35, 34, 36] investigated the dose calculation error connected to applying a conventional tissue-to-water conversion spotting the cases here such a deviation could be relevant as compared to other treatment typical uncertainties (HLUT calibration, etc.) Moreover, they suggested approximated methods accounting for the water nonequivalence of tissues in nuclear interactions have been proposed and recommended to be systematically applied to treatment planning in clinical practice (see Figure 11.11). In fact, the method developed in [33] is currently routinely used in the treatments with scanned carbon ions at NIRS. With this method, there is a conversion from a stopping effective density $\rho_S$ of the patient to a nuclear effective density $\rho_N$, defined as the ratio of the attenuation of primary carbon ions in a patient to that in water, through a semiempirical relationship

$$\rho_N/\rho_S = k\sum_i w_i Z_i^{-1/3}/Z_{water}^{-1/3} \tag{11.11}$$

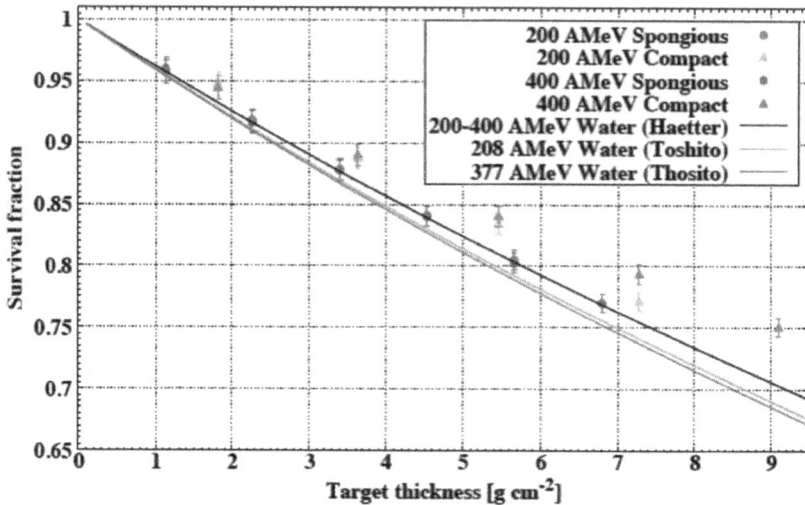

**Figure 11.12**   Measured attenuation of carbon beams of different initial energies for different types of synthetic bone material targets (spongious, compact), representing different anatomical regions. Figure from [10].

### 11.4.3   NOVEL EXPERIMENTAL MEASUREMENTS AND IMPACT ON TPS

Recent measurements [10] provided for the first time an experimental assessment of the impact of neglecting the explicit consideration of bone material induced nuclear fragmentation, instead of its density scaled water alias, in a treatment plan with carbon ion beams. There it was first measured the attenuation of different carbon ion beams with growing layers of bone materials of different compositions, and the corresponding production of lighter fragments, resolved in energy and angular distribution. This returned that a density scaling with water would overestimate up to a factor 5% the nuclear attenuation of the primary carbon particle, with an impact on dose (see Figure 11.12).

Further, the propagation of all the related deviations (attenuation of primary, production of secondaries, angular spreading of the latter fragments), on a treatment plan for a water phantom with a bone layer on the entrance has been measured, returning a major deviation in the falloff of the spread out Bragg peak.

### 11.5   SUMMARY AND OUTLOOK

We briefly reviewed the status of research in accounting for projectile and target nuclear fragmentation in particle beam therapeutic plans, including their biological impact. While projectile fragmentation has been extensively described, especially for carbon ions, the contribution of target fragments is recently being an object of study, especially for its role in the biological impact of high LET fragments. Different media may also contribute, through a different fragmentation pattern, in a non-negligible way to the overall dose and biological dose, with an effect which cannot be simply accounted for by scaling for the medium density, especially for the denser target regions, like bones. Ongoing and future research is then now committed to fill these gaps, i.e., by measuring the low-energy fragments produced in target fragmentation, like it is the plan of FOOT experiment [4], increasing the collection of data for Helium and Oxygen beams, and for bone-like targets. This will allow Monte Carlo codes to trustfully describe the complete radiation field generated in any region and type of clinical irradiation. At the same time, modern treatment planning should include the possibility to fully handle the nuclear impact of different materials.

# REFERENCES

1. Treatment planning for a scanned carbon beam with a modified microdosimetric kinetic model. *Physics in medicine and biology*, 55(22):6721–37, nov 2010.

2. U. Amaldi, W. Hajdas, S. Iliescu, N. Malakhov, J. Samarati, F. Sauli, and D. Watts. Advanced quality assurance for CNAO. *Nuclear Instruments and Methods in Physics Research Section A: Accelerators, Spectrometers, Detectors and Associated Equipment*, 617(1-3):248–249, 2010.

3. U. Amaldi and G. Kraft. Radiotherapy with beams of carbon ions. *Reports on Progress in Physics*, 68(8):1861–1882, aug 2005.

4. G. Battistoni, M. Toppi, V. Patera, and The FOOT Collaboration. Measuring the Impact of Nuclear Interaction in Particle Therapy and in Radio Protection in Space: the FOOT Experiment. *Frontiers in Physics*, 8, feb 2021.

5. E. V. Bellinzona, L. Grzanka, A. Attili, F. Tommasino, T. Friedrich, M. Krämer, M. Scholz, G. Battistoni, A. Embriaco, D. Chiappara, G. A. P. Cirrone, G. Petringa, M. Durante, and E. Scifoni. Biological Impact of Target Fragments on Proton Treatment Plans: An Analysis Based on the Current Cross-Section Data and a Full Mixed Field Approach. *Cancers*, 13(19):4768, sep 2021.

6. L. Burigo, I. Pshenichnov, I. Mishustin, and M. Bleicher. Comparative study of dose distributions and cell survival fractions for 1h, 4he, 12c and 16o beams using geant4 and microdosimetric kinetic model. *Physics in Medicine & Biology*, 60(8):3313, 2015.

7. D. J. Carlson, R. D. Stewart, V. Semenenko, and G. Sandison. Combined use of Monte Carlo DNA damage simulations and deterministic repair models to examine putative mechanisms of cell killing. *Radiation research*, 169(4):447–459, 2008.

8. R. Carlson. Proton-Nucleus Total Reaction Cross Sections and Total Cross Sections Up to 1 GeV. *Atomic Data and Nuclear Data Tables*, 63(1):93–116, may 1996.

9. Å. K. Carlsson, P. Andreo, and A. Brahme. Monte Carlo and analytical calculation of proton pencil beams for computerized treatment plan optimization. *Physics in Medicine and Biology*, 42(6):1033–1053, jun 1997.

10. S. Colombi, M. Rovituso, E. Scifoni, C. Schuy, A. Eichhorn, M. Kraemer, M. Durante, and C. La Tessa. Interaction of therapeutic 12 C ions with bone-like targets: physical characterization and dosimetric effect at material interfaces. *Physics in Medicine & Biology*, 66(18):185003, sep 2021.

11. A. Cometto, G. Russo, F. Bourhaleb, F. M. Milian, S. Giordanengo, F. Marchetto, R. Cirio, and A. Attili. Direct evaluation of radiobiological parameters from clinical data in the case of ion beam therapy: an alternative approach to the relative biological effectiveness. *Physics in Medicine and Biology*, 59(23):7393–7417, dec 2014.

12. F. A. Cucinotta, R. Katz, J. W. Wilson, L. W. Townsend, J. Shinn, and F. Hajnal. Biological effectiveness of high-energy protons: Target fragmentation. *Radiation Research*, 127(2):130–137, 1991.

13. M. Durante and F. A. Cucinotta. Physical basis of radiation protection in space travel. *Reviews of Modern Physics*, 83(4), 2011.

14. M. Durante and H. Paganetti. Nuclear physics in particle therapy: a review. *Reports on progress in physics. Physical Society (Great Britain)*, 79(9):096702, 2016.

15. T. Elsässer, W. K. Weyrather, T. Friedrich, M. Durante, G. Iancu, M. Krämer, G. Kragl, S. Brons, M. Winter, K.-J. J. Weber, and M. Scholz. Quantification of the relative biological effectiveness for ion beam radiotherapy: Direct experimental comparison of proton and carbon ion beams and a novel approach for treatment planning. *International Journal of Radiation Oncology Biology Physics*, 78(4):1177–1183, 2010.

16. A. Embriaco, A. Attili, E. Bellinzona, Y. Dong, L. Grzanka, I. Mattei, S. Muraro, E. Scifoni, F. Tommasino, S. Valle, et al. Fluka simulation of target fragmentation in proton therapy. *Physica Medica*, 80:342–346, 2020.

17. W. Enghardt, J. Debus, T. Haberer, B. G. Hasch, R. Hinz, O. Jäkel, M. Krämer, K. Lauckner, J. Pawelke, and F. Pönisch. Positron emission tomography for quality assurance of cancer therapy with light ion beams. *Nuclear Physics A*, 654(1 SUPPL. 1):1047c–1050c, 1999.

18. P. Fossati, S. Molinelli, N. Matsufuji, M. Ciocca, A. Mirandola, A. Mairani, J. Mizoe, A. Hasegawa, R. Imai, T. Kamada, R. Orecchia, and H. Tsujii. Dose prescription in carbon ion radiotherapy: a planning study to compare NIRS and LEM approaches with a clinically-oriented strategy. *Physics in medicine and biology*, 57(22):7543–54, nov 2012.

19. M. C. Frese, V. K. Yu, R. D. Stewart, and D. J. Carlson. A Mechanism-Based Approach to Predict the Relative Biological Effectiveness of Protons and Carbon Ions in Radiation Therapy. *Radiation Oncology Biology*, 83(1):442–450, 2012.

20. E. M. Friedlander and H. H. Heckman. Relativistic heavy-ion collisions: experiment. In *Treatise on heavy-ion science*, pages 401–562. Springer, 1985.

21. T. Friedrich, U. Scholz, T. Elssser, M. Durante, and M. Scholz. Calculation of the biological effects of ion beams based on the microscopic spatial damage distribution pattern. *International Journal of Radiation Biology*, 88(1-2):103–107, 2012.

22. A. Goldhaber and H. Heckman. High energy interactions of nuclei. *Annual Review of Nuclear and Particle Science*, 28(1):161–205, 1978.

23. C. Grassberger and H. Paganetti. Elevated LET components in clinical proton beams. *Physics in medicine and biology*, 56(20):6677–91, oct 2011.

24. R. Grün, T. Friedrich, E. Traneus, and M. Scholz. Is the dose-averaged LET a reliable predictor for the relative biological effectiveness? *Medical Physics*, 46(2):1064–1074, 2019.

25. K. Gunzert-Marx, H. Iwase, D. Schardt, and R. S. Simon. Secondary beam fragments produced by 200 MeV u-1 12C ions in water and their dose contributions in carbon ion radiotherapy. *New Journal of Physics*, 2008.

26. E. Haettner, H. Iwase, M. Krämer, G. Kraft, and D. Schardt. Experimental study of nuclear fragmentation of 200 and 400 MeV/u 12C ions in water for applications in particle therapy. *Physics in Medicine and Biology*, 58(23):8265–8279, 2013.

27. D. C. Hansen, A. Lühr, R. Herrmann, N. Sobolevsky, and N. Bassler. Recent improvements in the SHIELD-HIT code. *International journal of radiation biology*, 88(1-2):195–199, 2012.

28. R. B. Hawkins. A Statistical theory of Cell Killing by Radiation of Varying Linear Transfer Energy. *Radiation Research*, 140(3):366–374, 1994.

29. R. B. Hawkins. A microdosimetric-kinetic model for the effect of non-Poisson distribution of lethal lesions on the variation of RBE with LET. *Radiation research*, 160(1):61–9, jul 2003.

30. Y. Hirano, S. Kodaira, H. Souda, K. Osaki, and M. Torikoshi. Estimations of relative biological effectiveness of secondary fragments in carbon ion irradiation of water using CR-39 plastic detector and microdosimetric kinetic model. *Medical Physics*, 47(2):781–789, 2020.

31. M. E. Howard, C. Beltran, S. Anderson, W. C. Tseung, J. N. Sarkaria, and M. G. Herman. Investigating Dependencies of Relative Biological Effectiveness for Proton Therapy in Cancer Cells. *International Journal of Particle Therapy*, 4(3):12–22, 2017.

32. J. Hüfner. Heavy fragments produced in proton-nucleus and nucleus-nucleus collisions at relativistic energies. *Physics Reports*, 125(4):129–185, 1985.

33. T. Inaniwa, N. Kanematsu, Y. Hara, and T. Furukawa. Nuclear-interaction correction of integrated depth dose in carbon-ion radiotherapy treatment planning. *Physics in Medicine and Biology*, 60(1):421–435, 2015.

34. T. Inaniwa, N. Kanematsu, S. Sato, and R. Kohno. A dose calculation algorithm with correction for proton-nucleus interactions in non-water materials for proton radiotherapy treatment planning. *Physics in Medicine and Biology*, 61(1):67–89, jan 2016.

35. T. Inaniwa, N. Kanematsu, H. Tsuji, and T. Kamada. Influence of nuclear interactions in body tissues on tumor dose in carbon-ion radiotherapy. *Medical Physics*, 42(12):7132–7137, nov 2015.

36. T. Inaniwa, S. H. Lee, K. Mizushima, D. Sakata, Y. Iwata, N. Kanematsu, and T. Shirai. Nuclear-interaction correction for patient dose calculations in treatment planning of helium-, carbon-, oxygen-, and neon-ion beams. *Physics in Medicine & Biology*, 65(2):025004, jan 2020.

37. F. Kamp, D. J. Carlson, and J. J. Wilkens. Rapid implementation of the repair-misrepair-fixation (RMF) model facilitating online adaption of radiosensitivity parameters in ion therapy. *Physics in Medicine and Biology*, 62(13):N285–N296, jul 2017.

38. N. Kanematsu, T. Inaniwa, and M. Nakao. Modeling of body tissues for Monte Carlo simulation of radiotherapy treatments planned with conventional x-ray CT systems. *Physics in Medicine and Biology*, 61(13):5037–5050, jul 2016.

39. C. P. Karger and P. Peschke. RBE and related modeling in carbon-ion therapy. *Physics in Medicine & Biology*, 63(1):01TR02, dec 2017.

40. Y. Kase, T. Kanai, N. Matsufuji, Y. Furusawa, T. Elsässer, and M. Scholz. Biophysical calculation of cell survival probabilities using amorphous track structure models for heavy-ion irradiation. *Physics in medicine and biology*, 53(1):37–59, jan 2008.

41. Y. Kase, T. Kanai, Y. Matsumoto, Y. Furusawa, H. Okamoto, T. Asaba, M. Sakama, and H. Shinoda. Microdosimetric measurements and estimation of human cell survival for heavy-ion beams. *Radiat. Res.*, 166(4):629–638, 2006.

42. A. C. Kraan. Range verification methods in particle therapy: Underlying physics and Monte Carlo modelling. *Frontiers in Oncology*, 5(JUN):1–27, 2015.

43. G. Kraft. The radiobiological and physical basis for radiotherapy with protons and heavier ions. *Strahlentherapie und Onkologie : Organ der Deutschen Rontgengesellschaft ... [et al]*, 166(1):10–13, jan 1990.

44. G. Kraft. Tumor Therapy with Heavy Charged Particles. *Progress in Particle and Nuclear Physics*, 45(S473-S544):S473–S544, 2000.

45. M. Krämer, O. Jäkel, T. Haberer, G. Kraft, D. Schardt, and U. Weber. Treatment planning for heavy-ion radiotherapy: physical beam model and dose optimization. *Physics in Medicine and Biology*, 45(11):3299–3317, nov 2000.

46. M. Krämer and M. Scholz. Treatment planning for heavy-ion radiotherapy: calculation and optimization of biologically effective dose. *Physics in Medicine and Biology*, 45(11):3319–3330, nov 2000.

47. M. Krämer, E. Scifoni, C. Schuy, M. Rovituso, W. Tinganelli, A. Maier, R. Kaderka, W. Kraft-Weyrather, S. Brons, T. Tessonnier, K. Parodi, and M. Durante. Helium ions for radiotherapy? Physical and biological verifications of a novel treatment modality. *Medical Physics*, 43(4):1995–2004, mar 2016.

48. A. Lühr, D. C. Hansen, R. Teiwes, N. Sobolevsky, O. Jäkel, and N. Bassler. The impact of modeling nuclear fragmentation on delivered dose and radiobiology in ion therapy. *Physics in medicine and biology*, 57:5169–5185, 2012.

49. W. Lynch. Nuclear fragmentation in proton-and heavy-ion-induced reactions. *Annual Review of Nuclear and Particle Science*, 37(1):493–535, 1987.

50. A. Mairani, I. Dokic, G. Magro, T. Tessonnier, J. Bauer, T. T. Böhlen, M. Ciocca, A. Ferrari, P. R. Sala, O. Jäkel, J. Debus, T. Haberer, A. Abdollahi, and K. Parodi. A phenomenological relative biological effectiveness approach for proton therapy based on an improved description of the mixed radiation field. *Physics in Medicine and Biology*, 62(4):1378–1395, 2017.

51. A. Mairani, I. Dokic, G. Magro, T. Tessonnier, F. Kamp, D. J. Carlson, M. Ciocca, F. Cerutti, P. R. Sala, A. Ferrari, T. T. Böhlen, O. Jäkel, K. Parodi, J. Debus, A. Abdollahi, and T. Haberer. Biologically optimized helium ion plans: Calculation approach and its in vitro validation. *Physics in Medicine and Biology*, 61(11):4283–4299, 2016.

52. N. Matsufuji, M. Komori, H. Sasaki, K. Akiu, M. Ogawa, A. Fukumura, E. Urakabe, T. Inaniwa, T. Nishio, T. Kohno, and T. Kanai. Spatial fragment distribution from a therapeutic pencil-like carbon beam in water. *Physics in Medicine and Biology*, 50(14):3393–3403, jul 2005.

53. S. Muraro, G. Battistoni, and A. Kraan. Challenges in Monte Carlo Simulations as Clinical and Research Tool in Particle Therapy: A Review. *Frontiers in Physics*, 2020.

54. H. Paganetti. Nuclear interactions in proton therapy: dose and relative biological effect distributions originating from primary and secondary particles. *Physics in medicine and biology*, 47(5):747–64, mar 2002.

55. K. Parodi, H. Paganetti, E. Cascio, J. B. Flanz, A. A. Bonab, N. M. Alpert, K. Lohmann, and T. Bortfeld. PET/CT imaging for treatment verification after proton therapy: a study with plastic phantoms and metallic implants. *Medical Physics*, 34(2):419–435, 2007.

56. T. Pfuhl, F. Horst, C. Schuy, and U. Weber. Dose build-up effects induced by delta electrons and target fragments in proton Bragg curves-measurements and simulations. *Physics in medicine and biology*, 63(17):175002, aug 2018.

57. N. B. Remmes, M. G. Herman, and J. J. Kruse. Optimizing Normal Tissue Sparing in Ion Therapy Using Calculated Isoeffective Dose for Ion Selection. *International Journal of Radiation Oncology\*Biology\*Physics*, 83(2):756–762, jun 2012.

58. M. Rovituso and C. L. Tessa. Nuclear interactions of new ions in cancer therapy: Impact on dosimetry. *Translational Cancer Research*, 6(Suppl 5):S914–S933, 2017.

59. D. Schardt, T. Elsässer, and D. Schulz-Ertner. Heavy-ion tumor therapy: Physical and radiobiological benefits. *Reviews of Modern Physics*, 82(1):383–425, feb 2010.

60. M. Scholz, A. M. Kellerer, W. Kraft-Weyrather, and G. Kraft. Computation of cell survival in heavy ion beams for therapy. The model and its approximation. *Radiation and environmental biophysics*, 36:59–66, 1997.

61. R. Serber. Nuclear reactions at high energies. *Physical Review*, 72(11):1114–1115, 1947.

62. O. Sokol, E. Scifoni, W. Tinganelli, W. Kraft-Weyrather, J. Wiedemann, A. Maier, D. Boscolo, T. Friedrich, S. Brons, M. Durante, and M. Krämer. Oxygen beams for therapy: advanced biological treatment planning and experimental verification. *Physics in Medicine & Biology*, 62(19):7798–7813, sep 2017.

63. R. D. Stewart, D. J. Carlson, M. P. Butkus, R. Hawkins, T. Friedrich, and M. Scholz. A comparison of mechanism-inspired models for particle relative biological effectiveness (RBE). *Medical Physics*, 45(11):e925–e952, 2018.

64. F. Tommasino and M. Durante. Proton radiobiology. *Cancers*, 7(1):353–381, 2015.

65. F. Tommasino, E. Scifoni, and M. Durante. New Ions for Therapy. *International Journal of Particle Therapy*, 2(3):428–438, 2015.

66. R. Tripathi, F. Cucinotta, and J. Wilson. Accurate universal parameterization of absorption cross sections III – light systems. *Nuclear Instruments and Methods in Physics Research Section B: Beam Interactions with Materials and Atoms*, 155(4):349–356, sep 1999.

67. R. K. Tripathi, F. A. Cucinotta, and J. W. Wilson. Universal parameterization of absorption cross sections. Technical report, 1997.

68. J. J. Wilkens and U. Oelfke. Direct comparison of biologically optimized spread-out bragg peaks for protons and carbon ions. *International Journal of Radiation Oncology, Biology, Physics*, 70(1):262–266, 2008.

69. M. Zaider and H. Rossi. The synergistic effects of different radiations. *Radiation research*, pages 732–739, 1980.

70. C. Zeitlin and C. La Tessa. The role of nuclear fragmentation in particle therapy and space radiation protection. *Frontiers in Oncology*, 6(MAR):1–13, 2016.

# 12 Monte Carlo characterization of nanoparticle radio-enhancement for hadron therapy

*Martina Fuss*
GSI Helmholtzzentrum fur Schwerionenforschung, Darmstadt, Germany

*Susanna Guatelli*
University of Wollongong, Wollongong, Australia

## CONTENTS

After accumulating substantial experimental evidence for high atomic number nanoparticle (high-Z NP) sensitization of cells and tumors under photon irradiation, in the last few years more studies have focused on the combination of proton or ion radiation with NPs and observed large differences in biological endpoints, including cell survival, tumor progression and animal overall survival. This chapter illustrates how state-of-the-art Monte Carlo techniques can be used to investigate NP radio-enhancement to help to understand the fundamental mechanism behind it and the biological result, to guide upcoming studies.

## 12.1 INTRODUCTION

Since its beginnings, the field of NP radiosensitization has expanded rapidly. After the early discovery by Adams et al. [1] and Matsudaira et al. [2] that iodine-containing contrast media led to a sensitization of cell cultures to X-rays, the seminal studies of Herold et al. [3] and Hainfeld et al. [4] showed radioenhancement of cells and tumors by gold micro- and nanoparticles, respectively. The advantages of high-Z elements in NP shape were obvious and immediately nurtured expectations to improve the biological outcome of irradiation and, ultimately, radiation therapies:

**Tumor selectivity** Small-size NPs accumulate preferentially in tumors while being effectively cleared from normal tissues through the kidneys thanks to the enhanced permeability and retention (EPR) effect (see e.g. [5]).

**Dose enhancement** Physically, the basic advantage of high–Z materials lies in the much increased interaction probability, as compared to tissue, with incident radiation and thus an increased emission of secondary radiation that deposits an additional dose locally.

**Clinical use** Some types of NPs were already safely used as contrast agents for imaging purposes.

Since then, the interest in using high–Z NPs, in particular made of gold, gadolinium, bismuth, iodine, hafnium, silver, and iron, for radiation enhancement in radiotherapeutic applications has constantly grown. In combination with photons and there especially for X-rays up to a few hundred kV, effective radio-enhancement has been shown many times (c.f. [6, 7, 8, 9, 10]) and follows mostly from physical interaction cross sections, most prominently due to the production of long-range secondary electrons by photoelectric effect. Currently, the gadolinium-containing polymer nanoparticles AGuIX (NH TherAguix SAS, France) are in clinical trials as radioenhancers for X-rays [11] and show the slow but steady advance into the clinics [12].

For the case of hadron beams, experimental evidence is however more divergent and investigations ongoing, with protons receiving particular attention. One main reason for the more complex proton and heavy ion situation is that secondary electron ($\delta$–electron) distributions for charged particles peak below $100\,\mathrm{eV}$ independently of the atomic number of the NP and allow for only a relatively short range (few nm) in a biological target, if not entirely absorbed in the NP material itself. Additionally, the NPs are generally not internalized into the cell nucleus but often show a tendency to accumulate around the nuclear membrane. This combination strongly limits their radioenhancing potential in a traditional understanding, starting from physical dose enhancement and aiming for damage to nuclear DNA. Notwithstanding, a number of experiments show evidence of radiosensitization *in vitro* or *in vivo* [13, 14, 15, 16], while others don't. Different mechanisms which could explain the observed biological effects are currently under discussion.

In this research domain, Monte Carlo (MC) methods can be very helpful to shed more light on different aspects of the incident heavy ion–nanoparticle interaction. In providing a connection between the micro- and nano- scale processes taking place and the observable experimental endpoints, sometimes aided by biological models, Monte Carlo studies help us to differentiate and quantify different contributions to the radioenhancing effect. Applications include global as well as nano-scale dose enhancement and the impact of NP geometry and/or coating and cellular distribution on different scales. Some studies focus on the characterization of secondary radiation (e.g. electrons in general, particle-induced X-ray emissions and Auger electrons) emitted by the NPs. Other ones characterize also radiation chemical effects, in particular the changes in radiolytic radical or reactive species production which would affect the biological outcome. Finally, the micro-scale energy deposition characteristics can be evaluated with biological models such as the Local Effect Model, among others.

Several Monte Carlo codes have been used so far to combine proton (TRAX [17], Geant4–DNA [18, 19, 20], TOPAS [21, 22] or, less frequently, heavier ion (Geant4 [23], Geant4-DNA [24], TOPASnBio [25], TRAX [26, 27, 28]) beams with high-Z NPs, producing a substantial amount of theoretical results in this active topic.

In this chapter, we first introduce the distinctive technical features which are useful for simulating high–Z NP-enhanced radiation interactions and afterwards give a brief overview about the existing approaches and results and discuss other emerging research directions.

## 12.2   CORE CONCEPTS OF MONTE CARLO METHOD FOR NANOPARTICLE RADIOENHANCEMENT

### 12.2.1   SIMULATION OF PHYSICS INTERACTIONS

It is extensively recognized that Monte Carlo-based studies of physical dose enhancement by means of NPs involve the calculation of energy deposition at a sub-cellular scale, considering a specific NP configuration, modeled with realistic NP dimensions, concentration and distribution in the biological medium.

Condensed History (CH) approach physics models, which condense several physical interactions into a single simulated "step" [29] and use multiple scattering theory of elastic collisions to account for the change in direction after each simulated step, are recognized not to be adequate for NP-dose enhancement studies. This is due to the low dimensionality of the NPs and to the fact that the energy deposition pattern at sub-cellular level is the mechanism at the basis of NP-driven dose enhancement (see Section 12.2.3). Track Structure (TS) physics models, describing particle interactions, event by event, are instead recognized to be the state of the art for NP-dose enhancement description of the physics mechanisms [30].

Many TS physics models have been developed in the past decades for radiation biophysics applications. TS codes capable to model the electromagnetic interactions in the biological medium (approximated as liquid water), which can be used for NP radio-enhancement studies in hadrontherapy include PARTRAC [31], Geant4-DNA [24], TRAX [32], RITRACKS [33], among others (for other MC codes the reader can refer to Nikjoo et al. [29]).

Track Structure MC codes can have differences in terms of physics models used to describe specific physical processes in liquid water and we invite to read the specific physics models and implementation details in the documentation accompanying the specific Monte Carlo code used. Here, we would like to draw the attention towards the electromagnetic processes which are usually implemented. Electron processes include ionization, electronic excitation, elastic scattering, vibrational excitation and molecular attachment. Interactions of protons, neutral hydrogen, neutral helium and charged states of helium take into account ionization, electronic excitation, electron loss or capture and elastic scattering. Finally, regarding ions heavier than helium, only ionization is usually modeled. Atomic de-excitation should be modeled to study dose enhancement effects due to Auger electrons emitted by the NP.

As far as the authors of this chapter know, Geant4-DNA – and therefore TOPASnBio – are currently the only TS codes that allow to couple the TS electromagnetic interactions with hadronic processes of protons, $\alpha$ particles and heavier ions.

Beyond liquid water, Geant4-DNA offers TS physics models for Au [34, 30] and Si [35, 36], while TRAX can describe particle interactions in Fe, Ag, Gd, Pt and Au [17] among others. These TS models for solid state materials take into account low dimensionality effects, such as plasmon excitation, important when describing particle interactions in NPs.

In the lack of TS physics models describing particle interactions in specific NP materials, a hybrid approach can be used, which couples TS approach in the biological medium and CH physics models in the NP. For example, this is what is usually done when using Geant4 and Geant4–DNA.

### 12.2.2   SIMULATION OF THE CHEMICAL DAMAGE

In contrast to the direct (physical) radiation effects caused by primary or secondary radiation particles, indirect damage refers to the chemical modifications in biological cells or tissues inflicted by radiolytic chemical species following irradiation. Especially for low-LET radiation, up to 85% of total cell inactivation following irradiation [37] can be caused by indirect radiation damage.

The mechanism of dose enhancement due to NPs, e.g. gold NPs, in proton or heavy ion therapy is extremely different with respect to X-ray radiotherapy. The ionization interactions of the incident heavy ions have a weak dependence on the atomic number of the NP and the increase of $\delta$-electrons is due to the high density of the NP [38]. Monte Carlo simulations showed that this enhancement of secondary electrons produces a low physical dose enhancement ratio [38]. It seems instead that the enhanced production of reactive species via radiolysis due to the presence of GNPs plays a more significant role in the observed radiosensitization [20, 39].

This implies that for modeling the biological effects in a realistic fashion, the modeling of the radiation chemistry is a very important step to be taken into account. Several TS codes take advantage of the detailed information obtained on individual physical interaction events (see previous section) and subsequently derive the production yield of the various reactive radiolytic species in water targets (as a proxy for biological tissues) under different irradiation conditions. First codes including water radiolysis date back more than 30 years [40, 41, 42, 43], then evolved over time (c.f. [44, 45, 33]). The reader can find an updated overview in chapter 17. Among the current codes with extensive capability in the modeling of the chemical stage are Geant4-DNA, TOPASnBio, PARTRAC and TRAX-CHEM.

The radiation chemical influence of NP presence can be supposed to happen secondarily, through an increased or altered production of radiolytic species, which in turn originates from either a net dose enhancement or an increased production of secondary electrons (including Auger electrons). Applications of radiolysis modeling to NP enhancement have therefore limited the interactions with the actual heavy element NP material to physical processes. The simulation of the radiation chemistry after the physical events logically takes place in the surrounding water material, the target of the radiolysis, and differs to that in water without NPs essentially in the locally enhanced presence of some radical species, e.g. the hydrated electron $e_{aq}^-$ and the ensuing differences in track recombinations, e.g. $OH^\bullet + OH^\bullet \rightarrow H_2O_2$.

The evolution of the "chemical track" (see Figure 12.1), the totality of all radiation-induced radicals present at a given time that stem from an individual radiation particle, is generally described

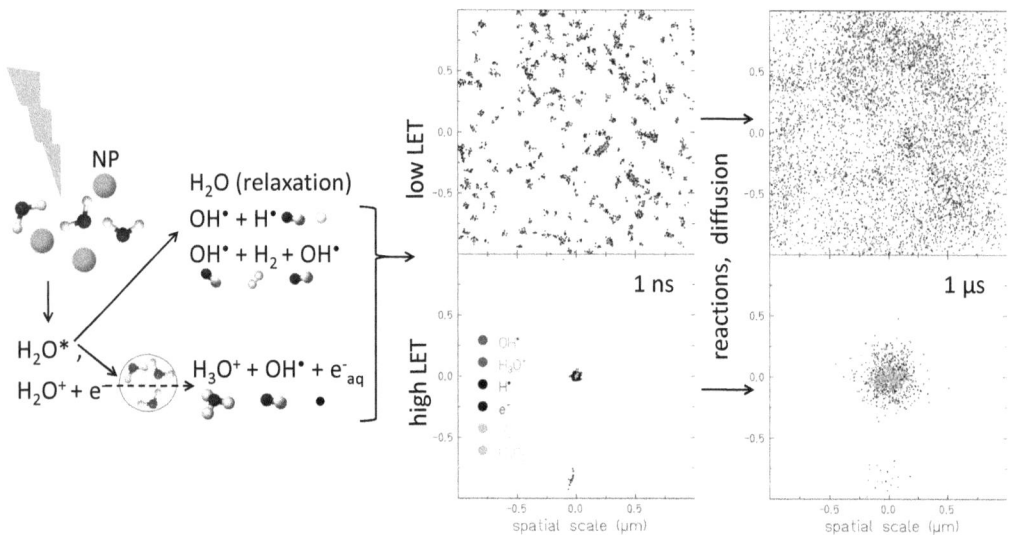

**Figure 12.1** Schematic of the simulation of pre-chemical and chemical stages of radiation interactions. On the left side, the main primary radical combinations produced through ionizations and electronic excitations are depicted. The right part shows a projection of the evolving chemical tracks at different time points (1 ns and 1 µs) of 1 MeV electrons (upper panels) and a 50 MeV/u C ion (lower panels). Both correspond to a dose of $\sim 1$ Gy.

in two stages which are characterized by a typical time scale. The shorter pre-chemical stage (up to $\sim 1$ ps) collects the positions and ionization or excitation levels of the physical stage, assigns the corresponding molecular dissociation results where appropriate, and thermalizes molecular fragments and sub-excitation (secondary) electrons alike to chemically reactive species (molecules, radicals and aqueous electrons). This stage is generally described via dissociation tables containing the probability of relaxation to the ground stage or specific dissociation channels. These can be obtained in principle from experimental studies, however in solvated conditions fast reactions such as proton transfers convert some of the physically generated ionic or radical species to an effective set of few important species to enter simulation: $OH^{\bullet}$, $H^{\bullet}$, $H_3O^+$, $e_{aq}^-$, $H_2$. Furthermore, it typically includes small (nanometric) random direction translocations of complementary fragments which originate in the repulsive potentials causing the dissociation and serve the practical purpose of preventing immediate recombination.

In the longer heterogenous chemical stage ($\leq 1\mu s$), these radiolytic species are tracked as they diffuse and react with each other, water, and sometimes selected additional solvents such as e.g. oxygen. There are two established MC methods for this transition from an initially heterogeneous, track-structure-determined dynamic to a quasi-homogeneous solution in chemical equilibrium (see Figure 12.1). The independent reaction time (IRT) approach is based on the initial separation of pairs of chemical species and the time evolution of their mutual (pair-wise) distance obtained from localization distribution functions, to give reaction times. This method is computationally fast but it does not keep track of the discrete, absolute positions of all the molecules as a function of time. The step by step approach is a more accurate method where all the chemical species and their reactions are followed individually during multiple simulation time steps. This approach is however computationally much heavier and thus slower than IRT methods. Typical outputs of the chemical stages consist of time-dependent G-values for all species, reaction statistics, or radial distributions of radicals and allow to study the new reaction dynamics with NPs.

### 12.2.3 BRIDGING THE GAP TO CALCULATE BIOLOGICAL ENDPOINTS

Nowadays there is a general consensus that DNA damage produced by ionising radiation is originated by the direct interaction of the particles with DNA molecules (physical stage, section 12.2.1) and indirect interaction of DNA with molecular species created during water radiolysis in the chemical stage (section 12.2.2). Despite the progress in the field, still a comprehensive understanding of how the direct/indirect interactions lead to biological endpoints is yet to be reached [46].

To answer to this need, different approaches are currently investigated and here we will introduce the so-called *chain*, the *Local Effect Model* (LEM), and the *Microdosimetric Kinetic Model* (MKM), which have been applied to Monte Carlo simulation results to predict biological endpoints of interest (e.g. cell survival curve), in hadrontherapy. The LEM and the MKM model have been adopted to quantify NP dose enhancement, while the *chain* model, including the modeling of the biological response, has never been applied to this problem domain but may be suitable.

The *chain*, the LEM and the MKM rely on the common hypothesis that the cellular damage is due to radiation effects in the nucleus of the cell. In other words, the nucleus is the sensitive target to radiation and other kinds of damages (e.g. damage to non-DNA targets, mitochondria function disruption and NP induced cellular stress [47]) are not considered.

#### 12.2.3.1 The *chain* model

The *chain* model consists of a realistic fully integrated Monte Carlo simulation to calculate the early DNA damage and subsequent biological responses with time, due to the exposure to protons with energies typical of the Spread Out Bragg Peak. The study was developed using Geant4–DNA, based on previous work performed by means of PARTRAC [48]. A semi-empirical biological repair model, developed by Belov et al. [49], has been applied to the early DNA damage calculated by means of the Monte Carlo simulation, to predict the foci accumulation yield along time, up to 25 hours after irradiation.

We invite to read the full paper of Sakata et al. 2020 [46] to have more details on this work. Here we would like to focus on some aspects of the study, which could be of interest to evaluate NP-enhancement in hadrontherapy.

In the simulation the fibroblast nucleus is described in detail, where chromatin fibers, including the nucleobases and the sugar-phosphate backbone, fill the volume of the nucleus. This geometry is computationally very demanding, therefore, if using Geant4–DNA, a user may evaluate the adoption of simplified geometries, which can for example be found in the extended Geant4 example *wholeNuclearDNA*.

The direct and indirect DNA damage calculations were derived from PARTRAC [48], and based on a model developed originally by Nikjoo et al. [50].

In summary, to calculate the probability of direct strand breaks (SBs), each energy deposition is assigned to the closest strand molecule when the position is within 3.5 Angstroms from the center of a strand molecule in the case of either sugar or phosphate. Once the simulation is completed, the total accumulated energy deposition in each strand molecule is used to calculate the probability of a direct SB. Based on a linearly increasing probability distribution, there is a 0% probability a break occurred when less than 5 eV was deposited, but a 100% probability a break occurred when over 37.5 eV.

The number of indirect SBs is evaluated by applying a probability of 40.5% that a chemical reaction between a hydroxyl radical and the sugar phosphate backbone leads to a single strand break (SSB).

The early DNA damage is then quantified by calculating the number of Double Strand Breaks (DSBs) and their complexity, following the scheme showed in Figure 12.2. DSBs and their complexity depend on the distance $d_{DSB}$, which is fixed equal to 10 base pairs.

In this simulation work, the early DNA damage is calculated following the free radical diffusion for 5 ns. Then, the total yield of DSBs as a function of time can be calculated based on the repair pathways, by applying the semi-empirical model developed by Belov and collaborators [49]. In particular, the repair model requires as input the yield of DSBs and the fraction of complex DNA damage.

The model described in the *chain* [46] may be used to calculate the early DNA damage and its evolution in time, with different configurations of NP distributions around the cell nucleus. This approach allows also to estimate the Radiobiological Effectiveness (RBE) calculated as ratio of

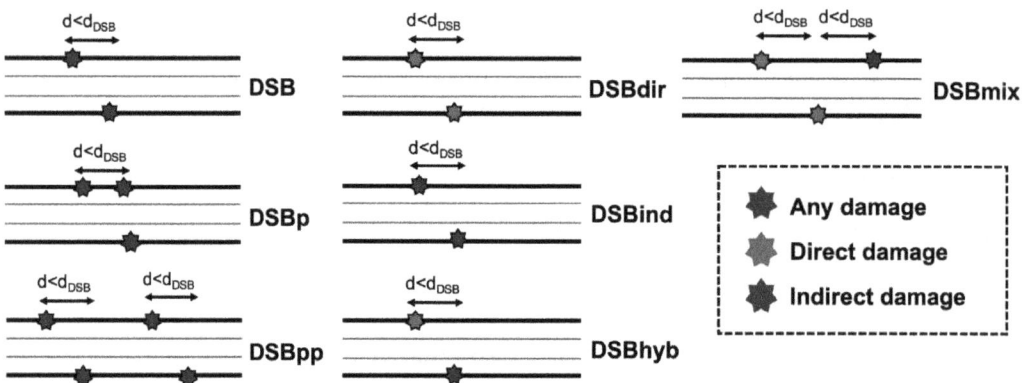

**Figure 12.2**  Scheme of classification to determine the complexity of the DSB (left side) and for the source of DSB (center/right). Figure courtesy of [46].

number of DSBs, obtained with the cell exposed to the radiation of interest and to a reference radiation (e.g. $^{60}$Co or $^{137}$Cs source).

### 12.2.3.2  The Local Effect Model

The Local Effect Model (LEM) [51], which is for example used clinically for carbon ion treatment planning at the Heidelberg Ion-Beam Therapy Center (Germany), relies on the determination of the biological effect of incident ions starting from the response of cells or tissues to photons.

The LEM relies on three assumptions [52, 53, 55]. The first one is that the survival fraction (SF) of a cell colony can be described via a linear-quadratic response model: $SF(D) = exp^{-\alpha \cdot D - \beta \cdot D^2}$. $D$ is the mean dose delivered to the colony, $\alpha$ and $\beta$ derive from in-vitro experiments and are characteristics of the target cell line. The second assumption is that the cell "inactivation," e.g. cell death, can be attributed to the creation of a number of lethal lesions (local modifications of the DNA produced by the incident radiation) within a sensitive small sub-cellular volume such as the cell nucleus. Finally, the contribution of sub-lethal damage at distances larger than the order of a few microns is ignored (third assumption).

The LEM has been refined over the years and a modified version of it has been used successfully to calculate the cell survival curve around a NP or a cluster of NPs, with a defined concentration and distribution in X-ray radiotherapy (e.g. [56], [57]). Here we will describe briefly the implementation of the LEM approach as adopted in [57], which was based on [56].

The LEM relates energy depositions on the nanoscale to the cell survival $S$, determined from in vitro experiments. $S$ can be expressed as function of the number of lethal events, $N$, following the Poisson statistics, as follows: $S = exp^{-N}$, where N is given by:

$$N = -\int_{V_S} \frac{ln(S(D(x,y,z)))}{V_S} dV, \qquad (12.1)$$

where $D(x,y,z)$ is the dose distribution in a nanometric volume $dV$, due to the incident radiation field; $S(D(x,y,z)) = exp^{-(\alpha D(x,y,z) + \beta D^2(x,y,z))}$; $V_S$ is the total volume of the sensitive region to radiation (e.g. the nucleus of the cell). $\alpha$ and $\beta$ are determined by means of experimental cell survival curves, without any NP in the biological medium. Equation 12.1 can then be used to compute the lethal events $N_{NP}$ due to the NP alone, after subtracting the dose calculated without NPs in water $D_{NP}(x,y,z) = D_{water+NP}(x,y,z) - D_{water}(x,y,z)$. The complete cell survival due to the NPs and the incident radiation field can then be evaluated with the number of lethal events created by the NPs alone ($N_{NP}$) and in water without the NPs ($N_{water}$), as follows: $S_{NP} = exp^{-(N_{NP}+N_{water})}$. $S_{NP}$ can then be compared to experimental survival curves in the presences of NPs to evaluate the quality of the model to reproduce experimental radiobiological results, as for example done in [56] and [57].

An emblematic study applying the LEM to study NP–radioenhancement in proton therapy is shown in Lin et al. [47]. The Monte Carlo simulations were performed with TOPAS [21] and were used to calculate the gold NP dose-enhancement in different configurations of NP distributions in the cell, in typical clinical kV and MV X-ray fields, and in proton therapy. The survival curves were calculated in-silico with the LEM, using $\alpha$ and $\beta$ values obtained in-vitro for different cell lines, when irradiated with X-rays. The study showed that gold NPs are more efficient to enhance the dose in the case of kV X-ray beams, when compared to MV and proton beams.

### 12.2.3.3  The Microdosimetric Kinetic Model

The Microdosimetric Kinetic Model (MKM) was firstly developed by Hawkins [58], [59], [60], [61]. In this approach the nucleus is divided into virtual spheres of radius $r_d$, called *domains*. The MKM model is described in detail in Kase et al. 2006 [62] and here it is briefly summarized.

The radiobiological endpoint estimated by means of the MKM is the $RBE_{10}$, which is calculated as the ratio of the dose required to achieve 10% cell survival using X-rays to that required when using the radiation of interest, assuming that the survival of cells $(S)$ is determined by the Linear Quadratic Model (LQM): $S = exp^{-(\alpha D + \beta D^2)}$, where $D$ is the dose, and $\alpha$ and $\beta$ are tissue radiosensitivity coefficients for the radiation of interest. The modified MKM relates the experimentally measured dose-mean lineal energy to the LQM parameter $\alpha$ for a particular radiation field. Using the LQM the $RBE_{10}$ can be expressed as:

$$RBE_{10} = \frac{2\beta D_{10,R}}{\sqrt{\alpha^2 - 4\beta \ln 0.1} - \alpha}, \tag{12.2}$$

$D_{10,R}$ is the dose corresponding to 10% when exposed to X-rays (e.g. 200 kVp X-rays), for the specific cell line considered. $\alpha$ is defined as:

$$\alpha = \alpha_0 + \frac{\beta}{\rho \pi r_d^2} y^*, \tag{12.3}$$

where $\alpha_0$ represents the initial slope of the survival fraction curve in the limit of zero LET, $\beta$ is a constant independent on LET, $\rho$ is the density of the biological medium $(1 \frac{g}{cm^3})$, $r_d$ is the radius of a sub-cellular domain. $y^*$ is the restricted dose-mean lineal energy which takes into account the cell overkilling effect for lineal energies above $> 150 \frac{keV}{\mu m}$ [62].

The MKM model has been adopted at the heavy ion therapy facility of HIMAC, National Institutes for Quantum and Radiological Science and Technology, Chiba, Japan, to determine the $RBE_{10}$, to calculate the RBE-weighted dose. Examples of Monte Carlo simulation studies using the MKM model to calculate the cell survival curve of specific cell lines in hadrontherapy are among others [63], [64], [65].

Kim et al. [66] applied for the first time the MKM model to investigate the NP radioenhancement in the case of an X-ray radiation field. In particular, the authors estimated the dose-mean lineal energy in the cell nucleus due to secondary radiation produced in the GNPs. It was found that both the MKM and the LEM can describe satisfactorily experimental cell survival curves.

As far as the authors of this chapter know, still, in the literature, there is not yet an in-silico study quantifying NP-radioenhancement in hadrontherapy using the MKM approach, and this is definitively a domain of further investigation.

## 12.3   MC SIMULATION STUDIES FOR NP RADIO-ENHANCEMENT

As mentioned before, existing MC approaches to NP radio-enhancement simulation cover different purposes, levels of detail and endpoints. Some studies first start from simpler models and neglect actual individual metallic particles in favor of a certain metal *concentration* in the material for the sake of simplicity [67]. This type of approach can work around limitations of CH calculations, since no nanometric material borders need to be accounted for, and approximates the macroscopic dosimetric effects of the presence of NPs which, especially for low LET radiation, can be compared to dosimetric measurements. To quantify the NP effect, the dose enhancement factor (DEF) defined as

$$DEF = \frac{D_{NPs}}{D_{no\,NPs}} \bigg|_{same\,irradiation\,conditions} \tag{12.4}$$

is often used. While this approach is simpler, it is nowadays widely recognized that it is not sufficient to gain meaningful insights in high-Z NP dose enhancement.

The local dose enhancement for different NP sizes in proton/ion radiation fields was covered in several research studies, including [17, 22, 68, 47, 19, 28, 38], with many works centering on gold NPs and a few comparing different NP materials [17, 68, 38]. Although the exact geometries considered differ in the set of studies under consideration, a strong physical dose enhancement is generally found very locally around irradiated NPs. Several-fold physical dose deposition can be

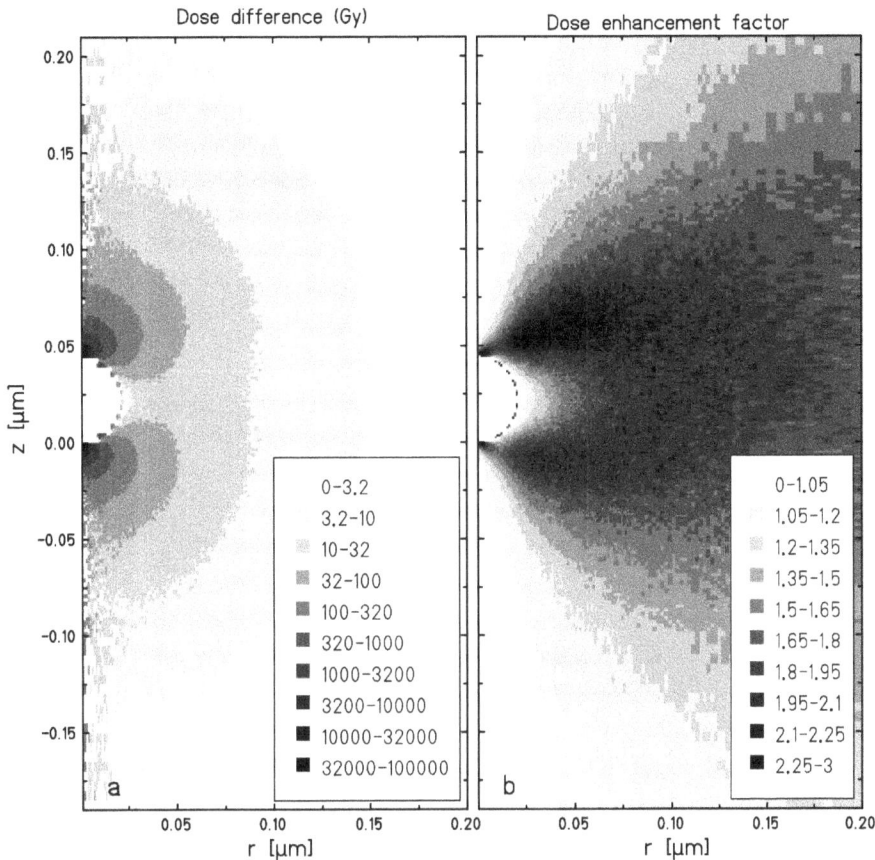

**Figure 12.3**   Nanoscale distribution in perpendicular ($r$) and longitudinal ($z$) direction of dose difference (a) and dose enhancement factor (b) for a water-embedded gold NP with respect to a uniform water volume for 53 MeV/u $^{16}$O ions. The ion path is along the $z$-axis in positive direction to centrally hit the 22 nm radius NP. Simulation carried out with TRAX [28].

found in the vicinity of a NP, and quantified as point-wise DEF in analogy to equation 12.4. An example for a gold NP hit by $^{16}$O ions can be found in Figure 12.3. The exact maximum values depend on the specific simulation set-up and the interaction cross sections and low-energy cut-off adopted. On the other hand, at a distance dose enhancement is significantly lower than that caused by kilovoltage photons (30 times lower at 10 micrometer from the gold NP surface in the simulation set-up of [47]). It should be noted that the global dose enhancement of a (water) target containing NPs vs. water only over a volume of e.g. cellular scale has found to be small to negligible for realistic NP concentrations under proton or ion irradiation due to the low interaction probability of projectile and NP [25, 28].

Some authors additionally consider the localization or distribution of the NPs either within a cell [47] or relative to each other, i.e. the effect of possible NP clustering [20, 25] which has been observed *in vitro* depending on NP size and coating. The available results for proton/ion beams show a decrease of dose enhancement for clustered NPs compared to dispersed ones [20, 25], because of the self-shielding of the NP aggregates. Note that for typical heavy ion irradiations, the average separation between individual tracks is relatively large and therefore the probability for two tracks to hit two contiguous (clustered) NPs is small.

Similar to equivalent work published earlier for photons as the incident radiation, a number of papers [e.g. 18, 47, 54] include biological modeling of DNA strand breaks or cell survival, see section 12.2.3, following the physical (dose) effects. In doing so, the expected biological effect caused by the highly inhomogeneous physical dose enhancement for hadrons can be characterized much more accurately. In the case of photon kV beams, secondary electrons produced in the GNP have a longer range, therefore contributing to the dose enhancement in a larger portion of the biological medium. Instead, as mentioned above, in proton or ion therapy the $\delta$-electrons have a very short range and can only contribute to the dose locally [47]. A consequence of this observation is that gold NPs can produce a biologically enhanced effect only when internalized in the cell nucleus in the case of proton therapy. The biological effects predicted are thus rather small particularly when NP localization is restricted to the cytoplasm, and do not seem to reach agreement with the sometimes encouraging experimental results.

Finally, new possibilities arise by including water radiolysis with chemical stage simulations. Up to date, a few studies combine hadron radiation with simulations of radiolysis [19, 25, 20, 69, 26] and aim typically for quantifying the enhancement (or decrease) of specific radical yields, most prominently for OH$^\bullet$. To that end, the radiolysis enhancement factor (REF)

$$\text{REF} = \left. \frac{G_{\text{total, NPs}}}{G_{\text{total, no NPs}}} \right|_{\text{same irradiation conditions}} \tag{12.5}$$

has been defined. The total REF (for the sum of all chemical species) appears to follow the behavior of DEF and yield a similar enhancement, but particular species can give different results especially for time points closer to the track dissolution (1 µs). An example for DEF and REF for different times into the chemical evolution is depicted in Figure 12.4. In this work [19], to calculate the probability of direct and indirect strand breaks, and DNA damage complexity [48] was adopted. Interestingly, for clustered NPs, increased OH$^\bullet$ G-values have been predicted [25].

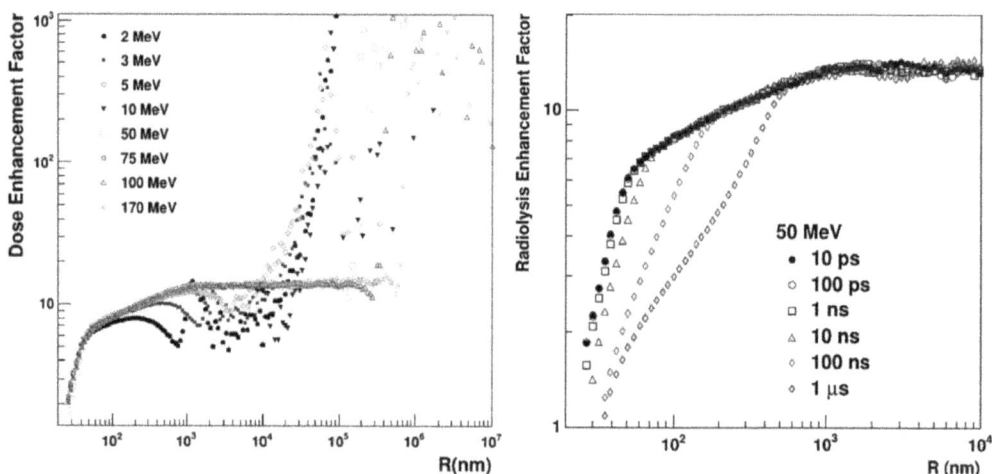

**Figure 12.4**    Dose enhancement factor and radiolysis enhancement factor for proton irradiation in presence of nanoparticles calculated with Geant4-DNA (Reprinted with permission from Tran et al. [19].)

## 12.4   RADIOENHANCERS BEYOND HIGH ATOMIC NUMBER NPS

In the case of hadron therapy, the use of high-Z NPs is not as efficient as in kV X-ray radiotherapy to cause radio-enhancement; the incident hadrons have a lower probability to interact with the NPs with respect to kV X-rays and the $\delta$-electrons have a short range. This means that the radio-enhancement happens only locally in the cell where the NPs are internalized [47].

Since few years ago, there is a strong interest in the scientific community to study a different mechanism of radio-enhancement, based on the amplification of the production of high-LET secondary particles via nuclear interactions, which increase the local energy deposition (within few micrometers) and the RBE.

One of the first studies in this direction, in proton therapy, is documented in [118], which proposed the so-called *proton boron fusion therapy*. The authors proposed as radio-enhancer $^{11}$B, which should be internalized preferentially in the tumor target. The incident protons can have a nuclear reaction with $^{11}$B, which produces a $^{12}$C nucleus in an excited state. This carbon nucleus is then split into an $\alpha$ particle of 3.76 MeV and a $^8$Be nucleus, which then breaks into two $\alpha$ particles of 2.74 MeV each. The three $\alpha$ particles have a high LET and therefore increase the dose locally and amplify the DNA damage. An interesting aspect is that the proton boron fusion reaction induces the emission of a prompt gamma ray, which can be used for imaging purposes.

Yoon and co-authors showed the potential of *proton boron fusion therapy* by means of Monte Carlo simulations, using MCNPX [71]. They found a dramatic increase of the dose in the tumor target (up to 50% the proton's maximum dose), induced by the presence of the boron. Nevertheless, it is important to note that the authors modeled the boron uptake region as a cylinder with a volume of approximately 23 cm$^3$ of pure $^{11}B$, with a density of 2.08 g/cm$^3$, in the tumor target, which is not realistic. While the merit of this work is to propose a new method to enhance the dose in proton therapy, it is then important to proceed with more realistic MC simulations or in-vitro experimental studies to demonstrate the applicability of *proton boron fusion therapy* in a more realistic scenario. This is what was done in Cirrone et al. [72].

The authors of this work irradiated samples of the prostate cancer line DU145 with a clinical proton beam, in the presence of sodium borocaptate (BSH), which is a common agent used clinically in Boron Neutron Capture Therapy (BNCT), to selectively deliver boron in cancer cells. In order to maximize the proton–boron fusion rate, the BSH was used with natural occurring boron isotopic abundance (i.e. about 80% $^{11}$B and 20% $^{10}$B). The BSH concentrations were equivalent to 40 ppm and 80 ppm of $^{11}$B. The cell lines were positioned in the middle of a 62 MeV clinical Spread-Out Bragg Peak (SOBP). The experiment was performed at the CATANA INFN-LNS facility (Catania, Italy). The radiobiological experiment showed a significant increase in terms of cell death, and of induction of DNA damage. As example, Figure 12.5 shows the result of the study in terms of cell survival curves. This work showed the potential of *proton boron fusion therapy* and, in general, of exploiting nuclear reactions in hadron therapy to amplify the dose and the DNA damage. It is important to observe that currently there is a debate on the mechanism of radio-enhancement observed in [72] (e.g. see [73]), aimed to understand more in depth the causes of the observed radio-enhancement, which could be beyond the nuclear reaction of proton–boron fusion, producing 3 $\alpha$ particles. Indeed, this scientific debate shows the interest in the scientific community on this type of radio-enhancers.

Another project in this research space is the Neutron Capture Enhanced Particle Therapy (NCEPT) [74], a method for increasing the radiation dose in proton and carbon ion therapy by enhancing the capture of thermal neutrons produced inside the treatment volume during irradiation. $^{10}$B and $^{157}$Gd-based drugs are proposed as agents to be internalized in the target of the treatment to increase neutron capture, due to the following nuclear reactions:

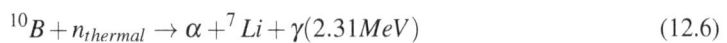

$$^{10}B + n_{thermal} \rightarrow \alpha + ^7Li + \gamma(2.31 MeV) \tag{12.6}$$

and

$$^{157}Gd + n_{thermal} \rightarrow ^{158}Gd^* \rightarrow ^{158}Gd + \gamma + 7.94 MeV \tag{12.7}$$

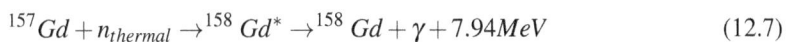

In the case of equation 12.6, high LET particles ($\alpha$ particles and Li nuclei) are emitted, with a range of few micrometers, similar to the cellular size. This increases the efficiency to kill cancer cells.

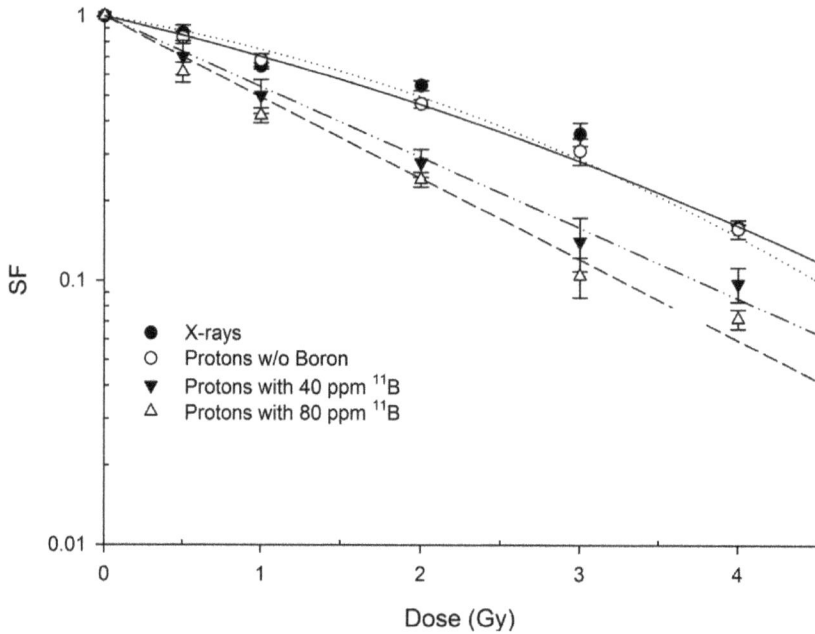

**Figure 12.5** Clonogenic dose response curves of prostate cancer cells DU145 irradiated with therapeutic protons in the presence or absence of BSH at mid-SOBP. Reprinted with permission from [72].

The same concept underlies BNCT. In the case of Gd (see equation 12.7), upon relaxation of the excited state, internal conversion (IC) and low-energy Auger electrons are produced, which then enhance the damage to DNA or other important cellular structures such as mitochondria, once they are internalized in the cell, close to these entities sensitive to radiation.

In this research domain, Monte Carlo simulations are an excellent tool to cast light on the mechanism of hadrontherapy boost as long as the effects of radiation are studied at the level of the DNA and/or of cellular structures, and the nuclear processes are modeled in detail in the Monte Carlo simulation. Similarly to the case of MC based studies for high-Z NPs, concentrations and distributions of the radio-enhancer should be modeled as accurately as possible.

## 12.5   DISCUSSION AND CONCLUSIONS

Nowadays there is a general consensus that radio-enhancement driven by high atomic number NPs is less efficient in hadron therapy, when compared to kV X-ray beams. This is due to a lower probability of the incident protons/carbon ions to interact with a NP, coupled with the short range of the $\delta$-electrons produced in the NPs [47]. In addition, due to the short range of the $\delta$-electrons, self-absorption effects within the high–Z NPs become more relevant. Altogether, the existing computational studies tend to rule out a sufficient physical enhancement of dose on cellular scales by electromagnetic processes (due to $\delta$-electrons, Auger electrons and characteristic X-rays).

In the case of protons and carbon ions, also radiolytic enhancement is very localized at the NP interface so that possibly [25], extra radical recombinations are favored, decreasing the net effect on the surrounding medium. For photons, oriented interfacial molecular layers of water around gold NPs have been proposed to have debilitated O-H bonds and suffer additional molecular dissociations by low-energy secondary electrons [75] at Au-water interfaces. Going into a similar direction and opening a way for a better understanding of NP radio-sensitization, a recent experimental study

[39] found an increase in OH$^\bullet$ yield for Au and Pt NPs with protons attributed to surface effects. No theoretical studies are however yet available on these aspects. Biological models coupled to MC calculations and taking into account typical cellular localizations of the NPs tend to show negligible effects for cell survival as an endpoint.

An increasing amount of experimental investigations have, however, found sensitizing effects under proton / ion irradiation. Some biological experiments observed some additional tenths in sensitizer enhancement ratio (SER $= (S_{\text{NPs}} - S_{\text{control}})/S_{\text{control}}|_{\text{same dose}}$, where $S$ is cell surviving fraction) or apparent RBE increase, or some tens of percent improvement of complete tumor regression (for a summary, see [76]). The large differences observed experimentally in these endpoints in presence of metal nanoparticles indicate that there is by no means a universal mechanism.

The NP effect for protons and heavier ions appears to be a combination of several aspects which individually depend on different properties not only of the incident radiation (mainly linear energy transfer) and cell line, but also of the NP – such as material, size / shape, concentration, and coating. The latter is particularly complex and has an influence both geometrically as an extra absorption layer, chemically for its possibility to stabilize and to prevent NP aggregation and possibly reacting with radiolytic products, and biologically in avoiding possible toxicities. The *enhancement* is now often regarded to have a much smaller, if any, role, as compared to actual *radio-sensitization* through biological pathways. Apart from a rather straightforward synergistic effect between possible selective cytotoxicity and radiation, oxidative stress especially of the mitochondria [77], and particularly depolarization of their membrane [78] has been discussed. For gold NPs and depending on the internalization route into the cytoplasm, hints for a signalling pathway triggered by gold ions that leads to an endogenous reactive oxygen species production have been obtained [79]. This means, however, that the most probable mechanisms for biological enhancement seem to become poorly addressable even with advanced MC capabilities.

Even if up to now, no reliable correlation has been achieved between MC predictions and the experimental results for radio-sensitization with NPs under ion irradiation, the multiple modeling directions triggered by the topic, as well as new funded collaborative research projects, have accelerated the technical development of MC tools. One example is the implementation [17, 34, 30] and sometimes test [69] of specific cross sections for discrete scattering models for the metals in question. Also the inclusion of the chemical stage of radiation interactions to current state-of-the-art MC codes has clearly benefited from an increased interest in radical generation related to NPs. These new features will certainly continue to be useful for many other future applications.

Finally, the emerging field of radio-enhancers, such as boron, which produce nuclear reaction products with high LET, preferentially in the tumor target, appears to be a very promising alternative approach for enhancing the effectiveness of particle therapy. The study of these type of radio-enhancers is only in its infancy and MC simulations can certainly be used as investigation tool to cast some light on the fundamental mechanism at the basis of the radio-enhancement.

## REFERENCES

1. Forrest H. Adams, Amos Norman, Renato S. Mello, and Doris Bass. Effect of radiation and contrast media on chromosomes. *Radiology*, 124:823–826, 1977.
2. Hiromichi Matsudaira, Akiko M Ueno, and Ikuko Furuno. Iodine contrast medium sensitizes cultured mammalian cells to X rays but not to $\gamma$ rays. *Radiat. Research*, 84:144–148, 1980.
3. D M Herold, I J Das, R V Iyer, and J D Chapman. Gold microspheres: a selective technique for producing biologically effective dose enhancement. *Int. J. Radiat. Biol.*, 76:1357–1364, 2000.
4. J F Hainfeld, Daniel N Slatkin, and Henry M Smilowitz. The use of gold nanoparticles to enhance radiotherapy in mice. *Phys. Med. Biol.*, 49:N309, 2004.
5. Dan Peer, Jeffrey M. Karp, Seungpyo Hong, Omid C. Farokhzad, Rimona Margalit, and Robert Langer. Nanocarriers as an emerging platform for cancer therapy. *Nature Nanotech.*, 2:751–760, 2007.

6. Devika B Chitrani, Salomeh Jelveh, Farid Jalali, Monique van Prooijen, Christine Allen, Robert G Bristow, Richard P Hill, and David A Jaffray. Gold nanoparticles as radiation sensitizers in cancer therapy. *Radiation Research*, 173:719–728, 2010.

7. Suneil Jain, Jonathan A.Coulter, Alan R.Hounsell, Karl T.Butterworth, S J McMahon, W B Hyland, M F Muir, Glenn R Dickson, Kevin M Prise, Fred J Currell, Joe M O'Sullivan, and David G Hirst. Cell-specific radiosensitization by gold nanoparticles at megavoltage radiation energies. *Int. J. Radiat. Oncol. Biol. Phys.*, 79:531–539, 2011.

8. F Xiao, Y Zheng, P CLoutier, Y He, D Hunting, and L Sanche. On the role of low-energy electrons in the radiosensitization of DNA by gold nanoparticles. *Nanotechnology*, 22:465101, 2011.

9. Karl T Butterworth, Stephen J McMahon, Laura E Taggart, and Kevin M Prise. Radiosensitization by gold nanoparticles: effective at megavoltage energies and potential role of oxidative stress. *Transl Cancer Res*, 2:269–279, 2013.

10. Lei Cui, Kenneth Tse, Payam Zahedia, Shane M Harding, Gaetano Zafarana, David A Jaffray, Robert G Bristow, and Christine Allen. Hypoxia and cellular localization influence the radiosensitizing effect of gold nanoparticles (AuNPs) in breast cancer cells. *Radiat. Research*, 182:475–488, 2014.

11. F. Lux et al. AGuIX from bench to bedside——Transfer of an ultrasmall theranostic gadolinium-based nanoparticle to clinical medicine. *The British Journal of Radiology*, 92(1093):20180365, 2019. PMID: 30226413.

12. J. Schuemann et al. Roadmap for metal nanoparticles in radiation therapy: current status, translational challenges, and future directions. *Phys. Med. Biol.*, 65:21RM02, 2020.

13. J-K Kim, S-J Seo, K-H Kim, T-J Kim, M-H Chung, K-R Kim, and T-K Yang. Therapeutic application of metallic nanoparticles combined with particle-induced x-ray emission effect. *Nanotechnology*, 21:425102, 2010.

14. Jerimy C Polf, Lawrence F Bronk, Wouter H P Driessen, Wadih Arap, Renata Pasquali, and Michael Gillin. Enhanced relative biological effectiveness of proton radiotherapy in tumor cells with internalized gold nanoparticles. *Appl. Phys. Lett.*, 98:193702, 2011.

15. J-K Kim, S-J Seo, H-T Kim, K-H Kim, M-H Chung, K-R Kim, and S-J Ye. Enhanced proton treatment in mouse tumors through proton irradiated nanoradiator effects on metallic nanoparticles. *Phys. Med. Biol.*, 57:8309–8323, 2012.

16. Sha Li, Sébastien Penninckx, Linda Karmani, Anne-Catherine Heuskin, Kassandra Watillon, Riccardo Marega, Jerome Zola, Valentina Corvaglia, Geraldine Genard, Bernard Gallez, Olivier Feron, Philippe Martinive, Davide Bonifazi, Carine Michiels, and Stéphane Lucas. LET-dependent radiosensitization effects of gold nanoparticles for proton irradiation. *Nanotechnology*, 27:455101, 2016.

17. C Wälzlein, E Scifoni, M Krämer, and M Durante. Simulations of dose enhancement for heavy atom nanoparticles irradiated by protons. *Phys. Med. Biol.*, 59:1141–1458, 2014b.

18. J C G Jeynes, M J Merchant, A Spindler, A-C Wera, and K J Kirkby. Investigation of gold nanoparticle radiosensitization mechanisms using a free radical scavenger and protons of different energies. *Phys. Med. Biol.*, 59:6431, 2014.

19. H N Tran, M Karamitros, V N Ivanchenko, S Guatelli, S McKinnon, K Murakami, T Sasaki, S Okada, M C Bordage, Z Francis, Z El-Bitar, M A Bernal, J I Shin, S B Lee, Ph Barberet, T T Tran, J M C Brown, T V Nhan Hao, and S Incerti. Geant4 Monte Carlo simulation of absorbed dose and radiolysis yields enhancement from a gold nanoparticle under mev proton irradiation. *Nucl. Instrum. Meth. Phys. Res. B*, 373:126–139, 2016.

20. D Peukert, I Kempson, M Douglass, and E Bezak. Gold nanoparticle enhanced proton therapy: Monte Carlo modeling of reactive species' distributions around a gold nanoparticle and the effects of nanoparticle proximity and clustering. *Int. J. Mol. Sci.*, 20:4280, 2019.

21. Schuemann J. Faddegon B. Perl J., Shin J. and Paganetti H. TOPAS: an innovative proton Monte Carlo platform for research and clinical applications. *Med. Phys.*, 39:6818–6837, 2012.

22. Y Lin, S McMahon, M Scarpelli, H Paganetti, and J Schuemann. Comparing gold nano-particle enhanced radiotherapy with protons, megavoltage photons and kilovoltage photons: a Monte Carlo simulation. *Phys. Med. Biol.*, 59:7675–7689, 2014.

23. S. Agostinelli et al. GEANT4 – a simulation toolkit. *Nucl. Instrum. Meth. A*, 506:250–303, 2003.

24. Bernal M. A. et al. Track structure modeling in liquid water: a review of the Geant4-DNA very low energy extension of the Geant4 Monte Carlo simulation toolkit. *Phys. Med.*, 31:157–178, 2015.

25. B Rudek, A McNamara, Jose Ramos-Mendez, H Byrne, Z Kuncic, and J Schuemann. Radio-enhancement by gold nanoparticles and their impact on water radiolysis for x-ray, proton and carbon-ion beams. *Phys. Med. Biol.*, 64:175005, 2019.

26. Daria Boscolo. *Nanoscale insights on hypoxia radiosensitization with ion beams*. PhD thesis, TU Darmstadt, 2018.

27. F Hespeels, A C Heuskin, T Tabarrant, E Scifoni, M Krämer, G Chêne, D Strivay, and S Lucas. Backscattered electron emission after proton impact on gold nanoparticles with and without polymer shell coating. *Phys. Med. Biol.*, 64:125007, 2019b.

28. M C Fuss, D Boscolo, M Durante, E Scifoni, and M Krämer. Systematic quantification of nanoscopic dose enhancement of gold nanoparticles in ion beams. *Phys. Med. Biol.*, 65:075008, 2020.

29. H. Nikjoo, S. Uehara, D. Emfietzoglou, and F.A. Cucinotta. Track-structure codes in radiation research. *Radiation Measurements*, 41(9):1052–1074, 2006. Space Radiation Transport, Shielding, and Risk Assessment Models.

30. D Sakata, I Kyriakou, S Okada, H N Tran, N Lampe, S Guatelli, M C Bordage, V N Ivanchenko, K Murakami, T Sasaki, D Emfietzoglou, and S Incerti. Geant4-DNA track-structure simulations for gold nanoparticles: the importance of electron discrete models in nanometer volume. *Med. Phys.*, 45:2230–2242, 2018.

31. Friedland W., Dingfelder M., Kundrát P., and Jacob P. Track structures, DNA targets and radiation effects in the biophysical Monte Carlo simulation code PARTRAC. *Mutat. Res.*, 711(1-2):28–40, 2011.

32. M. Krämer and G. Kraft. Calculations of heavy-ion track structure. *Radiation and Environmental Biophysics*, 33(2):91–109, 1994.

33. Plante I. and Cucinotta F. A. Monte-carlo simulation of ionizing radiation tracks. *Applications of Monte Carlo Methods in Biology, Medicine and Other Fields of Science*, 2011.

34. D Sakata, S Incerti, M C Bordage, N Lampe, S Okada, D Emfietzoglou, I Kyriakou, K Murakami, T Sasaki, H N Tran, S Guatelli, and V N Ivantchenko. An implementation of discrete electron transport models for gold in the Geant4 simulation toolkit. *J. Appl. Phys.*, 120:244901, 2016.

35. Valentin A., Raine M., Gaillardin M., and Paillet P. Geant4 physics processes for microdosimetry simulation: Very low energy electromagnetic models for protons and heavy ions in silicon. *NIM B*, 287:124–129, 2012.

36. Valentin A., Raine M., Gaillardin M., and Paillet P. Geant4 physics processes for microdosimetry simulation: Very low energy electromagnetic models for electrons in silicon. *NIM B*, 288:66–73, 2012.

37. Ryoichi Hirayama, Atsushi Ito, Miho Noguchi, Yoshitaka Matsumoto, Akiko Uzawa, Gen Kobashi, Ryuichi Okayasu, and Yoshiya Furusawa. OH radicals from the indirect actions of X-rays induce cell lethality and mediate the majority of the oxygen enhancement effect. *Radiation Research*, 180(5):514–523, 2013.

38. S. McKinnon et al. Local dose enhancement of proton therapy by ceramic oxide nanoparticles investigated with Geant4 simulations. *Physica Medica*, 32(12):1584–1593, 2016.

39. Sandra Zwiehoff, Jacob Johny, Carina Behrends, Alina Landmann, Florian Mentzel, Christian Bäumer, Kevin Kröninger, Christoph Rehbock, Beate Timmermann, and Stephan Barcikowski. Enhancement of proton therapy efficiency by noble metal nanoparticles is driven by the number and chemical activity of surface atoms. *Small*, 18(9):2106383, 2022.

40. Peter Clifford, Nicholas J. B. Green, Mark J. Oldfield, Michael J. Pilling, and Simon M. Pimblott. Stochastic models of multi-species kinetics in radiation-induced spurs. *J. Chem. Soc., Faraday Trans. 1*, 82:2673–2689, 1986.

41. Simon M. Pimblott and Jay A. LaVerne. Stochastic simulation of the electron radiolysis of water and aqueous solutions. *The Journal of Physical Chemistry A*, 101(33):5828–5838, 1997.

42. N. J. B. Green, M. J. Pilling, S. M. Pimblott, and P. Clifford. Stochastic modeling of fast kinetics in a radiation track. *The Journal of Physical Chemistry*, 94(1):251–258, 1990.

43. J. E. Turner, R. N., Hamm, H. A. Wright, R. H. Ritchie, J. L. Magee, A. Chatterjee, and Wesley E. Bolch. Studies to link the basic radiation physics and chemistry of liquid water. *Radiat. Phys. Chem.*, 32:503–510, 1987.

44. H. Nikjoo, P. O'Neill, D. T. Goodhead, and M. Terrisol. Computational modelling of low-energy electron-induced dna damage by early physical and chemical events. *Int. J. Radiat. Biol.*, 71:467–483, 1997.

45. F Ballarini, M Biaggi, M Merzagora, A. Ottolenghi, M. Dingfelder, W. Friedland, P. Jacob, and H. G. Paretzke. Stochastic aspects and uncertainties in the prechemical and chemical stages of electron tracks in liquid water: a quantitative analysis based on Monte Carlo simulations. *Radiation and Environmental Biophysics*, 39:179–188, 2000.

46. D Sakata, O Belov, M-C Bordage, D Emfietzoglou, S Guatelli, T Inaniwa, V Ivanchenko, M Karamitros, I Kyriakou, N Lampe, I Petrovic, Al Ristic-Fira, W-G Shin, and S Incerti. Fully integrated Monte Carlo simulation for evaluating radiation induced DNA damage and subsequent repair using Geant4-DNA. *Scientific Reports*, 10:20788, 2020.

47. Y Lin, S McMahon, H Paganetti, and J Schuemann. Biological modeling of gold nanoparticle enhanced radiotherapy for proton therapy. *Phys. Med. Biol.*, 60:4149–4168, 2015.

48. W. Friedland et al. Simulation of DNA damage after proton irradiation. *Radiation Research*, 159:401–410, 2003.

49. O. V. Belov et al. A quantitative model of the major pathways for radiation-induced dna double-strand break repair. *J. Theor. Biol.*, 366:115–130, 2015.

50. H. Nikjoo, P. O'Neill, W. E. Wilson, and D. T. Goodhead. Computational approach for determining the spectrum of dna damage induced by ionizing radiation. *Radiation Research*, 156:577–583, 2001.

51. Thilo Elsässer, Michael Krämer, and Michael Scholz. Accuracy of the local effect model for the prediction of biologic effects of carbon ion beams in vitro and in vivo. *International Journal of Radiation Oncology*Biology*Physics*, 71(3):866–872, 2008.

52. M. Scholz and G. Kraft. Track structure and the calculation of biological effects of heavy charged particles. *Adv. Space Res.*, 18(1):5–14, 1996.

53. M. Scholz and G. Kraft. The physical and radiobiological basis of the local effect model: a response to the commentary by R. Katz. Radiat Res.:612–620, 2004.

54. M. Sotiropoulos, N. T. Henthorn, J. W. Warmenhoven, R. I. Mackay, K. J. Kirkby, and M. J. Merchant. Modelling direct DNA damage for gold nanoparticle enhanced proton therapy Nanoscale, 2017.

55. Brown J. M. C and Currell F. J. A local effect model-based interpolation framework for experimental nanoparticle radiosensitisation data. *Cancer Nano*, 8:1–10, 2017.

56. McMahon S. et al. Biological consequences of nanoscale energy deposition near irradiated heavy atom nanoparticles. *Scientific Reports*, 1, 2011.

57. Engels E. et al. Advances in modelling gold nanoparticle radiosensitization using new geant4-dna physics models. *Physics in Medicine and Biology*, 65(22):225017, 2020.

58. Hawkins R B. A microdosimetric-kinetic model of cell death from exposure to ionizing radiation of any LET, with experimental and clinical applications. *Int J Radiat Biol*, 69:739–755, 1996.

59. Hawkins R B. A microdosimetric-kinetic theory of the dependence of the RBE for cell death on LET. *Medical Physics*, 25:1157–1170, 1998.

60. Hawkins R B. A microdosimetric-kinetic model for the effect of non-Poisson distribution of lethal lesions on the variation of RBE with LET. *Radiation Research*, 160:61–69, 2003.

61. Hawkins R B. The relationship between the sensitivity of cells to high-energy photons and the RBE of particle radiation used in radiotherapy. *Radiation Research*, 172:761–776, 2009.

62. Y. Kase, T. Kanai, Y. Matsumoto, Y. Furusawa, H. Okamoto, T. Asaba, M. Sakama, and H. Shinoda. Microdosimetric measurements and estimation of human cell survival for heavy-ion beams. *Radiation Research*, 166(4):629–638, 2006.

63. Sato T and Furusawa Y. Cell survival fraction estimation based on the probability densities of domain and cell nucleus specific energies using improved microdosimetric kinetic models. *Radiation Research*, 178:341–356, 2012.

64. D. Bolst, L.T. Tran, L. Chartier, D.A. Prokopovich, A. Pogossov, S. Guatelli, M.I. Reinhard, M. Petasecca, M.L.F. Lerch, N. Matsufuji, V.L. Perevertaylo, C. Fleta, G. Pellegrini, M. Jackson, and A.B. Rosenfeld. RBE study using solid state microdosimetry in heavy ion therapy. *Radiation Measurements*, 106:512–518, 2017.

65. L.T. Tran, D. Bolst, S. Guatelli, A. Pogossov, M. Petasecca, M.L.F. Lerch, L. Chartier, D.A. Prokopovich, M.I. Reinhard, M. Povoli, A. Kok, V.L. Perevertaylo, N. Matsufuji, T. Kanai, M. Jackson, and A.B. Rosenfeld. The relative biological effectiveness for carbon, nitrogen, and oxygen ion beams using passive and scanning techniques evaluated with fully 3D silicon microsimeters. *Medical Physics*, 45(5):2299–2308, 2018.

66. H Kim, W Sunga, and S-J Ye. Microdosimetric-kinetic model for radio-enhancement of gold nanoparticles: Comparison with LEM. *Radiat. Res.*, 195:293–300, 2021.

67. Jongmin Cho, Carlos Gonzalez-Lepera, Nivedh Manohar, Matthew Kerr, S Krishnan, and S H Cho. Quantitative investigation of physical factors contributing to gold nanoparticle-mediated proton dose enhancement. *Phys. Med. Biol.*, 61:2562–2581, 2016.

68. I Martínez-Rovira and Y Prezado. Evaluation of the local dose enhancement in the combination of proton therapy and nanoparticles. *Med. Phys.*, 42:6703–6710, 2015.

69. F Hespeels, S Lucas, T Tabarrant, E Scifoni, M Krämer, G Chêne, D Strivay, H N Tran, and A C Heuskin. Experimental measurements validate the use of the binary encounter approximation model to accurately compute proton induced dose and radiolysis enhancement from gold nanoparticles. *Phys. Med. Biol.*, 64:065014, 2019a.

70. Do-Kun Yoon, Joo-Young Jung, and Tae Suk Suh. Application of proton boron fusion reaction to radiation therapy: A Monte Carlo simulation study. *Applied Physics Letters*, 105:223507, 2014.

71. L. S. Waters et al. The MCNPX Monte Carlo radiation transport code. *AIP Conference Proceedings*, 896:81, 2007.

72. G. A. P. Cirrone et al. First experimental proof of proton boron capture therapy (PBCT) to enhance protontherapy effectiveness. *Scientific Reports*, 8:1141, 2018.

73. A. Mazzone et al. On the (un)effectiveness of proton boron capture in proton therapy. *Eur. Phys. J. Plus*, 134:361, 2019.

74. Safavi-Naeini M et al. Opportunistic dose amplification for proton and carbon ion therapy via capture of internally generated thermal neutrons. *Scientific Reports*, 8:16257, 2018.

75. Manon Gilles, Emilie Brun, and Cécile Sicard-Roselli. Quantification of hydroxyl radicals and solvated electrons produced by irradiated gold nanoparticles suggests a crucial role of interfacial water. *J. Colloid Interface Sci*, 525:31–38, 2018.

76. D Peukert, I Kempson, M Douglass, and E Bezak. Metallic nanoparticle radiosensitisation of ion beam radiotherapy: A review. *Physica Medica*, 47:121–128, 2018.

77. Y Pan, A Leifert, D Ruau, S Neuss, J Bornemann, G Schmid, W Brandau, U Simon, and W Jahnen-Dechent. Gold nanoparticles of diameter 1.4 nm trigger necrosis by oxidative stress and mitochondrial damage. *Small*, 5:2067–2076, 2009.

78. W W-Y Kam and R B Banati. Effects of ionizing radiation on mitochondria. *Free Rad. Biol. Med.*, 65:607–619, 2013.

79. S Penninckx, A-C Heuskin, C Michiels, and S Lucas. The role of thioredoxin reductase in gold nanoparticle radiosensitization effects. *Nanomedicine*, 13(22):2917–2937, 2018.

# 13 Increasing particle therapy biological effectiveness by nuclear reaction-driven binary strategies

*Lorenzo Manti*
University of Naples Federico II, Naples, Italy
Istituto Nazionale di Fisica Nucleare (INFN), Section of Naples, Naples, Italy

*Andrea Attili*
INFN National Institute for Nuclear Physics, Rome, Italy

*Pavel Bláha*
Nuclear Physics Institute, Czech Academy of Sciences, Prague, Czech Republic

*Silva Bortolussi*
Universitá degli studi di Pavia, Pavia, Italy
Istituto Nazionale di Fisica Nucleare, Pavia Section, Pavia, Italy

*Giacomo Cuttone*
Istituto Nazionale di Fisica Nucleare - Laboratori Nazionali del Sud, Catania, Italy

*Ian Postuma*
Istituto Nazionale di Fisica Nucleare-Sezione di Pavia, Pavia, Italy

## CONTENTS

DOI: 10.1201/9781003023920-13

## 13.1   INTRODUCTION

Charged particle inverted dose-depth profile represents the physical pillar of protontherapy. On the other hand, there is no obvious radiobiological advantage in the use of protons since their LET in the clinical energy range (a few keV/$\mu$m, at mid-Spread-Out Bragg Peak, SOBP) is too low to achieve a cell-killing effect significantly greater than in conventional radiotherapy. This currently prevents protontherapy from being useful against intrinsically radioresistant cancers. Radioresistance of cancer cells implies dose-escalation regimes to achieve tumor local control. .In theory, every tumor can be controlled if a sufficiently high dose can be delivered that is able to suppress the proliferative potential of all cancer cells. However, in clinical practice, the maximum radiation dose is unfortunately limited by the tolerance of the surrounding normal tissue. A well-known relationship links physical radiation quality (LET) and its biological effectiveness (RBE), based on the notion that cellular lethality increases with the degree of DNA damage clustering, i.e. complexity, which reflects the nano-scale model of radiation action. Therapeutic $^{12}$C ion beams show a LET at mid-SOBP of about 50 keV/$\mu$m, conferring these particles a greater RBE for tumor cell killing, which is the radiobiological justification for their use against radioresistant cancers. However, the non-negligible dose deposition beyond the SOBP due to nuclear fragmentation and economical issues encumber this form of hadrontherapy. Additionally, limited radiobiological data exist on long-term normal tissue radiotoxicity. It is already known from previous studies that many different factors are associated with radioresistance of cancer cells and multiple reviews have already described some of the possible mechanisms underlying radioresistance during conventional radiotherapy. Examples are cancer stem cells and hypoxia, as well as perturbations in survival pathways, DNA damage repair pathways, developmental pathways. Many molecular inhibitors have been tested in combination with conventional radiotherapy, while only very few have been tested in combination with protons or carbon ions. Since particle therapy is on the rise, this calls for further exploration of these combined therapies in a preclinical setting. Previously, particle radiation facilities provided limited access for biological experiments, which limited the time to perform such experiments. However, international consortia on particle therapy research are growing and now recognize the potential of radiobiological experimental work. Therefore, the European Particle Therapy Network is producing a considerable effort to form a network of research and therapy facilities in order to coordinate and standardize radiobiological experiments. For carbon ions specifically, limited data on combination therapies are available. This is mainly due to the high RBE of carbon ions by which the additional benefit of molecular inhibitors might be difficult to demonstrate. Furthermore, the use of carbon ions worldwide is limited, which could also explain why fewer studies have been published regarding combination treatment with carbon ions. In the next paragraph, combined molecular approaches targeting specific repair pathways will be briefly illustrated, together with an outlook of recently proposed systemic approaches where radiation may upregulate the fundamental anti-cancer response by the immune system. In the context of achieving greater RBE at cell tumor inactivation while maintaining reasonably low-dose levels in healthy tissues, the role of physics and, specifically of certain nuclear reactions, has recently re-gained center stage in the form of so-called binary strategies. Historically, the first approach to predict a tumor-confined increase of radiobiologically effective doses by irradiation with a primary beam is the Boron Neutron Capture Therapy (BNCT) which exploits the 10B(n,$\alpha$)7Li reaction. The BNCT is defined as a binary approach since an external neutron beam serves no therapeutic purpose by itself but is needed to trigger the secondary particles which bring about the radiobiologically effective action on the tumor A boron-10

(10B)-labeled carrier must deliver higher concentrations of 10B to target tumor cells compared to the concentrations uptaken by surrounding normal tissues. The administration of borated formulation is followed by irradiation with low-energy neutrons. When a neutron collides with 10B, high-LET particles, i.e., $\alpha$-particles and recoiling 7Li particles, are released within one cell's diameter by the 10B(n, $\alpha$)7Li neutron capture reaction, which occurs with a high cross section (3738 b) at thermal energy. These high-LET particles can destroy the 10B-containing cells without exerting hazardous effects on the adjacent normal cells. Therefore, if sufficient quantities of boron compounds can be made to accumulate selectively in tumor cells with enough contrast to surrounding normal cells, the BNCT becomes an ideal radiotherapy modality. The selective properties of BNCT make it a radiotherapy option potentially useful also for disseminated or infiltrated malignancies. BNCT requires: a) low-energy neutron beams, whose availability is not trivial; b) selectivity in boron uptake by tumor cells only; c) a complex dosimetry of the mixed-field arising from neutron interaction with the tissue elements. Recently another binary approach has been proposed that exploits the 11B(p, $\alpha$)8Be reaction, whose cross section resonates at 675 keV, hence being termed Proton-Boron Capture Therapy (PBCT). In protontherapy such energies are those of protons as they slow down across the tumor region. The latter eliminates the requirement for selective boron uptake by cancer cell as alpha particles will be not generated, in principle, in healthy tissues at the beam entrance channel where incident proton energy is too high from that of the cross section maximum; thus if proven viable, PBCT would elegantly bypass one of the most critical requirements of BNCT.

## 13.2 NOVEL FRONTIERS IN PARTICLE THERAPY: THE RADIOBIOLOGICAL POINT OF VIEW

### 13.2.1 OVERCOMING CANCER RADIORESISTANCE

The ultimate goal of any form of curative radiotherapy resides in achieving local tumor control by suppressing the proliferative ability of all clonogenic cancer cells. If, on the one hand, the dosimetric precision inherent to charged particle therapy, in principle, allows to reduce the risk of adverse effects due to unnecessary dose absorbed by healthy tissues and/or organs at risk, on the other hand cancer radioresistance continues to represent a cause for treatment failure, leading to local recurrence, metastases and poor prognostic outlook [70]. Most of the available knowledge on the molecular mechanisms underlying cancer radioresistance derives from the predominant experience with conventional radiotherapy [53], which has highlighted how tumor response to ionizing radiation is deeply influenced by the heterogeneity that characterizes the tumor microenvironment [59]. Such heterogeneity and the changes the tumor microenvironment undergoes during cancer progression and the course of a radiotherapy regime, contribute to a variety of tumor subpopulations exhibiting differing radiosensitivities [14, 2] and define what is referred to as intrinsic and acquired radioresistance, respectively [7, 73]. Hypoxia is arguably one of the most intensively studied factors contributing to cancer radioresistance [15, 37, 38, 40, 6]. Although the low Oxygen Enhancement Ratio (OER) presented by high-LET radiation is the obvious radiobiological pillar of 12C-ion based radiotherapy against hypoxia-induced cancer radioresistance, charged particle radiobiology still lacks a thorough knowledge on the impact that the different physical nature of radiation may have on the molecular signaling pathways encompassing radioresistance and tumor microenvironment. The need for a re-definition of cellular radiosensitivity to charged particles is exemplified by peculiar inconsistencies if observed radioresponse is compared against the expected behavior based solely on the known LET-RBE relationship, with reported instances of a greater effectiveness exhibited by protons compared to photons in sensitizing resistant glioma cancer cells, which was ascribed to proton-specific increased ROS levels [78, 3]. These findings, coupled with the observation of a greater proportion of clustered DNA damage left unrepaired in cells exhibiting defects in the Fanconi Anemia/BRCA repair pathway following proton irradiation compared to photons at comparable LET values [51], have led to the suggestion of a clinically useful "New Biology" of protons by Held et al. (2016). Thus, in line with the increasing awareness of a variable proton RBE as a function of physical parameters, the genetic heterogeneity of tumors with regard to their repair capabilities may be exploited to single out proton-susceptible tumors [25, 34, 22]. However, despite indications of a significantly high efficiency of 12C ions at killing cancer stem in hypoxic niches [60], overcoming cancer radioresistance is still an urgent necessity in charged particle therapy, hence various approaches to enhance its biological effectiveness are being explored.

## 13.2.2 EXPLOITING BIOMOLECULAR APPROACHES

Targeting specific molecular pathways involved in cancer radioresistance has been proposed as a potential avenue to sensitizing cancer cells to charged particles in approaches that are designed to combine the peculiar radiobiological properties of the latter with novel molecular inhibitors directed to suppress a number of cancer cell pro-survival mechanisms and/or counteract radioresistant cell niches [44]. In this context, few radiobiological and clinically relevant data exist. These strategies have in common the idea that charged particles may modulate or act on most of these potential targets in a different manner compared to photons [71, 72] and include the DNA Damage Response (DDR) machinery [53] as well as proliferation- and cell death-associated gene transcription signalling pathways [61], cancer stem cells [74] and, of course, hypoxia. In counteracting the latter by charged particles, their concomitant use with hypoxia inducible factor (HIF)-1 inhibitors has been proposed. This is because, in contrast with the fundamental role that physiological levels of oxygen play in the yield of photon irradiation-induced DNA damage, HIF-1 expression is strongly upregulated by photons in hypoxic cells and its activation is linked with neo-angiogenesis, tumor growth and metastasization. Whereas the use of HIF-1 inhibitors in conventional radiotherapy has yielded inconclusive results, their role in particle therapy is still unexplored and may be of potential interest for clinical protons, where OER is supposed to be similar to that of photons. Additionally, the use of vascular endothelial growth factor (VEGF) inhibitors is warranted, especially in combination with 12C-ion therapy, because of the importance of hypoxia-modulated angiogenesis via the HIF-1/VEGF signalling pathway [106] and the demonstrated efficacy of high-LET radiation against hypoxia. Closely linked with the presence of hypoxic niches within the tumor is the presence of the intrinsically radioresistant cancer stem cells [42, 24], whose functional properties including self-renewal capacity, long-term repopulation potential, and tumor initiation and progression capacity render them a determinant of cancer resilience to radiotherapy. A number of survival signaling pathways have been identified that contribute to cancer stem cell radioresistance (i.e., Wnt, Notch, Hedgehog, anti-apoptotic Bcl-2, TGF-beta, and PI3K/Akt/mTOR), for which several pharmacological inhibitors have been developed over the years, thereby representing as many potential targets for combined treatments [44, 59]. Finally, given the pivotal role that repair has in conferring radioresistance, targeting of DDR signalling pathways, such as those centered on Poly(ADP-ribose) polymerase (PARP), a key responder and effector of radiation-induced DNA breakage, or on the genome integrity regulator tumor suppressor protein p53, are an attractive strategy to explore in hadrontherapy [44]. For example,the PARP inhibitor, AZD2281, was shown to enhance DNA damage yield and cell-cycle arrest in the tumor-conformed SOBP for clinical proton beams by Hirai et al. (2016), while more recently [50] have shown an increased 12C-ion induced cancer cell sensitization when administered in combination with another PARP inhibitor, talazoparib. Similarly attractive appears the concomitant use in particle therapy of antagonists of the mouse double minute 2 and X (MDM2/X), negative regulators of p53 [56], based on promising pre-clinical findings on targeting the MDM2/X-p53 pathway for the treatment of glioblastomas shown by several inhibitors in co-therapy scenarios with drugs and photon irradiation [12].

## 13.2.3  EXPLOITING SYSTEMIC RESPONSES

In order to grow and spread, cancer cells develop mutations that allow them to escape recognition and elimination by the host's immune system [33]. Immunotherapy (IT) has gained importance in cancer treatment due to its potential to recover the individual patient's immune recognition of cancer and develop an acquired immune response against malignant cells in the entire body. Available IT agents are therefore designed to either re-activate the immune system or release its brakes to allow recognition of cancer cells as non-self, and successfully reject them. However, even in malignancies where IT has proven efficacy (e.g. melanoma, non-small cell lung cancer, and certain genitourinary malignancies), response rates remain low, highlighting the need for more effective agents or combined modalities [64, 10, 32]. There exists a revival of interest in the modulatory effects of ionizing radiation on the immune system as mounting evidence has consistently shown the ability of locally administered radiotherapy to induce a system-wide immune response [20, 21, 27] in addition to exerting its cytotoxic action on the tumor site, suggesting that radiation can work together with the immune system to eliminate cancer [27, 28, 32, 58]. As a result, historically established concepts have been revisited, such as those describing a mere immunosuppressive action by radiation whereas it is now accepted that radiation causes multiple immunostimulatory effects [21]. Furthermore, in-vitro radiobiological phenomena collectively known as Non-Targeted Effects (NTEs), specifically the bystander effect, have been re-assessed, in light of new reports of regression of tumors outside of radiation field, thereby bridging the conceptual gap with the abscopal responses sporadically reported in vivo [66, 28]. Unfortunately, due to various immune escape mechanisms put in place by the tumor, radiotherapy alone rarely results in a systemic response of metastatic disease sites, that is the abscopal effect. The rarity of radiotherapy-induced abscopal effects, with 46 reported cases in the literature from 1969 to 2014 [1], reflects the fact that, once metastases are detected, a sustained cancer-related immunosuppression has already been established [75]. In order to elicit the abscopal effects of RT in preclinical models mimicking metastatic disease, some of this concurrent immune suppression must be relieved. This concept was initially tested in a series of experiments that first linked the abscopal effects to an immune-mediated mechanism. In a clinical trial, where 41 patients with metastatic cancer were treated with a combination of local radiotherapy and administration IT factors, abscopal response occurred in a remarkable 26.8% of the patients [31]. The radiobiological rationale in support of a synergistic use of radiotherapy and immunotherapy relies on the fact that radiation induces "immunogenic cell death" (ICD), a process that involves the release of various cytokines and signals that modify the microenvironment of tumors and stimulate influx of immune cells to recognize tumor-specific antigens presented by dying cells as a result of therapeutic doses of radiation. This, in turn, cross-primes T-cells in draining lymph nodes, causing their activation and eventual increase in tumor infiltration by cells facilitated in recognizing the tumor cells. By such processes, radiotherapy has been shown to significantly modify the tumor microenvironment and to possess the potential to convert an irradiated tumor into an in-situ vaccine to provide systemic, long-lasting protection against cancer. [26, 27]. Thus, the view that radiation may indeed revert a host's suppressed immune status, not only by locally enhancing radiation-induced lethality in directly irradiated cancer cells through the (re)-activation of the innate and adaptive immune system, but also leading to out-of-field immune-mediated anti-metastatic responses, has been consolidating [21]. The idea that combining radiotherapy with immunotherapy may allow better local and systemic tumor controls, has naturally led to the proposal of exploring if, and to what extent, such immune system radiomodulation is influenced by radiation quality [23]. The possibility that charged particle exposure may elicit stronger immune responses than after photon irradiation is based on the aforementioned physical advantages and radiobiological peculiarities exhibited by protons and 12C ions [71]. Several pre-clinical and clinical trials are ongoing to experimentally verify whether charged particle therapy may potentiate the benefits brought by immunotherapy to overcome radioresistance and tumor invasiveness. For example, Gameiro et al. (2016) [30] have shown that proton irradiation is able to induce hallmarks of immunogenic modulation by upregulating the expression of calreticulin and other tumor cell-surface markers involved in immune recognition in stem-like breast cancer cells. Several studies are also examining the immunoadjuvant effects of protonther-apy against non-small cell lung cancer on the grounds of differential biological responses induced by protons, i.e. more immunogenicity and less immunosuppression if compared to photons [49]. Recently, in-vivo work by Takahashi et al. (2019) [52] for the first time showed that carbon ion irradiation combined with dual immune checkpoint blockade therapy enhanced local anti-tumor ef-ficacy and induced an abscopal effect by inhibiting distant metastases in a preclinical murine model of osteosarcoma. Equally promising are the results by Mirjolet et al. (2021), demonstrating for the first time in a clinical protontherapy setting and using an ectopic mouse model with a trans-planted colon carcinoma cell line, that a single proton dose of 16.4 Gy activated several immune response pathways, inducing intra-tumor infiltration of CD8+ T cells, CD4+ T cells and type 1 tumor associated-macrophage (TAM1). In conclusion, validation of a clinical advantage deriving from coupling of hadrontherapy and immunotherapy would arguably represent a strong argument in favor of a further expansion of anticancer therapies based on charged particles as they remain, overall, just a fraction of all radiotherapy modalities.

## 13.3   THE RADIOBIOLOGICAL RATIONALE OF PHYSICS-BASED STRATEGIES FOR CHARGED PARTICLE-MEDIATED RADIOSENSITIZATION

Strategies based on physical interaction between ionizing radiation and metallic nanoparticles or that exploit nuclear fusion reactions have gained momentum in recent years and shown promising results to achieve clinically effective radiosensitization. In the following sections, an overview of such methods to reverse cellular radioresistance is presented.

### 13.3.1   NANOPARTICLE-MEDIATED RADIOSENSITIZATION

The use of metallic complexes has been actively investigated as a means of enhancing tumor cyto-toxicity induced by high-energy photons based on amplification of primary processes as compre-hensively reviewed in Kobayashi et al. (2010) [43]. To avoid size-dependent poor diffusion of such active products into the cancer tissues, research was soon directed to developing metallic nanoparti-cles (MNPs) due to their ability to passively accumulate in higher concentrations in tumor tissue than in the surrounding normal tissues when injected into the bloodstream. The selective delivery of NPs occurs because of the enhanced permeability and retention effect (EPR), whereby systems that are small enough (diameter <200 nm) tend to permeate through the tumor blood vessel walls [55]. Tu-mors recruit their own blood supply by angiogenesis, and their vasculature has leaky capillary walls that allow for NPs to easily pass through the wall. The most commonly considered formulation has been traditionally gold nanoparticles (GNPs), i.e. particles of gold with a diameter of 100 nm or less. In addition to good biocompatibility because of their inert chemical nature, GNPs were mostly expected to be ideal photosensitizers for those reactions characterized by a strong dependence on Z, such as photoelectric and pair production interactions of X-rays [47]. Among the several emissions that occur, Auger electrons can play an important radiosensitizing role when produced by photon interaction with high-Z GNPs since they have much shorter range than fluorescent photons, with much higher ionization density, thereby deploying a highly localized clustered DNA damage (Ku et al., 2019). Generally, it is the high absorption of photons by NPs to augment secondary electrons, increasing the levels of DNA damage by physically enhancing the dose. However, high-Z metal NPs (MNPs) have also been shown to act through distinct biological mechanisms including higher levels of oxidative stress, increasing levels of reactive oxygen species (ROS) and inducing highly reactive hydroxyl radicals which go on to cause further DNA damage [16]. To improve tumor target-ing, then NPs may be functionalized with tumor specific agents such as antibodies or other peptides [29]. Other MNPs have been investigated over the years as radiosensitizers, and sophisticated NPs, composed of other heavy elements such as hafnium [54] and gadolinium [68], are already being considered for clinical usage and possible theranostic agents. Equally sophisticated is the theranostic use of Superparamagnetic Iron Oxide Nanoparticles (SPIONs) in light of the development of MR-Linacs, whose radiosensitising properties have recently assessed in combination with kVp X-rays over a panel of cancer cell lines in vitro, as well as for the first time, in vivo with a H460 lung xenograft model [67]. Although initially devised and long investigated for photons/electrons, the strategy based on the use of nano-radiosensitizers has been proposed and is being increasingly tested also for charged particles, mainly protons and, to a lesser extent, 12C ions. This approach was not initially regarded as capable of leading to significantly measurable radiosensitizing effects for proton and ion radiotherapy because of the decrease in collision stopping power of charged particles as a weak logarithmic function of Z in contrast with the high photoelectric absorption with strong Z-dependence exhibited by kV X-rays. However, as recently reviewed by Lacombe et al. (2017) [48] and by Peukert et al. (2018) [62], experimental evidence has been accumulated that seems to dispel this notion, although only limited in vitro and in vivo data are available and much remains to be understood about the underlying physical and radiobiological mechanisms responsible for the observed radiosensitizing effects such as those of proton irradiation in the presence of GNPs. Indeed, charged particles are able to give rise to a nonlinear avalanche of electron emissions from high-Z NPs through impact ionization and ensuing Auger cascades. Importantly, surface plasmon excitation can result in a large production of secondary electrons that can continue to excite and ionize surrounding biomolecules and neighboring nanoparticles, providing a solid rationale for proton-therapy radiosensitization [48] In addition, Coulomb nanoradiator (CNR) effects that produce burst emission of fluorescent X-rays and low-energy electron (LEEs) via Auger cascade and a generalized increase in chemical damage by reactive oxygen species (ROS) are thought as major players in the dose enhancement effects that are observed for high-Z NPs and high-energy proton beams as shown by Geant4-based simulations by Peukert et al. (2019) [63]. To confirm such theoretical predictions, a number of high-Z MPNs were tested by Rashid et al. (2019) [65] and all showed a radiosensitizing action compatible with an increased intracellular ROS production in a human colon carcinoma cell line exposed within the SOBP of a 150-MeV proton beam. More recently, increased induction of cytogenetic damage but lack of an LET dependence on the incident particle LET were shown in a proof-of-principle study aimed at investigating the radiosensitizing properties of large (50 nm diameter) GNPs on CHO-K1 cells exposed at varying depths along a 50-mm SOBP modulated from a 200-MeV clinical proton beam (Cunningham et al., 2021) [19]. Finally, Zhang et al. (2021) [79] were able to show for the first time evidence of in-vivo radiosensitization by GNPs of 12C ion irradiation in tumor-bearing mice, which also these authors attribute to an increased production of ROS and, more specifically, to the activation of the mitochondrial apoptotic pathway in line with cytoplasmic GNP localization of the incorporated GNPs. Though intriguing, these results warrant further radiobiological studies to unveil the full potential of nano-material radiosensitization of charged particle therapy.

### 13.3.2 BINARY APPROACHES BASED ON NUCLEAR PHYSICS REACTIONS

### 13.3.2.1 Boron-Neutron Capture Therapy (BNCT)

BNCT, as explained above, exploits the neutron capture reaction in 10B, carried into tumor cells by suitable drugs before low-energy neutron irradiation. The neutron capture reaction occurs with a cross section of 3837 b at thermal energy and has the following two branches:

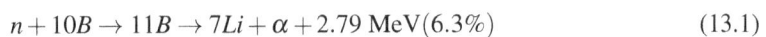

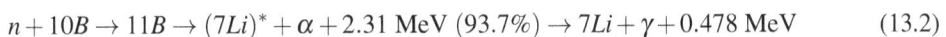

$$n + 10B \rightarrow 11B \rightarrow 7Li + \alpha + 2.79 \text{ MeV} (6.3\%) \tag{13.1}$$

$$n + 10B \rightarrow 11B \rightarrow (7Li)^* + \alpha + 2.31 \text{ MeV} (93.7\%) \rightarrow 7Li + \gamma + 0.478 \text{ MeV} \tag{13.2}$$

Suitable boron drugs have been developed for clinical use and many strategies are being followed to design new carriers able to guarantee a high boron concentration between tumor and normal tissues. Today, the only drug used for patients is Boronophenylalanine (BPA), ensuring tumor to healthy tissue concentration ratios of about 3.5:1 [8]. Albeit not high, this ratio is still useful for a safe and effective BNCT treatment.

BNCT was first applied to treat a patient affected by malignant glioma in 1951, using the Brookhaven Graphite Research Reactor [8]. Since then, it has been applied in institutions equipped with research nuclear reactors, where suitable neutron beams were designed according to the tumors to be treated: epithermal for deep-seated and thermal or hyperthermal for shallow cancer (i.e. nodular melanoma). A review of the clinical trials performed since the recent years is described in [120]. The pathologies that have been treated with a higher number of patients are Glioblastoma Multiforme (GBM), recurrent and newly diagnosed head and neck tumors and skin melanoma. In recent years, an important technological innovation has opened the way to more clinical applications, since suitable neutron beams can now be obtained with proton accelerators coupled to Be or Li targets. In Japan, clinical centers with neutron beams obtained by cyclotron and Be target are already applying BNCT to patients [121] ; all over the world new facilities based on accelerators are being projected and constructed.

BNCT is based on the emission of two high-LET particles following the neutron capture in 10B, having a much higher cross section compared to the interaction with other elements in biological tissues. Globally, neutron irradiation of biological tissues in the presence of 10B generates a mixed radiation field. Apart from 10B(n, alpha)7Li reaction, thermal neutrons are also captured in 14N, producing a proton. Alpha, lithium ions and protons have moderate to high ionization density values (164, 151 and 44 keV/mm, respectively), and short ranges in tissue (9, 5 and 11 $\mu$m, respectively). Moreover, epithermal neutrons thermalize in tissue mainly through elastic scattering in hydrogen, producing a recoil proton that deposits dose. Finally, there is a low-LET component of the dose, due to gamma generated by neutrons capture in hydrogen and by the structural photons, which is always present in a neutron beam. The only selective component of the absorbed dose is the one due to neutron capture in 10B, because there is a differential accumulation in tumor. The other components are a background which must be kept as low as possible. Due to this unavoidable dose absorbed by healthy tissues, BNCT treatment planning prescribes the dose to reach the maximum tolerated dose in the most radiosensitive tissue involved in the irradiation, and calculated tumor dose according to the known boron concentration.

From the radiobiological point of view, one of the most exploited models is the tumor cell culture irradiation in presence and in absence of boron. Survival of tumor cells as a function of the absorbed dose is a measure of the biological effectiveness of BNCT compared to a reference radiation, typically photons. As explained later with more details, the first model employed to express biologically-weighted BNCT dose, was multiplying each dose component by the RBE/CBE fixed factors, obtained by cell-survival curves [122]. The RBE measured for different cell lines show that BNCT is around 5 times more effective than photons in reducing tumor cell survival. Figure 13.1 shows a typical experiment irradiating rat osteosarcoma cells in a thermal neutron field in presence and in absence of BPA and using a 60Co source as the photon reference radiation [123]. These curves, opportunely fitted, allow the calculation of RBE for the neutron dose component of 2.2±0.5 and a CBE for the boron dose component of 5.3±1.5. It is important to note that BNCT poses an important requirement: in order to calculate properly the effectiveness, dose delivered to cell cultures must be calculated in detail, taking into account that equilibrium of charged particles may not hold, thus the Monte Carlo transport of each secondary charged component must be performed.

### 13.3.2.2   Proton-Boron Capture Therapy (PBCT)

PBCT, as aforementioned, is a novel binary approach, first theoretically proposed by Yoon et al. (2014) [118] with the aim of potentiating the efficiency of protontherapy, as to render it amenable to treat radioresistant cancers . Specifically, in order to increase the clinical RBE of protons, commonly assumed to be 1.1, the PBCT strategy is based on the exploitation of the nuclear fusion reaction between low-energy protons and 11B (p-B, in brief):

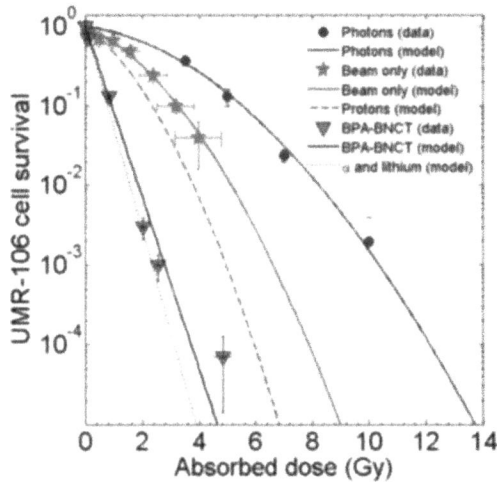

**Figure 13.1**    Rat osteosarcoma UMR-106 cell survival curves as a function of the absorbed dose

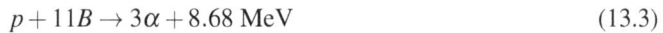

$$p + 11B \rightarrow 3\alpha + 8.68\,\text{MeV} \tag{13.3}$$

ensuing the simultaneous release of three high-LET alpha particles [11]. The average energy of the emerging alpha particles is between 3 and 4 MeV [39] , which translates to maximal ranges of approximately 18–27 μm, corresponding to the mean diameter of a cell nucleus. The high-LET of such particles provides thus the basic radiobiological rationale for the clinical use of PBCT since it would in principle allow for deployment of highly localized clustered damage in the hit 11B-containing cancer cells. The maximum for the reaction cross section is believed to occur for incident proton energies of around 700 keV (see Figure 13.2, hence the probability of PBCT increases with the protons slowing down within the SOBP, which corresponds to the region where the tumor is located.

Conversely, at the beam entrance, corresponding in vivo to the healthy tissues, the mean proton energy is far too high for the reaction to be triggered, hence physics would selectively drive and confine the radiobiological enhancement of protontherapy to the tumor volume. This would therefore eliminate one of the most stringent and limiting criteria for clinical viability of BNCT, that is the necessity that the boron carrier be uptaken almost exclusively by the cancer cells.

Besides theoretical considerations on the actual feasibility of such an approach, it was only with the work by Cirrone et al. (2018) [17] that the first experimental proof by radiobiological measurements was provided by showing that irradiation in the presence of an 11B carrier resulted in a significant increase of the effectiveness of a clinical 62-MeV proton beam at inducing cell killing in a prostate cancer cell line (Figure 13.3). The dose-modifying factor at 10 % survival (DMF10) at the middle position of the SOBP was $1.46 \pm 0.12$ for cells irradiated in the presence of BSH (sodium mercaptododecaborate, $Na_2B_{12}H_{11}SH$) at a concentration of 80 ppm of 11B.

These results were attributed to the expected increase in cell lethality due to the high-LET radiation generated by the p-B reaction as theoretically predicted [118, 39] as well as inferred experimentally [77]. That the putative radiosensitizing action of the p-B reaction is brought about by high-LET alpha particle and, more importantly, that the PBCT could represent a viable approach in the high-energy clinical protontherapy scenario are supported by recent work studying the yield and level of complexity of radiation-induced chromosome aberrations (CAs) in normal mammary epithelial MCF-10A cells irradiated at the clinical proton beam (131.5-164.8 MeV) of the Centro

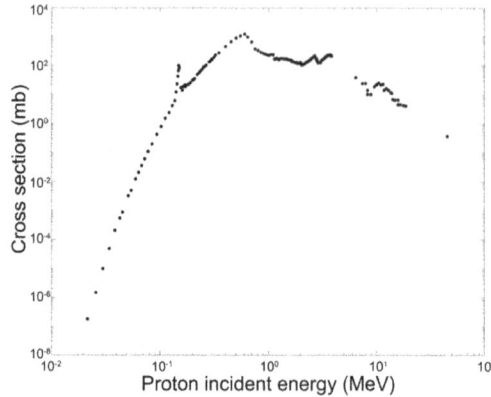

**Figure 13.2**   Total p-B experimental reaction cross section for the most probable $\alpha 1$ channel decay from EXFOR database

Nazionale di Adroterapia Oncologica (CNAO), Pavia, Italy [13]. In this study, while DU 145 cells cells irradiated in the presence of the 11B carrier BSH underwent increased clonogenic cell death along the SOBP but not at the entrance, MCF-10A cells displayed substantially increased fractions of complex CAs (Figure 13.4), which are a well-documented biomarker of high-LET exposure [5].

To gain further radiobiological evidence on the involvement of the alpha particles in the observed PBCT-based radiosensitization, the degree of CA complexity was examined – here presented as frequencies of chromosomes and breaks per complex exchange (Figure 13.5) and resulted greater in boron-treated cells compared to the samples irradiated by protons alone.

Following the research already performed for BNCT, the 11B carriers being evaluated in PBCT studies are BSH (described above) and BPA (boronophenylalanine, $C_9H_{12}BNO_4$), which are currently being used in the BNCT treatment, with others being under consideration [7] [35]. The PBCT binary approach may be a promising way how to overcome radioresistance of some types of tumors (e.g. hypoxic, such as pancreatic) as a possible alternative to the use of heavier particles (i.e. 12C ions) and the related issues, such as high cost, fragmentation, and/or radiobiological uncertainties connected with late toxicity, while maintaining the inherent benefits of charged particle therapy in the form of healthy tissue sparing. In spite of the accumulating experimental evidence from a radiobiological point of view [17] [13] the exact mechanisms remain to be properly elucidated. The discrepancy between the yield of alpha particles and the observed biological effects remains a source of controversy [88] [2] [41]. Possible explanations currently being investigated include the contribution of concomitant bystander effects. A modality that conceptually stems from PBCT is another binary approach utilizing the reaction between protons and 19F atoms:

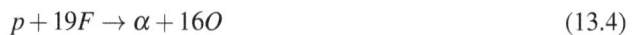

$$p + 19F \rightarrow \alpha + 16O \tag{13.4}$$

where the created alpha particle as well as the recoiled 16O atom would lead to increase in cancer cell killing The cross section maximum for the p-F reaction is reached for proton energies of around 2-3 MeV, hence comparable to those of the PBCT, thus offering the same advantage of being effective exclusively in the tumor region, which would be strengthened by the high affinity for tumor cells of the 19F carriers, such as 19FDG (19Fluorodeoxyglucose) whose isotopic analog, 18FDG, is commonly used during positron emission tomography [9]. Indeed, a possible advantage over PBCT offered by the use of the p-F reaction is its theranostic potential. warranting experimental investigation on this binary approach.

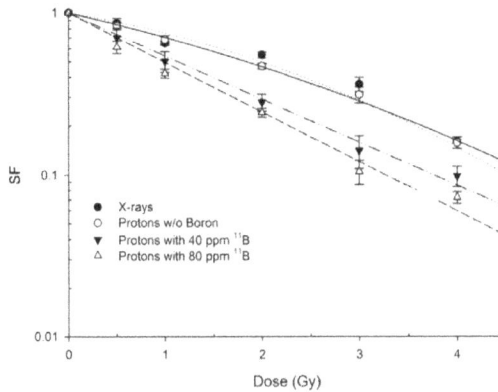

**Figure 13.3**   Boron-mediated increase in proton irradiation-induced cell death. Clonogenic dose response curves of prostate cancer cells DU145 irradiated with therapeutic protons in the presence or the absence of BSH at mid-SOBP. Data are weighted mean values plus standard error from four independent experiments in the case of proton irradiation in the absence of BSH (open circles) and in the presence of the compound at the highest concentration used (80 ppm, open triangles). X ray-irradiation survival data are also shown for comparison (from Cirrone et al., 2018)

## 13.4    MONTE CARLO SIMULATIONS STUDIES FOR THE EVALUATION OF THE RADIOBIOLOGICAL EFFECT ENHANCEMENT IN NUCLEAR REACTION-DRIVEN BINARY STRATEGIES

### 13.4.1    MONTE CARLO SIMULATIONS FOR THE EVALUATION OF RADIOBIOLOGICAL EFFECT IN BNCT

The theoretical advantage of BNCT compared to fast neutrons or, in general, to external beam therapies is the possibility to localize the absorbed dose to the tumor by selective incorporation of 10B. Suitable neutron beams are produced at research nuclear reactors and, recently, by high-current proton accelerators coupled with beryllium or lithium targets [124] Neutron beams of suitable energy to treat deep-seated tumors are obtained with proper beam shaping assemblies (BSA) [124]. In tissue the neutrons are thermalized, causing the neutron capture reaction 10B(n,$\alpha$)7Li, producing 7Li (average LET: 190 keV/$\mu$m) and alpha particles (160 keV/$\mu$m), both of them are of short range and highly damaging to cells. The energy deposition of such particles is limited within a short range (¡10 $\mu$m). The remaining contribution to the absorbed dose is given by 580 keV protons (38 keV/$\mu$m) ejected following the 14N(n,p)14C reaction, as well as by gamma rays.

Several models have been developed to calculate the absorbed dose of the 10B(n,$\alpha$)7Li reaction to the nuclei of cells exposed to boron localized to different cellular locations. Although analytical models have been used in the past [106, 107], the Monte Carlo (MC) technique allows a more realistic simulation of cell and tissue geometry [94, 119]. At present, one of the main reference MC codes for BNCT is MCNP [95, 85], which was also used for treatment planning. More recently also PHITS [111, 115] has been used for this purpose [107]. Other general purpose codes, such as Geant4 [81, 82] and Fluka [92, 83] are also used. A comparison between these two codes for BNCT evaluations is reported in [89]. One of the complications in the evaluation of the biological effect following the neutron capture reaction arises from the fact that the tissues targeted with boron are exposed to a mixed radiation field composed by particles with different radiobiological effectiveness [105]. The first strategy to calculate a photon-equivalent dose was proposed by J. Coderre, and it consisted in multiplying each component of the BNCT dose by fixed Relative Biological

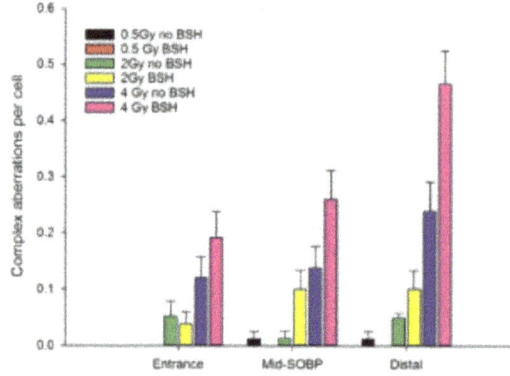

**Figure 13.4** Evidence for the action of high-LET radiation generated by clinical protons via the p-B reaction. Frequency of complex CAs as revealed by mFISH as a function of dose and position along the CNAO proton beam SOBP for samples irradiated in the presence or the absence of BSH (from Bláha et al., 2021).

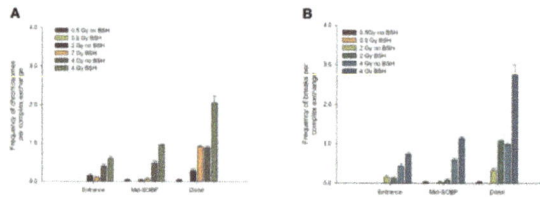

**Figure 13.5** Classification of complex exchanges revealed by mFISH analysis in terms of frequencies of number of chromosomes, left panel (A), and number of breaks (right panel (B)) involved; for MCF-10A cells irradiated at entrance, mid, and distal positions of the CNAO clinical proton beam.

Effectiveness factors, obtained from radiobiological in vitro and in-vivo studies. The boron component was weighted by a Compound Biological Factor, which considered that different borated formulations may cause different biological effects at the same dose [122]. More recently, it has been demonstrated that this approach, albeit still used in clinical dose reporting, gives artificially high doses in the tumor. For this reason, new, more refined models have been proposed. One of these is the Photon Iso-Effective dose model [125, 126]. Photon iso-effective dose is defined as the reference dose that produces the same level of cell survival as a given combination of the absorbed dose components of a mixed field BNCT radiation. Dedicated radiobiological experiments provide the dose-response relationship, choosing proper in-vitro or in-vivo models, irradiated with neutrons, neutrons in presence of boron, and reference radiation (typically photons from 60Co or from conventional radiotherapy facility). A mathematical expression quantifying the effect of interest under both photon and BNCT treatment conditions is necessary, considering also important biological phenomena such as synergism between different radiations and sublethal damage repair. The general expression for the photon isoeffective dose, when both synergism and repair mechanism are considered, and using survival-dose curves obtained with in-vitro experiments is:

$$\alpha_R D_R + G_R(\theta')\beta_R D_R^2 = \sum_{i=1}^{4} \alpha_i D_i + \sum_{i=1}^{4}\sum_{j=1}^{4} G_{ij}(\theta)\sqrt{\beta_i\beta_j}D_i D_j \tag{13.5}$$

In this case, the survival curves are fitted with the generalized Linear Quadratic Model, where $\alpha$ and $\beta$ are the parameters of the fit for the reference radiation and for the 4 dose components in BNCT and Gij($\theta$) is the generalized Lea-Catcheside factor which modifies the quadratic term of LQ model by taking into account the probability of repair ($\theta$ is the irradiation time) [127]. In [126], the same concept has been described using radiobiological data in-vivo, i.e. using as the effect to be compared the Tumor Control Probability. The Photon Iso-effective dose model has been proved as a more realistic tool to interpret the clinical outcome of patients treatment in different clinical trials in the light of the dosimetry re-calculated with this method. Another strategy that has been proved useful to account the different radiobiological effect of the dose components in the same framework is to base the biological computations on microdosimetric evaluations [100], such as in the Microdosimetric Kinetic Model [96, 97, 98]. Using the MKM the cell survival of various charged particles can be estimated from the probability of specific energies deposited in subvolumes (domains) of the cell nucleus. Following the LQ formalism (McMahon 2019) the dependence of linear parameter to the microdosimetric spectra can be expressed as

$$\alpha = \alpha_0 + \beta z_{*1D} \tag{13.6}$$

where $\alpha_0$ is a constant parameter that represents the initial slope of the surviving fraction curve in the limit of LET = 0, $\beta$ is the quadratic term, assumed to be independent on radiation type and LET, and z*1D is the saturation-corrected dose-mean specific energy of the domain delivered in a single event [103]. While $\alpha_0$ and $\beta$ depend on the specific cell line and biological endpoint and are usually phenomenologically determined from survival curves of a low-LET reference radiation, the physical dependence on the radiation is completely encapsulated in $z_{*1D}$, which can be evaluated from

$$z_{*1D} = \frac{\int_0^\infty z_{sat} z f_1(z) dz}{\int_0^\infty z f_1(z) dz} \tag{13.7}$$

where f1(z) is the probability density of energy z deposited by a single deposition event in the domain, and $z_{sat}$ represents the saturation-corrected specific energy defined as follows

$$z_{sat} = \frac{z_0^2}{z}(1 - exp(-z^{''}/z_0^2)) \tag{13.8}$$

where $z_0$, the saturation coefficient, indicates the energy above which the saturation correction due to the overkilling effect became important. This coefficient is usually determined phenomenologically. A strategy to fix the value of this parameter is given in [103].

MC codes, such as PHITS used in [100], are exploited to determine the microscopic probability f1(z) tracking main particle components ($\alpha$ particles, 7Li, protons and gammas) and secondary electrons that are generated from the neutron capture. An example of these microdosimetric evaluations is reported in Figure 13.6.

Another microdosimetric approach has been described by Sato et al. in [115]. The model is based on the Stochastic Microdosimetric Model [128] and calculates the photon iso-effective BNCT dose considering the intra- and intercellular heterogeneity in 10B distribution. The dose distributions in domains are calculated by the microdosimetric function implemented in PHITS, taking into account the 10B distribution inside cells and the dose rate effect. The SMK model approximates the dose by their mean value, which is important in BNCT because of the higher heterogeneity of the absorbed dose in each cell nucleus due to the stochastic nature of the intercellular 10B distribution.

### 13.4.2 MONTE CARLO SIMULATIONS FOR THE EVALUATION OF THE RADIOBIOLOGICAL EFFECT ENHANCEMENT IN PBFT AND NCEPT

Other topics in which MC simulation can be important in the context of radiobiology of binary radiotherapy, is the comprehension of possible mechanisms leading to the enhancement of radiobiological effectiveness the additions of specific radioisotopes (like 11B or 19F) to exploit nuclear

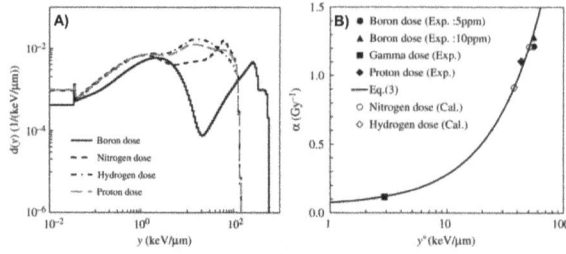

**Figure 13.6** A) Probability densities of lineal energy, d(y), for the "boron" (10B(n, $\alpha$)7Li re-action), "nitrogen" (14N(n, p)14C reaction), "hydrogen" (1H(n, n)1H) and "proton" (1H(n, $\gamma$)2H reaction) doses calculated using the microdosimetric function in the PHITS code. B) Measured $\alpha$ value (V79 cells) for each of the four major BNCT dose components as a function of calculated y*. The solid line and open markers denote the relationship between $\alpha$ and y* expected from Equation (mkm-bnct). Figures taken from (Horiguchi et al. 2015).

reactions triggered by protons on these nuclei [17, 13]. In analogy to the BNCT, these reactions can generate short- range high-LET alpha particles inside the tumors, thereby allowing a highly localized DNA-damaging action. In the case of Proton-Boron Fusion Therapy (PBFT) with 11B, an open question that MC studies have been done to determine the potential role of the p+11B $\rightarrow$ 3 $\alpha$reactions in the biological enhancement of proton therapy effectiveness. The alpha particles produced in the reaction have an average of 4 MeV kinetic energy and are generated at the point of interaction of the proton and the 11B. The breakup of the boron is not prompt in most cases but usually an unstable 12C is created thanks to a resonance at 675 keV [11]. This nucleus mostly decays $\alpha$, emitting a first alpha particle, and then the 8Be decays $\alpha$ as well, splitting in another pair of alpha particles. The experimental total cross section for p-11B reaction can be seen in Figure 13.7. The upper curve in the figure clearly shows a resonance pattern: cross section is peaked at proton energies about 675 keV where it reaches a maximum of 0.8 b. This resonance has been highlighted to be exploited for therapeutic use in combination with proton therapy: if boron is located preferentially inside the tumor region, the proton effect would be enhanced where proton energy is low, i.e. at the end of their range inside the tumor, improving the therapeutic index [118].

The Monte Carlo simulations studies have been carried out using mainly MCNPX [109, 99] and Geant4 [81, 82]. These studies suggest that this contribution is basically negligible in ordinary clinical irradiation conditions [88, 87] and that the observed enhancement in the radiobiological effectiveness of the PBFT is not related to the alpha particles produced in the abovementioned nuclear reactions. Some studies [114] have proposed an alternative nuclear process for the production of secondary low-energy particles by capturing thermal neutrons produced inside the treatment volume during irradiation in presence of boron-10 and gadolinium-157-based drugs, the Neutron Capture Enhanced Particle Therapy (NCEPT). During particle therapy, such as proton and carbon ion therapy, a fraction of the primary particles undergo non-elastic collisions with nuclei in the target. This results in the production of a range of nuclear fragments at the target site (see also Section Mixed field approaches for evaluating biological impact of projectile and target fragmentation), including a mixture of fast and thermal neutrons. In presence of 10B or 157Gd, the thermal neutron component can exploited through the nuclear reactions:

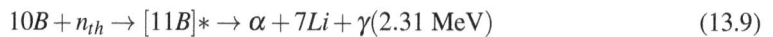

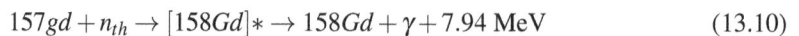

$$10B + n_{th} \rightarrow [11B]* \rightarrow \alpha + 7Li + \gamma(2.31 \text{ MeV}) \tag{13.9}$$

$$157gd + n_{th} \rightarrow [158Gd]* \rightarrow 158Gd + \gamma + 7.94 \text{ MeV} \tag{13.10}$$

In the case of 10B, the the capture mechanism results in the production of several high LET products and , while, in the case of 157Gd, it results in high energy and the production of low-energy

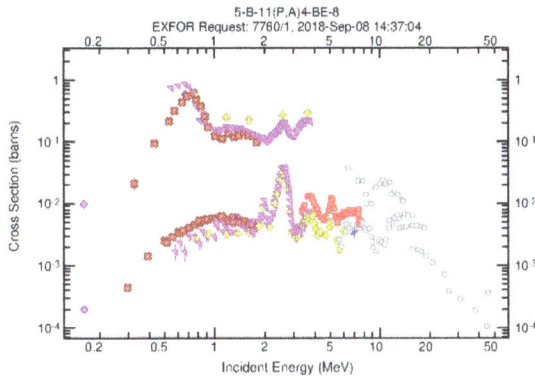

**Figure 13.7** Experimental data for the proton-boron fusion reaction (p+11B $\alpha$3). Data Taken from EXFOR database [113]. Different colors correspond to different experimental campaigns. Two curves can be seen: the one with higher cross section relates to the channel known as *alpha*$_0$: after the carbon decay the 8Be is created in its fundamental state, while the latter relates to the *alpha*$_1$ channel, where the beryllium is created in one of its excited states.

Auger electrons, the latter exploitable for therapeutic effects. A comparative analysis between PBFT and NCEPT has been carried out using both MCNPX and GEANT4 based MC simulations in [117], showing a lower effectiveness of the NCEPT approach, although the excess dose rate from both the methods are about more than several orders of magnitude lower than the dose rate from proton beam therapy even when using 1000 ppm of boron (see Figure 13.8).

We remark however that at present, the results of these studies are somewhat contradictory, depending on the used Monte Carlo implementations and assumptions. Furthermore, the majority of them are simply based on the valuation of the yield of alpha particles and other high-LET particles produced from the nuclear reaction, and the corresponding physical dose amplification. A study with a proper biological insight based on a quantitative radiobiological modeling to evaluate the expected increase in the tumor killing effectiveness is still missing. An exception is the study carried out in [88] that also suggest a negligible radiobiological role of the alpha particles in the case of the (p+11B $\rightarrow$ 3$\alpha$) reaction. However, even in this case, the radiobiological evaluations are based on simplified models that account the mixed-field irradiation through the evaluation of a dose-averaged LET that does not properly account for the mixed contribution of proton and low-energy nuclear products (Se also Sections Monte Carlo to link RBE with radiation quality quantities and Mixed field approaches for evaluating biological impact of projectile and target fragmentation).

### 13.4.3    ISSUES IN THE EVALUATION OF THE BIOLOGICAL EFFECT OF SLOW SECONDARY PARTICLES

At present, the radiobiological models clinically used to predict the RBE in high-LET external beam charged particle therapy are the Local Effect Model (LEM) [116, 91, 93] and the MKM (see previous section). These models often rely on MC codes for the macroscopic tracking of the particle beams, including the secondary particles generated from nuclear fragmentation, coupled with a simplified analytical models for the description of the track structure at a nanometric level (amorphous track models) [90, 104, 101]. One of the basic assumptions of this approach is the so-called track-segment condition, in which the particles are assumed to have enough energy to completely cross the cell nucleus, assumed to be the radiosensitive part of the cell, without a significant change in kinetic energy. In general, the track-segment condition is not verified in a binary radiotherapy process, due

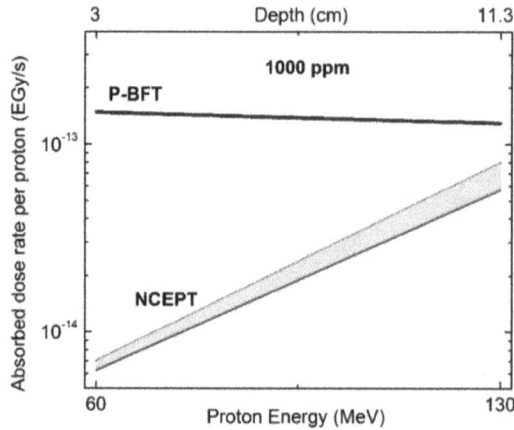

**Figure 13.8**   A comparative evaluation for NCEPT and PBFT in terms excess dose rate transfer to the tumor site when 1000 ppm of 10B and 11B has been applied respectively. The PBFT has been evaluated through an approximated analytical calculation while, in NCEPT, MCNPX and GEANT4 have been used (defining the lower and upper limits).

to the presence of very low-energy particles in the mixed field. This is particularly relevant in the case of alpha particles generated in both neutron and proton capture nuclear reactions. The most part of the energy of these particles is released in the same cell where they are produced, and often only in a subvolume of the cell. An approximate correction to account the partial cell nucleus crossing of slow particles can be applied through a corrective weighting in the mixed field formalism for the LQ parameters:

$$\alpha = \sum_i \alpha_i D_i \Delta L_i / \sum_i D_i \Delta L_i \tag{13.11}$$

$$\sqrt{\beta} = \sum_i \sqrt{\beta_i} D_i \Delta L_i / \sum_i D_i \Delta L_i \tag{13.12}$$

Where the index i is the track index, $D_i$ is the dose contribution of the track, $(\alpha_i, \beta_i)$ are the LQ parameters of the track and $\Delta L_i$ is the length of the track in the cell nucleus. The high local energy density found in the track results in complex DNA damage. In principle, a more precise evaluation of these effects should rely on the complete spatial knowledge of the track structure. MC codes capable of simulating the track structure down to a nano-scale level can also be used for these evaluations. Examples of these codes are Geant4-DNA [102, 112] or Trax [108, 84]. Due to their relevance for the evaluation of radiobiological effects in the case of complex mixed radiation fields, attempts to include nanometric evaluations in treatment planning simulation and optimization have also been made. An example of these studies is reported in [86], where, exploiting the Geant4-DNA code, a treatment plan has been optimized using a cost function based on nanodosimetric quantities scored in cell sub-volumes, such as the ionization cluster size, the probability distribution $P(v,Q)$ of the number of ionizations per particle of quality radiation Q, and other derived quantities.

## REFERENCES

1. Abuodeh, Y., Venkat, P., Kim, S. (2016). Systematic review of case reports on the abscopal effect. *Curr Probl Cancer*, 40(1), 25

2. Ahmadi Ganjeh, Z., Eslami-Kalantari, M. (2020). Investigation of Proton–Boron Capture Therapy vs. proton therapy. *Nucl. Instruments Methods Phys. Res. Sect. A Accel. Spectrometers, Detect. Assoc. Equip.*, 977, 164340

3. Alan Mitteer, R., Wang, Y., Shah J, Gordon, S., Fager, M., Butter, P.P., Jun Kim, H., Guardiola-Salmeron, C., Carabe-Fernandez, A., Fan, Y. (2015). Proton beam radiation induces DNA damage and cell apoptosis in glioma stem cells through reactive oxygen species. *Sci Rep*, 5:13961.

4. Alfonso, J.C.L., Berk. L. (2019). Modeling the effect of intratumoral heterogeneity of radiosensitivity on tumor response over the course of fractionated radiation therapy. Radiat Oncol, 14(1), 88.

5. Anderson, R. M., Stevens, D. L., Goodhead, D. T. (2002). M-FISH analysis shows that complex chromosome aberrations induced by $\alpha$-particle tracks are cumulative products of localized rearrangements. *Proc. Natl. Acad. Sci.*, 99, 12167.

6. Bader, S.B., Dewhirst, M.W., Hammond, E.M. (2021). Cyclic Hypoxia: An Update on Its Characteristics, Methods to Measure It and Biological Implications in Cancer. *Cancers*, 13, 23.

7. Balmukhanov, S.B., Yefimov, M.L., Kleinbock, T.S. (1967). Acquired radioresistance of tumor cells. Nature, 216, 709.

8. Barth, R.F., Mi, P., Yang, W. (2018). Boron delivery agents for neutron capture therapy of cancer. *Cancer Commun*, 38, 35.

9. Bastiannet, E., Groen, H., Jager, P.L., Cobben, D.C.P., Graaf van der, W.T.A., Vaalburg, W., Hoekstra, H.J. (2004). The value of FDG-PET in the detection, grading and response to therapy of soft tissue and bone sarcomas; a systematic review and meta-analysis. Cancer treatment reviews, 30.1: 83-101.

10. Bayraktar, S., Batoo, S., Okuno, S., Glück, S. (2019). Immunotherapy in breast cancer. J Carcinog., 18, 2.

11. Becker, H. W., Rolfs, C., Trautvetter, H. P. (1987). Low-energy cross sections for 11B(p,3alpha). Zeitschrift fur Phys. A At. Nucl., 327, 341.

12. Berberich, A., Kessler, T., Thomé, C.M., Pusch, S., Hielscher, T., Sahm, F., Oezen, I., Schmitt, L.M., Ciprut, S., Hucke, N., Ruebmann, P., Fischer, M., Lemke, D., Breckwoldt, M.O., von Deimling, A., Bendszus, M., Platten, M., Wick, W. (2019). Targeting Resistance against the MDM2 Inhibitor RG7388 in Glioblastoma Cells by the MEK Inhibitor Trametinib. Clin Cancer Res., 25(1), 253.

13. Bláha, P., Feoli, C., Agosteo, S., Calvaruso, M., Cammarata, F.P., Catalano, R., Ciocca, M., Cirrone, G.A.P., Conte, V., Cuttone, G., Facoetti, A., Forte, G.I., Giuffrida, L., Magro, G., Margarone, D., Minafra, L., Petringa, G., Pucci, G., Ricciardi, V., Rosa, E., Russo, G., Manti, L. (2021). The Proton-Boron Reaction Increases the Radiobiological Effectiveness of Clinical Low- and High-Energy Proton Beams: Novel Experimental Evidence and Perspectives. Front Oncol, 11:682647.

14. Brown, J.M. (2000). Tumor radiosensitivity: it's the subpopulations that count. Int J Radiat Oncol Biol Phys., 47(3), 549.

15. Brown, J. M. (2007). Tumor hypoxia in cancer therapy. Methods Enzymol., 435, 297.

16. Butterworth, K.T., McMahon, S.J., Currell, F.J., Prise, K.M. (2012). Physical basis and biological mechanisms of gold nanoparticle radiosensitization. Nanoscale., 4(16), 4830.

17. Cirrone, G.A.P., Manti, L., Margarone, D., Petringa, G., Giuffrida, L., Minopoli, A., Picciotto, A. Russo, G., Cammarata, F., Pisciotta, P., Perozziello, F.M., Romano, F., Marchese, V., Milluzzo, G., Scuderi, V., Cuttone, G., Korn, G. (2018). First experimental proof of Proton Boron Capture Therapy (PBCT) to enhance protontherapy effectiveness. Sci. Rep., 8, 1141

18. Cirrone, G.A.P., Petringa, G., Attili, D., Chiappara, D., Manti, L., Bravatá, V., Margarone, D., Mazzocco, M, Cuttone, G. (2019). Study of the discrepancy between analytical calculations

and observed biological effectiveness in proton boron caputre therapy (PBCT). RAD Assoc. J., 3, 147–151.

19. Cunningham, C., Maryna De Kock, M., Engelbrecht, M., Xanthene Miles, X., Slabbert, J. Vandevoorde, C. (2021). Radiosensitization effect of gold nanoparticles in proton therapy. Front Public Health., In press.
20. Demaria, S., Kawashima, N., Yang, A.M., Devitt, M.L., Babb, J.S., Allison, J.P., Formenti, S.C. (2005). Immune-mediated inhibition of metastases after treatment with local radiation and CTLA-4 blockade in a mouse model of breast cancer. Clin Cancer Res., 11(2), 728.
21. Demaria, S., Coleman, C.N,, Formenti, S.C. (2016) Radiotherapy: Changing the Game in Immunotherapy. Trends Cancer., 2(6), 286.
22. Deycmar, S., Faccin, E., Kazimova, T., Knobel, P.A., Telarovic, I., Tschanz, F., Waller, V., Winkler, R., Yong, C., Zingariello, D., Pruschy, M. (2020). The relative biological effectiveness of proton irradiation in dependence of DNA damage repair. Br J Radiol, 93(1107), 20190494.
23. Durante, M., Formenti, S. (2020). Harnessing radiation to improve immunotherapy: better with particles? Br J Radiol, 93, 20190224.
24. Emami Nejad, A., Najafgholian, S., Rostami, A., Sistani, A., Shojaeifar, S., Esparvarinha, M., Nedaeinia, R., Haghjooy Javanmard, S., Taherian, M., Ahmadlou, M., Salehi, R., Sadeghi, B., Manian, M. (2021). The role of hypoxia in the tumor microenvironment and development of cancer stem cell: a novel approach to developing treatment. Cancer Cell Int, 21(1), 62.
25. Fontana, A.O., Augsburger, M.A., Grosse, N., Guckenberger, M., Lomax, A.J., Sartori, A.A., Pruschy, M.N. (2015). Differential DNA repair pathway choice in cancer cells after proton- and photon-irradiation. Radiother Oncol, 116(3):374.
26. Formenti, S.C., Demaria, S. (2009) Systemic effects of local radiotherapy. Lancet Oncol., 10(7), 718.
27. Formenti,S.C., Demaria, S. (2012). Radiation therapy to convert the tumor into an in situ vaccine. Int J Radiat Oncol Biol Phys, 84(4), 879.
28. Formenti, S.C., Rudqvist, N.P., Golden, E., Cooper, B.,Wennerberg, E., Lhuillier, C., Vanpouille-Box, C., Friedman, K., Ferrari de Andrade, L., Wucherpfennig,K.W., Heguy, A., Imai,N., Gnjatic, S., Emerson, R.O., Zhou, X.K., Zhang, T., Chachoua, A., Demaria, S. (2018). Radiotherapy induces responses of lung cancer to CTLA-4 blockade. Nat Med, 24, 1845.
29. Friedman, A.D., Claypool, S.E., Liu, R. (2013). The smart targeting of nanoparticles. Curr Pharm Des, 19, 631.
30. Gameiro, S.R., Malamas, A.S., Bernstein, M.B., Tsang, K.Y., Vassantachart, A., Sahoo, N., Tailor, R., Pidikiti, R., Guha, C.P., Hahn, S.M., Krishnan, S., Hodge, J.W. (2016). Tumor Cells Surviving Exposure to Proton or Photon Radiation Share a Common Immunogenic Modulation Signature, Rendering Them More Sensitive to T Cell-Mediated Killing. Int J Radiat Oncol Biol Phys, 95(1), 120.
31. Golden, E.B., Chhabra, A., Chachoua, A., Adams, S., Donach, M., Fenton-Kerimian, M., Friedman, K., Ponzo, F., Babb, J.S., Goldberg, J., Demaria, S., Formenti, S.C. (2015). Local radiotherapy and granulocyte-macrophage colony-stimulating factor to generate abscopal responses in patients with metastatic solid tumors: a proof-of-principle trial. Lancet Oncol., 16(7),795.
32. Hader, M., Frey, B., Fietkau, R., Hecht, M., Gaipl, U.S. (2020). Immune biological rationales for the design of combined radio- and immunotherapies. Cancer Immunol Immunother, 69(2), 293.
33. Hanahan, D., Weinberg, R.A. (2000). The Hallmarks of Cancer. Cell, 100(1),
34. Held, K.D., Kawamura, H., Kaminuma, T., Paz, A.E.S., Yoshida, Y., Liu, Q., Willers, H., Takahashi, A. (2016). Effects of Charged Particles on Human Tumor Cells. Front. Oncol., 6, 23.

35. Hideghéty, K., Brunner, S., Cheesman, A., Szabó, E.R., Polanek, R., Margarone, D., Tökés, T., Mogyorósi, K. (2019). 11Boron Delivery Agents for Boron Proton-capture Enhanced Proton Therapy. Anticancer Res., 39 (5), 2265.

36. Hirai, T., Saito, S., Fujimori, H., Matsushita, K., Nishio, T., Okayasu, R., Masutanim M. (2016). Radiosensitization by PARP inhibition to proton beam irradiation in cancer cells. Biochem Biophys Res Commun, 478(1):234.

37. Horsman, M.R., Wouters, B.G., Joiner, M.C., Overgaard, J. (2009). The oxygen effect and fractionated radiotherapy. In Basic Clinical Radiobiology; Joiner, M., van der Kogel, A., Eds.; Hodder Arnold: London, UK; pp. 207–216.

38. Hsieh, C.H., Lee C.H., Liang J.A., Yu, C.Y., Shyu, W.C. (2010). Cycling hypoxia increases U87 glioma cell radioresistance via ROS induced higher and longterm HIF-1 signal transduction activity. Oncol Rep, 24:1629.

39. Jung, J.-Y., Yoon, D.-K., Barraclough, B., Lee, H.C., Suh, T.S., Lu, B. (2017). Comparison between proton boron fusion therapy (PBFT) and boron neutron capture therapy (BNCT): a Monte Carlo study. Oncotarget, 8, 39774–39781.

40. Kato, Y., Yashiro, M., Fuyuhiro, Y., Kashiwagi, S., Matsuoka, J., Hirakawa, T., Noda, S., Aomatsu, N., Hasegawa, T., Matsuzaki, T., Sawada, T., Ohira, M., Hirakawa, K. (2011). Effects of Acute and Chronic Hypoxia on the Radiosensitivity of Gastric and Esophageal Cancer Cells. Anticancer Res, 31, 3369.

41. Khaledi, N., Wang, X., Hosseinabadi, R. B., Samiei, F. (2020). Is the proton–boron fusion therapy effective? J. Radiother. Pract., 1–5.

42. Kim, H., Lin, Q., Glazer, P.M., Yun, Z. (2018). The hypoxic tumor microenvironment in vivo selects the cancer stem cell fate of breast cancer cells. Breast Cancer Res, 20(1), 16.

43. Kobayashi, K., Usami, N., Porcel, E., Lacombe, S., Le Sech, C. (2010). Enhancement of radiation effect by heavy elements. Mutat Res/Rev Mutat Res, 704(1-3), 123.

44. Konings, K., Vandevoorde, C., Baselet, B., Baatout, S., Moreels, M. (2020). Combination Therapy With Charged Particles and Molecular Targeting: A Promising Avenue to Overcome Radioresistance. Front Oncol. 10, 128.

45. Ku, A., Facca, V.J., Cai, Z., Reilly, R.M. (2019). Auger electrons for cancer therapy – a review. EJNMMI Radiopharm Chem, 4, 27.

46. Kuncic, Z., Lacombe, S. (2018). Nanoparticle radio-enhancement: principles, progress and application to cancer treatment. Phys Med Biol, 63(2), 02TR01.

47. Kwatra, D., Venugopal, A., Anant, S. (2013). Nanoparticles in Radiation Therapy: A Summary of Various Approaches to Enhance Radiosensitization in Cancer. Transl Cancer Res, 2, 330.

48. Lacombe, S., Porcel, E., Scifoni, E. (2017). Particle therapy and nanomedicine: state of art and research perspectives. Cancer Nanotechnol, 8(1), 9.

49. Lee Jr., H. J., Zeng, J., Rengan, R. (2018). Proton beam therapy and immunotherapy: an emerging partnership for immune activation in non-small cell lung cancer. Transl Lung Cancer Res, 7(2), 180.

50. Lesueur, P., Chevalier, F., El-Habr, E.A., Junier, M.P., Chneiweiss, H., Castera, L., Müller, E., Stefan, D., Saintigny, Y. (2018). Radiosensitization Effect of Talazoparib, a Parp Inhibitor, on Glioblastoma Stem Cells Exposed to Low and High Linear Energy Transfer Radiation. Sci Rep, 8(1), 3664.

51. Liu, Q., Ghosh, P., Magpayo, N., Testa, M., Tang, S., Gheorghiu, L., Biggs, P., Paganetti, H., Efstathiou, J.A., Lu, H.M., Held, K.D., Willers, H. (2015). Lung cancer cell line screen links Fanconi anemia/BRCA pathway defects to increased relative biological effectiveness of proton radiation. Int J Radiat Oncol Biol Phys, 91(5):1081.

52. Ma, H., Takahashi, A., Yoshida, Y., Adachi, A., Kanai, T., Ohno, T., Nakano, T. (2015). Combining carbon ion irradiation and non-homologous end-joining repair inhibitor NU7026 efficiently kills cancer cells. Radiat Oncol, 10, 225.

53. Maier, P., Hartmann. L.,Wenz, F., Herskind, C. (2016). Cellular pathways in response to ionizing radiation and their targetability for tumor radiosensitization. Int J Mol Sci,

54. Maggiorella, L., Barouch, G., Devaux, C., Pottier, A., Deutsch, E., Bourhis, J., Borghi, E., Levy, L., (2012). Nanoscale radiotherapy with hafnium oxide nanoparticles. Future Oncol, 8(9), 1167.

55. Matsumura, Y., Maeda, H. (1986). A new concept for macromolecular therapeutics in cancer chemotherapy: mechanism of tumoritropic accumulation of proteins and the antitumor agent smancs. Cancer Res, 46(12 Pt 1), 6387.

56. Miles, X., Vandevoorde, C., Hunter, A., Bolcaen, J. (2021). MDM2/X Inhibitors as Radiosensitizers for Glioblastoma Targeted Therapy. Front Oncol, 11, 703442.

57. Mirjolet, C., Nicol, A., Limagne, E., Mura, C., Richard, C., Morgand, V., Rousseau, M., Boidot, R., Ghiringhelli, F., Noel, G., Burckel, H. (2021). Impact of proton therapy on antitumor immune response. Sci Rep, 11(1), 13444.

58. Mondini, M., Levy, A,, Meziani, L., Milliat, F., Deutsch, E. (2020) Radiotherapy-immunotherapy combinations-perspectives and challenges. Mol Oncol, 14(7), 1529.

59. Olivares-Urbano, M.A., Carmen Griñán-Lisón, C., Marchal, J.A., Núñez, M.I. (2020). CSC Radioresistance: A Therapeutic Challenge to Improve Radiotherapy Effectiveness in Cancer. Cells, 9, 1651.

60. Oonishi, K., Cui, X., Hirakawa, H., Fujimori, A., Kamijo, T., Yamada, S., Yokosuka, O., Kamadam T. (2012). Different effects of carbon ion beams and X-rays on clonogenic survival and DNA repair in human pancreatic cancer stem-like cells. Radiother Oncol, 105, 258.

61. Park, H.J., Oh, J.S., Chang, J.W., Hwang,S.G., Kim, J.S. (2016). Proton irradiation sensitizes radioresistant non-small cell lung cancer cells by modulating epidermal growth factor receptor-mediated DNA repair. Anticancer Res, 36, 20.

62. Peukert, D., Kempson, I., Douglass, M., Bezak, E. (2018). Metallic nanoparticle radiosensitisation of ion radiotherapy: A review. Phys Med, 47,121.

63. Peukert, D., Kempson, I,, Douglass, M., Bezak, E. (2019). Gold Nanoparticle Enhanced Proton Therapy: Monte Carlo Modeling of Reactive Species' Distributions Around a Gold Nanoparticle and the Effects of Nanoparticle Proximity and Clustering. Int J Mol Sci, 20(17), 4280.

64. Pu, X., Wu, L., Su, D., Mao, W., Fang, B. (2018). Immunotherapy for non-small cell lung cancers: biomarkers for predicting responses and strategies to overcome resistance. BMC Cancer, 18, 1082.

65. Rashid, R.A., Abidin, S.Z., Anuar, M.A.K., Tominaga, T., Akasaka, H., Sasaki, R., Kie, K., Razak, K.A., Pham, B.T.T., Hawkett, B.S., Carmichael, M.-A., Geso, M., Rahman, W.N. (2019). Radiosensitization effects and ROS generation by high Z metallic nanoparticles on human colon carcinoma cell (HCT116) irradiated under 150 MeV proton beam. OpenNano, 4, 100027.

66. Reynders, K., Illidge, T., Siva, S., Chang, J.Y., De Ruysscher, D. (2015). The abscopal effect of local radiotherapy: using immunotherapy to make a rare event clinically relevant. Cancer Treat Rev, 41(6), 503.

67. Russell, E., Dunne, V., Russell, B., Mohamud, H., Ghita, M., McMahon, S.J., Butterworth, K.T. Schettino, G., McGarry, C.K., Prise, K.M.. (2021). Impact of superparamagnetic iron oxide nanoparticles on in vitro and in vivo radiosensitisation of cancer cells. Radiat Oncol, 16, 104

68. Sancey, L., Lux, F., Kotb, S., Roux, S., Dufort, S., Bianchi, A., Crémillieux, Y., Fries, P., Coll, J.L., Rodriguez-Lafrasse, C., Janier, M., Dutreix, M., Barberi-Heyob, M., Boschetti, F., Denat, F., Louis, C., Porcel, E., Lacombe, S., Le Duc, G., Deutsch, E., Perfettini, J.L., Detappe, A., Verry, C., Berbeco, R., Butterworth, K.T., McMahon, S.J., Prise, K.M., Perriat, P., Tillement,

O. (2014). The use of theranostic gadolinium-based nanoprobes to improve radiotherapy efficacy. Br J Radiol, 87(1041), 20140134.

69. Takahashi, Y., Yasui, T., Minami, K., Tamari, K., Hayashi, K., Otani, K., Seo, Y., Isohashi, F., Koizumi, M., Ogawa, K. (2019). Carbon ion irradiation enhances the antitumor efficacy of dual immune checkpoint blockade therapy both for local and distant sites in murine osteosarcoma. Oncotarget, 10(6), 633.

70. Tang, L., Wei, F., Wu, Y., He, Y., Shi, L., Xiong, F., Gong, Z., Guo, C., Li, X., Deng, H., Cao, K., Zhou, M., Xiang, B., Li, X., Li, Y., Li, G., Xiong, W., Zeng, Z. (2018). Role of metabolism in cancer cell radioresistance and radiosensitization methods. J Exp Clin Cancer Res, 37(1), 87.

71. Tinganelli, W., Durante, M. (2020). Carbon Ion Radiobiology. Cancers (Basel), 12(10), 3022.

72. Vanderwaeren, L., Dok, R., Verstrepen, K., Nuyts, S. (2021). Clinical Progress in Proton Radiotherapy: Biological Unknowns. Cancers (Basel), 13(4), 604.

73. West, C.M., Davidson, S.E., Elyan, S.A., Swindell, R., Roberts, S.A., Orton, C.J., Coyle, C.A., Valentine, H., Wilks, D.P., Hunter, R.D., Hendry, J.H. (1998). The intrinsic radiosensitivity of normal and tumor cells. Int J Radiat Biol, 73, 409.

74. Wozny, A. S., Vares, G., Alphonse, G., Lauret, A., Monini, C., Magné, N., Cuerq, C., Fujimori, A., Monboisse, J. C., Beuve, M., Nakajima, T., Rodriguez-Lafrasse, C. (2019). ROS Production and Distribution: A New Paradigm to Explain the Differential Effects of X-ray and Carbon Ion Irradiation on Cancer Stem Cell Migration and Invasion. Cancers, 11(4), 468.

75. Ye, J.C., Formenti, S.C. (2018). Integration of radiation and immunotherapy in breast cancer - Treatment implications. Breast, 38, 66.

76. Yoon, D.-K., Jung, J.-Y., Suh, T. S. (2014). Application of proton boron fusion reaction to radiation therapy: A Monte Carlo simulation study. Appl. Phys. Lett., 105, 223507.

77. Yoon, D.-K., Nganawa, N., Kimura, M., Choi, M.-G., Kim, M.-S., Kim, Y.-J., Law, M.W.-M., Djeng, S.-K., Shin, H.-B., Choe, B.-Y., Suh, T.S. (2019). Application of proton boron fusion to proton therapy: Experimental verification to detect the alpha particles. Appl. Phys. Lett., 115, 223701.

78. Zhang, X., Lin, S.H., Fang, B., Gillin, M., Mohan, R., Chang, J.Y. (2013). Therapy Resistant cancer stem cells have differing sensitivity to photon versus proton beam radiation. J Thorac Oncol, 8:1484.

79. Zhang, P., Yu, B., Jin, X., Zhao, T., Ye, F., Liu, X., Li, P., Zheng, X., Chen, W., Li, Q. (2021). Therapeutic Efficacy of Carbon Ion Irradiation Enhanced by 11-MUA-Capped Gold Nanoparticles: An in vitro and in vivo Study. Int J Nanomedicine, 16, 4661.

80. Zhu, H., Zhang, S. (2018). Hypoxia inducible factor-1$\alpha$/vascular endothelial growth factor signaling activation correlates with response to radiotherapy and its inhibition reduces hypoxia-induced angiogenesis in lung cancer. J Cell Biochem, 119(9), 7707.

81. Agostinelli, S., Allison, J., Amako, K., Apostolakis, J., Araujo, H., Arce, P., Asai, M., Axen, D., Banerjee, S., Barrand, G., Behner, F., Bellagamba, L., Boudreau, J., Broglia, L., Brunengo, A., Burkhardt, H., Chauvie, S., Chuma, J., Chytracek, R., ... Zschiesche, D. (2003). GEANT4 - A simulation toolkit. Nuclear Instruments and Methods in Physics Research, Section A: Accelerators, Spectrometers, Detectors and Associated Equipment.

82. Allison, J., Amako, K., Apostolakis, J., Arce, P., Asai, M., Aso, T., Bagli, E., Bagulya, A., Banerjee, S., and Barrand, G. (2016). Recent developments in Geant4. Nuclear Instruments and Methods in Physics Research Section A: Accelerators, Spectrometers, Detectors and Associated Equipment, 835, 186–225.

83. Böhlen, T. T., Cerutti, F., Chin, M. P. W., Fassò, A., Ferrari, A., Ortega, P. G., Mairani, A., Sala, P. R., Smirnov, G., and Vlachoudis, V. (2014). The FLUKA Code: Developments and challenges for high energy and medical applications. Nuclear Data Sheets, 120, 211–214. https://doi.org/10.1016/j.nds.2014.07.049

84. Boscolo, D., Krämer, M., Durante, M., Fuss, M. C., and Scifoni, E. (2018). TRAX-CHEM: A pre-chemical and chemical stage extension of the particle track structure code TRAX in water targets. Chemical Physics Letters, 698, 11–18. https://doi.org/10.1016/j.cplett.2018.02.051

85. Brown, F. B., Barrett, R. F., Booth, T. E., Bull, J. S., Cox, L. J., Forster, R. A., Goorley, T. J., Mosteller, R. D., Post, S. E., and Prael, R. E. (2002). MCNP version 5. Trans. Am. Nucl. Soc, 87(273), 2–3935.

86. Casiraghi, M., and Schulte, R. W. (2015). Nanodosimetry-Based Plan Optimization for Particle Therapy. Computational and Mathematical Methods in Medicine, 2015, 1–13.

87. Chiniforoush, T. A., Hadadi, A., Kasesaz, Y., and Sardjono, Y. (2021). Evaluation of effectiveness of equivalent dose during proton boron fusion therapy (PBFT) for brain cancer: A Monte Carlo study. Applied Radiation and Isotopes, 170(January), 109596.

88. Cirrone, G. A. P., Petringa, G., Attili, A., Chiappara, D., Manti, L., Bravatà, V., Margarone, D., Mazzocco, M., and Cuttone, G. (2019). STUDY OF THE DISCREPANCY BETWEEN ANALYTICAL CALCULATIONS AND THE OBSERVED BIOLOGICAL EFFECTIVENESS IN PROTON BORON CAPTURE THERAPY (PBCT). RAD Association Journal, 3(3).

89. Chen, Z., Yang, P., Lei, Q., Wen, Y., He, D., Wu, Z., and Gou, C. (2019). Comparison of Bnct Dosimetry Calculations Using Different Geant4 Physics Lists. Radiation Protection Dosimetry, 187(1), 88–97.

90. Elsässer, T., and Scholz, M. (2007). Cluster effects within the local effect model. Radiation Research, 167, 319–329.

91. Elsässer, T., Weyrather, W. K., Friedrich, T., Durante, M., Iancu, G., Krämer, M., . . . Scholz, M. (2010). Quantification of the relative biological effectiveness for ion beam radiotherapy: Direct experimental comparison of proton and carbon ion beams and a novel approach for treatment planning. International Journal of Radiation Oncology Biology Physics, 78(4), 1177–1183.

92. Ferrari, A, Sala, P. R., Fasso, A., and Ranft, J. (2005). FLUKA: A Multi-Particle Transport Code. In Slac.

93. Friedrich, T., Scholz, U., Elssser, T., Durante, M., and Scholz, M. (2012). Calculation of the biological effects of ion beams based on the microscopic spatial damage distribution pattern. International Journal of Radiation Biology, 88(1–2), 103–107.

94. Gabel, D., Foster, S., and Fairchild, R. G. (1987). The Monte Carlo simulation of the biological effect of the 10B (n, $\alpha$) 7Li reaction in cells and tissue and its implication for boron neutron capture therapy. Radiation Research, 111(1), 14–25.

95. Goorley, T., James, M., Booth, T., Brown, F., Bull, J., Cox, L. J., Durkee, J., Elson, J., Fensin, M., Forster, R. A., Hendricks, J., Hughes, H. G., Johns, R., Kiedrowski, B., Martz, R., Mashnik, S., McKinney, G., Pelowitz, D., Prael, R., . . . Zukaitis, T. (2012). Initial MCNP6 release overview. Nuclear Technology, 180(3), 298–315.

96. Hawkins, R. B. (1994). A Statistical theory of Cell Killing by Radiation of Varying Linear Transfer Energy. Radiation Research, 140(3), 366–374.

97. Hawkins, R. B. (1996). A microdosimetric-kinetic model of cell death from exposure to ionizing radiation of any LET, with experimental and clinical applications. International Journal of Radiation Biology, 69, 739–755.

98. Hawkins, R. B. (2003). A microdosimetric-kinetic model for the effect of non-Poisson distribution of lethal lesions on the variation of RBE with LET. Radiation Research, 160(1), 61–69.

99. Hendricks, J. S., McKinney, G. W., Waters, L. S., Roberts, T. L., Egdorf, H. W., Finch, J. P., . . . Swinhoe, M. T. (2005). MCNPX extensions version 2.5. 0. Los Alamos National Laboratory, 15.

100. Horiguchi, H., Sato, T., Kumada, H., Yamamoto, T., and Sakae, T. (2015). Estimation of relative biological effectiveness for boron neutron capture therapy using the PHITS code coupled with a microdosimetric kinetic model. Journal of Radiation Research, 56(2), 382–390.

101. Inaniwa, T., Furukawa, T., Kase, Y., Matsufuji, N., Toshito, T., Matsumoto, Y., Furusawa, Y., and Noda, K. (2010). Treatment planning for a scanned carbon beam with a modified microdosimetric kinetic model. Physics in Medicine and Biology, 55(22), 6721–6737.

102. Incerti, S., Baldacchino, G., Bernal, M., Capra, R., Champion, C., Francis, Z., Guatelli, S., Guèye, P., and Mantero, A. (2010). The Geant4-DNA project. Int. J. Model. Simul. Sci. Comput.

103. Kase, Y., Kanai, T., Matsumoto, Y., Furusawa, Y., Okamoto, H., Asaba, T., Sakama, M., and Shinoda, H. (2006). Microdosimetric measurements and estimation of human cell survival for heavy-ion beams. Radiat. Res., 166(4), 629–638.

104. Kase, Y., Kanai, T., Matsufuji, N., Furusawa, Y., Elsässer, T., and Scholz, M. (2008). Biophysical calculation of cell survival probabilities using amorphous track structure models for heavy-ion irradiation. Physics in Medicine and Biology, 53(1), 37–59.

105. Kiger, J. L., Kiger, W. S., Riley, K. J., Binns, P. J., Patel, H., Hopewell, J. W., Harling, O. K., Busse, P. M., and Coderre, J. A. (2008). Functional and histological changes in rat lung after boron neutron capture therapy. Radiation Research, 170(1), 60–69.

106. Kitao, K. (1975). A Method for Calculating the Absorbed Dose near Interface from Reaction. Radiation Research, 61(2), 304–315. Kobayashi, T., and Kanda, K. (1982). Analytical calculation of boron-10 dosage in cell nucleus of neutron capture therapy. Radiation Research, 91(1), 77–94.

107. Kumada, H., Yamamoto, K., Matsumura, A., Yamamoto, T., and Nakagawa, Y. (2007). Development of JCDS, a computational dosimetry system at JAEA for boron neutron capture therapy. Journal of Physics: Conference Series, 74(1).

108. Krämer, M., and Kraft, G. (1994). Calculations of heavy-ion track structure. Radiation and Environmental Biophysics, 33(2), 91–109.

109. Mascia, A., DeMarco, J., Chow, P., and Solberg, T. (2004). Benchmarking the MCNPX nuclear interaction models for use in the proton therapy energy range. In Proc. of the 14th Int. Conf. on Computers in Radiotherapy (Seoul, Korea, May 2004) (pp. 478–481).

110. McMahon, S. J. (2019). The linear quadratic model: Usage, interpretation and challenges. Physics in Medicine and Biology, 64(1).

111. Niita, K., Sato, T., Iwase, H., Nose, H., Nakashima, H., and Sihver, L. (2006). PHITS-a particle and heavy ion transport code system. Radiation Measurements, 41(9–10), 1080–1090.

112. Okada, S., Murakami, K., Incerti, S., Amako, K., and Sasaki, T. (2019). MPEXS-DNA, a new GPU-based Monte Carlo simulator for track structures and radiation chemistry at subcellular scale. Medical Physics, 46(3), 1483–1500.

113. Otuka, N., Dupont, E., Semkova, V., Pritychenko, B., Blokhin, A. I., Aikawa, M., . . . Dunaeva, S. (2014). Towards a more complete and accurate experimental nuclear reaction data library (EXFOR): international collaboration between nuclear reaction data centres (NRDC). Nuclear Data Sheets, 120, 272–276.

114. Safavi-Naeini, M., Chacon, A., Guatelli, S., Franklin, D. R., Bambery, K., Gregoire, M.-C., and Rosenfeld, A. (2018). Opportunistic dose amplification for proton and carbon ion therapy via capture of internally generated thermal neutrons. Scientific Reports, 8(1), 16257.

115. Sato, T., Iwamoto, Y., Hashimoto, S., Ogawa, T., Furuta, T., Abe, S. ichiro, Kai, T., Tsai, P. E., Matsuda, N., Iwase, H., Shigyo, N., Sihver, L., and Niita, K. (2018). Features of Particle and Heavy Ion Transport code System (PHITS) version 3.02. Journal of Nuclear Science and Technology, 55(6), 684–690.

116. Scholz, M., Kellerer, A. M., Kraft-Weyrather, W., and Kraft, G. (1997). Computation of cell survival in heavy ion beams for therapy. The model and its approximation. Radiation and Environmental Biophysics, 36, 59–66.

117. Tabbakh, F., and Hosmane, N. S. (2020). Enhancement of Radiation Effectiveness in Proton Therapy: Comparison Between Fusion and Fission Methods and Further Approaches. Scientific Reports, 10(1), 1–12.

118. Yoon, D. K., Jung, J. Y., and Suh, T. S. (2014). Application of proton boron fusion reaction to radiation therapy: A Monte Carlo simulation study. Applied Physics Letters, 105(22).

119. Zamenhof, R., Redmond, E. 2nd, Solares, G., Katz, D., Riley, K., Kiger, S., and Harling, O. (1996). Monte Carlo-based treatment planning for boron neutron capture therapy using custom designed models automatically generated from CT data. International Journal of Radiation Oncology, Biology, Physics, 35(2), 383–397.

120. Malouff Timothy D., Seneviratne Danushka S., Ebner Daniel K., Stross William C., Waddle Mark R., Trifiletti Daniel M., Krishnan Sunil, Boron Neutron Capture Therapy: A Review of Clinical Applications, Frontiers in Oncology, 2021, 11:351

121. Shinji Kawabata, Minoru Suzuki, Katsumi Hirose, Hiroki Tanaka, Takahiro Kato, Hiromi Goto, Yoshitaka Narita, and Shin-Ichi Miyatake, Accelerator-based BNCT for patients with recurrent glioblastoma: a multicenter phase II study, Neuro-Oncology Advances 3(1), 1–9, 2021

122. J.A. Coderre and G.M. Morris. The radiation biology of boron neutron capture therapy. Radiation research, 151(1):1–18, 1999.

123. Silva Bortolussi, Ian Postuma, Nicoletta Protti, Lucas Provenzano, Cinzia Ferrari,Laura Cansolino, Paolo Dionigi, Olimpio Galasso, Giorgio Gasparini, Saverio Altieri,Shin-Ichi Miyatake and Sara J. González. Understanding the potentiality of acceleratorbased-boron neutron capture therapy for osteosarcoma: dosimetry assessment basedon the reported clinical experience. (2017) 12:130

124. Kreiner, A.J.; Bergueiro, J.; Cartelli, D.; Baldo,M.; Castell,W.; Asoia, J.G.; Padulo, J.; Sandín, J.C.S.; Igarzabal, M.; Erhardt, J.; others. Present status of accelerator-based BNCT. Reports of Practical Oncology amd Radiotherapy 2016, 21, 95–101.

125. S. J. González and G. A. Santa Cruz. The photon-isoeffective dose in boron neutron capture therapy. Radiation research, 178(6):609–621, 2012.

126. S. J. González, E.C.C. Pozzi, A. Monti Hughes, L. Provenzano, H. Koivunoro, D.G. Carando, S.I. Thorp, M.R. Casal, S. Bortolussi, V.A. Trivillin, et al. Photon iso-effective dose for cancer treatment with mixed field radiation based on dose-response assessment from human and an animal model: clinical application to boron neutron capture therapy for head and neck cancer. Physics in Medicine & Biology, 62(20):7938, 2017.

127. Lea DE, Catcheside DG. The mechanism of induction by radiation of chromosome aberration in Tradescandia, J Genet 1942 44:216–45

128. Sato, T. and Furusawa, Y. Cell Survival Fraction Estimation Based on the Probability Densities of Domain and Cell Nucleus Specific Energies Using Improved Microdosimetric Kinetic Models. Radiat. Res. 178, 341–356 (2012).

# 14 Monte Carlo simulations for targeted alpha therapy

*Susanna Guatelli and David Bolst*
University of Wollongong, Wollongong, Australia

*Eva Bezak*
University of South Australia, Adelaide, Australia
The University of Adelaide, Adelaide, Australia

## CONTENTS

## 14.1 INTRODUCTION

Targeted alpha therapy (TAT) is a form of radiotherapy currently being trialed and developed, with the first human clinical trial in 1997. TAT consists of delivering an $\alpha$-emitting isotope directly to a tumor, sparing surrounding healthy cells. Similar to other radiotherapy treatments, Monte Carlo (MC) radiation physics simulations have been used for internal dosimetry estimates in TAT. In addition, MC simulations have been used to study more efficient methods to produce $\alpha$-emitters in nuclear facilities, with the goal of improving the viability of this treatment in the clinics.

This chapter provides a description of the fundamental physics mechanisms at the basis of TAT (Section 2) and an overview of the clinical perspective of TAT (Section 3), to contextualize the use of MC simulations in this therapeutic space. Section 4 follows with an overview of examples of MC simulations aimed to support the development of $\alpha$-emitter production processes and radiation detectors of interest for TAT. Particular attention is devoted to the use of MC codes for TAT internal dosimetry, subject of Section 5, and for radiobiological studies in Section 6. Finally, Section 7

DOI: 10.1201/9781003023920-14

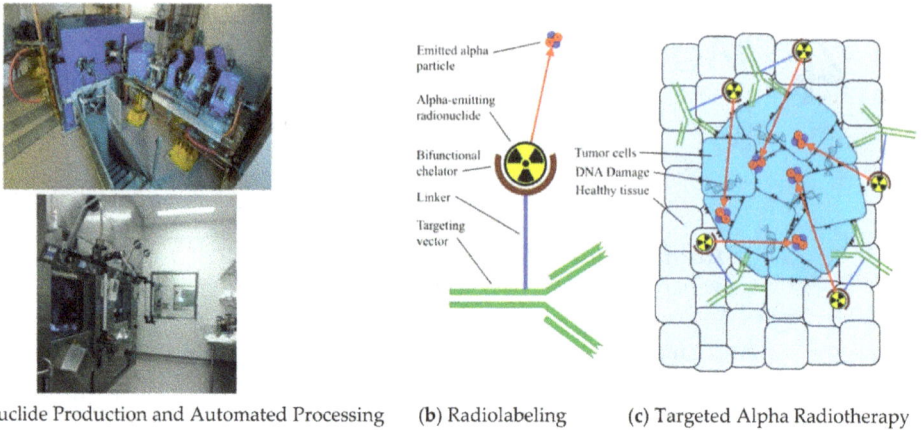

(a) Radionuclide Production and Automated Processing     (b) Radiolabeling     (c) Targeted Alpha Radiotherapy

**Figure 14.1**   Key aspects of targeted alpha therapy: (a) radionuclide production in a nuclear facility, and shielded automated processing; (b) radiolabelling the $\alpha$-emitting radionuclide to a suitable targeting vector to form a bioconjugate; and (c) targeted alpha radiotherapy destroys tumor cells while sparing surrounding healthy tissue. Figure and caption courtesy of [1].

provides simple MC examples for TAT internal dosimetry, using a multi-scale approach. We conclude the chapter with some final remarks in Section 8.

## 14.2   TAT: FUNDAMENTAL PHYSICS MECHANISMS

Targeted alpha therapy consists of delivering an $\alpha$-emitter directly to tumor cells or to its microenvironment, while sparing the healthy surrounding tissues [1]. Candidate TAT radioisotopes are 212Pb, 211At, 213Bi, 225Ac, 233Ra, 149Tb and 227Th [2] (their decay chains are fully described in [3]). Besides the approved bone-seeking $\alpha$-emitter $^{223}$Ra, the radioisotopes that have been more extensively studied in a clinical environment are $^{225}$Ac and its short-lived daughter nuclide $^{213}$Bi [4].

The TAT radioisotopes are produced by means of nuclear interactions, via cyclotrons, nuclear reactors or generator decays [1]. The $\alpha$-emitter is then conjugated with a targeting vector, e.g. monoclonal antibodies (mAb), biomolecules, peptides, nanocarriers, or small-molecule inhibitors, and delivered to the body via injection [1]. The radioisotope then congregates preferentially around tumor cells, delivering therapeutic radiation dose while decaying and emitting ionizing $\alpha$ particles.

The emitted $\alpha$ particles have a kinetic energy between 2 and 10 MeV, a high initial linear energy transfer (LET) of 60–100 keV/$\mu$m, and a short range (50 $\mu$m–80 $\mu$m), therefore producing large localized energy depositions in the targeted cancerous cells, causing complex DNA double strand breaks, which then lead to cell death [5].

TAT is more effective than targeted radionuclide therapy by means of $\beta^-$ particles, because the lethality is not dependent on the cell cycle or oxygenation and the DNA damage is more complex and therefore more difficult to repair. This is due to the higher LET of $\alpha$ particles. It has been estimated that to attain a single cell kill probability of 99.99%, tens of thousands of $\beta$-decays are required, whereas only a few $\alpha$-decays at the cell membrane achieve the same kill probability. Ultimately, a single $\alpha$ particle transversal can kill a cell [1]. In addition, the shorter range of $\alpha$-particles when compared to $\beta$ electrons make the treatment more localized to the targeted cancer cells.

Figure 14.1 shows the key aspects of TAT, from $\alpha$-emitter production to the physical mechanisms of cancer treatment.

## 14.3   CLINICAL PERSPECTIVES OF TAT

The first clinical trial of TAT employed $^{213}$Bi as the alpha emitter, conjugated to the anti-leukemia antibody, HuM195, and was reported in 1997 [6, 7]. Since then, numerous clinical trials have been performed with $^{211}$At, $^{223}$Ra, $^{224}$Ra, $^{225}$Ac, $^{212}$Pb, and $^{227}$Th [8, 1], for therapy of recurrent brain and ovarian cancers, colon, prostate, gastric, blood, breast, lung and bladder cancers, myelogenous leukemia, neuroendocrine tumors, non- Hodgkin lymphoma, glioblastoma, metastatic melanoma, skeletal metastases and others [Seidl et al. 2014] [9, 10, 1]. For a recent clinical review, the reader may refer to [10].

The development of clinical trials using TAT has been justified by the *in vitro* and *in vivo* pre-clinical studies showing a consistent trend of targeted cancer cell toxicity.

Monoclonal antibodies to target specific antigens or receptors have been used effectively to control the progression of different cancers. However, cancer specific antibodies alone can be insufficient to control cancer progression. Monoclonal antibodies labeled with radionuclides form radioimmunoconjugates (RIC), which can deliver high dose radiation directly to the cancer cells [11]. It was demonstrated that radioisotopes that emit $\alpha$ radiation are also effective in the killing of isolated cancer cells in transit and in the vascular and lymphatic systems as well as in inducing tumor regression by killing tumor capillary endothelial cells [11].

With respect to other radiotherapy treatments, TAT has the advantage to potentially treat both primary and metastatic diseases, including disseminated cancer cells and small tumor cell clusters that are not detected by positron emission tomography (PET), single-photon emission computerized tomography (SPECT) or magnetic resonance imaging (MRI) [2, 5, 3], coupled with a high radiobiological effectiveness.

In section 3.1 we report an example of clinical trial of TAT.

### 14.3.1   TAT FOR CASTRATE-RESISTANT PROSTATE CANCER

While metastatic castrate-resistant prostate cancer (mCRPC) is fatal for most men, recent clinical trials using three radionuclide-based therapies demonstrate improved control of mCRPC. The common RICs include: a) $\alpha$-emitting radionuclide $^{223}$RaCl$_2$ (Xofigo®) for palliation, b) beta-emitting $^{177}$Lu labeled anti-PSMA antibody J591, and c) $\alpha$-emitting $^{225}$Ac labeled PSMA617 ligand. These different approaches indicate the real, yet different benefits of $\alpha$ and $\beta$ radiotherapy for advanced prostate cancer and all have limitations with respect to curative therapy. $^{223}$RaCl$_2$ targets osteoblasts, not prostate cancer cells, and is primarily used to treat metastatic lesions in the bone. While $^{177}$Lu improves survival of mCRPC, it does not achieve cure at the maximum tolerance dose, and there is little room for improvement as the fatal disease progresses. On the other hand, $^{225}$Ac-PSMA617 is highly toxic to prostate cancers. It is, however, also toxic to the salivary glands (as they express PSMA), causing severe xerostomia. So while clinical data might suggest that TAT (using conjugates that directly target cancer cells) is better suited for both palliative and radical therapies, vectors, that target receptors on cancer cells only, are a must to avoid normal tissue complications.

## 14.4   MONTE CARLO SIMULATION STUDIES FOR TAT ASSOCIATED TECHNOLOGY

### 14.4.1   RADIOISOTOPE PRODUCTION

Securing a constant, efficient and economically viable supply of clinically relevant amounts of $\alpha$-emitting radionuclides remains a challenge, since their production requires complex nuclear infrastructures. Examples of nuclear techniques for the generation of TAT radioisotopes are cyclotrons, accelerating and bombarding targets with an incident beam of protons, $\alpha$ particles, lithium and carbon ions, nuclear reactors and "generator" systems, where the radioisotope is produced from a radionuclide decay [1]. A significant international effort is devoted towards the development of more efficient nuclear techniques to respond to this challenge.

In this context, MC simulations can be a very useful tool to investigate and optimize nuclear physics techniques to produce $\alpha$-emitters. For example, Kim and co-authors [12] used MCNPX [13] to determine the thickness of an aluminium target to degrade the energy of an $\alpha$ beam, emerging from the Korea Institute of Radiological and Medical Sciences (KIRAMS) cyclotron, from 45 MeV to approximately 29 MeV, before bombarding a natural bismuth target to produce At isotopes. The study was motivated by the need to obtain an $\alpha$ beam with a kinetic energy of 29 MeV, in order to maximize the cross section of production of $^{211}$At via the reaction $^{209}$Bi$(\alpha,2n)^{211}$At, peaking at around $\sim$30 MeV, while minimizing the production of $^{210}$At ($^{209}$Bi$(\alpha,3n)^{210}$At, peaking at $\sim$40 MeV, which is associated with an unwanted bone marrow toxicity.

Another very interesting study has been reported in [14], where the production of 38 nuclides, including $^{225}$Ac, deriving from the proton-induced spallation of thorium at TRIUMF's 500 MeV Isotope Production Facility, was studied. In particular, the team measured the nuclide production cross sections from irradiation of thorium by 438 MeV protons and compared the experimental results to FLUKA [15] and Geant4 [16] simulation results. The study found that FLUKA and Geant4 agreed reasonably well with the experimental measurements, in terms of total nuclide mass yield, especially in the spallation and peak fission curve regions. However, they showed differences with the experimental measurements at the edges of the fission yield and the evaporation regions. This work shows, that beyond specific MC simulation codes for radiation physics, there is an urgent need to refine the models describing nuclear processes, in order to be able to model the process of medical radioisotope production more accurately.

### 14.4.2 SIMULATION OF QUALITY ASSURANCE DETECTORS

Since the start of the use of MC codes in medical physics, MC simulations have been extensively used to design, investigate and optimize novel detector technology, for both diagnostic and therapeutic quality assurance applications, because they allow to solve some design problems efficiently and in an inexpensive way.

MC-based studies have been performed in the scientific community to develop novel quality assurance technology for TAT as well, to monitor the radioisotope distributions of both the parent and daughter isotopes (if decay chains are involved), including Compton and Cherenkov luminescence imaging systems.

#### 14.4.2.1 Compton imaging in TAT

[Lee at al 2019] [17] used GATE 7.0, a MC simulation platform [18] based on Geant4 [16], to evaluate the performance of a Compton SPECT system for *in vivo* monitoring of the position and distribution of $^{225}$Ac. Utilising the 218 and 440 keV gamma rays, emitted in the decay chain of $^{225}$Ac by daughters $^{221}$Fr and $^{213}$Bi, the photoelectric and Compton scattering events can be used for image reconstruction, increasing thus the SPECT detection efficiency. The SPECT's performance, using four gantry heads of a 100×100 array of 3 mm×3 mm×6 mm virtual Frisch-grid CZT detectors, was evaluated for various phantoms and compared with physical in-phantom measurements. The authors concluded that the Compton SPECT imaging performed better than conventional SPECT imaging, offering higher quality of reconstructed images and that the position and distribution of the $^{225}$Ac radionuclide in the reconstructed images matched well with the simulation conditions [17].

### 14.4.2.2 Cherenkov imaging in TAT

In the work of Ackerman and Graves [19], Geant4 was used to estimate the Cerenkov light (CL) output from α-emitting radionuclides, including $^{225}$Ac, $^{230}$U, $^{213}$Bi, $^{212}$Bi and $^{212}$At. CL can be detected by optical imaging systems, rendering this type of monitoring for *in vitro* and small animal dosimetry imaging. The energy of α particles produced in radioactive decay is, however, well below the threshold for producing CL. As such, the CL (similar to the Compton SPECT method above) utilizes the gamma rays and β particles (i.e. electrons) produced in the decay chain from the parent isotope to a stable daughter. If the energies of the gamma rays are high enough, they can produce secondary electrons of high enough energies (above 263 keV) to produce Cerenkov light. However, this also means that there can be a significant delay between the α decay and CL emission. It is expected that the CL intensity is proportional to the radioisotope activity. Three simulation geometries were used in the work of Ackerman and Graves [19]: a simple cube of water, a six-well plate and a small centrifuge tube to estimate the CL yields. The authors conclude that $^{212}$Bi and $^{213}$Bi isotopes can be imaged using CL resulting from β decay of daughters. Nevertheless, the accompanied emission of high energy gamma rays will dilute the information. $^{230}$U and $^{211}$At do not produce enough CL on clinically useful timescales. Finally, $^{225}$Ac can be imaged due to the $\beta^-$-emitters in its decay chain, but the interpretation of the imaging data is complex due to time effects.

## 14.5 TAT INTERNAL DOSIMETRY

Accurate dosimetric calculations are required for the success of all types of radiotherapy techniques. Due to the sub-millimeter range of α particles and being located within the patient, real time dosimetry of TAT is especially difficult. Measurements of the emitted characteristic gamma rays can give an estimate of the macroscopic α dose but this is not necessarily relevant. As direct measurements are difficult, if not impossible, theoretical approaches, such as MC calculations, can be employed to estimate the dose delivered in TAT to entire organs or, at the microscopic level, to cells. MC calculations at nanoscale level can be used to evaluate the direct and indirect damage to DNA and its complexity.

In term of internal dosimetry calculations for radiopharmaceuticals, it is important to start with the formalism proposed by the Medical Internal Radiation Dose (MIRD) Committee. The MIRD committee was formed within the Society of Nuclear Medicine in 1965, with the aim of standardizing internal dosimetry calculations, improving emission data for radionuclides, and enhancing data on pharmacokinetics for radiopharmaceuticals [20]. The MIRD Pamphlet No. 1 was published in 1968 and described a unified approach for internal dosimetry, which has since been updated several times [20].

The MIRD Pamphlet 21 [21, 8], deriving from multiple revisions of the MIRD formalism, has been extensively used in the scientific community for internal dosimetry calculations. In this formalism, the absorbed dose, $D$, to a target volume region $r_T$ from a source region $r_S$ is calculated as follows:

$$D(r_T) = \int A(r_S,t)\, dt \bullet S(r_T \leftarrow r_S),$$

where $A(r_S,t)$ is the activity of the radioisotope distributed homogeneously in $r_S$ , integrated over time, usually from the moment of the radiopharmaceutical administration to infinity. The S-value is the mean absorbed dose to the target region $r_T$, due to the radioisotope distributed in $r_S$, per unit activity.

S-values are calculated by means of MC simulations and tabulated [22]. They are specific to the radionuclide and depend on the anatomical model chosen to represent the patient (e.g. whole-body mathematical phantoms, voxelised phantoms based on CT/MR images, organs, parts of organs, cell populations).

A method to calculate dose distributions with higher spatial resolution due to radionuclides is based on dose point kernels (DPKs). DPKs describe the deposited energy as a function of distance from the site of emission of the radiation and are calculated by means of MC simulations [22]. The anatomical information of the patient can be provided by CT scans (as voxelised phantoms) and the activity distribution by SPECT scans [23]. The convolution of a DPK of a specific radionuclide and the activity distribution at a certain time after the injection provides the absorbed dose rate [22]. The main advantage of this method is that it provides a quick dose rate calculation in voxels, taking into account the anatomical detail of the patient. One drawback is that DPKs are calculated in homogeneous media of unit density soft tissue [22].

Various research groups have developed software tools for radioisotope internal dosimetry, which require two key components: a phantom, and the biokinetics/biodistribution of the radionuclide through the body. Human phantoms have evolved in details over the years, from early stylized mathematical phantoms, to realistic reference voxel phantoms, to patient-specific voxel phantoms generated from CT/MRI scans. There is also growing interest in using phantoms based on non-uniform rational B-spline (NURBS) or meshes. [24] provides a very informative review of computational phantoms.

Software tools that use reference phantoms include MIRDose [25], OLINDA/EXM [26] (created as a replacement for MIRDose), MABDOSE [27], and IDAC-Dose 2.1 [Anderson et al. (2017)]. The software packages OLINDA/EXM and IDAC-Dose 2.1 provide realistic voxel-based reference phantoms and calculate the absorbed doses to organs. Biokinetic data of the radionuclide of interest is input by the user, and tabulated specific S-values, are generated on the reference phantom and used to determine mean doses to organs.

The dosimetric approach is affected by severe limitations when applied to TAT because the concept of dose, which is a deterministic physical quantity, averaged over a "large" volume, fails when the range of the incident radiation is similar to a few cells. In addition, the average number of $\alpha$-particle cell-nucleus traversals required to kill a cell, ranges from as low as 1 to as high as 20 [8]. Consideration of realistic spatial and temporal distributions of the radionuclide in the biological medium, at intracellular level, could offer an important insight. It is the microscopic $\alpha$ radiation effect that is required to determine both the treatment efficacy and the toxicity.

Based on these observations, a microdosimetric approach, which takes into account the stochastic nature of particle interactions (see Chapter 9), offers a powerful methodology to investigate the physics mechanisms of TAT at cellular level [8]. It is important to note that it is essential to describe the spatial and temporal distribution of the $\alpha$-emitter in the biological medium as accurately as possible. There have been multiple microdosimetry studies using MC approaches in TAT, for example, using Geant4 [16], and PHITS [28].

[Sato et al. 2021] [29] developed a patient-specific dosimetry system for TAT based on PHITS coupled with a microdosimetric kinetic model [Hawkins et al. 1996]

[Huang et al. 2012] [30] used Geant4 and Geant4-DNA and a microdosimetric approach to demonstrate the hypothesis of underlying antivascular $\alpha$ therapy (TAVAT), in the case of $^{213}$Bi radionuclide. The tested hypothesis was that the therapeutic efficacy of TAVAT relates to the extravasation of the $\alpha$-immunoconjugates through porous tumor vascular walls and widened endothelial junctions into the perivascular space in the solid tumor. Geant4 and Geant4-DNA were used to calculate the specific energy deposited in the nucleus of endothelial cells (ECs), using intraluminal and perivascular models to represent normal tissue and tumor ECs, respectively. It was found that an intravenous injection of 25 mCi of 3.2 mCi/mg $\alpha$-immunoconjugate was able to deliver a cytotoxic dose to the tumor capillary endothelial cells (3.2 Gy) but not a significant dose to normal tissue endothelial cells (1.8 cGy), with a therapeutic gain of 180. This study is emblematic to show that it is very important to consider more realistic distributions of the $\alpha$ emitter at cellular level. To consider a homogeneous distribution of the $\alpha$-emitter in the biological medium could be a very limiting factor when investigating the physics mechanisms at the basis of TAT.

Thanks to the development of more sophisticated and powerful MC codes, it is nowadays possible to study the effectiveness of TAT at DNA level. An example is shown in [31], where Geant4-DNA [Incerti et al. 2010] was used to calculate double strand break yields in an atomic-resolution DNA geometrical model, and then the radiobiological effectiveness (RBE), in order to compare the effectiveness of $^{225}$Ac and $^{212}$Pb radioisotopes when used to treat brain micrometastases.

In conclusion, thanks to the development of more powerful computing processors and the availability of extensive computing infrastructures (supercomputers), nowadays it is possible to use MC simulations for a multi-scale approach in TAT internal dosimetry.

## 14.6    MC SIMULATIONS FOR *IN-VITRO* AND *IN-VIVO* STUDIES

MC methods can be used and have been proven beneficial at all levels of TAT research, including in preclinical studies (both *in vitro* and *in vivo* research).

In the work of [32] the trajectory of $\alpha$ particles (resulting from the decay of $^{149}$Tb (initial energy 3.97 MeV) and $^{211}$At (average initial energy 6.87 MeV) through human hemopoietic stem cells were modeled using MC methods. Cell survival, for each $\alpha$ particle passage through the cell's nucleus, was calculated as a function of LET. The modeled data was compared with the results of a corresponding *in vitro* experimental study. In their model, the cell survival was a function of exp(-⌣/✧), where ⌣ is the chord length through the nucleus and ✧ is the $\alpha$ particle's mean free path between two lethal events in the nucleus and is a function of LET. Another adopted assumption was that the cell survival was exponential as a whole (i.e. following the linear quadratic model), while the kill of an individual cell depended on a single lethal event. Three different scenarios were simulated, including non-targeted distribution of radioisotope through the simulated volume and isotope labelling on the surface of isolated cells. The authors [32] conclude that the spatial modeling of $\alpha$ particles relative to the target volume is essential to predict radiation effects. For targeted decays, the lower energy $\alpha$ particles (such as those from $^{149}$Tb) were more detrimental (up to 5 times more effective in cell killing) than $\alpha$ particles resulting from $^{211}$At decay. This is directly related to the LET of respective $\alpha$ particles.

In the work of Frelin-Labalme et al. 2020 [33], MC methods were used to simulate the spatial distribution of $^{212}$Pb-?VCAM-1 radioimmunoconjugate and the resultant dose deposition in a culture medium. The spatial distribution, as a function of time, was determined experimentally using silicon detectors positioned above and below the culture dishes. MC simulations were then used to analyze the measured spectra, as a function of different decay positions in the medium. Finally, the simulated spectra were in turn used to deconvolve the measured spectra to determine the RIC's distribution. Once the distribution was known, absorbed dose to cells could be calculated. The authors confirmed some variation in the spatial distribution of $^{212}$Pb-?VCAM-1 between the top and the bottom of the culture dishes, which varied with time and could be a consequence of gravitational and electrostatic forces. As such, assumptions about uniform and non-changing RIC distributions in *in vitro* experiments can lead to significant errors in dosimetry calculations [33].

In another interesting example [34], clonogenic assay *in vitro* experiments (Chinese hamster V79 lung fibroblasts) were correlated with MC simulations to predict cell survival from a combined therapy of chemotherapy (doxorubicin or daunomycin) and TAT ($^{210}$Po-citrate). In their work, MC simulations of cell survival were based on fluorescent intensities of individual cells as measured by flow cytometry. Additionally, in this complex scenario, a cell may die due to chemotherapy drug and TAT working independently or synergistically, with lognormal distribution of cellular uptake of both therapeutic agents assumed. The authors concluded that their model was capable of predicting the treatment response on a cell-by-cell basis and may be useful for testing multimodality therapies.

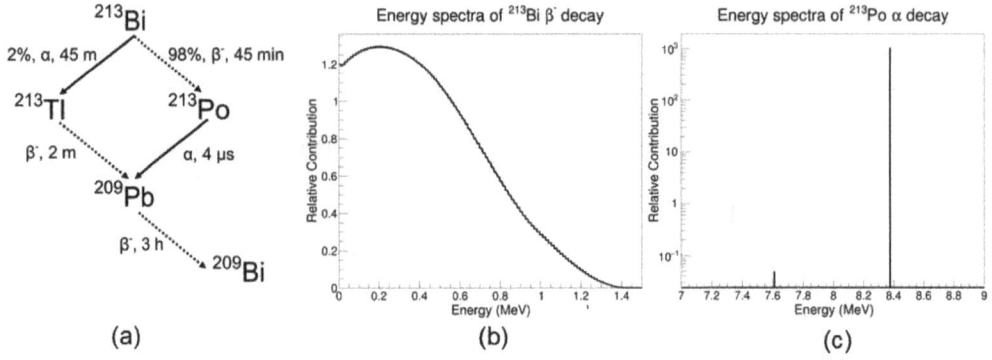

**Figure 14.2** (a) Decay scheme of $^{213}$Bi to $^{209}$Bi, (b) the energy spectra of electrons generated via $\beta^-$ decay of $^{213}$Bi and (c) the energy spectra of $\alpha$ generated via the decay of $^{213}$Po. The energy spectra were generated with Geant4 10.6.p02.

## 14.7 MONTE CARLO SIMULATIONS FOR TAT MULTI-SCALE DOSIMETRIC CALCULATIONS: A GUIDE FOR BEGINNERS

The following section showcases some MC-based calculations of fundamental physical quantities of interest in TAT internal dosimetry using Geant4 (version 10.6.p2). This section is intended as a starting point for beginners, who would like to use MC codes for dosimetry, micro- and nano-dosimetry calculations in TAT. It is suggested to attempt to reproduce the results shown in this section with either Geant4 or any other MC radiation physics code of interest.

$^{213}$Bi was used as the $\alpha$ source for these calculations, a diagram of its decay scheme is shown in Figure 14.2(a) and energy spectra of selected electrons and $\alpha$ particles are shown in Figure 14.2(b) and (c). Since $^{213}$Bi undergoes beta decay 98% of the time, with its daughter $^{213}$Po undergoing $\alpha$ decay entirely, the majority of $\alpha$ particles from a $^{213}$Bi source comes from its $^{213}$Po daughter, which has a significantly shorter half-life of 4 $\mu$s compared to its parent's 45 minute half-life.

### 14.7.1 CALCULATION OF DOSE POINT KERNEL

DPKs are radial energy deposition profiles in water from isotropic sources of particles emitted from a radionuclide. In the simulation shown here, the DPKs were calculated for an electron and $\alpha$-particle of energies 0.2 and 8.376 MeV, respectively, using the *TestEM12* Geant4 extended example. The choice of 0.2 MeV is due to it being the most probable energy of electrons from the decay of $^{213}$Bi and 8.376 MeV being the most probable $\alpha$ energy from a $^{213}$Bi source, coming from its $^{213}$Po daughter (see Figure 14.2). The *G4EMPhysicsList_option4* constructor was used to describe the particle electromagnetic (EM) interactions as it is deemed to be the most accurate Geant4 EM constructor for medical physics applications [35]. Figure 14.3 shows the results of the simulation, averaging over $10^6$ primary particles.

### 14.7.2 MICRODOSIMETRY CALCULATIONS

Microdosimetry is the study of the stochastic energy depositions from particles in micron-sized volumes. One of the fundamental quantities in microdosimetry is the lineal energy, $y$, which is the energy deposited in a volume, $\varepsilon$, divided by the sensitive volume's mean chord length, $<l>$. For more details on the microdosimetric approach, the reader can refer to Chapter. Microdosimetry in particle radiotherapy: Monte Carlo simulations and its verification.

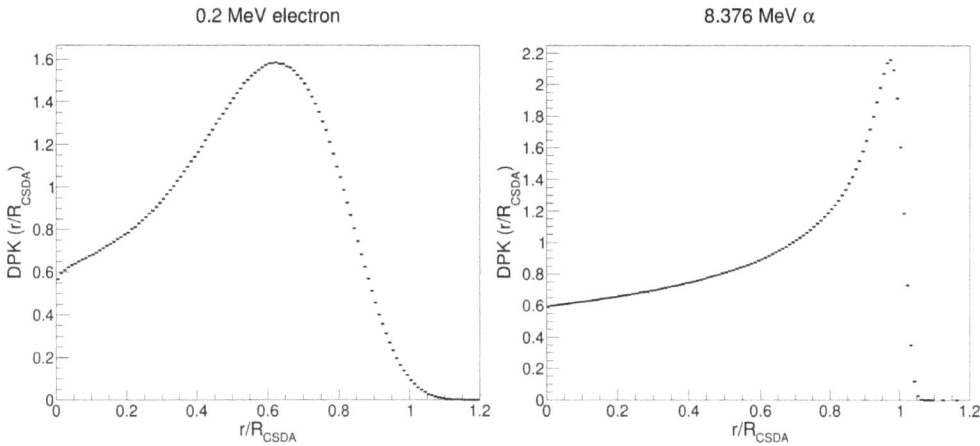

**Figure 14.3** Examples of dose point kernels (DPKs) obtained for a 0.2 MeV electron (left) and a 5.885 MeV α particle (right) in water. Calculations by means of Geant4 10.6.p02.

Here we show an example of microdosimetric calculation, using a $^{213}$Bi radioisotope, to estimate the radiation effect on a cell nucleus. The advanced Geant4 example *Radioprotection* was modified and used here to calculate microdosimetric quantities of interest.

Figure 14.4(a) shows the setup of the Geant4 simulation used to calculate the energy deposition from $^{213}$Bi in the biological medium. The simulation consists of a 100 μm diameter water sphere, representing a cell. At the center of this sphere is a water sphere with a 10 μm diameter, representing a cell nucleus. In this simulation study, it is assumed that $^{213}$Bi is homogenously distributed around the cell nucleus, for simplicity. To reduce the execution time of the simulation, the $^{213}$Bi is distributed as a sphere with an outer diameter of 30 μm and inner diameter of 10 μm. Figures 14.4(b) and (c) show the resulting microdosimetric spectra within the 10 μm water sphere (cell nucleus). The left plot shows the relative frequency of lineal energy events within the sphere, while the right plot displays the dose weighted lineal energy, *yd(y)*, distribution.

These plots distinguish between particle tracks from α decay (predominately from $^{213}$Po) as well as from β decay (mostly from $^{213}$Bi). The left plot shows that β-events are more prevalent for lineal energies below ~5 keV/μm, while α particle events dominate above this lineal energy value. The right plot shows that the majority of dose deposited within the cell nucleus comes from the higher lineal energy, more lethal, α events, as expected.

## 14.7.3 NANODOSIMETRIC CALCULATIONS

In MC codes there are two methods of transporting particles through matter, the "condensed history" (CH) and the "track structure" (TS) approach. General purpose MC codes use the CH approach, this "condenses" multiple physical interactions into a single one, greatly reducing the required time to track a certain particle through matter. The CH approach is typically accurate for energy deposition in volumes larger than a few microns. For smaller volumes, a TS approach is required. Specialized MC codes which focus on micron and nanometer sized volumes adopt the TS approach, which models all interactions the particle takes individually, at the cost of greater computational requirements. TS codes such as PARTRAC [36] or Geant4-DNA [37] are more suitable than CH based MC codes to describe particle interactions at nanometer scales, allowing DNA strand breaks and their complexity to be calculated. This method can offer a very useful insight to understand more in-depth radiobiological results, as demonstrated in the application of Geant4-DNA to other treatments (e.g. [38]).

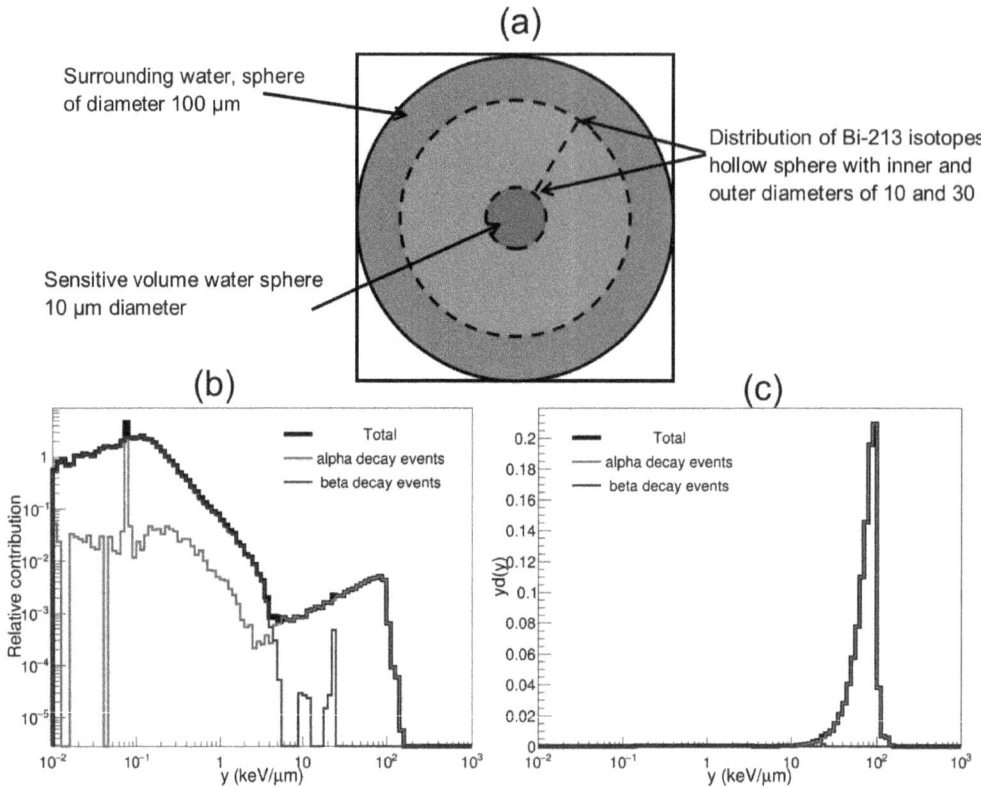

**Figure 14.4** (a) Geometrical configuration of the Geant4 simulation to calculate the microdosimetric spectra in a cell nucleus of 10 μm diameter (sensitive volume), when $^{213}$Bi is homogenously distributed in a spherical shell, surrounding the nucleus, with an external radius of 30 μm. The biological medium is modeled with a sphere of diameter 100 μm. (b) and (c) The resulting microdosimetric spectra calculated within the 10 μm water sphere. The simulation includes all decay channels of $^{213}$Bi.

Example track structures calculated by means of Geant4-DNA of an electron and an α particle with energies of 0.2 and 8.376 MeV, respectively, in water are shown in Figure 14.5. These track structures were generated using the Geant4 extended example *microdosimetry*, which provides a detailed description of particle interactions below the micron scale. These track structures are generated in a 1 micrometer water cube, with each black dot representing a point in the cube where the particle has undergone an interaction, for example via ionization, excitation or elastic scattering. In these two example cases, the electron produces approximately 100 secondary electrons via ionization while the α particle generates approximately 4000 electrons.

## 14.8 DISCUSSION AND CONCLUSIONS

MC simulations are used in TAT for a range of applications, from the investigation of more efficient nuclear techniques to produce TAT radionuclides and the development of quality assurance detector technology for TAT, to internal dosimetry. In the last few decades, extensive progress has been done in MC codes for radiation physics. To perform TAT internal dosimetric calculations, increasingly more realistic phantoms have been developed, representing entire bodies, organs, cell populations, etc. In the last ten years, it has been clearly emerging that to couple dosimetry with MC based

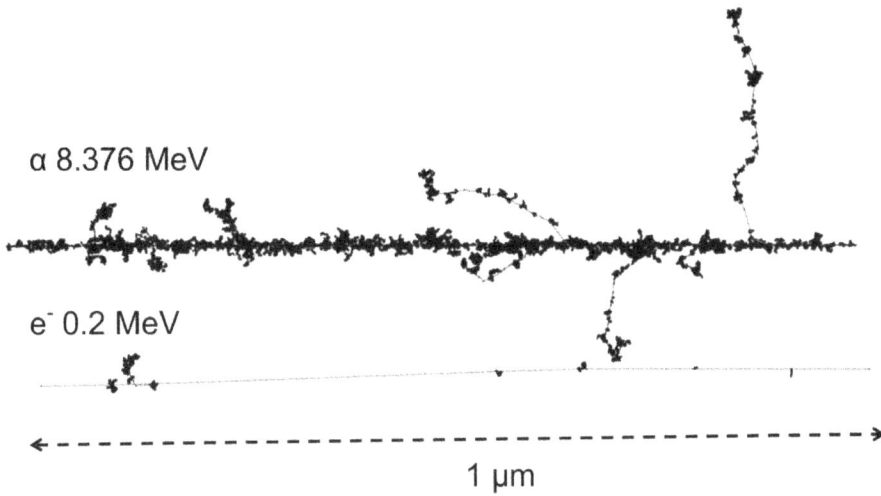

**α 8.376 MeV**

**e⁻ 0.2 MeV**

1 μm

**Figure 14.5**   Example track structures of a 0.2 MeV electron and 8.376 alpha particle in water, generated by using the track structure code Geant4-DNA [37].

micro- and nano- dosimetry, may offer a unique insight to improve clinical outcomes of TAT. Nowadays, a multi-scale approach is possible thanks to the development of increasingly more sophisticated MC codes, and the viability of more powerful computing processors and infrastructures.

## REFERENCES

1. Nelson, B. J. B., Andersson, J. D., Wuest, F. (2021) Targeted Alpha Therapy: Progress in Radionuclide Production, Radiochemistry, and Applications, *Pharmaceutics, Basel*, 13(1): 49.
2. Penfold, S., et al. (2014) MC simulations of dose distributions with necrotic tumor targeted radioimmunotherapy. *Applied Radiation and Isotopes*, 90: 40-45.
3. Seidl, C. (2014) Radioimmunotherapy with α-particle-emitting radionuclides. *Immunotherapy; London,* 6(4): 431-58.
4. Morgenstern, A., et al. (2018) An Overview of Targeted Alpha Therapy with $^{225}$Actinium and $^{213}$Bismuth. *Current Radiopharmaceuticals*, 11: 200-208.
5. Allen, B. (2006) Internal high linear energy transfer (LET) targeted radiotherapy for cancer, *Phys. Med. Biol.* 51: R327–R341.
6. Jurcic, J. G., et al. (1997) Targeted alpha-particle therapy for myeloid leukemias: a phase I trial of bismuth-213-HuM195 (anti-CD33). *Blood*, 90:2245.
7. Jurcic, J. G., et al. (2002) Targeted alpha particle immunotherapy for myeloid leukemia. *Blood*, 100(4): 1233-1239.
8. Sgouros, G., et al. (2010) MIRD Pamphlet No. 22: radiobiology and dosimetry of alpha-particle emitters for targeted radionuclide therapy. *J. Nucl Med.,* 51: 311-328.
9. Elgqvist, J., et al. (2014). The potential and hurdles of targeted alpha therapy—Clinical trials and beyond. *Front. Oncol.*, 3: 324.
10. Marcu, L., et al. (2018) Global comparison of targeted alpha vs targeted beta therapy for cancer: in vitro, in vivo and clinical trials. *Critical Reviews in Oncology / Hematology*, 123:7-20.
11. Allen, B. (2011) Future prospects for targeted alpha therapy, *Curr Radiopharm*; 4 (4):336-42.
12. Kim, G., et al. (2014), Production of α-particle emitting 211At using 45 MeV α-beam. *Phys. Med. Biol.* 59: 2849–2860.

13. Waters, L. S., et al. (2005) MCNPX version 2.5.0, Los Alamos National Laboratory, Los Alamos, US.
14. Robertson, A. K H., et al. (2020) Nuclide production cross sections from irradiation of thorium by 438 MeV protons and a comparison to FLUKA and GEANT4 simulations. *Physical Review C*, 102: 044613.
15. Ferrari, A., et al. (2005), FLUKA: A multiparticle transport code, *Technical Report No. SLAC-R-773*, CERN, Geneva, Switzerland.
16. Allison, J., et al. (2016) Recent developments in GEANT4, *Nucl. Instr. Methods Phys. Res. A*, 835: 186.
17. Lee, T., et al. (2019) Performance evaluation of a Compton SPECT imager for determining the position and distribution of 225Ac in targeted alpha therapy: A MC simulation based phantom study. *Applied Radiation and Isotopes*: 154, 108893.
18. Jan, S, et al. (2004) GATE: a simulation toolkit for PET and SPECT. *Phys Med Biol.*, 49(19):4543-4561.
19. Ackerman, N.L. & Graves, E.E. (2012) The potential for Cerenkov luminescence imaging of alpha-emitting radionuclides. *Physics in Medicine & Biology*, 57: 771–783.
20. Hindorf, C. (2014) Chapter 18, IAEA publication ISBN 92-0-107304-6: Nuclear Medicine Physics: A Handbook for Teachers and Student.
21. Bolch, W.E., et al. (2009) MIRD pamphlet No. 21: a generalized schema for radiopharmaceutical dosimetry–standardization of nomenclature, *J. Nucl. Med.* 50: 477-484.
22. Bailey, D. L., et al. (2014) Nuclear Medicine Physics, A Handbook for Teachers and Students, IAEA Publication.
23. Thierens, H. M., et al. (2001) Dosimetry from organ to cellular dimensions. *Comput Med Imaging Graph*, 25(2): 187-193.
24. Xu, et al. (2020) Technical Note: The development of a multi-physics simulation tool to estimate the background dose by systemic targeted alpha therapy. *Medical Physics*, 47(6): 2550-2557.
25. Stabin, M. G., (1996) Mirdose: personal computer software for internal dose assessment in nuclear medicine. *Journal of Nuclear Medicine*, 37(3): 538-546.
26. Stabin, M. G., et al. (2005) Olinda/exm: the second-generation personal computer software for internal dose assessment in nuclear medicine. *Journal of Nuclear Medicine*, 46(6): 1023-1027.
27. Johnson, T. K., et al. (1999) Mabdose.I: Characterization of a general purpose dose estimation code. *Medical Physics*, 26(7): 1389-1395.
28. Sato, T., et al. (2018) Features of particle and heavy ion transport code system (phits) version 3.02. *Journal of Nuclear Science and Technology*, 55(6): 684-690.
29. Sato, T., et al. (2021) Individual dosimetry system for targeted alpha therapy based on phits coupled with microdosimetric kinetic model. *EJNMMI Physics*, 8(1).
30. Huang, C-Y, et al. (2012), MC calculation of the maximum therapeutic gain of tumor antivascular alpha therapy, *Med. Phys.* 39 (3).
31. Ackerman, N. L., et al. (2018) Targeted alpha therapy with $^{212}$Pb or $^{225}$Ac: Change in RBE from daughter migration, *Physica Medica*, 51: 91-98.
32. Charlton, D. E., et al. (1998) Theoretical treatment of human haemopoietic stem cell survival following irradiation by alpha particles. *International Journal of Radiation Biology*, 74(1): 111-118.
33. Frelin-Labalme, A.-M., et al. (2020) Radionuclide spatial distribution and dose deposition for in vitro assessments of $^{212}$Pb-$\alpha$VCAM-1 targeted alpha therapy. *Medical Physics*, 47(3): 1317-1326.
34. Akudugu, J. M., et al. (2012) A method to predict response of cell populations to cocktails of chemotherapeutics and radiopharmaceuticals: Validation with daunomycin, doxorubicin, and the alpha particle emitter $^{210}$Po. *Nuclear Medicine and Biology*, 39(7): 954-961.

35. Arce, P., et al. (2021) Report on G4-Med, a Geant4 benchmarking system for medical physics applications developed by the Geant4 Medical Simulation Benchmarking Group, *Medical Physics*, https://doi.org/10.1002/mp.14226.
36. Friedland, W., et al. (2011), Track structures, DNA targets and radiation effects in the biophysical MC simulation code PARTRAC, *Mutation Research/Fundamental and Molecular Mechanisims of Mutagenesis*, 711(1-2).
37. Incerti, S, et al. (2018) Geant4-DNA example applications for track structure simulations in liquid water: A report from the Geant4-DNA Project. *Med. Phys.* 45 (8): e722-e739.
38. Sakata, D., et al. (2020) Fully integrated MC simulation for evaluating radiation induced DNA damage and subsequent repair using Geant4-DNA. *Scientific Reports*, 10(1), 20788.

# 15 Experimental and modelling challenges in FLASH radiotherapy with Monte Carlo methods

*Daria Boscolo, Martina Fuss, and Walter Tinganelli*
GSI Helmholtzzentrum fur Schwerionenforschung Darmstadt,
Germany

*Pankaj Chaudary*
Queen's University Belfast, Belfast, UK
National Physical Laboratory, England, UK

## CONTENTS

## 15.1 INTRODUCTION

Building upon pioneering work carried out from the late 1950s on, a current revival of experimental investigations into the so-called FLASH effect (see [1, 2] and references therein) is successfully demonstrating a differential tissue sparing effect. A reduced radiation induced toxicity in the normal tissue while maintaining tumor cytotoxicity has been shown both in vitro and in vivo for different animal models and endpoints when delivering the dose at high intensity. Typically, dose rates are $> 40$Gy/s for FLASH applications compared to $\sim 5$ Gy/min in conventional radiotherapy. The exceptional FLASH radiation tolerance can potentially widen the therapeutic window between tumor control and normal tissue complication probability for future use in patients. With most studies showing a FLASH effect being performed with electron and X-ray radiation, much less is known about proton and ion radiation. This is mainly due to technological limitations and to the limited amount of accelerator centers able to deliver sufficiently large doses to sufficiently large volumes under the FLASH dose rate constrains. However the combination of the physical and biological advantages of ion and proton therapy with the FLASH dose rates could give rise to a new and more efficient way to treat cancer. Based on this concept and on the first *in vitro* and *in vivo* results, the First-in-Human FLASH Research Trial is ongoing at the Proton Therapy Center of the Cincinnati

DOI: 10.1201/9781003023920-15

**228**

Children's hospital with ten patients to be treated in a single treatment session of less than one-second radiation exposure.

Despite the striking experimental evidences, no conclusive mechanistic explanation underlying the FLASH effect has been found until now and some studies employing accepted FLASH dose rates could not confirm any sparing effect, particularly *in vitro*. Possibly, for a the proper understanding of the biological effects and the mechanisms at their base, it is important to consider the large variability of dose rate ranges investigated up to now. While the more recent studies have been carried out at dose rates ranging from 40 to 1000 Gy/s, the very early studies are mostly performed at sensibly larger dose rates, between $10^7$ and $10^{10}$ Gy/s, compared to those achieved using laser-driven ion acceleration. Here, we will refer to the first ones as "FLASH" dose rates, and the second group as "ultra-high dose rates." Under these two very different conditions it is likely that different mechanisms contribute to the tissue sparing effect.

Monte Carlo studies can be of great help on their own or in combination with other modelling approaches to clarify the feasibility or quantitative impact of several of these proposed mechanisms and to facilitate clinical application of FLASH irradiation. We discuss how physical, radiation chemical and biological predictions can be obtained based on Monte Carlo calculations, which differences exist between different radiation qualities, and give an overview about the current results.

## 15.2  EXPERIMENTAL EVIDENCES

### 15.2.1  ELECTRONS AND PHOTONS

#### 15.2.1.1  In vitro effects

Vozenin and Wilson et al. have provided a detailed overview of the *in vitro* effects of FLASH electrons [1, 2]. Cellular effects of ultra-high dose rates were reported as early as the 1970s and indicated some evidence of reduced cell killing at such dose rates. Berry between 1972–1973 compared the effects of radiation dose rate from protracted, continuous irradiation to ultra-high dose rates of $10^9$ Gy/sec from pulsed accelerators [5], noticed some non-predictable effects and discussed the impact of these dose rates on responses under hypoxia. A later study conducted using pulsed electron beam at a dose rate of 380 Gy/sec reported no significant variations in the cell killing RBE or OER at FLASH and conventional dose rate electrons using V79 cells [6]. Only recently Adrian et al. [7] have reported that DU145 cancer cells irradiated either under normoxic conditions or hypoxic conditions present a significant difference in the cell survival at doses higher than 18 Gy, however the dose response between 5–10 Gy at FLASH or conventional dose rate were similar. Fouillade et al. [8] showed the effect of FLASH electrons on the biomarkers of DNA DSB damage TRP53BP1 and $\gamma$-H2AX foci recently.

#### 15.2.1.2  In vivo effects

Favaudon et al. in 2014 [11] revived the interest in FLASH radiotherapy by reporting the normal tissue sparing effects of FLASH electrons in mouse lung tumor models. An account of the in vivo effects of FLASH electrons in mice is provided in table 15.1, where all parameters studied are listed. After the success of FLASH effects in rodent or mouse models, it is also important to understand whether such normal tissue sparing effects are translated in higher mammals, as the ultimate goal is to use FLASH for human treatment. In this direction, the first study reporting the efficacy of FLASH electrons was reported by Vozenin et al.[12] in 2018, where the dose escalation studies with FLASH electrons were conducted in Goettingen mini pig skin and nasal plenum tumors of cats. Based on the dose escalation potential achieved with FLASH radiotherapy in these higher mammals, first evidence of clinical translation of FLASH radiotherapy feasibility in human patient was reported in 2019 [13]. In this study, 75 year old patient presented with CD30+ T-cell cutaneous lymphoma disseminated throughout the skin surface and was treated with 15 Gy FLASH electron dose in a 3.5

**Table 15.1**

**Normal and tumor tissue effects after FLASH irradiation in *in vivo* pre-clinical studies: from mice to large mammals. Adapted from [10].**

| Organ/Tumor Evaluated | Radiation Quality and Delivery Parameters | Normal Tissue Effects/Tumor Control |
|---|---|---|
| Lung (mice) | Dose rate:<br>- FLASH: >40 Gy/s;<br>- CONV: 0.03 Gy/s.<br>Total dose: 15 Gy. | No complications with FLASH below 20 Gy at 36-weeks follow-up. Better normal tissue protection than CRT and comparable tumor control. |
| Whole brain (mice) | Pulsed electron beam.<br>Dose rate:<br>- FLASH: >100 Gy/s;<br>- CONV: 0.1 Gy/s.<br>Total dose: 10 Gy. | Memory and neurogenesis preservation in the hippocampus after FLASH; Electron FLASH is superior at brain function preservation to conventional delivery. CONV led to permanent alterations in neurocognitive end points 6 months post treatment, while FLASH did not cause neuroinflammation, learning/memory deficits. |
| Whole brain (juvenile mice) | Pulsed electron beam.<br>Dose rate:<br>- FLASH: $4.4 \times 10^6$ Gy/s;<br>- CONV: 0.077 Gy/s.<br>Total dose: 8 Gy. | FLASH therapy was found to preserve the neurogenic niche, neurogenesis in the hippocampus and normal growth hormone levels post irradiation which were all degraded by CRT. FLASH was also found to result in normal or near normal results in learning, memory and socialization tests at 4 months post treatment, while CRT caused major deficits. |
| Whole brain (mice) | Syncrotron X-rays.<br>Dose rate: 37 Gy/s (12,000 Gy/s in the slice). | No memory deficit (preservation of spatial memory); reduced impairment of hippocampal cell division; induction of less reactive astrogliosis. |
| Whole brain (mice) | High energy electrons (16-20 MeV).<br>Dose rate:<br>- FLASH: 300Gy/s (16 MeV) and 200 Gy/s (20MeV);<br>- 0.13 Gy/s.<br>Single dose of 30 Gy. | FLASH showed reduced pro-inflammatory cytokines and less loss of dendritic spine density in the hippocampus, also reduced cognitive impairment and neurodegeneration compared to conventional therapy. |
| Total body irradiation (mice) | Dose rate:<br>- FLASH: 200 Gy/s;<br>- CONV: <0.072 Gy/s.<br>Total dose: 4 Gy. | FLASH therapy was found to result in greater killing of Leukemia cells as well as longer remission delays and survival than CRT. FLASH therapy was found to preserve partial hematopoietic stem/progenitor cell function which was completely destroyed by CONV. |

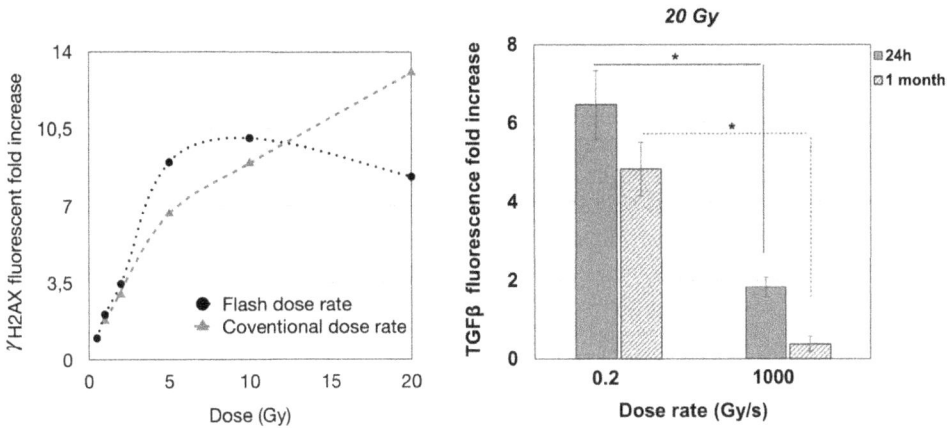

**Figure 15.1** (A) Effect of proton dose rate on DNA DSB damage as revealed through fold change in the intensity of $\gamma$-H2AX foci in human lung fibroblasts (IMR 90) cells, adapted from [9]. (B) Effect of dose rate on the expression of inflammation marker-TGF $\beta$ shown as fold increase in the intensity at 24 hrs and 1 month after exposure to 20 Gy FLASH protons or 20 Gy conventional dose rate protons. Reprinted with permission from Buonanno et al. [9].

cm diameter spot on the arm in 90 milliseconds. All of these in-vivo studies indicate a similar tumor cell killing effect of FLASH electrons to conventional dose rate radiotherapy whereas the normal tissue sparing effects of FLASH electrons were superior to the conventional radiotherapy.

Most of the *in vitro* studies with FLASH X-rays were conducted at ultra-high dose rate in the period between 1960–1970. Prempree et al. [14] for the first time studied the in-vitro effects of ultra-high dose rate X-rays on the repair time of chromosome breaks delivered at a dose rate of $4.5 \times 10^8$ Gy/sec in human lymphocytes. Later Berry et al. [5] also studied how FLASH X-rays affect the cell survival; other than these studies not much information is available for the *in vitro* effects of FLASH photons. Radiobiological studies with FLASH photons mainly employed synchrotron generated X-rays. In a recent study Montay-Gruel et al. [15] have confirmed that FLASH X-rays can also produce normal tissue sparing effects similar to FLASH electrons. Authors report that a 10 Gy X-ray dose delivered at a dose rate of 37 Gy/sec did not induce memory deficit and it reduced hippocampal cell division impairment and astrogliosis otherwise increased by conventional dose rate radiotherapy.

### 15.2.2 PROTON AND CARBON IONS

#### 15.2.2.1 In vitro effects

Only one over ten in vitro studies using a FLASH proton radiation demonstrates a significant difference with proton beam, delivered with a conventional dose rate, in reducing the cells' damage [16]). However, it is important to point out that most of the in vitro studies have been done at ambient oxygenation, where no FLASH effect is expected. Cells in vitro are cultivated at abient oxygenation (21% of oxygen), while in tissues, the normal oxygenation (physioxia) is between 4 and 7% approximately [17]. The dramatic increase in radioresistance occurs with oxygen concentrations ranging from 0% to 3% [18]. Thus, small changes in oxygen levels in tissues that are at low oxygen concentrations may result in an increase in radioresistance. In contrast, decreases in oxygen concentration, even by several percentage points, starting at oxygen concentrations of 21%, will not lead to a radioresistance increase. FLASH dose rate, $>100$ Gy/s, reduces the chronic but not the acute effects of normal lung fibroblast cells compared to the cells irradiated with a conventional dose rate [9], as shown in Figure 15.1. Indeed, FLASH radiation produces a lower number of senescent cells and a significant reduction of Transforming Growth Factor (TGF-$\beta$), released after radiation, suggesting FLASH's role in the chronic inflammatory process. No significant acute effects, for example, DNA double-strand breaks (DSBs) or $\gamma$H2AX foci, have been found [9].

Although most particle therapy centers use protons to irradiate deep-seated tumors, a strong culture of heavy-ion using carbon ion beams is developing in many countries. While FLASH-RT has been studied in the context of the electron, photon, and proton therapies, the efficacy of heavy ions, such as carbon ions, under FLASH conditions remains unclear.

In vitro studies to verify an eventual FLASH effect with carbon ion radiation are still ongoing. However, as discussed in section 15.3.3, the peculiar physical and biological properties of carbon ion radiations could lead to different outcomes compared to what has been observed with proton radiation. To verify if oxygen depletion occurs with carbon ion irradiation, a first in vitro FLASH experiment has been done. The investigators' hypothesis was based on the assumption that the $O_2$ level would reduce if oxygen depletion occurs [18], increasing cell survival. Indeed, existing models suggest that a slight drop in oxygenation might lead to a noticeable increase in the oxygen enhancement ratio (OER), especially at oxygen concentrations between 0.5 and 4%, which would lead to a measurable increase in cell survival. Meanwhile, this hypothesis also suggests no significant OER changes either at higher oxygen levels, like the 21% of oxygen (21% is the standard cell cultures' oxygen level in the biology laboratory) and at 0% of oxygen (since no depletion can occur in this condition). Normal tissue cells cultivated at different oxygen conditions and irradiated with 8 Gy of a carbon ion beam have been then analyzed with a clonogenic assay to investigate the cell survival. As hypothesized, the results show no differences in the surviving fractions of cells irradiated with $^{12}$C in the plateau region (dose-averaged linear energy transfer (LET) of approx. 13 keV/$\mu$m), cultivated in normoxia (21 %) and anoxia (0 %). In comparison, a significant difference in cell survival is shown for cells cultivated at 0.5 % of $O_2$, suggesting an increased sparing effect of FLASH for a higher $O_2$ of 4 %.

### 15.2.2.2  In vivo effects

Contrary to the in vitro results, in vivo studies investigating the FLASH proton beam radiation have shown positive findings by obtaining a FLASH sparing effect and, in one study, even better tumor control than conventional radiation [16]. Clear and significant results have been found in the induction of lung fibrosis in mice (C57BL/6J) after FLASH (40 Gy/s) compared to conventional (1 Gy/s) radiation [19]. The FLASH irradiated mice showed 30% less lung fibrosis, chronic effect and reduced skin dermatitis. Moreover, a general improved overall survival in the FLASH PBT treated mice have been found [19]. To investigate the mechanisms behind the FLASH effect process, gene expression studies have been done. The results demonstrate that the main mechanisms involved in this complex process are DNA repair, inflammation, and immune response pathways [19]. Further studies have been done investigating the proliferative ability of nine weeks mice (C57BL/6J) intestinal crypt cells after 15 Gy of whole abdominal FLASH (78 Gy/s) and conventional irradiation (0.9 Gy/s) [20]. Three days after treatment, significantly reduced cell proliferation was found for the conventionally irradiated animals but not for the FLASH irradiated ones. Moreover, mice irradiated with 18 Gy protons focused on the intestines and harvested eight weeks post-irradiation revealed that conventional dose-rate-irradiated mice had considerably increased fibrosis compared to the FLASH-irradiated mice that showed a degree of fibrosis comparable to that of un-irradiated mice [20]. Moreover, compared to the conventional radiation, after FLASH radiation TGF-beta is strongly reduced, attenuating the chronic inflammation after radiation. In general, FLASH, compared to conventional radiation, modifies the blood's cytokine expression in the irradiated animals' blood, which may reflect and perhaps reduce toxicity. In a murine model irradiated in the limb with FLASH and conventional radiation, between 45 and 55 days after radiation, mice treated with FLASH dose rate have a significant delay in desquamation and an accelerated resolution compared to those irradiated with the conventional dose rate. Moreover, less than half of the animals

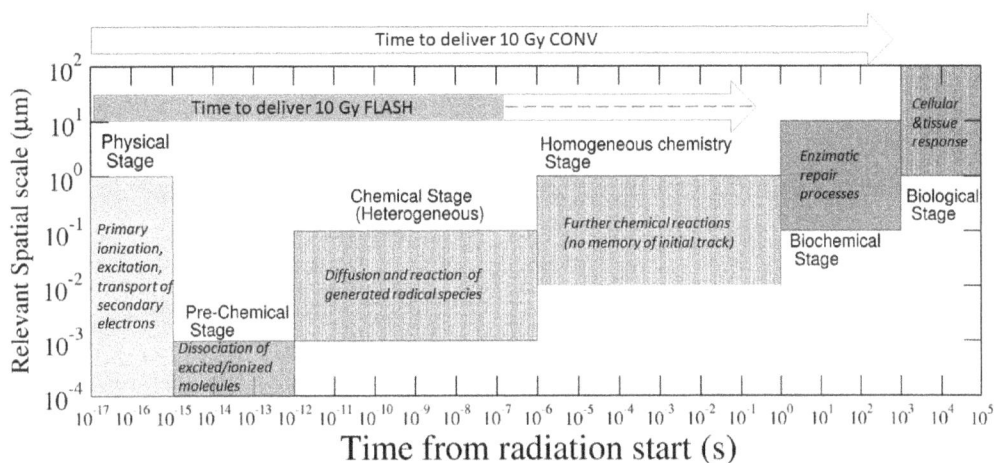

**Figure 15.2**    Scheme illustrating the time and spatial scales relevant for the subsequent steps of radiation interactions / effects in biological targets. Adapted from Weber et al. [21].

exhibited desquamation compared with 100% of the conventionally treated animals. The proton beam in vivo experiment seems to confirm that a dose of radiation delivered with a FLASH, compared to a conventional dose rate, offers the advantage of less severe soft tissue damage and skin toxicity. The immune system is a necessary ally in the battle against cancer. It plays a vital role in containing the tumor and counteracting it by preventing its progression and spread via metastasis. FLASH radiation is also as efficient as conventional radiation in controlling tumor growth in immunocompetent mice. FLASH irradiation appears to be, just like conventional irradiation, able to activate an immune response and give the same tumor control [16]. In one study, however, FLASH irradiation surprised even the experimenters. The tumor growth was reduced more in the FLASH irradiated animal than the ones treated conventionally [2]. The C57BL/6J mice lung tumors (induced by injection of Lewis lung carcinoma cells (LLC)) growth was measured after 18 Gy of particle beam whole thorax irradiation. FLASH PBT irradiated tumors were significantly smaller than those of the animals irradiated with the conventional treatment.

## 15.3    MONTE CARLO AND MODELING APPROACHES

### 15.3.1    MODELS INVESTIGATING MICROSCOPIC MECHANISM

Although the fundamental mechanism of FLASH is still far from fully understood, a significant effort has been made by many international modelling research groups in order to justify the striking experimental evidences accumulated over the years. Since the early observations, many authors have pointed towards the early chemical stage of radiation damage as the crucial time frame, guided by the duration of the irradiation itself (see schematic overview in Figure 15.3). Another argument in favor of a radiation chemical explanation is the fact that, especially for low-LET radiation, up to 85% of total cell inactivation following irradiation can be caused by indirect radiation damage. (In contrast to the direct effects, indirect damage refers to the molecular lesions in biological cells or tissues inflicted chemically following irradiation.) The theoretical range for a possible dose-modulating effect is therefore very large. A purely physical explanation can be excluded with high probability, however a biological mechanism behind the FLASH effect seems possible.

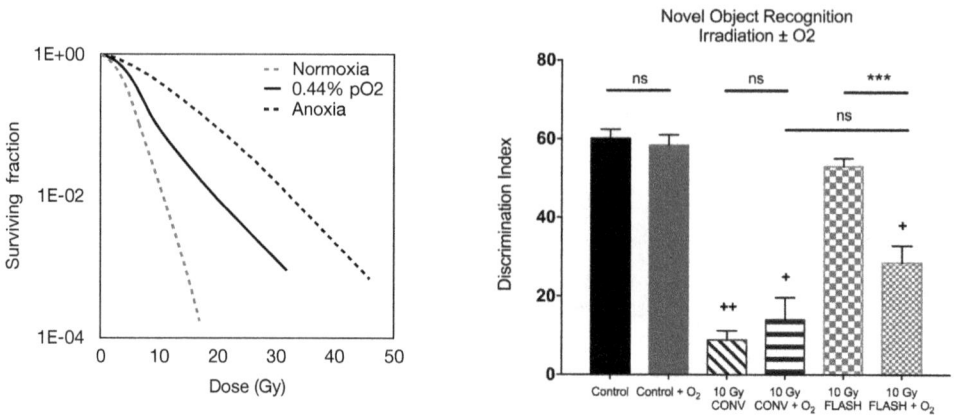

**Figure 15.3** (A) Survival of CHO cells irradiated with single electron pulses at ultra high dose rates ($\sim 10^9$ Gy/s) at various oxygenation conditions. The low oxygenation curve exhibits the "anoxic slope" from a threshold on. Data from [3]. (B) Impact of varying tissue oxygenation through carbogen breathing on appearance of FLASH effect. Reprinted with permission from Montay-Gruel et al. [4].

The radiation chemistry community has investigated several possible mechanisms on the very early stages of the radiation damage, often with the help of Monte Carlo techniques. In particular, Monte Carlo track structure codes able to describe the passage of radiation including the heterogeneous chemical stage demonstrated to be very useful for quantifying the production yield of the various reactive radiolytic species in water targets under different irradiation conditions and have been widely used for studying different possible mechanisms suspected to play a role in the FLASH effect. In these codes the track evolution, until reaching the chemical equilibrium, is generally modeled as a three step process where each stage is characterized by a typical time scale: the physical, the pre-chemical and the (homogeneous) chemical stage.

- The physical stage corresponds to the direct effect of radiation. During this stage the ionization and excitation processes are described based on cross sections. This stage lasts $10^{-15}$ s and is the core part of all track structure codes.
- The pre-chemical stage (from $10^{-15}$ s to $10^{-12}$ s) consists in the dissociation and thermalization process of all ionized and excited water molecules and electrons produced earlier through dissociation tables for the particular ionization type or excitation states.
- The chemical stage consists in the diffusion and reaction of the newly produced chemical species with themselves and with the target material. This stage is considered to be concluded when the radicals are diffused enough to reach an equilibrium state (the radical yields in water reach a constant value) and the initial radiation track structure stops to play a role in the chemical dynamic, generally at 1 $\mu$s.

Most of these codes are only able to simulate water targets and only few of them can include other solutes in the target material, e.g. molecular oxygen which is in this case particularly relevant for studying FLASH applications, or another type of scavenger. Due to the many interactions to be considered these codes are generally computationally expensive and in most of the cases the solute material is described as a continuum and the interaction probability is sampled based on concentration approaches. In the following sections, some of the main possible FLASH mechanisms that have been studied and can be explored by the use of these techniques will be reviewed.

### 15.3.1.1   Oxygen depletion hypothesis

This hypothesis has been intensely discussed and for some time considered to be the most plausible explanation for the FLASH effect. It originates from the very early investigations with ultra-high dose rate irradiation, where the impact of the initial target oxygenation was for the first time observed together with the measurement of "breaking" survival curves (displaying a slope corresponding to anoxia after a threshold [2]) under low oxygenations at ultra-high dose rate ($10^9$ Gy/s), as shown in Figure 15.3.

According to this hypothesis, under FLASH irradiation regimes a large part of the dissolved oxygen is removed by interacting with radiolytic species in a time scale short enough to exclude any possibility of oxygen re-diffusion from the surrounding non-irradiated volume or blood vessels. The irradiated volume could thus experience a transient hypoxia which results in an increased tissue radioresistance according to the well-known sensitizing effect of oxygen. In particular, the main formulation of this hypothesis holds that the oxygen removal takes place in the heterogeneous chemical stage of radiation (time scales in the order some 100 ns).

When interacting with biological media (often approximated as pure water), radiation leads to the production of reactive chemical species, among them hydrated electrons $e_{aq}^-$ and hydrogen radicals $H^\bullet$. In oxygenated targets these two radiolytic products can interact with the dissolved molecular oxygen and produce the cytotoxic superoxide anion and its protonated form, perhydroxyl.

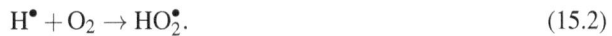

$$e_{aq}^- + O_2 \rightarrow O_2^{\bullet -} \tag{15.1}$$

$$H^\bullet + O_2 \rightarrow HO_2^\bullet. \tag{15.2}$$

Recent Monte Carlo studies and basic oxygen consumption experiments, however, demonstrated that for typical doses and oxygenation levels, used in pre-clinical experiments, the amount of oxygen depleted is not sufficient to justify an increased radioresistance. In water targets indeed a depletion of only 2.1-2.5% $pO_2$ is expected per 100 Gy. A noticeable increase in the hypoxia-induced radioresistance can then only be expected at extremely high doses and dose rates and in very low oxygenated systems (typically in the tumor region). At extremely high dose rates, due to the higher instantaneous radical concentrations produced, recombination among these compete with reactions (15.1) and (15.2) and decrease oxygen consumption further.

Larger consumption yields are expected in more complex and biologically relevant solutions for larger time scale. An increased oxygen depletion of a factor 4/3 is e.g. expected in cell culture medium. In this case additional products such as carbon centered radicals can contribute to a larger oxygen consumption yield. As explained in the next session 15.3.1.3, different biological processes must be studied in these saptio-temporal scales and in this respect Monte Carlo track structure codes become highly inefficient. The full tracking of each species becomes computationally very costly and combinations with concentration based approaches seem indeed more suitable.

### 15.3.1.2   Intertrack effects

One possibility often cited as a candidate mediator of the FLASH effect is the so-called intertrack effect. *Inter*track recombination (in contrast to *intra*track, the radical recombination which takes place within each single radiation track and depends highly on LET) means the reactivity of the primary radiolytic radicals belonging to one radiation track with the ones from a neighboring track within the heterogeneous chemical stage (see above). A noticeable effect is enabled by a simultaneously high dose rate and high total absorbed dose, so that two or more radiation tracks become spatially and temporally close enough each other to overlap. This leads to a partial suppression of the radical yields due to the mutual stabilization and thus to generally less reactive / toxic species surviving the track stage: the amount of indirect radiation damage decreases.

Intertrack effects have been predicted only for an extreme range of dose rates and doses. Monte Carlo study on water radiolysis by electrons shows that, for a standard time point of 1 $\mu$s, the radical numbers per dose, especially of OH$^\bullet$, decrease for large doses: a 10 Gy instantaneous electron dose can reduce OH$^\bullet$ number by 8% while a 80 Gy suppress it by as much as 36% [22]. In typical "FLASH" dose rate conditions these requirements are not fulfilled or close to reach. Single pulse doses are normally below a few Gy, and the overall times needed to deliver 10 Gy exceed the track chemistry stage considerably. A classical intertrack effect does not provide a straightforward explanation there. However, it is important to point out that ultra-high dose rate as employed in the early experimental observations of FLASH in the 1960s (making use of the Febetron accelerator), reached conditions to warrant a considerable biological impact of intertrack reactions. Similar conditions (e.g. almost 50 Gy in 3 ns with electrons) guarantee that all tracks develop simultaneously over the largest part of the chemical track expansion, and lead to an estimated OH$^\bullet$ yield decrease up to 25% for this example.

### 15.3.1.3   Radical-radical recombination

Radical-radical recombinations have also been mentioned sometimes as a possible origin of the FLASH effect. In this context, the recombinations refer to the homogeneous chemistry stage, after the chemical tracks of individual radiation particles (and spurs) are mostly dispersed ($\geq$1 $\mu$s ), and therefore to a phenomenon which depends essentially on the chemical species' concentrations. When aiming to interpret radiation effects in biological materials (cells, tissues), at this stage a pure water model cannot represent all the necessary competing reactions any more, and additional organic molecules and biomolecules in the target should be incorporated for a more realistic description.

Some important reactions known to take place are the scavenging of primary radicals (OH$^\bullet$, e$_{aq}^-$, H$^\bullet$) by organic molecules (here indicated with the generic symbol RH) to give R$^\bullet$ in competition to their reaction with O$_2$, but also the slow disproportionation of intermediate species (mainly O$_2^{\bullet-}$ + HO$_2^\bullet$ + H$_2$O to H$_2$O$_2$ + OH$^-$ + O$_2$). Furthermore, the R$^\bullet$ formed will be subject to fast peroxidation, producing large amounts of organic peroxyl radicals ROO$^\bullet$. Especially in the case of lipid-rich environments (such as membranes), ROO$^\bullet$ can even go on to abstract hydrogen from further RH giving ROOH + R$^\bullet$, which continues a chain reaction. It has been argued that this mechanism might contribute substantially to a FLASH effect via a hugely increased oxygen depletion [23], see section 15.3.1.1, at FLASH dose rates. On the other hand, enhanced recombinations among the organic radicals in the homogeneous chemical stage [24] could reduce either the effective radical toxicity, possible toxicity from accumulated organic peroxides ROOH, and / or the indirect damage. The interesting study by Labarbe et al. [24] starts from known MC-calculated radical yields at 1 $\mu$s and a reduced reaction scheme (with one typified biomolecule and a radical scavenger) as an input for an analytical calculation of the time evolution of the reactive species. Up to date there is however no full MC code including a comprehensive reaction table and thus able to follow up the fate of the radicals escaping the track chemistry to the point where they cause damage to the relevant target molecules or are scavenged and "neutralized," or recombine. Such implementations are however under development and could much enhance our understanding about the detailed changes in the radical reaction pathways under FLASH conditions. It is important to underline that all of the reaction paths mentioned above depend on the presence of oxygen, even where the focus is not on its depletion. This is in full agreement with the pivotal importance of oxygenation as proven in experiments.

### 15.3.2   RADIOBIOLOGICAL MODELS

Since the mechanisms behind FLASH are not currently understood, the specific biological aspects to be modeled following radiation are unfortunately not clear. The differential macroscopic effects observed experimentally (typically *in vivo* and consisting in late effects of normal tissue) are elusive to standard Monte Carlo simulations even when combined with extended biological models such as dose response, RBE modelling, or enhancement by oxygen via OER. Nevertheless, interesting approaches have been studied to link radiobiological effects to the underlying physical events/principles in a meaningful way and are summarized in what follows.

As introduced before, transient hypoxia can in principle render biological tissues more radioresistant, even if the magnitude of this effect, and its possibility to induce the desired differential effect, are under discussion.

A series of studies have investigated the effects on cell survival of an estimated or ab-initio-calculated yield of oxygen depletion per dose when linking it to OER and sometimes including rediffusion kinetics depending on dose rate, blood vessel properties, and metabolic oxygen consumption. Among them only one of these models is based on Monte Carlo methods and its application is at the moment limited to sparsely ionizing radiation [25]. In this model the cellular responce to radiation is calculated from DSB production and repair probabilities. The DSB yield positioning and repair probability are sampled with Monte Carlo techniques based on cell line dependent lethality parameters obtained by fitting experimental data. The oxygen dependent radiobiological response is calculated under the assumption that the only effect of the system oxygenation is a modification of the total yields of DSB by a fixed factor HRF (Hypoxia reduction factor) obtained either by fitting experimental data or by OER modeling approaches. The impact of oxygen depletion as a function of dose rate can be described introducing a dynamical oxygen concentration accounting for oxygen depletion and target re-oxygenation.

It has to be acknowledged that ultimately, the application of OER models stemming from *in vitro* survival data can be less reliable and has a convincing predictive value only for similar experiments, not necessarily normal tissue late effects. However, taken together these studies indicate conclusively that oxygen depletion will only lead to considerable sparing for samples oxygenated less than 0.8–1.9% $pO_2$ (15–25 $\mu M$), lower than typical in normal tissues, and call for alternative explanations. Furthermore, oxygen depletion should not depend strongly on pulse microstructure, in contrast to findings from biology experiments.

A particularly interesting interpretation is the one offered in Pratx & Kapp [26] who sustain that a determining aspect of oxygen depletion might be that NT stem cells in extremely hypoxic microenvironments could be the ones really benefiting from the transient hypoxia (not the main share of differentiated cells in a tissue) and subsequently aid tissue recovery.

The immune system has been the target of a further FLASH hypothesis. A mathematical approach presented by Jin et al. [27] shows how the different exposure distribution among circulating lymphocytes could lead to a striking immune sparing effect triggered directly by irradiation time, in additional dependence of blood volume and share of cardiac output irradiated. While high-intensity irradiation will kill few peripheral blood lymphocytes with excessive doses, the same overall dose given at conventional dose rate exposes many more blood cells to a lower but still lethal dose. Intriguingly, this pathway could naturally explain volume (target field size) effects, and it predicts a lower dose rate threshold for a FLASH effect in humans than for rodents.

### 15.3.3   EXPECTED FLASH EFFECTS FOR PROTON AND ION RADIATION

When considering the possibility of combining FLASH with ion and proton therapy, it is necessary to consider the large variability of LET values involved in typical clinical scenarios. For ion beam therapy the radiation quality changes drastically not only when considering different particle beams but also when looking at differential effects between normal tissues (mainly in the entrance channel) and tumor (high LET towards the Bragg peak).

The radiation effect (at the same dose) in this case is not only determined by the different tissue responses but also by radiobiological quantities, such as RBE or OER, which are known to have a strong dependence on the radiation quality. For instance, the impact of the indirect effect of radiation and the yields of radiation induced radiolytic production, for a fixed amount of energy deposited, anti-correlate with the LET. As an example, the radiolytic yield for solvated electrons drops about a factor between 5 to 10 when the LET is increased from 0.1 to 100 keV/$\mu$m. This LET dependency on the radical production on the radiation quality affects the impact of the indirect effect and as a consequence also leads to a reduced oxygen consumption for higher LET radiations (see eq. 15.1). A lower sparing effect for proton and ions compared to electrons and photons and in the tumor region respect to the entrance channel is thus predicted under FLASH irradiation condition. Also the well known anti-correlation of the OER with radiation LET could combine very well with FLASH application, leading to an enhanced normal tissue radio-resistance while preserving the same anti-tumor efficacy. Also the increased oxygen production along the ion track for very high LET values has been considered as a possible mechanism contributing to enhance the differential FLASH effect in carbon irradiation [28]. According to this hypothesis, following a particular dissociation channel typical of multiple ionization events, molecular oxygen can be produced by radical recombination along the track of very densely ionizing radiations and locally enhance the radiation effect especially in the tumor region.

## REFERENCES

1. M-C Vozenin, J H Hendry, and CL Limoli. Biological benefits of ultra-high dose rate flash radiotherapy: sleeping beauty awoken. *Clinical oncology*, 31(7):407–415, 2019.
2. J D Wilson, E M Hammond, G S Higgins, and K. Petersson. Ultra-high dose rate (flash) radiotherapy: Silver bullet or fool's gold? *Front Oncol.*, 9:1563, 2020.
3. H B Michaels, E R Epp, C C Ling, and E C Peterson. Oxygen sensitization of CHO cells at ultrahigh dose rates: Prelude to oxygen diffusion studies. *Radiation Research*, 76:510–521, 1978.
4. P Montay-Gruel et al. Long-term neurocognitive benefits of flash radiotherapy driven by reduced reactive oxygen species. *Proc. Nat. Ac. Sci.*, 116:10943–10951, 2019.
5. RJ Berry. Effects of radiation dose-rate: from protracted, continuous irradiation to ultra-high dose-rates from pulsed accelerators. *British medical bulletin*, 29(1):44–47, 1973.
6. BU Zackrisson, U Håkan Nyström, and P Ostbergh. Biological response in vitro to pulsed high dose rate electrons from a clinical accelerator. *Acta Oncologica*, 30(6):747–751, 1991.
7. G. Adrian, E. Konradsson, M. Lempart, S. Bäck, C. Ceberg, and K. Petersson. The flash effect depends on oxygen concentration. *Brit. J. Radiol.*, 93:20190702, 2020.
8. C. Fouillade et al. Flash irradiation spares lung progenitor cells and limits the incidence of radio-induced senescence. *Clinical Cancer Research*, 26(6):1497–1506, 2020.
9. M Buonanno, V Grilj, and D J Brenner. Biological effects in normal cells exposed to flash dose rate protons. *Radiotherapy and Oncology*, 139:51–55, 2019.
10. L G Marcu, E Bezak, D D Peukert, and P Wilson. Translational research in flash radiotherapy—from radiobiological mechanisms to in vivo results. *Biomedicines*, 9(2):181, 2021.
11. V. Favaudon et al. Ultrahigh dose-rate FLASH irradiation increases the differential response between normal and tumor tissue in mice. *Sci. Transl. Med.*, 6:245ra93, 2014.
12. M.-C. Vozenin et al. The advantage of FLASH confirmed in mini-pig and cat-cancer patients. *Clin. Canc. Res.*, 25:35–42, 2019.
13. J. Bourhis et al. Treatment of a first patient with FLASH-radiotherapy. *Radiother. Oncol.*, 139:18–22, 2019.
14. T Prempree, A Michelsen, and T Merz. The repair time of chromosome breaks induced by pulsed x-rays of ultra-high dose-rate. *International Journal of Radiation Biology and Related Studies in Physics, Chemistry and Medicine*, 15(6):571–574, 1969.
15. P Montay-Gruel et al. X-rays can trigger the flash effect: Ultra-high dose-rate synchrotron light source prevents normal brain injury after whole brain irradiation in mice. *Radiotherapy and Oncology*, 129(3):582–588, 2018.

16. J R Hughes and J L Parsons. Flash radiotherapy: Current knowledge and future insights using proton-beam therapy. *International journal of molecular sciences*, 21(18):6492, 2020.
17. J E Dennis, G A Whitney, J Rai, R J Fernandes, and T J Kean. Physioxia stimulates extracellular matrix deposition and increases mechanical properties of human chondrocyte-derived tissue-engineered cartilage. *Frontiers in bioengineering and biotechnology*, 8, 2020.
18. W Tinganelli et al. Kill-painting of hypoxic tumours in charged particle therapy. *Scientific reports*, 5(1):1–13, 2015.
19. S Cunningham et al. Flash proton pencil beam scanning irradiation minimizes radiation-induced leg contracture and skin toxicity in mice. *Cancers*, 13(5):1012, 2021.
20. E Diffenderfer et al. Design, implementation, and in vivo validation of a novel proton flash radiation therapy system. *International Journal of Radiation Oncology\* Biology\* Physics*, 106(2):440–448, 2020.
21. Uli Andreas Weber, Emanuele Scifoni, and Marco Durante. Flash radiotherapy with carbon ion beams. *Medical Physics*, 49(3):1974–1992, 2022.
22. R Watanabe and K Saito. Monte Carlo simulation of water radiolysis in oxygenated condition for monoenergetic electrons from 100 eV to 1 MeV. *Rad. Phys. Chem.*, 62:217–228, 2001.
23. D Spitz et al. An integrated physico-chemical approach for explaining the differential impact of flash versus conventional dose rate irradiation on cancer and normal tissue responses. *Radiotherapy and Oncology*, 2019.
24. R Labarbe, L Hotoiu, J Barbier, and V Favaudon. A physicochemical model of reaction kinetics supports peroxyl radical recombination as the main determinant of the flash effect. *Radiotherapy and Oncology*, 153:303–310, 2020.
25. H Liew et al. Deciphering time-dependent dna damage complexity, repair, and oxygen tension: A mechanistic model for flash-dose-rate radiation therapy. *International Journal of Radiation Oncology\*Biology\*Physics*, 2021.
26. G Pratx and D S Kapp. Ultra-high-dose-rate FLASH irradiation may spare hypoxic stem cell niches in normal tissues. *Int. J. Rad. Oncol. Biol. Phys.*, 105:P190–P192, 2019.
27. Jian-Yue Jin, Anxin Gu, Weili Wang, Nancy L. Oleinick, Mitchell Machtay, and Feng-Ming (Spring) Kong. Ultra-high dose rate effect on circulating immune cells: A potential mechanism for flash effect? *Radiotherapy and Oncology*, 149:55–62, 2020.
28. N W Colangelo and E I Azzam. The importance and clinical implications of flash ultra-high dose-rate studies for proton and heavy ion radiotherapy. *Radiation research*, 193(1):1–4, 2020.

# 16 Towards multiple ion applications in particle therapy

*Taku Inaniwa*
Institute for Quantum Medical Science, Chiba, Japan

*Michael Kramer*
GSI Helmholtz Centre for Heavy Ion Research GmbH, Darmstadt, Germany

*Andrea Mairani*
Heidelberg Ion-Beam Therapy Center (HIT), Heidelberg, Germany
Medical Physics, National Centre of Oncological Hadrontherapy (CNAO), Pavia, Italy
Clinical Cooperation Unit Radiation Oncology, German Cancer Consortium (DKTK) Core-Center Heidelberg, National Center for Tumor Diseases (NCT), Heidelberg University Hospital (UKHD) and German Cancer Research Center (DKFZ), Heidelberg, Germany
Heidelberg University, Heidelberg, Germany

*Emanuele Scifoni*
TIFPA-INFN Trento Institute for Fundamental Physics and Applications, Trento, Italy

*Olga Sokol*
GSI Helmholtzzentrum für Schwerionenforchung, Darmstadt, Germany

## CONTENTS

MULTIPLE ION treatments are being considered as a possible outlook of the use of different particle beams, exploiting at once their different physical and radiobiological features. While technical feasibility of multi-ion facilities with fast particle switching seems not to be prohibitive, different planning approaches to exploit the potential benefits of such treatments, and thus

DOI: 10.1201/9781003023920-16

justifying their cost, have been developed in Europe and Japan, and are summarized in the present chapter.

## 16.1  INTRODUCTION

A new frontier for particle therapy is now represented by multiple ion treatments [3]. While particle therapy with ions heavier than protons is still representing a small portion as compared to the number of patients receiving and facilities applying proton therapy, a steadily growing trend in both numbers is evident as reported by the PTCOG continuously updated statistics [12].

Beside the established use of carbon $^{12}$C ion beams, now reaching an extensive application especially in Japan (7 centers) and in Europe (4 centers) and a solid collection of clinical results [32, 31], and while the indications for specific use of $^{12}$C or protons in selected patient cases are arising, the studies of other ions are emerging. The idea behind those is to enhance the "palette" of nuclear projectiles, exploiting the different and sometime complementary peculiar physical and biological properties of such particle beams [30]. This is in particular the case of helium $^{4}$He ions, which after the initial exploratory studies in Berkeley from the 80s, was returning as a subject of intensive studies for research purposes [18, 28, 21] and is now in clinical application at HIT [20]. The advantages of $^{4}$He beams are the more limited multiple Coulomb scattering, and thus a superior quality of lateral penumbra, as compared to the protons, and a lower impact of fragmentation, especially in the tail region, as compared to the $^{12}$C beams, which places this modality as an attracting alternative solution to both beams, not only for the intermediate LET distribution values. Different isotopic choices for helium are also evaluated: beside the broader studies in play with $^{4}$He, in fact interesting parallel investigations are in course for $^{3}$He [8].

Another quite importantly explored option is the use of oxygen $^{16}$O beams. Proposed from Tobias in the 80s at Berkeley, it was later considered as an alternative candidate to $^{12}$C for the pilot project started at GSI in late 90s, since the importance of high LET radiation for contrasting hypoxic tumors emerged from several in vitro and in vivo studies. The main rationale for $^{16}$O fields is, in fact, the broader region covered by a high LET distribution, over a threshold able to significantly reduce the impact of the hypoxia, and thus of the oxygen enhancement ratio (OER). Specifically, as compared to even heavier particles, oxygen ions are only slightly larger than carbons and thus the improvement in LET is not so dramatically counterbalanced by a larger fragmentation impact in the normal tissue, and thus in a trade-off pays not a huge price as recently demonstrated [26]. Other isotopic species of both carbon and oxygen ($^{11}$C and $^{15}$O), are nowadays considered in the context of radioactive beams studies, uniting the advantage of PET emission based range monitoring (see the dedicated chapter in this book) are completing the palette of explored projectiles.

Since in the past decade our knowledge on the differential physical and radiobiological properties of several particle beams has greatly expanded, there comes immediately a question, whether we could "mix the colors" of the palette, i.e., can we exploit to the full the different peculiarities of the available particles, by delivering an intensity modulated distribution of multiple ion beams?

This novel approach, of course, might face several issues. The first being clearly the technical feasibility, i.e. the possibility not only to dispose of different sources of species, but also of a fast beam switching, so that the multi-ion treatment can be really delivered in a single fraction, without eliciting complex radiobiological responses induced by a split dose application. This issue, however, seems to be surmountable: the typical switching time at HIT is on the order of minutes, while the new Toshiba systems which are designed in Japan can do it in pulse by pulse of synchrotron operation. Another issue and, at the same time a novel opportunity, is the treatment planning. Obviously, an inverse planning approach is tremendously complicated by such an additional degree of freedom; however, several approaches are in play in this connection and will be described in the following sections of this chapter. In Section 2, the IMPACT (Intensity modulated particle therapy with composite ion beams) method based on radiation quality optimization will be reported. Part 3 will describe the Combined Ion-Beam with Constant RBE (CICR) approach dedicated to maintaining a uniform RBE on the compound plan using different ions. Finally, in the last Part the MIBO (Multi-Ion full Biological Optimization) approach, specifically designed for hypoxia, will be summarized. We finally will draw some overall conclusions and perspective of this new field, in particular in connection to Monte Carlo dedicated enhancements.

## 16.2 RADIATION QUALITY OPTIMIZATION

In ion-beam therapy treatment planning, a biological dose, which is defined as the product of absorbed dose and relative biological effectiveness (RBE), is optimized for the individual clinical cases. The RBE is a ratio of dose for a reference radiation to that for the radiation of interest to yield a defined biological effect. The RBE depends on various factors such as radiation quality, dose, dose rate, oxygen pressure, tissue type, immune status, and endpoint. Ideally, all these factors should be incorporated into the RBE model [24]. However, that is difficult due to the complexity of the mechanism causing the biological effect. The generic RBE of 1.1 has been thus clinically used in proton therapy independent of these factors. Even in carbon-ion therapy, simplified RBE models have been used in clinical treatments, where survival of specific cell lines is used as the endpoint [13, 6]. The radiation quality of therapeutic carbon-ion beams is considered in the RBE calculations. However, the radiation quality has been considered as an unadjustable physical quantity that is uniquely determined by the ion type, target size, and target depth. Therefore, the goal of radiation therapy, i.e., to control the tumors while preserving the normal tissues, has been generally achieved by the design of the dose distribution. A highly-localized dose distribution by ion beams is useful to deliver a large enough dose to the tumor while sparing the organs at risk (OARs). In actual treatments, however, the planning target volume (PTV) occasionally overlaps the OARs. For such clinical cases, the treatment planners have to choose a compromised dose level in the overlapped region. In addition, the cancer cells can coexist with the normal cells within the PTV. For such clinical cases, also, the treatment planners have to choose a compromised dose level for cancer cells and normal cells. Since the radiation response of tissues (cells) depends differently on radiation quality, there must be an optimum value of radiation quality which effectively kills the cancer cells while maintaining the normal cells. It is thus desirable to control the distribution of radiation quality within the patient independently, in addition to the dose distribution. The multi-ion therapy in which two or more ion species with different radiation qualities are delivered in one treatment session can be used for this purpose. In this subsection, the multi-ion therapy for dose and radiation quality optimization is reported.

The dose-averaged LET has been primarily used to describe the radiation quality of ion beams, and many biological data such as the RBE and oxygen enhancement ratio (OER) have been accumulated as a function of this quantity [4, 27]. Thus, it seems reasonable to optimize the dose-averaged LET of therapeutic ion beams in multi-ion therapy. The contradictory discussions exist that the dose-averaged LET is not an ideal index for expressing the biological effectiveness of radiations. Instead, microdosimetric quantities such as specific energy may be better indices for expressing the RBE of radiations, as they directly relate to ionizing densities in microscopic sites.

In the microdosimetric kinetic (MK) model, the biological effectiveness of radiations is predicted from the dose mean specific energy per event $z_{dD}$ [7]. The overkill effects overserved in high LET radiation exposures can be accounted for by introducing the saturation corrected dose-mean specific energy per event $z_{dD}^*$ [14]. The $z_{dD}^*$-based MK model referred to as the modified MK model has been used in clinical treatments of carbon-ion therapy in Japan [9, 10], and that will be used in helium-ion therapy in Germany [19]. As representative physical quantities describing the radiation quality of ion beams, we thus selected dose-averaged LET L and the saturation corrected dose-mean specific energy per event $z_{dD}^*$ in this report. The dose distribution of the multi-ion therapy $D$ at $\mathbf{x}$ can be calculated as

$$D = \sum_j d_j \cdot w_j \qquad (16.1)$$

where $d_j$ is the dose deposited by the scanned pencil beam at the $j$th spot ($j$th beamlet) to $\mathbf{x}$, and $w_j$ is the number of incident ions referred to as the weight required for the $j$th beamlet. The distribution of radiation quality $Q$, e.g., $L$ or $z^*_{dD}$, at $\mathbf{x}$ in the multi-ion fields are described as

$$Q = \frac{\sum_j q_j \cdot d_j \cdot w_j}{\sum_j d_j \cdot w_j} \tag{16.2}$$

where $q_j$ is the dose-averaged LET $l_j$ or the saturation corrected dose-mean specific energy per event $z^*_{dDj}$ deposited by the $j$th beamlet to $\mathbf{x}$. In multi-ion therapy treatment planning, the beam weights $\mathbf{w}$ (the vector notation of the weights $w_j$) for all beamlets are determined by minimizing the following dose- and radiation quality-based cost function

$$f(w) = \sum_{\mathbf{x} \in T} \left[ \zeta_T \left( \frac{D(\mathbf{x}, \mathbf{w}) - D_T}{D_T} \right)^2 + \widehat{\zeta}_T \left( \frac{Q(\mathbf{x}, \mathbf{w}) - Q_T}{Q_T} \right)^2 \right]$$
$$+ \sum_{\mathbf{x} \in O} \left[ \zeta_O \Theta \left( \frac{D(\mathbf{x}, \mathbf{w}) - D_O^{max}}{D_O} \right)^2 + \widehat{\zeta}_O \Theta \left( \frac{Q(\mathbf{x}, \mathbf{w}) - Q_O^{max}}{Q_O} \right)^2 \right] \tag{16.3}$$

where the first and second sum are running over the target T and the OAR O modified by the Heavyside step function $\Theta$. $D_T$, $\zeta_T$, $D_O^{max}$, $\zeta_O$ are the prescribed dose to the target, the penalty constant for the dose deviation from $D_T$, the maximum allowed dose to the OAR, and the penalty constant for the overdosage in the OAR, respectively. Similarly, $Q_T$, $\widehat{\zeta}_T$, $Q_O^{max}$, $\widehat{\zeta}_O$ are the prescribed radiation-quality value to the target, the penalty constant for the deviation from $Q_T$, the maximum allowed radiation-quality value, and the penalty constant for the excess of the radiation quality value in the OAR, respectively.

To show the proof of principle of dose and radiation-quality optimization with multi-ion beams in clinical situation, we made a dose and dose-averaged LET optimized multi-ion therapy plan with an opposing-field geometry for a prostate case. In this example case, the PTV partially overlaps the rectum. Here, protons, and helium, carbon, and oxygen ions were selected as ion species. We set $D_T$ = 2 Gy to the PTV, $Q_T$ = 80 keV/μm to the prostate and $Q_T$ = 50 keV/μm to the remaining region in the PTV, $Q_O^{max}$ = 30 keV/μm to the rectum. The resultant dose and dose-averaged LET distributions of the multi-ion therapy plan are shown in Figure 16.1. In accordance with the prescriptions, dose-averaged LETs in the prostate, PTV, and rectum could be adjusted at 80 keV/μm, 50 keV/μm, and below 30 keV/μm, respectively, while keeping the dose across the PTV at 2 Gy uniformly.

In the modified MK model, the biological effectiveness of radiations is uniquely determined by $z^*_{dD}$ of the radiations. The multi-ion therapy plan to achieve uniform dose and $z^*_{dD}$ distributions across the target are, thus, equivalent to the constant RBE optimization (Böhlen et al. 2012, Kopp et al. 2020), see the following part. Ideally, all the factors affecting the biological effectiveness of radiations should be incorporated into the RBE model, and taken into account in biological/clinical optimization for the individual clinical cases. In this sense, the kill-painting [29] or the multiple ion full biological optimization (MIBO) [25] tackling the partially hypoxic tumors may be advanced treatment methods we should aim for as personalized treatments. However, there are still several challenges to overcome to realize these treatments, such as the accumulation of in vivo tumor response data to hypoxia and the developments of imaging modalities providing proper and sufficiently resolved oxygen-concentration map of a tumor. The dose and radiation-quality optimized treatments may be an appropriate method as a first step of clinical implementation of multi-ion therapy.

## 16.3 CONSTANT RBE OPTIMIZATION

Carbon ion beams provide high-precision dose delivery accompanied by lower LET in the entrance channel and higher LET increasing exponentially towards the distal-end. In general, carbon ion

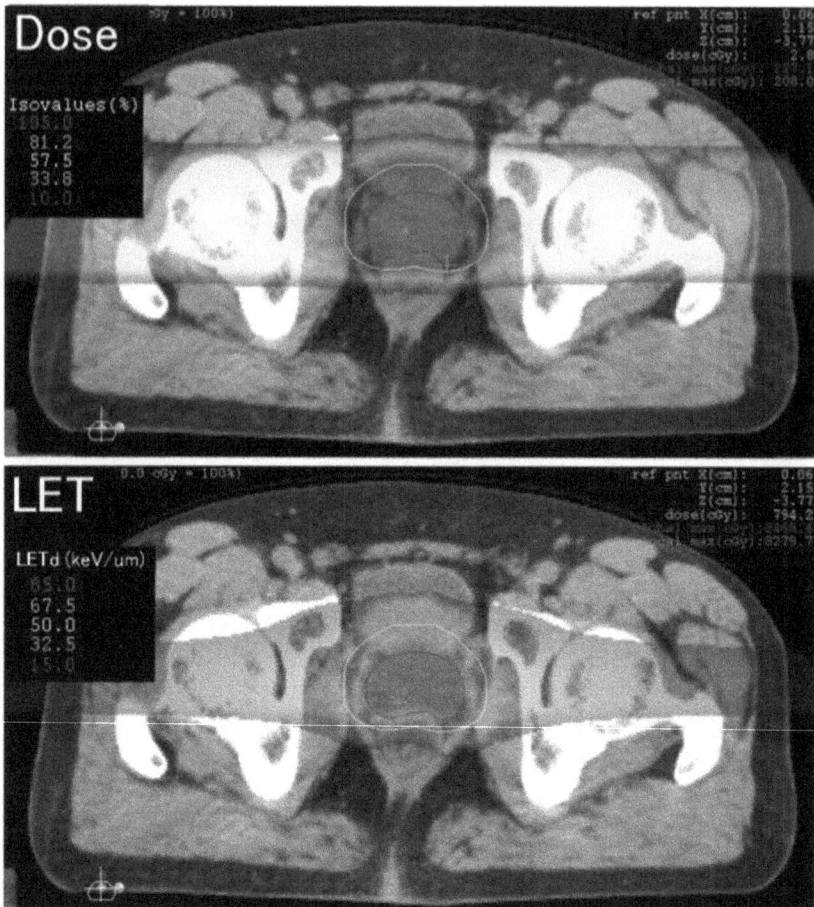

**Figure 16.1**  Dose (upper panel) and dose-averaged LET (lower panel) distributions for a prostate cancer case by the multi-ion therapy with protons, and helium, carbon, and oxygen ions. Please refer to [11] for the color version.

LET compared to protons is higher, yielding more complex DNA damage, increased cell-kill per unit dose and hence potential for improved tumor control, especially for radio-resistant indications. This radio-resistance is overcome by a highly localized ionization increasing along the particle track which maximizes at the Bragg region. Nevertheless, this introduces a variable RBE effect that is dependent on multiple dimensions and factors that are not completely understood. Therefore, these variations must be modeled by sophisticated biological models tuned for specific tissue types defined by each facility, which involves assumptions/approximations for model-specific input parameters and reference conditions for tissue response such as $\frac{\alpha}{\beta}$ (tissue fractionation parameter in the framework of the linear-quadratic (LQ) model) as well as variation assumption on cell characteristics. Since these characteristics vary between tumor types and even patients, the biological effect can only be estimated prior to facility start-up using a single definition/procedure for RBE-weighted dose optimization. Compared to protons, which clinically neglect well-known RBE variations and globally accept an "average" RBE of 1.1, the RBE of carbon ions shows variation between $\tilde{1}.3$ and 4 on average along beam path. These variations in RBE are accompanied by substantial uncertainty in delivered biological effect in the patient, which is typically estimated as a 20–30% uncertainty within the literature [22]. For instance, surveying the impact of biophysical model and key tissue

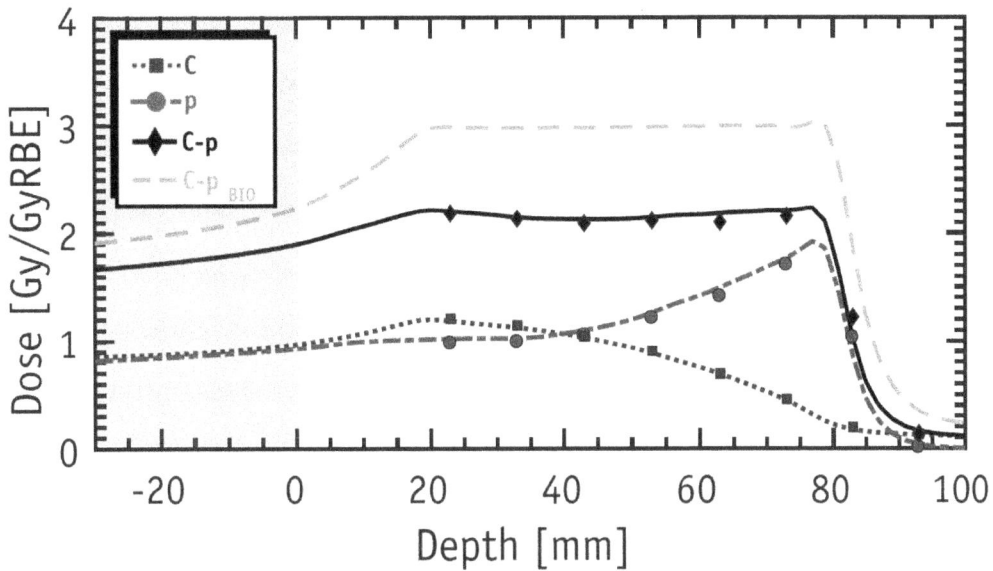

**Figure 16.2** A CICR single field arrangement using carbon ions (dotted line) and protons (dash-dotted line). In addition to single physical dose contributions, total physical dose (solid line) and biologically weighted dose (dashed line) distributions are displayed. Please refer to [15] for the color version.

input parameters (considering clinically acceptable uncertainty) showed variations in the target dose predictions on the order of 20–40% depending on beam arrangement and tumor type, location, etc., largely because of variations in the RBE prediction methods.

That said, the usage of multiple ions in a single fraction and field arrangement has been proposed to mitigate these RBE uncertainties in the clinic [2, 15]. For example, protons and carbon ions are the two major clinical particle beams that could readily combine at multiple centers worldwide to create multi-ion field treatment plans. Furthermore, other novel ions such as helium and oxygen at HIT as well as neon at QST could be applied as demonstrated in the prior section to further elevate LET and therapeutic window. The approach applied at HIT for multi-ion therapy involves combining low and high LET particle beams within the same treatment delivery session to homogenize several physical and biological aspects of the treatment field characteristics. This includes physical dose, RBE, LET and in turn RBE-weighted dose. Therefore, within the necessary additions to treatment planning optimization procedures, RBE, LET and physical dose gradients could be nearly eliminated within the target volume as opposed to those delivered in conventional carbon ion therapy using single field or multi-field arrangements. Within the combined ion-beam with constant RBE (CICR) concept, individual branches of the treatment field (e.g., proton and carbon ion branches) are treated individually with almost no constraints. Recent studies showed that best results were achieved when using a forward and reverse wedge configuration for the proton and carbon ion beam branch, respectively, overlapping in the center of the target. An experimentally delivered CICR plan with carbon ions and protons is shown in Figure 16.2, detailing both branches as well as physical and biologically weighted dose using an anthropomorphic phantom. In the context of current clinical optimization procedures in particle therapy, multi-ion treatment optimization adds further mathematical and computational requirements to an already complex optimization regime. Therefore, dedicated efforts to develop, investigate and establish optimal techniques for treatment design and definition of primary optimization goals are warranted.

Comparing single field treatment plans with protons, helium ions, and carbon ions and CICR plans combining protons/carbon ions and helium/carbon ions are shown in Figure 16.3. Highly conformal RBE and physical dose distributions can be seen for the CICR plan with carbon ions and protons, although also the carbon ion and helium ions showed reduced gradients in the target compared to the single field carbon ion alone. Due to their low LET range, protons also feature less heterogeneous physical dose distribution than single particle heavy ion treatments; carbon ion and helium ion fields show gradients in both RBE and LETd in the target.

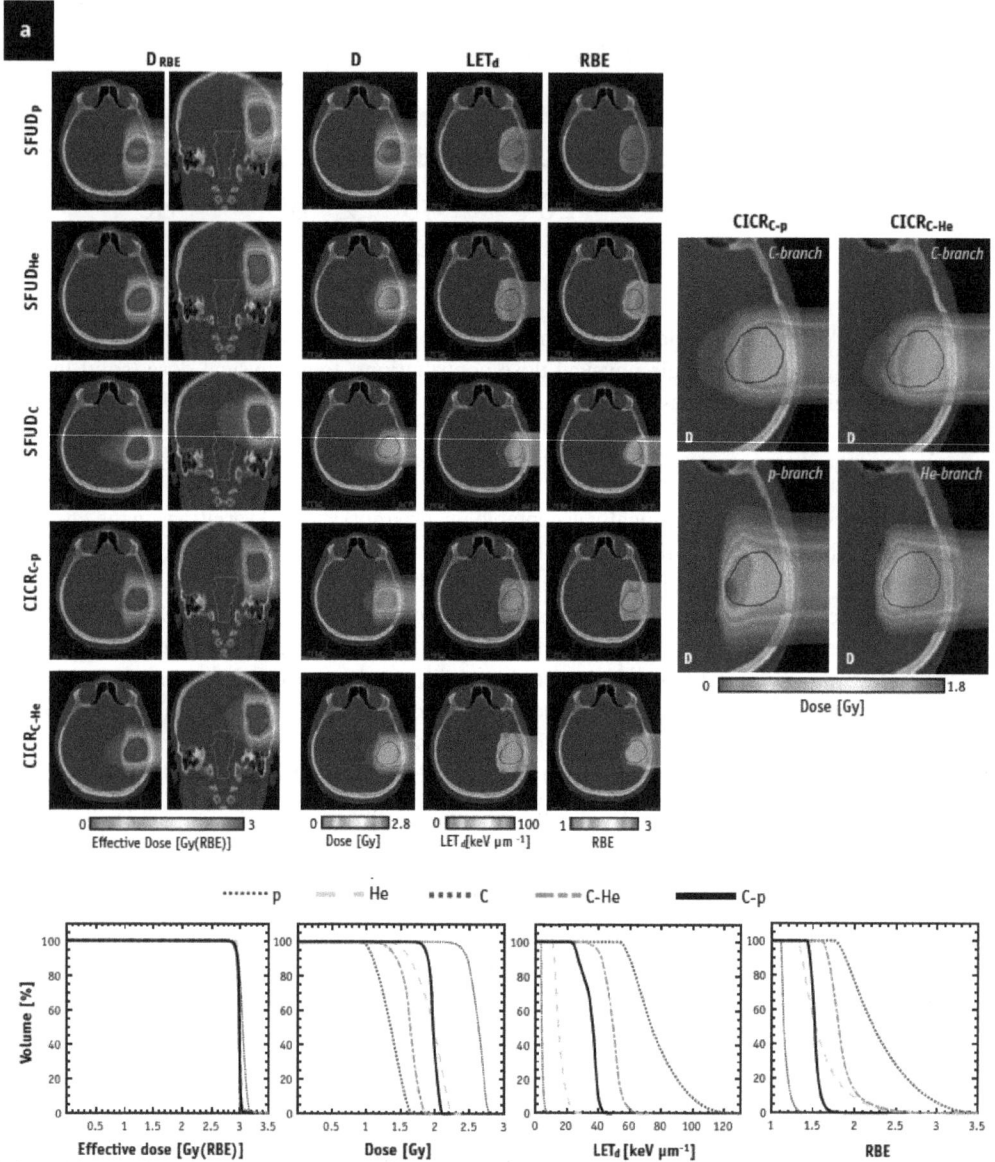

**Figure 16.3**  Single field arrangements for protons, carbon ions, helium ions and CICR fields combining carbon ions with protons and carbon ions and helium ions in a patient study. Volume histograms for RBE, DRBE, Dose and LET are displayed for the target. Please refer to [15] for the color version.

However, there are structural challenges for multi ion therapy. Despite increasing interest in carbon ion therapy in the US, there are few centers in the world that deliver more than a single ion. This limits the number of facilities that can currently develop and potentially apply multi ion therapy. There are also challenges with the branch delivery itself that have to be resolved. Fast ion source switching has been proposed to mitigate potential tumor motion or treatment delay effects e.g. reductions in RBE and physical dose homogeneity in the patient that stem from the exact optimization of multiple ions in one spot. More specifically, the multi-ion treatment branches can be susceptible to Inter-fractional deviations from prescribed plan. Therefore, reduction in total treatment delivery, especially when delivery of more than 2 particle species in a multi-ion treatment should be considered. It should be investigated whether the usage of robust optimization of RBE and DRBE in parallel could be clinically beneficial and with increasing biophysical modeling and planning complexity, further investigations of multi-ion treatment should focus on robustness aspects of treatment delivery. Moreover, ideal mixtures of 2 or more particle species should be investigated and whether boosting LET with O/Ne provides further clinical advantages.

Future visions of particle therapy impicture more personalized, patient-specific treatment regimes. For instance, the concept introduced alongside the HIT approach to multi-ion therapy, known as PRECISE, involves clinical consideration of all available treatment modalities under the aspects of target coverage, LET distribution, and other relevant clinical end points.

## 16.4  MULTI-ION FOR HYPOXIA

Hypoxia, induced by the poor vascularization, is considered as one of the factors increasing the resistance of the tumors to the radiotherapy treatment. The most accredited explanation for this effect is a so-called oxygen fixation phenomenon at the chemical stage of the radiation interaction with tissue. Hydroxyl radicals R*, produced during the interaction of radiation with water, can further interact with molecular oxygen, forming peroxyl radicals RO2* and inducing a difficult to repair ("fixed") DNA damage. Meanwhile, with the lack of O2 in the tissue, the damage would be mainly caused by the R* radicals and mainly restored. High-LET ion beam therapy is considered to be a promising solution for tackling hypoxic tumors. Heavier ions have denser ionization tracks which increases the chances for the radicals to interact between themselves, as well as for the molecular oxygen production in the track region.

The idea behind the MIBO (Multi-Ion full Biological Optimization) approach [25] is taking benefit from the simultaneous use of heavy ions, directed to the hypoxic tumor cores, and lighter ions, targeted at remaining normoxic areas. This way, one would benefit from the increased total biological effect in the hypoxic areas and, on the other hand, lower fragmentation and RBE values in normoxic regions, which in turn would lead to a better sparing of surrounding residual tissue.

Currently, this approach is realized in the recent version of TRiP98, the research treatment planning system of GSI [16, 5]. It handles the oxygenation distribution by importing the voxelized maps for PET-tracer (e.g., fluoromisonidazole) uptake distribution and the associated look-up table for converting the uptake values into $pO_2$ values. The optimization is performed following the kill-painting approach [29] where the optimized quantity is a desired uniform survival level in the target, and accounting for tissue oxygenation is done by including the OER values in the calculation of the biological effects in both forward and inverse planning.

The absorbed dose in water can be expressed as

$$D(Gy) = C \times F_\eta (\text{mm}^{-2}) \times \overline{LET} \left( \frac{\text{MeV}}{\text{g cm}^{-2}} \right) \tag{16.4}$$

where $F_\eta$ is a particle fluence, $C = 1.602189 \times 10^8$, and $\overline{LET}$ is the dose-averaged linear transfer resulting from the contributions of all the primary beams:

$$\overline{LET} = \langle LET \rangle_D = \frac{\sum_i LET_i D_i}{\sum_i D_i} = \frac{\sum_i LET_i^2 F_i}{\sum_i LET_i F_i} \tag{16.5}$$

with $D_i$ dose and $F_i$ fluence of the radiation component $i$.

The biological response (cell survival) following the dose $D$ can be calculated using the low-dose approximation [17]:

$$-\ln S = \begin{cases} D(\beta D + \alpha), & D \le D_{cut} \\ D_{cut}(\beta D_{cut} + \alpha) + (D - D_{cut})S_{max}, & D > D_{cut} \end{cases} \tag{16.6}$$

with $D_{cut}$, $S_{cut}$ being the linear-quadratic-linear model [1] parameters controlling in LEM the transition to exponential dose-effect relation at high doses, and $s_{max} = 2\beta \cdot D_{cut} + \alpha$ being the corresponding slope. Here, $\alpha$ and $\beta$ are the dose-weighted averages for radiobiological coefficients for the mixed field calculated based on the knowledge of $\alpha_l$ and $\beta_l$ of each of the mixed field components. Introducing the OER as a dose-modifying factor $D' = D/OER$ and considering the contributions from all the primary beams in the dose-averaged LET calculation, the equation 16.6 can be further rewritten as

$$-\ln(S) = \begin{cases} \dfrac{D}{OER}\left(\beta\dfrac{D}{OER} + \alpha\right), & D \le D_{cut} \\ \dfrac{D_{cut}}{OER}\left(\beta\dfrac{D_{cut}}{OER} + \alpha\right) + (D - D_{cut}) \cdot s_{max} & D > D_{cut} \end{cases} \tag{16.7}$$

and the biological dose can be calculated as

$$D_{bio} = \begin{cases} \sqrt{-\ln S / \beta_X + (\alpha_X / 2\beta_X)^2} - (\alpha_X / 2\beta_X), & D \le D_{cut} \\ (-\ln S + \ln S_{cut}) / S_{max} + D_{cut} & D > D_{cut} \end{cases} \tag{16.8}$$

with $\alpha_X$ and $\beta_X$ being the photon response parameters.

The dose optimization in TRiP98 is done with gradient-based methods, and to accounting for the oxygenation, these gradients at modified are accordingly:

$$\nabla\alpha'\left(\overline{LET}, pO_2\right) = \frac{\nabla\alpha}{OER\left(\overline{LET}, pO_{2,i}\right)} - \alpha\frac{\nabla OER\left(\overline{LET}, pO_2\right)}{\overline{OER}^2} \tag{16.9}$$

$$\nabla\sqrt{\beta'}\left(\overline{LET}, pO_2\right) = \frac{\nabla\sqrt{\beta}}{OER\left(\overline{LET}, pO_2\right)} - \sqrt{\beta}\frac{\nabla OER\left(\overline{LET}, pO_2\right)}{\overline{OER}^2} \tag{16.10}$$

The concept of MIBO is demonstrated in Figure 16.4, where the treatment plan was optimized on a box target with hypoxic (0.15% $pO_2$) central part (a). Two pairs of opposite $^4$He and $^{16}$O beams were used for optimizing the plan for a uniform isoeffective dose of 6.5 Gy(RBE,OER). The one-dimensional cuts along the central line of a modeled CT for the optimized dose and dose-averaged LET are shown in subfigures (b) and (c), respectively. As one can see, while both ions contribute to the dose in a similar proportion in the normoxic parts of the target, the dose in the hypoxic core is primarily delivered by oxygen beams. The LET profile in the hypoxic part has high values about 80 keV/μm, reaching almost 100 keV/μm at the border regions, while the high-LET values are avoided in the normoxic margins.

A similar trend can be observed for the MIBO realization for a patient plan for chordoma tumor as shown in Figure 16.5. The plan was optimized for a uniform dose of 2 Gy(RBE,OER) to the PTV, delivered with two pairs of opposing fields of $^4$He and $^{16}$O. The hypoxia map (Figure 16.5a)

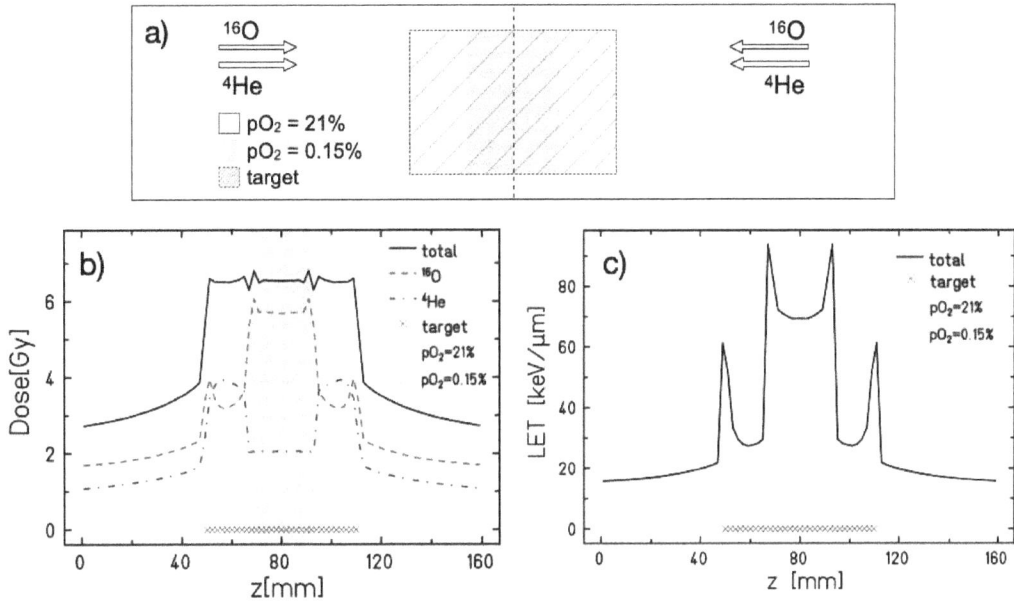

**Figure 16.4** MIBO optimization on a simple geometry. a) A sketch of the geometry: a rectangular 60 mm long target is at the center of a 160 mm long water CT; $pO_2 = 0.15\%$ in the central 28 mm region, and 21% in the remaining volume. Plan was optimized for two pairs of parallel-opposed fields of $^4$He and $^{16}$O. b) RBE- and OER- weighted total dose distribution profile and single-ion contributions. (b) Dose-averaged LET profile. Adapted from [25].

was emulated by the uniform shrinking the target contours and assigning gradually decreasing $pO_2$ values to the respective areas. Helium beams contribute to the dose distribution only in the outer parts of the tumor, while most of the dose in the hypoxic part, as well as the high LET values in the hypoxic core are produced by the oxygen beams.

The examples given here, were using the emulated hypoxia maps. One of the limitation of the MIBO approach that needs to be resolved is the difficulty to obtain a sufficiently resolved oxygenation map of a tumor, and to robustly account for its fast temporal variation in the course of a treatment, considering the limitation of the currently available techniques (functional PET and MRI).

## 16.5 OVERVIEW AND OUTLOOK

Simultaneous use of several ions and optimal combination of their physical and radiobological properties within one treatment plan is expected to greatly increase the flexibility of ion beam treatment planning. However, to transfer the above-mentioned approaches into clinical practice, further simulation and experimental studies are highly required. These would be needed, first to complete characterising in detail the different species employed (for example the fragmentation of Oxygen beam is still far to be fully characterized experimentally [23]) but even more, in particular, to ensure the correct prediction of the biological response of different tissues to the combined treatment, or to understand, which combination of ions and respective LET range would be the most beneficial for a wide range of tumors. Monte Carlo methods in these context could be extremely useful for having all particle species combined in one planning engine. However, an additional challenge is represented by the increased computational need, opened by the additional degrees of freedom introduced by such an approach.

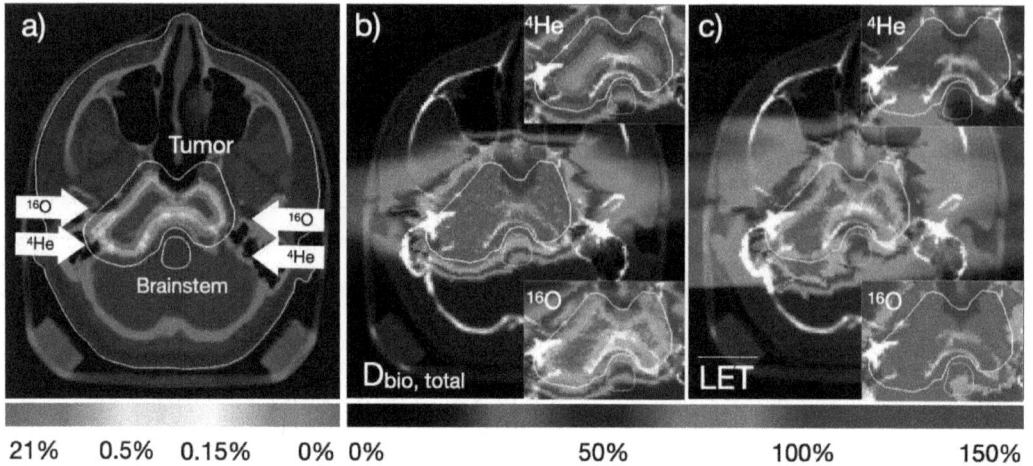

**Figure 16.5** MIBO optimization on a chordoma patient plan. a) Emulated hypoxia map and field arrangement. b) Resulting total RBE-OER-weighted dose (relative compared to the prescribed PTV dose of 2 Gy). c) Dose-averaged LET distribution (relative compared to the LET of 60 keV/μm). Insets correspond to the partial contributions from $^4$He and $^{16}$O fields. Please refer to [25] for the color version.

## REFERENCES

1. Melvin Astrahan. Some implications of linear-quadratic-linear radiation dose-response with regard to hypofractionation. *Medical Physics*, 35(9):4161–4172, 2008.
2. T T Böhlen, S Brons, M Dosanjh, A Ferrari, P Fossati, T Haberer, V Patera, and A Mairani. Investigating the robustness of ion beam therapy treatment plans to uncertainties in biological treatment parameters. *Physics in Medicine and Biology*, 57(23):7983–8004, nov 2012.
3. D K. Ebner, S J Frank, T Inaniwa, S Yamada, and T Shirai. The emerging potential of multi-ion radiotherapy. *Frontiers in Oncology*, 11:27, 2021.
4. Y Furusawa, K Fukutsu, M Aoki, H Itsukaichi, K Eguchi-Kasai, H Ohara, F Yatagai, T Kanai, and K Ando. Inactivation of Aerobic and Hypoxic Cells from Three Different Cell Lines by Accelerated $^3$He-, $^{12}$C- and $^{20}$Ne-Ion Beams. *Radiation Research*, 154(5):485–496, 2000.
5. A Gemmel, B Hasch, M Ellerbrock, W K Weyrather, and M Krämer. Biological dose optimization with multiple ion fields. *Phys. Med. Biol.*, 53:6991–7012, 2008.
6. C Gillmann, O Jäkel, I Schlampp, and C P Karger. Temporal lobe reactions after carbon ion radiation therapy: Comparison of relative biological effectiveness–weighted tolerance doses predicted by local effect models i and iv. *International Journal of Radiation Oncology\*Biology\*Physics*, 88(5):1136–1141, 2014.
7. R B Hawkins. A microdosimetric-kinetic model of cell death from exposure to ionizing radiation of any let, with experimental and clinical applications. *International Journal of Radiation Biology*, 69(6):739–755, 1996.
8. F Horst, D Schardt, H Iwase, C Schuy, M Durante, and U Weber. Physical characterization of 3he ion beams for radiotherapy and comparison with 4he. *Physics in Medicine & Biology*, 66(9):095009, apr 2021.
9. T Inaniwa, T Furukawa, Y Kase, N Matsufuji, T Toshito, Y Matsumoto, Y Furusawa, and K Noda. Treatment planning for a scanned carbon beam with a modified microdosimetric kinetic model. *Physics in Medicine and Biology*, 55(22):6721–6737, oct 2010.
10. T Inaniwa, N Kanematsu, N Matsufuji, T Kanai, T Shirai, K Noda, H Tsuji, T Kamada, and H Tsujii. Reformulation of a clinical-dose system for carbon-ion radiotherapy treatment

planning at the national institute of radiological sciences, japan. *Physics in Medicine and Biology*, 60(8):3271–3286, mar 2015.

11. T Inaniwa, N Kanematsu, K Noda, and T Kamada. Treatment planning of intensity modulated composite particle therapy with dose and linear energy transfer optimization. *Physics in Medicine and Biology*, 62(12):5180–5197, may 2017.

12. M Jermann. Particle therapy patient statistics (per end of 2019), 2020. [Online; accessed 6-July-2021].

13. T Kanai, M Endo, S Minohara, N Miyahara, H Koyama-ito, H Tomura, N Matsufuji, Y Futami, A Fukumura, T Hiraoka, Y Furusawa, K Ando, M Suzuki, F Soga, and K Kawachi. Biophysical characteristics of himac clinical irradiation system for heavy-ion radiation therapy. *International Journal of Radiation Oncology\*Biology\*Physics*, 44(1):201–210, 1999.

14. Y Kase, T Kanai, Y Matsumoto, Y Furusawa, H Okamoto, T Asaba, M Sakama, and H Shinoda. Microdosimetric measurements and estimation of human cell survival for heavy-ion beam. *Radiation Research*, 166(4):629–638, 2006.

15. B Kopp, S Mein, I Dokic, S Harrabi, T T Böhlen, T Haberer, J Debus, A Abdollahi, and A Mairani. Development and validation of single field multi-ion particle therapy treatments. *International Journal of Radiation Oncology\*Biology\*Physics*, 106(1):194–205, 2020.

16. M Krämer, O Jäkel, T Haberer, G Kraft, D Schardt, and U Weber. Treatment planning for heavy-ion radiotherapy: physical beam model and dose optimization. *Phys. Med. Biol.*, 45(11):3299, 2000.

17. M Krämer and M Scholz. Rapid calculation of biological effects in ion radiotherapy. *Physics in Medicine and Biology*, 51(8):1959–1970, mar 2006.

18. M Krämer, E Scifoni, C Schuy, M Rovituso, W Tinganelli, A Maier, R Kaderka, W Kraft-Weyrather, S Brons, T Tessonnier, K Parodi, and M Durante. Helium ions for radiotherapy? physical and biological verifications of a novel treatment modality. *Medical Physics*, 43(4):1995–2004, 2016.

19. A Mairani, G Magro, T Tessonnier, T T Böhlen, S Molinelli, A Ferrari, K Parodi, J Debus, and T Haberer. Optimizing the modified microdosimetric kinetic model input parameters for proton and4he ion beam therapy application. *Physics in Medicine and Biology*, 62(11):N244–N256, may 2017.

20. A Mairani, S Mein, B Kopp, J Besuglow, I Dokic, J Naumann, S Harrabi, A Abdollahi, T Haberer, and J Debus. Back to the future: Helium ion therapy 2020. *International Journal of Radiation Oncology Biology Physics*, 108, 2020.

21. S Mein, I Dokic, C Klein, T Tessonnier, T T Böhlen, G Magro, J Bauer, A Ferrari, K Parodi, T Haberer, J Debus, A Abdollahi, and A Mairani. Biophysical modeling and experimental validation of relative biological effectiveness (rbe) for $^4$he ion beam therapy. *Radiat. Oncol.*, 14(1):123, 2019.

22. S Mein, C Klein, B Kopp, G Magro, S Harrabi, C P Karger, T Haberer, J Debus, A Abdollahi, I Dokic, and A Mairani. Assessment of rbe-weighted dose models for carbon ion therapy toward modernization of clinical practice at hit: In vitro, in vivo, and in patients. *International Journal of Radiation Oncology\*Biology\*Physics*, 108(3):779–791, 2020.

23. A Rucinski, G Traini, A Baratto Roldan, G Battistoni, M De Simoni, Y Dong, M Fischetti, PM Frallicciardi, E Gioscio, C Mancini-Terracciano, et al. Secondary radiation measurements for particle therapy applications: Charged secondaries produced by 16o ion beams in a pmma target at large angles. *Physica Medica*, 64:45–53, 2019.

24. M Scholz and G Kraft. Track structure and the calculation of biological effects of heavy charged particles. *Advances in Space Research*, 18(1):5–14, 1996. Physical, Chemical, Biochemical and Biological Techniques and Processes.

25. O Sokol, M Krämer, S Hild, M Durante, and E Scifoni. Kill painting of hypoxic tumors with multiple ion beams. *Phys. Med. Biol.*, 64:045008, 2019.

26. O Sokol, E Scifoni, W Tinganelli, W Kraft-Weyrather, J Wiedemann, A Maier, D Boscolo, Th Friedrich, S Brons, M Durante, and M Krämer. Oxygen beams for therapy: advanced biological treatment planning and experimental verification. *Phys. Med. Biol.*, 62:7798–7813, 2017.

27. B S Sørensen, J Overgaard, and N Bassler. In vitro rbe-let dependence for multiple particle types. *Acta Oncologica*, 50(6):757–762, 2011.

28. T Tessonnier, A Mairani, S Brons, P Sala, F Cerutti, A Ferrari, T Haberer, J Debus, and K Parodi. Helium ions at the heidelberg ion beam therapy center: comparisons between fluka monte carlo code predictions and dosimetric measurements. *Physics in Medicine and Biology*, (16):6784–6803, 2017.

29. W Tinganelli, M Durante, R Hirayama, M Krämer, A Maier, W Kraft-Weyrather, Y Furusawa, T Friedrich, and E Scifoni. Kill-painting of hypoxic tumours in charged particle therapy. *Scientific Reports*, 5(1), 2015.

30. F Tommasino, E Scifoni, and M Durante. New Ions for Therapy. *International Journal of Particle Therapy*, 2(3):428–438, 2015.

31. H Tsujii and T Kamada. A Review of Update Clinical Results of Carbon Ion Radiotherapy. *Japanese Journal of Clinical Oncology*, 42(8):670–685, 07 2012.

32. H Tsujii, J Mizoe, T Kamada, M Baba, H Tsuji, H Kato, S Kato, S Yamada, S Yasuda, T Ohno, T Yanagi, R Imai, K Kagei, H Kato, R Hara, A Hasegawa, M Nakajima, N Sugane, N Tamaki, R Takagi, S Kandatsu, K Yoshikawa, R Kishimoto, and T Miyamoto. Clinical Results of Carbon Ion Radiotherapy at NIRS. *Journal of Radiation Research*, 48(Suppl A):1–13, 03 2007.

# 17 Monte Carlo for chemistry in radiation biology

*Ianik Plante*
Human Health and Performance Contract, Houston, TX, USA

## CONTENTS

## 17.1  INTRODUCTION

### 17.1.1  IMPORTANCE OF RADIATION PHYSICS AND CHEMISTRY IN RADIOBIOLOGY

The events resulting from the absorption of ionizing radiation in matter are conventionally divided into four temporal stages ([1, 2]); the first three stages, the physical, physico-chemical, and non-homogeneous chemical stages, are depicted in Figure 17.1. During the *physical* stage, the incident radiation ionizes and excites the molecules of the medium, creating secondary electrons. The resulting species are unstable and undergo fast rearrangement in the *physicochemical* stage. These two processes produce radical and molecular products of radiolysis that are distributed in a highly non-homogeneous track structure. Secondary electrons slow down to sub-excitation energies, thermalize, become trapped ($e_{tr}^-$) and eventually hydrated ($e_{aq}^-$). These are reactants present within $\sim 10^{-12}$ s, and during the *non-homogeneous chemical* stage they diffuse and react with one another or with the environment, until most intra-track reactions are complete ($\sim 10^{-6}$ s). Finally, in a biological system, a *biological* stage follows and the biological responses of the system to radiation exposure begin during this transient stage ($\sim 10^{-3}$ s or longer). Because the radiation physics and chemistry precede the biological stage, they have been of crucial importance in understanding the biological effects of ionizing radiation ([3]).

DOI: 10.1201/9781003023920-17

| Physical stage (<$10^{-15}$ s) | Physico-chemical stage ($10^{-15}$-$10^{-12}$ s) | Non-homogeneous chemical stage ($10^{-12}$-$10^{-6}$ s) |
|---|---|---|

**Proton transfer**

$H_2O^{\cdot+} + H_2O \rightarrow H_3O^+ + \ ^{\cdot}OH$

**Ionization**

$H_2O^{\cdot+} + e^-$

**Electron thermalization**

$e^-_{dry} \rightarrow e^-_{th} \rightarrow e^-_{tr} \longrightarrow e^-_{aq}$

$H_2O$

**Non-dissociative deexcitation**

$H_2O$+ thermal energy

**Excitation**

$H_2O^*$

**Dissociative deexcitation**

$\begin{cases} H^{\cdot} + \ ^{\cdot}OH \\ 2H^{\cdot} + O(\ ^3P) \\ H_2 + O(\ ^1D) \end{cases}$

**Auto-ionization**

$H_2O^{\cdot+} + e^-$

Non-homogeneous chemical stage reactions:

$H^{\cdot} + H^{\cdot} \rightarrow H_2$

$H^{\cdot} + \ ^{\cdot}OH \rightarrow H_2O$

$H^{\cdot} + e^-_{aq} \rightarrow H_2 + OH^-$

$H^{\cdot} + O(\ ^3P) \rightarrow \ ^{\cdot}OH$

$^{\cdot}OH + \ ^{\cdot}OH \rightarrow H_2O_2$

$^{\cdot}OH + OH^- \rightarrow H_2O + e^-_{aq}$

$^{\cdot}OH + e^-_{aq} \rightarrow OH^-$

...

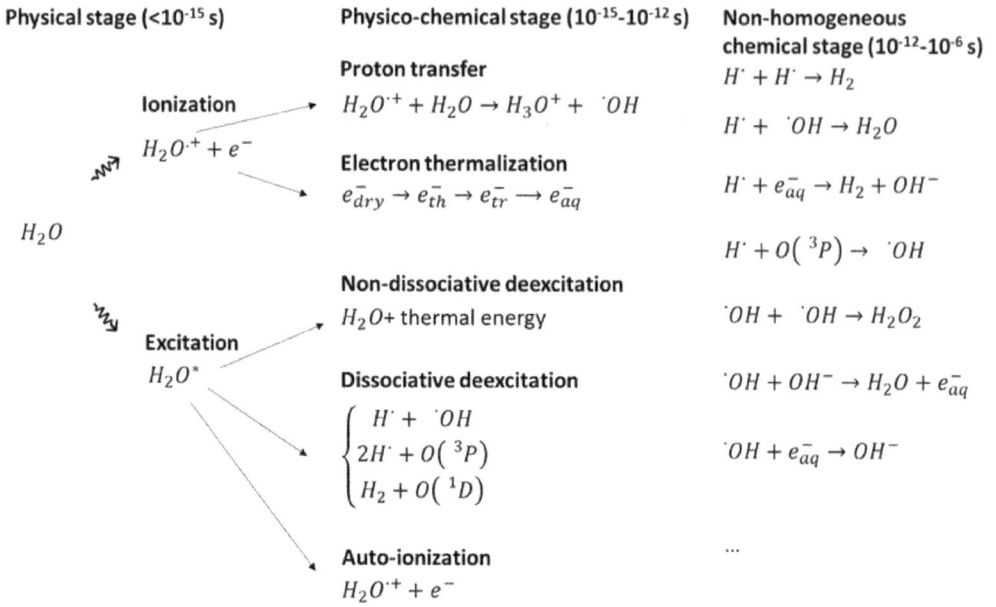

**Figure 17.1** Overview of water radiolysis, illustrating the events in the physical, physico-chemical and non-homogeneous chemical stages. In biological systems, a fourth stage, the biological stage, follows the chemical stage.

## 17.1.2 THE RADIATION TRACK STRUCTURE

There are several types of ionizing radiations; however, the types considered in this book chapter are electron, ions, and energetic photons (x-rays or γ-rays). All these radiation types lead to ionized electrons. The locations where the interactions between the radiation and the medium take place are determined by the physical properties of the radiation and the medium, resulting in energy being deposited non-homogeneously, i.e. the radiation track structure (Figure 17.2).

*The physical stage*

An ionization leads to an ionized molecule and an electron. In water, this is written as

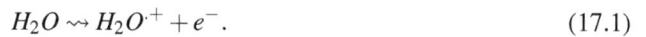

$$H_2O \rightsquigarrow H_2O^{\cdot+} + e^-. \tag{17.1}$$

Because electrons occupy different orbitals, there are several ionization levels in the water molecule, usually named $1b_1$, $3a_1$, $1b_2$, $2a_2$ and $1a_1$ ([4]). The ionization of the $1a_1$ level, which is an inner orbital, is much rarer than the other superficial orbitals, and results in the emission of a 500 eV Auger electron ([5]) and the formation of a doubled charged ion $H_2O^{2+}$. Multiple ionizations are also possible, with probability of occurrence decreasing for each additional ionization ([6]). In some interactions, the energy transfer is insufficient to ionize the molecule. This leads to an excited state, noted as $H_2O^*$:

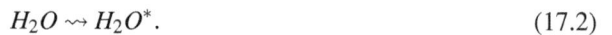

$$H_2O \rightsquigarrow H_2O^*. \tag{17.2}$$

Many excited states of the water molecule are known ([7]) (Table 17.1). Those considered for the radiolysis of water are usually the states $\tilde{A}^1B_1$, $\tilde{B}^1A_1$ and the excitation of vibrational and rotational levels, $H_2O^*_{vib}$. In radiation transport codes, the probabilities of occurrence of ionization and excitations are obtained from cross sections, which can be an be calculated using the dielectric theory ([8, 9], and others); however, this topic is beyond the scope of this book chapter.

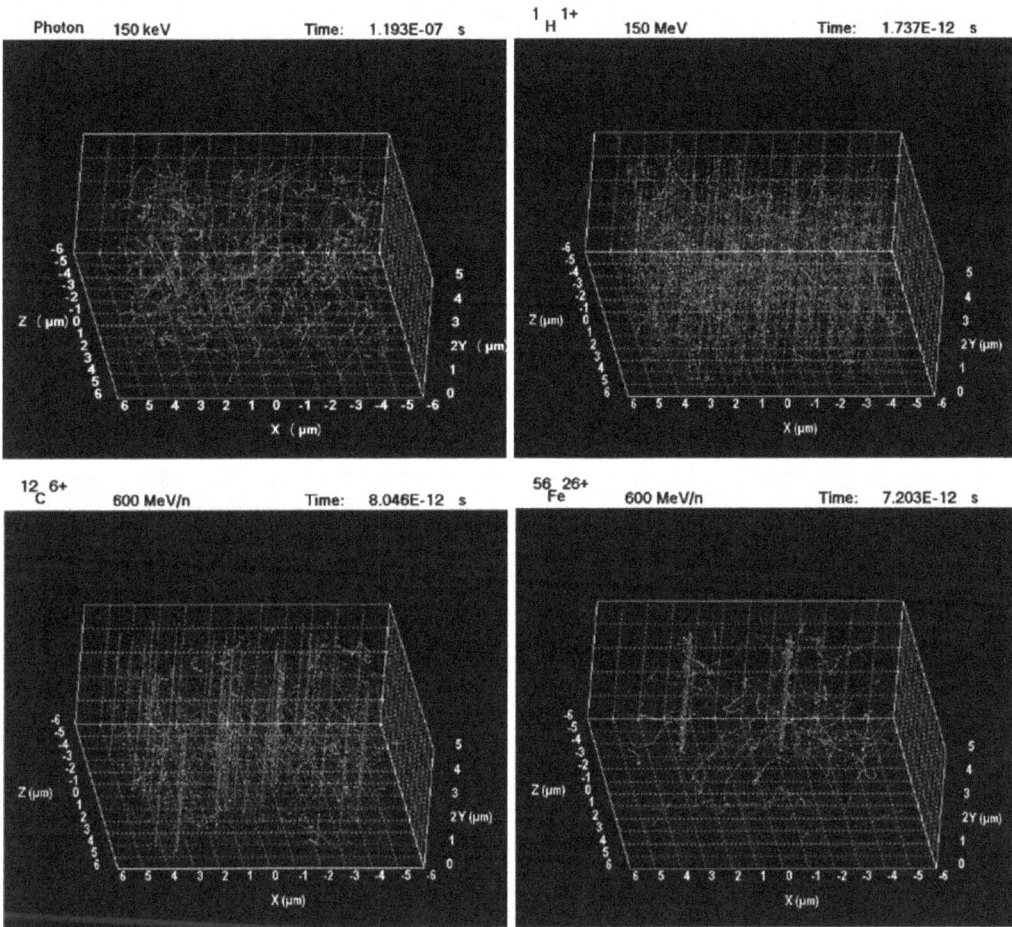

**Figure 17.2** Simulation of the irradiation of a 10 μm x 10 μm x 5 μm volume by $^{137}Cs$ photons, 150-MeV protons, 600 MeV/n carbon ions, and 600 MeV/n iron ions. Each dot represents a radiolytic specie. In all cases, the dose to the irradiated volume is ∼0.5 Gy, and periodic boundary conditions were used.

*The physicochemical stage*

The species created during the physical stage are unstable, and they rearrange by different mechanisms during the physicochemical stage, which lasts about 10–12 s. At the end of the physical stage, the following species are present in the medium:

1. Singly ionized water molecules ($H_2O^{\bullet+}$)
2. Multiple ionized water molecules ($H_2O^{2+}$, $H_2O^{3+}$, etc.)
3. Excited water molecules ($H_2O^*$)
4. Dry electrons ($e_{dry}^-$)

The water cations $H_2O^{\bullet+}$ undergo a random walk during their very short lifetime (∼10 fs) by means of a sequence of electron transfers from neighboring water molecules to the $H_2O^{\bullet+}$ hole, until a proton transfer occurs ([10]):

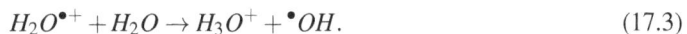

$$H_2O^{\bullet+} + H_2O \rightarrow H_3O^+ + {}^\bullet OH. \qquad (17.3)$$

This yields a cation $H_3O^+$ and a hydroxyl radical (${}^\bullet OH$) ([11]).

**Table 17.1**

**Branching ratios for excited states of the water molecule ([6])**

| State | | Mechanism | Ratio | | Result | |
|---|---|---|---|---|---|---|
| $H_2O^{\bullet+} + e^-$ | $\rightarrow$ | Electron recombination | N/A | $\rightarrow$ | $H_2O^*_{vib}$ | |
| $H_2O^*_{vib}$ | $\rightarrow$ | Non-dissociative deexcitation | 45% | $\rightarrow$ | $H_2O$+ thermal energy | |
| | $\rightarrow$ | Dissociative deexcitation | 55% | $\rightarrow$ | $H^\bullet + {}^\bullet OH$ | 79.8% |
| | | | | | $2H^\bullet + O(^3P)$ | 5.5% |
| | | | | | $H_2 + O(^1D)$ | 14.8% |
| $H_2O^*\,(\tilde{A}^1B_1)$ | $\rightarrow$ | Non-dissociative deexcitation | 45% | $\rightarrow$ | $H_2O$+ thermal energy | |
| | $\rightarrow$ | Dissociative deexcitation | 55% | $\rightarrow$ | $H^\bullet + {}^\bullet OH$ | |
| $H_2O^*\,(\tilde{B}^1A_1)$ | $\rightarrow$ | Auto-ionization | 50% | $\rightarrow$ | $H_2O^{\bullet+} + e^-$ | |
| | $\rightarrow$ | Non-dissociative deexcitation | 22.5% | $\rightarrow$ | $H_2O$+ thermal energy | |
| | $\rightarrow$ | Dissociative deexcitation | 27.5% | $\rightarrow$ | $H^\bullet + {}^\bullet OH$ | 78% |
| | | | | | $2H^\bullet + O(^3P)$ | 12% |
| | | | | | $H_2 + O(^1D)$ | 10% |

A dry electron ($e^-_{dry}$) loses its energy until it become thermalized (i.e. in thermal equilibrium with the medium) ($e^-_{th}$), trapped ($e^-_{tr}$) and eventually hydrated ($e^-_{aq}$) (i.e. surrounded by water molecules oriented so that the electron cannot escape). The sequence can be written as

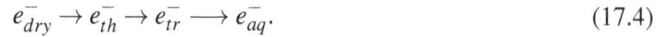

$$e^-_{dry} \rightarrow e^-_{th} \rightarrow e^-_{tr} \longrightarrow e^-_{aq}. \tag{17.4}$$

## 17.2 SIMULATION MODELS AND APPROACHES

The non-homogeneous chemical stage follows the physicochemical stage ($\sim 10^{-12}$ s) and continues until the reactants are distributed homogeneously ($\sim 10^{-6}$ s). At the end of the physicochemical stage, the radiolytic species $H^\bullet$, $^\bullet OH$, $H_2$, $H^+$, $OH^-$, etc. are present in the medium. The radiolytic species are highly reactive and distributed non-homogeneously, depending of the radiation type.

### 17.2.1 DIFFUSION MODEL

In general, individual particles in solution evolve according to the diffusion equation (DE):

$$\frac{\partial}{\partial t} p(r, t \mid r_0) = D\nabla^2 p(r, t \mid r_0), \tag{17.5}$$

where $t$ is the time, $r_0$ and $r$ are the position vectors[1], and $D$ and is the diffusion coefficient. With the initial condition $p(r, t \rightarrow 0 \mid r_0) = \delta(r - r_0)$ and the boundary condition $p(|r| \rightarrow \infty, t \mid r_0) = 0$, the solution, which is the Green's function of the diffusion equation (GFDE), is given by

$$p(r, t \mid r_0) = \frac{1}{(4\pi Dt)^{3/2}} exp\left[ -\frac{(r - r_0)^2}{4Dt} \right]. \tag{17.6}$$

The diffusion constants of main radiolytic species are shown in Table 17.2.

---

[1] Here $r = (x, y, z)$ and $r_0 = (x_0, y_0, z_0)$. Through the chapter, bold quantities in equations are used to indicate vectors.

**Table 17.2**

**Diffusion coefficients ($D$) and radii of radiolytic species ([13])**

| Species | $D$ ($10\,nm^2s^{-1}$) | Radius (nm) | Species | $D$ ($10\,nm^2s^{-1}$) | Radius (nm) |
|---|---|---|---|---|---|
| $H^\bullet$ | 7.0 | 0.19 | $O_2^{\bullet-}$ | 1.75 | 0.22 |
| $^\bullet OH$ | 2.2 | 0.22 | $HO_2^\bullet$ | 2.3 | 0.21 |
| $H_2O_2$ | 2.3 | 0.21 | $HO_2^-$ | 1.4 | 0.25 |
| $H_2$ | 4.8 | 0.14 | $O(^3P)$ | 2.0 | 0.20 |
| $e_{aq}^-$ | 4.9 | 0.50 | $O^{\bullet-}$ | 2.0 | 0.25 |
| $H^+$ | 9.46 | 0.25 | $O_3^{\bullet-}$ | 2.0 | 0.20 |
| $OH^-$ | 5.3 | 0.33 | $O_3$ | 2.0 | 0.20 |
| $O_2$ | 2.4 | 0.17 | | | |

## 17.2.2   REACTION MODEL

In the diffusion-reaction model, two particles react when the interparticle distance is smaller than their reaction radius and certain conditions are met. Indeed, the interparticle diffusion vector can be described by two independent diffusion processes ([14]). The first process corresponds to the diffusion of the particles weighted by their diffusion coefficients, analogous to the diffusion of the center of mass. The second process is the interparticle diffusion vector, of which the length determines the occurrence of a chemical reaction during a time interval. This process is analogous to a particle diffusing freely around a spherical object (in 3D), with boundary conditions at the surface that are determined by the reaction rate constant. Several types of chemical reactions are considered. The theory described in this section is the framework of the GFDE, which is used in radiation chemistry codes.

## 17.2.3   TYPES OF CHEMICAL REACTIONS

The reactions can be either fully or partially diffusion-controlled, and they involve neutral or charged particles. This gives four classes of reactions that were introduced by [15] and used by several investigators ([16, 17]). An additional type of reaction considers the reaction with the species present in solution (background reactions). These reactions are necessary to simulate the effect of scavengers and dosimeters, which are important topics in radiation chemistry ([18]). All reactions are included in tables in the Appendix.

### 17.2.3.1   Diffusion-controlled and partially diffusion-controlled reactions

For diffusion-controlled (type I) reactions, the rate constant $k_a$ is considered infinite, meaning that the particles react whenever they collide. The inner boundary condition is given by $p(|r| = \sigma, t \mid r_0) = 0$, where $\sigma$ is the reaction radius. It is also called the Smoluchowski boundary condition ([19]). The initial condition is $p(r,t \mid r_0) = \delta(r - r_0)$. For these reactions, $p_I(r,t \mid r_0)$ is

$$4\pi r r_0 p_I(r,t \mid r_0) = \frac{1}{\sqrt{4\pi Dt}}\,exp\left[-\frac{(r-r_0)^2}{4Dt}\right] - exp\left[-\frac{(r+r_0-2\sigma)^2}{4Dt}\right]. \qquad (17.7)$$

As for free diffusion, $p_I(r,t \mid r_0)$ is the probability distribution for the interparticle vector to be $r$ at time $t$, given that it was $r_0$ at $t=0$. Integrating $p_I(r,t \mid r_0)$ over the 3D space, assuming angular symmetry, yields the probability of survival (or not reacting) of the pair of particles with an interparticle distance $r_0$ at time $t$. The probability of reaction $P_I(r,t \mid r_0)$, is, therefore

$$P_I(t \mid r_0) = 1 - \int_\sigma^\infty 4\pi r^2 p_I(r,t \mid r_0)\,dr = \frac{\sigma}{r_0}Erfc\left(\frac{r_0-\sigma}{\sqrt{4Dt}}\right), \qquad (17.8)$$

where $Erfc(z)$ is the complementary error function

$$Erfc(z) = \frac{2}{\sqrt{\pi}} \int_z^\infty \exp\left(-t^2\right) dt. \tag{17.9}$$

In partially diffusion-controlled (type II) reactions, the reaction rate $k_a$ is finite, meaning that a collision of two particles does not necessarily mean that the particles will react. Thus, the inner boundary condition, which is also called the radiation[2] boundary condition is ([20]):

$$4\pi\sigma^2 D \frac{\partial}{\partial r} p(r,t \mid r_0)\Big|_{r=\sigma} = k_a p(|r| = \sigma, t \mid r_0). \tag{17.10}$$

For partially diffusion-controlled reactions, the radial GFDE $p_{II}(r,t \mid r_0)$ is

$$4\pi r r_0 p_{II}(r,t \mid r_0) = \frac{1}{\sqrt{4\pi Dt}} exp\left[-\frac{(r-r_0)^2}{4Dt}\right] + exp\left[-\frac{(r+r_0-2\sigma)^2}{4Dt}\right]$$
$$+ \alpha W\left(\frac{r+r_0-2\sigma}{\sqrt{4Dt}}, -\alpha\sqrt{Dt}\right). \tag{17.11}$$

where $W(x,y) = \exp\left(2xy+y^2\right) Erfc(x+y)$, and $\alpha = -(k_a + 4\pi\sigma D)/(4\pi\sigma^2 D)$. The probability of reaction, $P_{II}(r,t \mid r_0)$, is:

$$P_{II}(t \mid r_0) = 1 - \int_\sigma^\infty 4\pi r^2 p_{II}(r,t \mid r_0) dr = \frac{\sigma\alpha+1}{r_0\alpha}\left[Erfc\left(\frac{r_0-\sigma}{\sqrt{4Dt}}\right) - W\left(\frac{r_0-\sigma}{\sqrt{4Dt}}, -\alpha\sqrt{Dt}\right)\right]. \tag{17.12}$$

### 17.2.3.2 Reactions involving charged particles

The theory describing diffusion and reaction of particles is more complex when there is an interaction potential between the particles. If the particles interact via a force[3] vector $F(r)$, a term is added to the DE:

$$\frac{\partial}{\partial t} p(r,t \mid r_0) = D\nabla^2 p(r,t \mid r_0) - D\beta\nabla\bullet(p(r,t \mid r_0)F(r)), \tag{17.13}$$

Where $\beta = 1/k_B T$, $k_B$ is Boltzmann's constant, and $T$ is the temperature. This is the Debye-Smoluchowski equation (DSE). For charged particles with electrostatic interaction, the Coulomb potential can be expressed as $\beta U(r) = r_c/r$, where $r_c = e^2/(4\pi\varepsilon_0 k_B T)$ is Onsager's radius. The radial component of the DSE can be written as

$$\frac{\partial}{\partial t} p(r,t \mid r_0) = D\frac{1}{r^2}\frac{\partial}{\partial r}\left[r^2 e^{-r_c/r}\frac{\partial}{\partial r}e^{r_c/r}\right]p(r,t \mid r_0). \tag{17.14}$$

As for non-interacting particles, reactions involving charged particles correspond to diffusion-controlled (type III) reactions ($k_a \to \infty$), and partially diffusion-controlled (type IV) reactions ($0 < k_a < \infty$) for particles with an electrostatic interaction. For the DSE, the exact Green's functions for the radial interparticle distance are known only in the Laplace space ([21]). In water, in which $r_c$ is small, the probability of reaction can be expressed in a form similar to diffusion-controlled reactions ([22]):

$$P_{III}(t \mid r_0) = \frac{\sigma_{eff}}{r_{0_{eff}}} Erfc\left(\frac{r_{0_{eff}} - \sigma_{eff}}{\sqrt{4Dt}}\right), \tag{17.15}$$

[2]Here, "radiation" refers to the radiation of heat at the boundary, not ionizing radiation.
[3]$F(r) = -\nabla U(r)$, where $U(r)$ is the potential energy.

where the distances are replaced by effective distances $r_{0_{eff}}$ and $\sigma_{eff}$:

$$r_{0_{eff}} = \frac{-r_c}{1 - \exp(r_c/r_0)} \text{ and } \sigma_{eff} = \frac{-r_c}{1 - \exp(r_c/\sigma)}. \tag{17.16}$$

The effective distances are always positive for $r$ or $\sigma > 0$. When $r_c \longrightarrow 0$ (no electric field between particles), $r_{0_{eff}} \longrightarrow r$ and $\sigma_{eff} \longrightarrow \sigma$. These reactions are given in Table 5.

For partially diffusion-controlled reactions of particles with electrostatic interactions, the DSE with an electrostatic potential is used (Equation 13). The inner boundary condition is

$$De^{r_c/r} \frac{\partial}{\partial r} \left[ e^{-r_c/r} p(r,t \mid r_0) \right] = k_a p(r,t \mid r_0), \tag{17.17}$$

The probability of reaction is approximately given by ([15]):

$$P_{IV}(t \mid r_0) = \frac{\sigma''_{eff}}{r_{0_{eff}}} \left[ Erfc(b) - W(b,a) \right], \tag{17.18}$$

where

$$a = \frac{4\sigma^2 \alpha}{r_c^2} \sqrt{\frac{t}{D}} \sinh(\frac{r_c}{2\sigma}), \tag{17.19}$$

$$b = \frac{r_c}{4\sqrt{Dt}} \left[ coth\left(\frac{r_c}{2r}\right) - coth\left(\frac{r_c}{2\sigma}\right) \right]. \tag{17.20}$$

In this case, $k_{dif} = 4\pi D\sigma_{eff}$ and $k_a$ is found by using $1/k_{obs} = 1/k_{dif} + 1/k_a$. Furthermore,

$$\alpha = v + \frac{r_c D}{\sigma^2(1 - \exp(-r_c/\sigma))}; v = \frac{k_a}{4\pi\sigma^2}; \tag{17.21}$$

$$\sigma''_{eff} = \frac{r_c}{\exp\left(\frac{r_c}{\sigma}\right) \left(1 + \frac{Dr_c}{\sigma^2 v}\right) - 1}. \tag{17.22}$$

When $r_c \to 0$ (no electric field between particles), $P_{IV}(t \mid r_0) \to P_{II}(t \mid r_0)$ Similarly, when $v \to \infty$ (totally diffusion-controlled reactions), $P_{IV}(t \mid r_0) \to P_{III}(t \mid r_0)$.

### 17.2.3.3 Other types of reactions

Type V reactions are those where a spin statistical factor of 1/4 affects the calculated diffusion-controlled reaction rate coefficient, because, for two radicals, only the singlet configuration of their combined spins allows the occurrence of the reaction (in contrast to the unreactive triplet configuration). These reactions are $H^\bullet + H^\bullet \to H_2$, $H^\bullet + e_{aq}^- \to H_2 + OH^-$, and $e_{aq}^- + e_{aq}^- \to H_2 + 2OH^-$.

The reactions with the background (type VI) are those for which one of the reactants (the species B) is in a known homogeneous concentration in the solution. For example, the concentration of $H_2O$, $H^+$ and $OH^-$ in pure liquid water at 25 oC are 55.3 M, $9.9 \times 10^{-8}$ M, and $9.9 \times 10^{-8}$ M, respectively. The reactions of the radiolytic species with $H_2O$, $H^+$ and $OH^-$ are considered type VI. First-order reactions (i.e. reactions comprising one reactant) are also considered as type VI, because the same approach is used to simulate them. Assuming that [B] is constant, the equation $d[A]/[A] = -k[B]dt$ is obtained from classical reaction kinetics. Therefore, the probability of reaction during the timestep $\Delta t$ is $P_{VI}(\Delta t) = 1 - \exp(-k[B]\Delta t)$, which can be approximated by $k[B]\Delta t$ for small time steps. Although the calculation of the probability of occurrence of type VI reactions is very simple, their role is nevertheless very important, because they allow the simulation of chemical systems of interest such as chemical dosimeters.

### 17.2.4   THE STEP-BY-STEP (SBS) SIMULATION METHOD

In this method, all the particles generated by the radiolysis are followed in time.

#### 17.2.4.1   Simple particle diffusion

The motion of the particles in solution is viewed as a random walk, or "jumps," due to collisions with molecules of the surrounding medium. In most codes, this is simulated as follows:

$$x_i(t + \Delta t) = x_i(t) + \sqrt{2D\Delta t}N_1, (23a) \tag{17.23a}$$

$$y_i(t + \Delta t) = y_i(t) + \sqrt{2D\Delta t}N_2, (23b) \tag{17.23b}$$

$$z_i(t + \Delta t) = z_i(t) + \sqrt{2D\Delta t}N_3, (23c) \tag{17.23c}$$

where $x_i(t)$, $y_i(t)$, and $z_i(t)$ are the coordinates of the particle $i$ at time $t$, $\Delta t$ is the time step, $D$ is the diffusion coefficient, and $N_1$, $N_2$ and $N_3$ are three standard normal random numbers[4]. This simple approach is important because it is used in several codes. At each time step, some particles in the system may collide, i.e., their interparticle distance is smaller than their reaction radii. In diffusion-controlled reactions, each collision is expected to result in a chemical reaction. In partially diffusion-controlled reactions, the reaction happens with a certain probability that is a function of the rate constant, and often of the specific code. If there is no reaction, the particles separate at a distance greater than the reaction radius.

#### 17.2.4.2   Diffusion-controlled reactions

For a two-particles system with diffusion-controlled reactions, Algorithm 1 can be used to sample the interparticle distance for the particles that have not reacted during the interval $\Delta t$. This algorithm is mathematically exact for the type I GFDE. Two cases are considered. For $(r_0 - \sigma) \geq \sqrt{D\Delta t}$, Algorithm 1a is used. Otherwise, Algorithm 1b is used.

| **Algorithm 1a. Sampling of $4\pi r^2 p_I(r, t \mid r_0)$ for $(r_0 - \sigma) \geq \sqrt{D\Delta t}$** |
|---|
| REPEAT { |
| GENERATE $U$ and $V$ uniform on [0,1] |
| IF $V < \dfrac{\sqrt{\pi}r_0}{\sqrt{\pi}r_0 + \sqrt{D\Delta t}}$ { |
| $R \leftarrow r_0 + \sqrt{2D\Delta t}N$, where $N$ is standard normal |
| } ELSE { |
| $R \leftarrow r_0 + \sqrt{4D\Delta t E}$, where $E$ is standard exponential |
| } |
| } UNTIL $R \geq \sigma$ and $U[(R - r_0)_+ + r_0] \leq R[1 - \exp(-(r_0 - \sigma)(R - \sigma)/D\Delta t)]$ |
| RETURN $R$ |

The function $(x)_+ = x$ if x>0, or 0 otherwise.

| **Algorithm 1b. Sampling of $4\pi r^2 p_I(r, \Delta t \mid r_0)$ for $(r_0 - \sigma) \leq \sqrt{D\Delta t}$** |
|---|
| DEFINE $W_1 = \sqrt{\pi/2}$; $W_2 = (2r_0 - \sigma)/\sqrt{2D\Delta t}$; $W_3 = r_0(r_0 - \sigma)\sqrt{2\pi}/(2D\Delta t)$ |
| $S = W_1 + W_2 + W_3$ |
| REPEAT { |
| GENERATE $U$ and $V$ uniform on [0,1] |
| IF $(0 \leq V < W_1/S)$, $R \leftarrow r_0 + \sqrt{2D\Delta t(2E + N^2)}$, where $E$ and $N$ are std. exponentials and normals |
| IF $(W_1/S \leq V < (W_1 + W_2)/S)$, $R \leftarrow r_0 + \sqrt{4D\Delta t E}$, where $E$ is standard exponential |
| IF $(V \geq (W_1 + W_2)/S)$, $R \leftarrow r_0 + \sqrt{2D\Delta t}N$, where $N$ is standard normal |
| }    UNTIL    $2U(r_0 - \sigma)\left[(R - r_0)_+^2 + (2r_0 - \sigma)(R - r_0) + r_0(r_0 - R)\right]/(2D\Delta t) \leq R[1 -$ |
| $\exp(-\frac{(r_0 - \sigma)(R - \sigma)}{D\Delta t})]$ and $R \geq \sigma$ |
| RETURN R |

---

[4]The terminology used in [23] for random numbers is used in the text and in the algorithms. The cases that are considered are 1) $U$: uniformly distributed between 0 and 1; 2) $E$: standard exponential; and 3) $N$: standard normal.

### 17.2.4.3  Partially diffusion-controlled reactions

The algorithm for sampling the interparticle distance for partially diffusion-controlled reactions (Equation 11) was presented in [24]. It is recalled in Algorithm 2.

---
**Algorithm 2. Sampling of $4\pi r^2 p_{II}(r, \Delta t \mid r_0)$**

CALCULATE $p_1 = \sqrt{D\Delta t / \pi r_0^2}$, $p_2 = \sqrt{D\Delta t / \pi r_0^2} \exp[-(r_0 - \sigma)^2 / 4D\Delta t]$ and

$p' = \Phi\left[\frac{(r_0 - \sigma)}{\sqrt{2D\Delta t}}\right] + \left(\frac{2\sigma}{r_0} - 1\right) \Phi\left[\frac{(\sigma - r_0)}{\sqrt{2D\Delta t}}\right] 1_{[r_0 \leq 2\sigma]}$

SET $s = p_1 + p_2 + p'$

REPEAT {

GENERATE $U$ and $V$ uniform on [0,1]

IF $sU \in [0, p_1]$, SET $R \leftarrow r_0 + \sqrt{4D\Delta t E}$, where $E$ is standard exponential.

IF $sU \in (p_1, p_1 + p_2]$, SET $R \leftarrow 2\sigma - r_0 + \sqrt{(r_0 - \sigma)^2 + 4D\Delta t E}$, where $E$ is std. exponential.

IF $sU \in (p_1 + p_2, s]$ {

REPEAT {

GENERATE $N$ as standard normal, $W$ uniform on [0,1]

SET $R \leftarrow r_0 + \sqrt{2D\Delta t} N$

} UNTIL $Y > \sigma$, or jointly $Y < \sigma$, $D\Delta t < 2\sigma^2$ and $W \leq (2\sigma - r_0)/r_0$

In the former case, SET $R \leftarrow Y$

In the latter case, SET $R \leftarrow 2\sigma - Y$

} UNTIL $Vh(R) \leq f(R)$

RETURN $R$

---

In algorithm 2, $\Phi(x)$ is the normal distribution function:

$$\Phi\left(x\sqrt{2}\right) = 1 - Erfc(x)/2, \tag{17.24}$$

and $1_{[condition]}$ is 0 if condition is false, or 1 if condition is true. The function $h(r) = 4\pi r^2 p_{max}(r)$, $f(r) = 4\pi r^2 p_{II}(r, \Delta t \mid r_0)$ and $p_{max}(r)$ is defined as:

$$p_{max}(r) = \frac{1}{4\pi r r_0 \sqrt{4\pi D\Delta t}} \; exp\left[-\frac{(r + r_0 - 2\sigma)^2}{4D\Delta t}\right] + exp\left[-\frac{(r - r_0)^2}{4D\Delta t}\right], \tag{17.25}$$

### 17.2.4.4  Reactions involved charged particles

The Green's functions of the DSE for reactions involving charged particles are known only in the Laplace space; therefore, how to sample these Green's functions for the interparticle distance is not known. As an approximation, Algorithms 1 and 2 previously described can be used, replacing $r_0$, $r$ and $\sigma$ by $r_{0_{eff}}$, $r_{eff}$ and $\sigma_{eff}$ (Equation 30). The sampled value (noted $r_{eff}$) is then transformed to r by inverting Equation 30.

### 17.2.4.5  Reactions with background

For the reactions with background species, the probability of reaction is $P_{VI}(\Delta t) = 1 - \exp(-k[B]\Delta t)$, where $[B]$ is the concentration of the species in uniform concentration in solution and $k$ is the reaction rate constant.

### 17.2.5  THE INDEPENDENT REACTION TIMES (IRT) METHOD

This simulation method was initially proposed by Prof. Masanori Tachiya ([25]), and further developed by others ([26, 15]). The IRT method provides a fast way to calculate the radiolytic yields from an initial track that does not require simulating the full random walk of all particles in the system. For $N$ particles, the number of pairs is $N(N-1)/2$, so that the calculation time increases as $O(N^2)$. In an SBS diffusion-reaction approach, these pairwise interactions need to be calculated at each time step. Therefore, the calculation time becomes prohibitive for relatively small N, even with modern computers. In the IRT approach, a reaction time is generated for each pair of particles present in the system. After the reaction times are generated for all pairs in the system, they are sorted. The program then goes over all reaction times and performs the reactions, removing the reactants and replacing by the products. New reaction times are sampled between the remaining particles present in the system and the newly generated particles. The reaction times are then added in the sorted list, and the program then proceeds to the next pair of particles. Therefore, competition between possible reactions is accounted for by the reaction times. In this section, the generation of reaction times for each type of reaction is discussed.

### 17.2.5.1 Diffusion-controlled reactions

The probability of reaction $P_I(t \mid r_0)$ is the cumulative probability of $dP_I(t \mid r_0)/dt$ in time. This function is normalized as

$$W_\infty = \int_0^\infty \frac{dP_I(t \mid r_0)}{dt} dt = \frac{\sigma}{r_0}. \tag{17.26}$$

Since $r_0 > \sigma$ (the initial interparticle distance is greater than the reaction radius), $W_\infty < 1$, and the fraction of pairs that reacts is $W_\infty$. Random time values can be generated by assigning uniformly distributed random numbers $U$ to the probability of reaction, i.e.,

$$U = \frac{\sigma}{r_0} Erfc\left(\frac{r_0 - \sigma}{\sqrt{4Dt}}\right). \tag{17.27}$$

Time values are obtained by solving Equation 28 for $t$ ([15]):

$$t = \frac{1}{4D}\left[\frac{r_0 - \sigma}{Erfc^{-1}(r_0 U/R)}\right]^2 \text{ for } U < W_\infty \tag{17.28a}$$

$$t = \infty \text{ (no reaction) for } U \geq W_\infty \tag{17.28b}$$

A different algorithm can be developed by writing $dP_I(t \mid r_0)/dt$ explicitly ([27]):

$$\frac{dP_I(t \mid r_0)}{dt} = \frac{D\sigma(r_0 - \sigma)}{2\sqrt{\pi}r_0(Dt)^{3/2}} exp\left[-\frac{(r - r_0)^2}{4Dt}\right]. \tag{17.29}$$

Since $dP_I(t \mid r_0)/dt$ is proportional to a "Type V Pearson density," i.e.,

$$Cx^{-b}exp(-c/x)b > 1; c > 0; x \in [0, \infty), \tag{17.30}$$

random time values distributed as $dP_I(t \mid r_0)/dt$ can be obtained as $c/X$, where $X$ is distributed as Gamma(b-1), with $b = 3/2$. Gamma distributed random numbers can be generated by several techniques ([23]). Therefore, time values can be generated by using Algorithm 4. As random variates generated by Equation 29 or by Algorithm 4 are distributed as $dP_I(t \mid r_0)/dt$, the number of reactions predicted by the IRT method for 2-particles with diffusion-controlled reactions have the same distribution than those generated by the step-by-step method, provided that the time steps are sufficiently small.

---

**Algorithm 4: Generation of time values for $dP_I(t \mid r_0)/dt$ (diffusion-controlled reactions)**

SET $W_\infty = \sigma/r_0$
GENERATE $W$ uniform on [0,1]
IF ($W < W_\infty$) {
REPEAT {
GENERATE $U$ and $V$ uniform on [0,1]
} UNTIL $(U^2 + V^2) < 1$
GENERATE $E$ standard exponential
$G = EU^2/(U^2 + V^2)$
RETURN $T = (r_0 - \sigma)^2/(4DG)$
}
ELSE {
RETURN $\infty$ (no reaction)
}

---

## 17.2.5.2 Partially diffusion-controlled reactions

As for diffusion-controlled reactions, $P_{II}(t \mid r_0)$ is the cumulative probability of the distribution $dP_{II}(t \mid r_0)/dt$. The normalization is:

$$W_\infty = \int_0^\infty \frac{dP_{II}(t \mid r_0)}{dt} dt = \frac{1+\alpha}{r_0 \alpha}. \tag{17.31}$$

One way to generate random time values is by assigning a random number $U$ to $P_{II}(t \mid r_0)$:

$$U = \frac{\sigma\alpha+1}{r_0\alpha} \left[ Erfc\left(\frac{r_0-\sigma}{\sqrt{4Dt}}\right) - W\left(\frac{r_0-\sigma}{\sqrt{4Dt}}, -\alpha\sqrt{Dt}\right) \right] \text{ for } U < W_\infty \tag{17.32a}$$

$$t = \infty \text{ (no reaction) for } U \geq W_\infty \tag{17.32b}$$

In this case, Equation 33a has to be solved numerically for $t$. Alternatively, a sampling algorithm can be developed by writing $dP_{II}(t \mid r_0)/dt$ explicitly:

$$\frac{dP_{II}(t \mid r_0)}{dt} = \frac{-D(1+\sigma\alpha)}{r_0\sqrt{\pi Dt}} exp\left[-\frac{(r_0-\sigma)^2}{4Dt}\right] + \alpha\sqrt{\pi Dt}W\left(\frac{r_0-\sigma}{\sqrt{4Dt}}, -\alpha\sqrt{Dt}\right). \tag{17.33}$$

Using the explicit form of $dP_{II}(t \mid r_0)/dt$, an efficient algorithm (Algorithm 5) for sampling the values of $t$ can be used.

---

**Algorithm 5a. Generation of times values for $dP_{II}(t \mid r_0)/dt$ (partially diffusion-controlled reactions)**

SET $W_\infty = (\alpha'-1)/r_0\alpha'$
GENERATE $W$ uniform on [0,1]
IF ($W < W_\infty$) {
REPEAT {
GENERATE $X$ distributed as g* (Algorithm 5b)
GENERATE $U$ uniform on [0,1]
} UNTIL ($X \leq 2\beta/\alpha'$ and $U \leq \lambda(X)$) or ($X \geq 2\beta/\alpha'$ and $UM/X \leq \lambda(X)$)
RETURN $T = X/D$
}
ELSE {
RETURN $\infty$ (no reaction)
}

---

The second part of the algorithm is:

---

**Algorithm 5b.**

GENERATE $U$ uniformly on [0,1]
IF $U < p/(p+qM)$, SET $V \leftarrow U(p+qM)/p$ and $X \leftarrow (pV/2)^2$
ELSE SET $V \leftarrow (1-U)(p+qM)/qM$ and $X \leftarrow (2/qV)^2$
RETURN $X$

---

The quantity $\alpha'=-\alpha$, and $\beta = (r_0 - \sigma)/2$, $p = 2\sqrt{2\beta/\alpha'}$, $q = 2/\sqrt{2\beta/\alpha'}$ and $M = Max\left(1/\alpha'^2, 3\beta/\alpha'\right)$. The function $\lambda(X)$ is defined as:

$$\lambda(X) = e^{-\beta^2/X}\left[1 - \alpha'\sqrt{\pi X}\Omega(\frac{\beta}{\sqrt{X}} + \alpha'\sqrt{X})\right]. \tag{17.34}$$

where $\Omega(x) = \exp(x^2)\,Erfc(x)$.

### 17.2.5.3 Reactions involved charged particles

The reaction times for Type III reactions are simulated by using Algorithm 4 or by inversion (Equation 29), replacing $r_0$, $r$ and $\sigma$ by $r_{0eff}$, $r_{eff}$ and $\sigma_{eff}$ (Equation 16). Because $P_{III}(t \mid r_0)$ has a form similar to $P_I(t \mid r_0)$, so does $dP_{III}(t \mid r_0)/dt$, which is obtained by doing the same variable substitutions. Type IV reactions are simulated by using Algorithm 5, replacing the time coefficients in $a$ and $b$ as given by Equations 19 and 20. In this case, the distribution of times $dP_{IV}(t \mid r_0)/dt$ is

$$\frac{dP_{IV}(t \mid r_0)}{dt} = \frac{\sigma''_{eff}a}{r_{0eff}\sqrt{\pi t}}\,exp\left[-b^2\right] - a\sqrt{\pi}W(b,a). \tag{17.35}$$

Since $a \propto \sqrt{t}$ and $b \propto 1/\sqrt{t}$, the approaches used for type II reactions can be used with the appropriate modifications in the code.

### 17.2.5.4 Reactions with continuous background

For reactions with continuous background, the reaction time is obtained by $t = -\log(U)/k[B]$, where $U$ is a uniformly distributed random number between 0 and 1.

### 17.2.6 POSITION OF NEW PARTICLES AFTER A CHEMICAL REACTION HAS OCCURRED

When two particles initially at positions $r_1'$ and $r_2'$ react, the position of the new species (products) should be determined. The GFDE theory does not provide this information. As a first approximation, since the mean square displacement $r^2 \cong 6Dt$, the position of the reaction site $r_r$ is located between the two old particles, weighted by the diffusion coefficients ([28]):

$$r_r = \frac{\sqrt{D_2}}{\sqrt{D_1}+\sqrt{D_2}}r_1' + \frac{\sqrt{D_1}}{\sqrt{D_1}+\sqrt{D_2}}r_2'. \tag{17.36}$$

If there is one reaction product, it is placed at the position $r_r$. If there are two or more products, they are placed randomly around the reaction site $r_r$, separated by a distance equal to the reaction radius. Clifford et al. [26] developed another approach for the IRT method to calculate the position of two products after a chemical reaction. This method is also used for the SBS simulations and is recalled briefly here. Two vectors $S_1$ and $S_2$ are defined:

$$S_1 = r_1 - r_2; S_2 = r_1 + br_2. \tag{17.37}$$

The constant $b = \sigma_1^2/\sigma_2^2$, where $\sigma_i^2 = 2D_it$, and i=1,2, is chosen such that the vector $S_2$ diffuses independently from the separation vector $S_1$, meaning their covariance is equal to 0. Such a vector $S_2$ is generated by sampling a Gaussian random vector of mean 0 and variance $\sigma_1^2(1 + \sigma_1^2/\sigma_2^2)$:

$$S_2 = \left(r_1 + \frac{\sigma_1^2}{\sigma_2^2}r_2\right) + N_3\left[0, \left(\sigma_1^2 + \frac{\sigma_1^4}{\sigma_2^2}\right)1\right]. \tag{17.38}$$

The length of the vector $S_1$ is equal to the reaction radius $\sigma$. Thus, only its direction (described by the angles $\Theta$ and $\vartheta$ in a spherical coordinate system) is needed. Due to the cylindrical symmetry around $r'$, the angle $\vartheta$ can be generated by a uniform random number between 0 and $2\pi$ ($\vartheta = 2\pi U_1$) and the angle $\Theta$ is generated the following way:

$$\Theta = Cos^{-1} \left[ 1 + \frac{1}{\alpha} ln \left[ 1 - U_2(1 - \exp(-2\alpha)) \right] \right]. \tag{17.39}$$

Here $U_1$ and $U_2$ are two independent random numbers between 0 and 1, $r'$ is the initial distance between reactants, and $\alpha = Rr'/2Dt$. Then, the position vectors $r_1$ and $r_2$ of the new particles are obtained from $S_1$ and $S_2$ by inversion of Eq. 37:

$$r_1 = \frac{D_1 S_1 + D_2 S_2}{D_1 + D_2}; r_2 = \frac{D_2(S_2 - S_1)}{D_1 + D_2} \tag{17.40}$$

### 17.2.7  SIMULATION CODES

The radiation track structure and radiation chemistry has been simulated using many different codes: PARTRAC ([29]), KURBUC (Kyushu University and Radiobiology Unit Code) ([30]), Radamol ([31]), GEANT4-DNA ([32]), gMicroMC ([33]), IONLYS-IRT ([16]), RITRACKS (Relativistic Ion Tracks), and others. A discussion of the specifics of these codes is given in Plante 2021. However, many of these codes use similar approaches.

## 17.3  APPLICATIONS OF RADIATION CHEMISTRY SIMULATIONS

### 17.3.1  CALCULATION OF RADIOLYTIC YIELDS

One of the main endpoints calculated by radiation chemistry codes are the radiolytic yields. The yield for the species X is noted G(X), and is given as

$$G(X) = \frac{Number\ of\ species\ X\ created\ (or\ destroyed)}{100\ eV\ of\ deposited\ energy}. \tag{17.41}$$

This unit uses 100 eV as denominator, which corresponds to the energy deposited in a radiation spur.

#### 17.3.1.1  Time evolution

The time evolution of the radiolytic yields is the primary quantity calculated by radiation chemistry codes. For example, the radiolytic yields for 300-MeV protons tracks were calculated in earlier work (Plante 2011). More recently, the time evolution of the yields for 5 MeV protons have been calculated by the codes PARTRAC, GEANT4-DNA, and gMicroMC. The comparison with corresponding results from RITRACKS is shown in Figure 17.3.

With time, radical products (H. and $^\bullet OH$) decrease while molecular products ($H_2$ and $H_2O_2$) increase, indicating that chemical reactions are occurring. There are several differences between codes. The yields of the radiolytic species given by different codes are already different at $10^{-12}$s, which indicates that the track structures are calculated differently in the physical and physicochemical stages. The SBS and IRT methods, as calculated by RITRACKS, are in relatively good agreement, but some cases the discrepancy between methods grow with time.

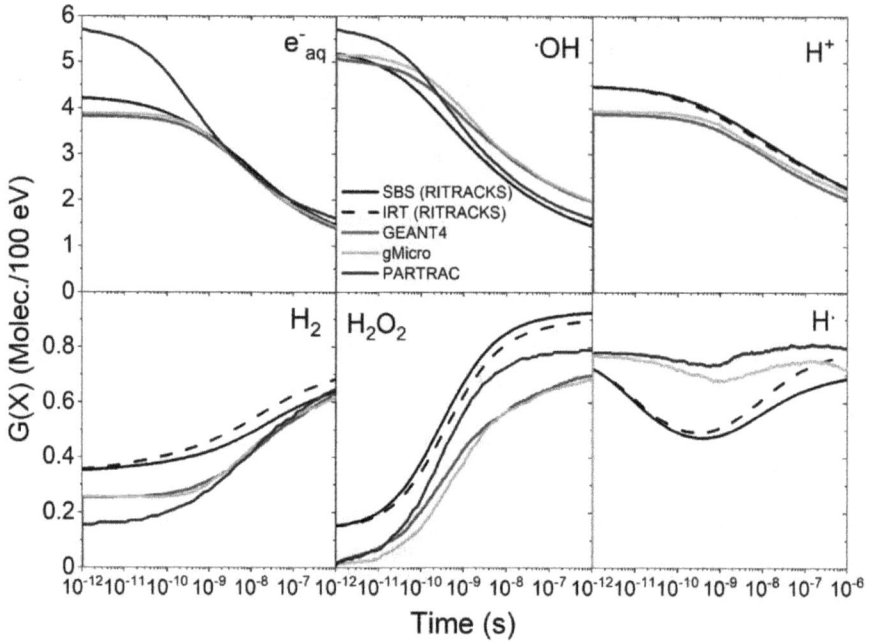

**Figure 17.3**   Time evolution of the yields of $H^\bullet$, $^\bullet OH$, $H_2$, $H_2O_2$, $e_{aq}^-$ and $H^+$ for 5-MeV protons, as calculated by the codes RITRACKS (SBS and IRT methods), GEANT4-DNA, gMicroMC, and PARTRAC. In some cases, the IRT and SBS results for RITRACKS are superimposed.

#### 17.3.1.2   Escape yields

The particles created in the track structure diffuse and react. Usually, the reactive species are distributed somewhat homogeneously about one microsecond after the passage of ionizing radiation. Therefore, the yields at one microsecond are considered important in radiation chemistry and radiobiology. The escape yield of species X is noted $G_X$. The escape yields of $H^\bullet$, $^\bullet OH$, $H_2$, $H_2O_2$, $e_{aq}^-$ and $H^+$ at $10^{-6}$ s have been calculated for 1–1000 MeV protons, with corresponding linear energy transfer (LET) 26.94–0.22 keV/μm, and α particles, of energies 0.25 to 1000 MeV/n, with LET 199.7–0.88 keV/μm. Results are shown in Figure 17.4, and compared to the results calculated by GEANT4, KURBUC, and experimental data.

The general trend of the results is as expected. The molecular yields increase and the radical yields decrease with LET due to the closer proximity of the radicals in the track structure. The results are also in agreement with experimental data and similar calculation results. The calculations obtained by the SBS and the IRT methods are slightly different. This difference was observed in former calculations ([27]). Some discrepancies exist between the GEANT4 and RITRACKS calculations; slightly more molecular products were calculated by GEANT4 than RITRACKS. For the molecular yields, KURBUC results are lower than those calculated by GEANT4 or RITRACKS.

### 17.3.2   CHEMICAL DOSIMETERS

Chemical dosimeters are interesting because they are relatively simple chemical systems that can be used to test theories and programs developed for radiation chemistry.

A very important system used in radiation chemistry is the Fricke dosimeter, developed in the 1920s ([40]Fricke and Morse 1927). This dosimeter typically includes a solution of 0.4 M $H_2SO_4$,

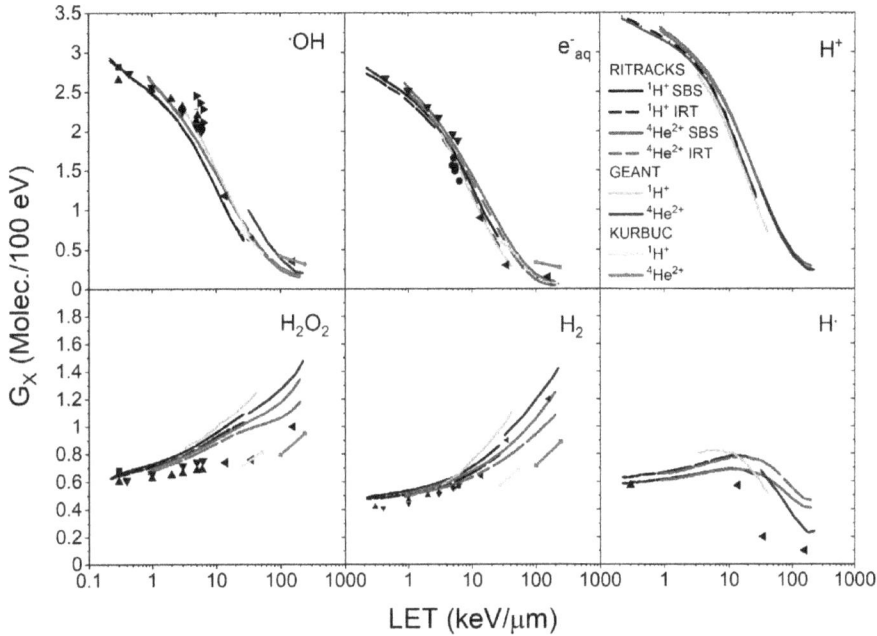

**Figure 17.4**    Primary yields of $H^\bullet$, $^\bullet OH$, $H_2$, $H_2O_2$, $e_{aq}^-$, and $H^+$ in neutral liquid water irradiated by protons (1000–1 MeV, LET 0.2–26.9 keV/μm) and alpha particles (1000-0.25 MeV/n, LET 199.7–0.88 keV/μm). Calculations by RITRACKS (SBS and IRT methods), GEANT4-DNA, and KURBUC. In some cases, the IRT and SBS results for RITRACKS are superimposed. Experimental values: Elliot et al. [34] (■), McCracken et al. [35] (▼), Burns and Sims [36] (▲), Naleway et al. [37] (●), Pastina and LaVerne [38] (◄), Sauer et al. [39] (►).

5 mM $FeSO_4$, with or without 0.25 mM $O_2$. In this dosimeter, the $Fe^{2+}$ ions react with the radicals, which leads to formation of $Fe^{3+}$. For low-LET radiation, in oxygenated medium, $G\left(Fe^{3+}\right) = 15.6$ Molec./100 eV. In deoxygenated medium, $G\left(Fe^{3+}\right) = 8.2$ Molec./100 eV. Molecular hydrogen is also produced $G\left(H_2\right) = 4.1$ Molec./100 eV. Simulations including relevant reactions were able to explain those yield values and the decrease of $G\left(Fe^{3+}\right)$ with increasing LET ([41]).

Another chemical dosimeter of interest is the ceric dosimeter. This dosimeter has played a significant role in the development and the understanding of radiation chemistry of water and aqueous solutions ([42]). Theoretical and experimental investigations have shown that the ceric-cerous dosimeter is sufficiently accurate and reproducible for reference dosimetry. Experimentally, optimal results are obtained by using a solution of 0.4 M $H_2SO_4$, $3\times10^{-5}$ M of $Ce^{4+}$ and $1\times10^{-5}$ M of $Ce^{3+}$ ([43]), with or without oxygen (0.25 mM). For this dosimeter, $G\left(Ce^{3+}\right) = 2.4$, regardless of the presence or absence of oxygen. Simulations were able to reproduce those yield values, including the dependencies with LET and concentration of $Ce^{3+}$ ([44, 45]).

### 17.3.3   DNA DAMAGE

Cellular DNA is damaged by both the direct and the indirect effects of ionizing radiation. In the "direct effect", the DNA itself is ionized, whereas the "indirect effect" involves the radiolysis of the solution surrounding the DNA and the subsequent reaction of the DNA with the radical products ([46]). Some types of damage are more biologically relevant because of the challenges they present to cellular repair mechanisms. These include DNA double strand breaks (DSBs) and other multiple damages that can be converted to DSB during attempted repair. The presence of a DSB can lead to loss of base sequences and/or can permit the two ends of a break to separate and rejoin with the wrong partner ([47]).

Extensive literature is now dedicated to radiation-induced DNA damage, notably simulated with the codes KURBUC, PARTRAC, and GEANT4. This topic is beyond the scope of this review; however, the theory described in this book chapter can be used to simulate indirect effects. Indeed, the rate constants are known for reactions between the radiolytic species $e_{aq}^-$, $^\bullet OH$ and $H^\bullet$ and the DNA bases (adenine, cytosine, guanine and thymine), and the sugar-phosphate backbone of DNA ([48]). Therefore, it is possible to simulate DNA that is damaged by radicals.

## 17.4  CONCLUSIONS

Radiation chemistry is of great importance in understanding radiation biology. Modeling approaches have been very successful in simulating the detailed chemical reactions induced by different types of ionizing radiations, notably those involved in chemical dosimeters. However, developing Monte-Carlo codes that simulate radiation interactions with matter is not easy. One prerequisite for radiation chemistry codes is a code that simulates the radiation track structure. This topic has been extensively studied, but some of the physics involved is still not well understood. A recent study (Peukert et al. 2019) has shown that all codes studied led to similar trends in yields, although the values are often significantly different. This also includes the yields at the beginning of the chemistry stage, which means that the track structures that are used as a starting point are different for each code. This shows that many topics pertaining to radiation track structure, notably on cross sections, still need to be investigated.

Regarding the simulation methods in radiation chemistry, the results obtained by SBS and IRT are slightly different. This difference was noted previously in model systems comprising one or two types of particles, notably those comprising charged particles ([27]). The difference between the IRT and SBS results, however, is smaller in acidic media (Plante 2011). Therefore, because hydrated electrons are quickly scavenged in acidic media, these results indicate that some improvements may be needed in the methods used to simulate the effects of charged particles. The effect of the reversibility of the reactions on results could also be studied. Of particular interest for reversible reactions is that the GFDE provides a distribution of interparticle distance of the products ([49]). A Green's function for the Debye-Smoluchowski equation for reversible reactions between charged particles could be useful to improve simulations, notably by providing a distribution of distances for the products. Several unsolved problems also exist regarding the GFDE. A closed form analytical expression for all GFDE expressions would be ideal, rather than an expansion on Legendre polynomials. Another topic of interest is to reconcile the results of the GFDE theory with the classical reaction kinetics. The GFDE theory presented in this chapter are based diffusion in an infinite medium. On the contrary, classical reaction kinetics are based on uniform concentrations of particles and imply closed systems. This is more similar to biological systems, in which the radiolytic species are generated in small compartments such as cellular organelles. This may strongly influence radiation chemistry at the cellular scale.

Writing radiation track structure and chemistry simulation codes from scratch does not appear to be a good investment of time nowadays. These codes require a tremendous amount of time and effort to build and validate, and many of the existing codes have a long history and have attained a high level of sophistication. Furthermore, many of the codes use very similar approaches, and several graduate students and researchers are therefore working on radiobiology projects building on open source codes. However, using open source codes can introduce several potential issues. First, it leaves the impression that the physics behind the radiation track structure, and the chemistry of water radiolysis and radiation, are fully understood, which may discourage research in this field. Secondly, because most users have not written the code themselves, without proper training, they may not fully understand the results that they obtain. Finally, it is more difficult to justify the creation of alternative codes, which reduces the diversity of available codes. Because the radiolysis of water is a complex problem with many aspects that are not fully resolved, it is good to have different approaches and perspectives to address it.

## ACKNOWLEDGMENTS

This work was supported by NASA grant number NNJ15HK11B.

## REFERENCES

1. Platzman R 1958 The physical and chemical basis of mechanisms in radiation biology *Radiation Biology and Medicine. Selected Reviews in the Life Sciences* ed W Claus (Addison-Wesley, Reading, MA) pp. 15–72.
2. Azzam E I, Jay-Gerin, J-P and Pain D 2012 Ionizing radiation-induced metabolic oxidative stress and prolonged cell injury *Cancer let.* **327** 48-60.
3. O'Neill P and Wardman P 2009 Radiation chemistry comes before radiation biology. *Int. J. Radiat. Biol.* **85** 9-25.
4. Aung S, Pitzer R M and Chan S I 1968 Approximate Hartree–Fock wave functions, one-electron properties, and electronic structure of the water molecule *J. Chem. Phys.* **49** 2071-2080.
5. Siegbahn H, Asplund L and Kelfve P 1975 The Auger electron spectrum of water vapour *Chem. Phys. Lett.* **35** 330-335.
6. Meesungnoen J and Jay-Gerin J-P 2005 High-LET radiolysis of liquid water with $^1$H$^+$, $^4$He$^{2+}$, $^{12}$C$^{6+}$, and $^{20}$Ne$^{9+}$ ions: effects of multiple ionization *J. Phys. Chem. A* **109** 6406-6419.
7. Goddard III W A and Hunt W J 1974 The Rydberg nature and assignments of excited states of the water molecule *Chem. Phys. Lett.* **24** 464-471.
8. Dingfelder M, Hantke D, Inokuti M and Paretzke H G 1998 Electron inelastic-scattering cross sections in liquid water *Radiat. Phys. Chem.* **53** 1-8.
9. Emfietzoglou D, Papamichael G and Nikjoo H 2017 Monte Carlo electron track structure calculations in liquid water using a new model dielectric response function *Radiat. Res.* **188** 355-368.
10. Ogura H and Hamill W H 1973 Positive hole migration in pulse-irradiated water and heavy water *J. Phys. Chem.* **77** 2952-2954.
11. Mozumder A and Magee J L 1975 The early events of radiation chemistry *Int. J. Radiat. Phys. Chem.* **7** 83-93.
12. Mozumder A 1988 Conjecture on electron trapping in liquid water. *Int. J. Radiat. Appl. Instr. Part C. Radiat. Phys. Chem.* **32** 287-291.
13. Elliot A J 1994 Rate constants and G-values for the simulation of the radiolysis of light water over the range 0-300 °C. Report AECL-11073. Atomic Energy of Canada Limited, Chalk River, Ontario
14. van Zon J S and ten Wolde P R 2005 Green's-function reaction dynamics: A particle-based approach for simulating biochemical networks in time and space *J. Chem. Phys.* **123** 234910.
15. Green N J B, Pilling M J, Pimblott S M and Clifford P 1990 Stochastic modeling of fast kinetics in a radiation track *J. Phys. Chem.* **94** 251-258.
16. Frongillo Y, Goulet T, Fraser M-J, Cobut V, Patau J-P and Jay-Gerin J-P 1998 Monte Carlo simulation of fast electron and proton tracks in liquid water - II. Nonhomogeneous chemistry *Radiat. Phys. Chem.* **51** 245-254.
17. Tomita H, Kai M, Kusama T, and Ito A 1997 Monte Carlo simulation of physicochemical processes of liquid water radiolysis *Radiat. Environ. Biophys.* **36** 105–116.
18. LaVerne J A, Štefanič I, and Pimblott S M 2005 Hydrated electron yields in the heavy ion radiolysis of water *J. Phys. Chem A* **109** 9393-9401.

19. von Smoluchowski M 1917 Mathematical theory of the kinetics of the coagulation of colloidal solutions *Z Phys. Chem.* **92** 129-168.

20. Collins F C and Kimball G E 1949 Diffusion controlled reaction rates *J. Colloid. Sci.* **4** 425-437.

21. Hong K M and Noolandi J 1978 Solution of the Smoluchowski equation with a Coulomb potential. I. General results *J. Chem. Phys.* **68** 5163-5171.

22. Clifford P, Green N J B and Pilling M J 1984 Analysis of the Debye-Smoluchowski equation. Approximations for the high-permittivity solvents *J. Phys. Chem.* **88** 4171-4176.

23. Devroye L 1986 Non-Uniform Variate Generation. (New York: Springer-Verlag).

24. Plante I, Devroye L and Cucinotta F A 2013 Random sampling of the Green's functions for diffusion-influenced reactions *J. Comput. Phys.* **242** 531-543.

25. Tachiya M 1983 Theory of diffusion-controlled reactions: Formulation of the bulk reaction rate in terms of the pair probability *Radiat. Phys. Chem.* **21** 167-175.

26. Clifford P, Green N J B, Oldfield M, Pilling M J and Pimblott S M 1986 Stochastic models of multi-species kinetics in radiation-induced spurs *J Chem Soc Faraday Trans 1* **82** 2673-2689.

27. Plante I and Devroye L 2017 Considerations for the independent reaction times and step-by-step methods for radiation chemistry simulations *Radiat. Phys. Chem.* **139** 157-172.

28. Bolch W E, Turner J E, Yoshida H, Bruce Jacobson K, Hamm R N, Wright H A, Ritchie R H and Klots C E 1988 Monte Carlo simulation of indirect damage to biomolecules irradiated in aqueous solution: The radiolysis of glycylglycine *Report No. ORNL/TM-10851* (Oak Ridge, TN: Oak Ridge National Lab).

29. Friedland W, Dingfelder M, Kundrát P and Jacob P 2011 Track structures, DNA targets and radiation effects in the biophysical Monte Carlo simulation code PARTRAC. *Mutat. Res. - Fund. Mol. M.* **711** 28-40.

30. Uehara S, Nikjoo H and Goodhead D T 1993 Cross-sections for water vapour for the Monte Carlo electron track structure code from 10 eV to the MeV region *Phys. Med. Biol.* **38** 1841.

31. Michalik V, Begusová M and Bigildeev E A 1998 Computer-aided stochastic modeling of the radiolysis of liquid water *Radiat. Res.* **149** 224-236.

32. Ramos-Méndez J, Perl J, Schuemann J, McNamara A, Paganetti H and Faddegon B 2018 Monte Carlo simulation of chemistry following radiolysis with TOPAS-nBio *Phys. Med. Biol.* **63** 105014.

33. Xun J 2017 Accelerated Monte Carlo simulation on the chemical stage in water radiolysis using GPU *Phys. Med. Biol.* **62** 3081–3096

34. Elliot A J, Chenier M P and Ouellette D C 1993 Temperature dependence of g values for $H_2O$ and $D_2O$ irradiated with low linear energy transfer radiation *J. Chem. Soc. Faraday Trans.* **89** 1193-1197.

35. McCracken D R, Tsang K T and Laughton P J 1998 Aspects of the physics and chemistry of water radiolysis by fast neutrons and fast electrons in nuclear reactors *Report AECL-11895* (Atomic Energy of Canada Ltd., Chalk River, Ontario).

36. Burns W G and Sims H E 1981 Effect of radiation type in water radiolysis. *J. Chem. Soc. Faraday Trans. 1* **77** 2803-2813.

37. Naleway C A, Sauer M C Jr, Jonah C D, and Schmidt K H 1979 Theoretical analysis of the LET dependence of transient yields observed in pulse radiolysis with ion beams *Radiat. Res.* **77** 47–61.

38. Pastina B and LaVerne J A 2001 Effect of molecular hydrogen on hydrogen peroxide in water radiolysis *J. Phys. Chem.* **105** 9316–9322.

39. Sauer M C, Schmidt K H, Hart E J, Naleway C A and Jonah C D 1977 LET dependence of transient yields in the pulse radiolysis of aqueous systems with deuterons and a Particles *Radiat. Res.* **70** 91–106.

40. Fricke H and Morse S 1927 The chemical action of roentgen rays on dilute ferrosulphate solutions as a measure of dose *Am. J. Roentgenol. Radium Therapy Nucl. Med.* **18** 430-432.

41. Autsavapromporn N, Meesungnoen J, Plante I and Jay-Gerin J-P 2007 Monte Carlo simulation study of the effects of acidity and LET on the primary free-radical and molecular yields of water radiolysis - Application to the Fricke Dosimeter *Can. J. Chem.* **85** 214-229.
42. Matthews R W 1971 An evaluation of the ceric-cerous system as an impurity-insensitive megarad dosimeter. *Int. J. Appl. Radiat. Isotopes* **22** 199-207.
43. Ferradini C and Pucheault J 1983 Biologie de l'Action des Rayonnements Ionisants (Paris: Masson)
44. Kohan L M, Meesungnoen J, Sanguanmith S, Meesat R and Jay-Gerin J-P 2014 Effect of temperature on the low-linear energy transfer radiolysis of the ceric-cerous sulfate dosimeter: A Monte Carlo simulation study *Radiat. Res.* **181** 495-502.
45. Plante I, Tippayamontri T, Autsavapromporn N, Meesungnoen J, and Jay-Gerin J-P 2012 Monte Carlo simulation of the radiolysis of the ceric sulfate dosimeter by low linear energy transfer radiation *Can. J. Chem.* **90** 717-723.
46. Jones G D D, Boswell T V, Lee J, Milligan J R, Ward J F and Weinfeld M 1994 A comparison of DNA damages produced under conditions of direct and indirect action of radiation *Int. J. Radiat. Biol.* **66** 441-445.
47. Ward J F 1994 The complexity of DNA damage: relevance to biological consequences *Int. J. Radiat. Biol.* **66** 427-432.
48. Martic C 2003 Modélisation des sommages radioinduits sur l'ADN : prise en compte des radicaux libres et des réparations primaires. PhD Thesis, Université de Toulouse III
49. Plante I and Devroye L 2015 On the Green's function of the partially diffusion-controlled reversible ABCD reaction for radiation chemistry codes *J. Comput. Phys.* **297** 515-529
50. Plante I 2020 A review of simulation codes and approaches for radiation chemistry. *Phys. Med. Biol.*

# 18 Recent developments in the TRAX particle track structure code

*Michael Kraemer*
GSI Helmholtz Centre for Heavy Ion Research GmbH, Darmstadt,
Germany

*Daria Boscolo and Martina Fuss*
GSI Helmholtzzentrum f. Schwerionenforschung Darmstadt,
Germany

*Emanuele Scifoni*
Emanuele Scifoni TIFPA-INFN Trento Institute for Fundamental
Physics and Applications, Trento, Italy

## CONTENTS

TRAX is a Monte Carlo particle track structure code realized in the early nineties. It was one of the first event by event radiation transport codes dedicated to particle beams for the nanoscale description of the specific dose deposition pattern. The code was continuously expanded and extended during the last 30 years at GSI, and applied in a series of different contexts. The main structure and methods of TRAX as well as its chemical extension TRAX-CHEM are here reviewed as an exemplary framework for treating physico-chemical processes on multiple scales, with a focus on its more recent extensions and applications, namely the study of high-Z material radioenhancement effects, and oxygen-radiation interplay at the nanoscale.

## 18.1 THE TRAX CODE

Among the several Monte Carlo codes for radiation transport, track structure codes are designed for nanoscopic description of a radiation track on an event by event basis. The major difference from the

DOI: 10.1201/9781003023920-18

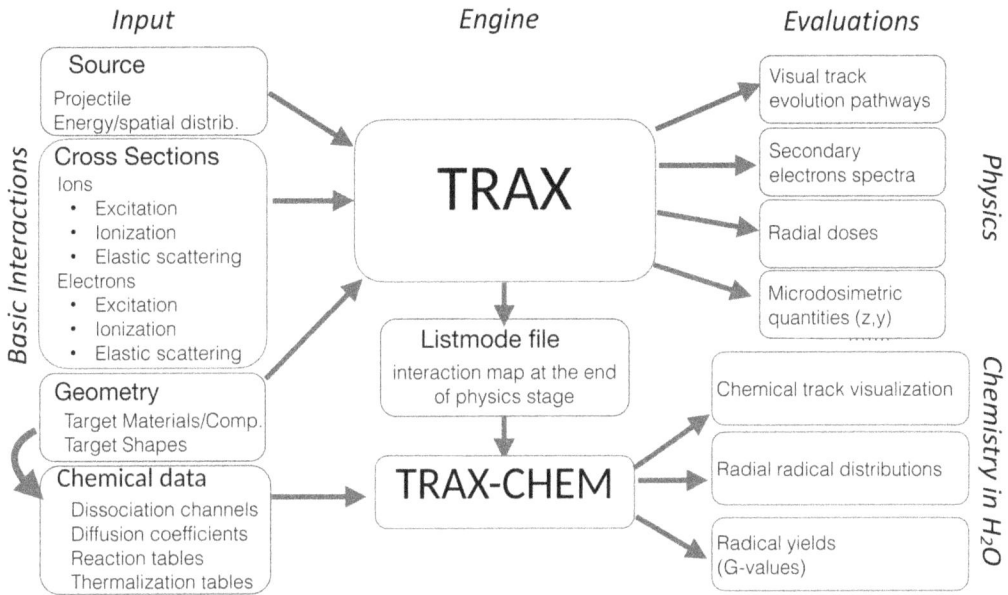

**Figure 18.1** Overview of the main structure of TRAX, including its extension module TRAX-CHEM.

"condensed history" codes is the detailed description of all interactions, without cut-off thresholds for electron energy propagation [1], at a price, on the other hand, of a larger computational cost. These codes don't allow the simulation of a complete beam, but rather focus on a specific "track segment" of the primary radiation. In this connection, TRAX, developed at GSI (Helmholtzzentrum für Schwerionenforschung), Darmstadt, in the early nineties, was one of the first codes dedicated to the description of charged particle tracks, with a focus to ion beams. This development was motivated especially by the need to understand the nanoscale features of energy deposition related to the "new" radiation explored in those years at GSI (the starting of the carbon ion scanning pilot project) and their impact on radiobiology and dosimetry [2]. From its first release in 1994 [3], TRAX was constantly expanded and extended during the last thirty years [2, 4, 5, 6].

The program has been designed (see Figure 18.1) to describe the propagation of electrons and ions (in all the possible charge states) through several different materials, ranging from simple atomic gases over molecules (compounds) to high-Z metals. All the trajectories are followed interaction by interaction, evaluating the different particles/species positions and energy depositions.

Several physical quantities may be straightforwardly evaluated by the program output, such as electron backscattering, transmission coefficients, electron energy and angular spectra and ionization distributions. Moreover, it is possible to compute other indirect quantities with high relevance for radiation type characterization and for dosimetry, such as radial dose and depth dose distributions and W-values. Finally, also micro-dosimetric quantities such as the lineal (y) and specific (z) energy transfer can be calculated.

The program covers a broad energy range, from a lower threshold between 1 and 10 eV (depending on the target material) for electrons, up to a few hundred MeV/u for ion beams. An example of TRAX calculation for protons and carbons is reported in Figure 18.2. Such a range is convenient for different applications ranging from dosimetric devices to biological systems. One of the key advantage of the code is its modular structure which makes it particularly suitable to different extensions, including different types of interactions, and even more advanced stages of radiation effect (see following section on TRAX-CHEM).

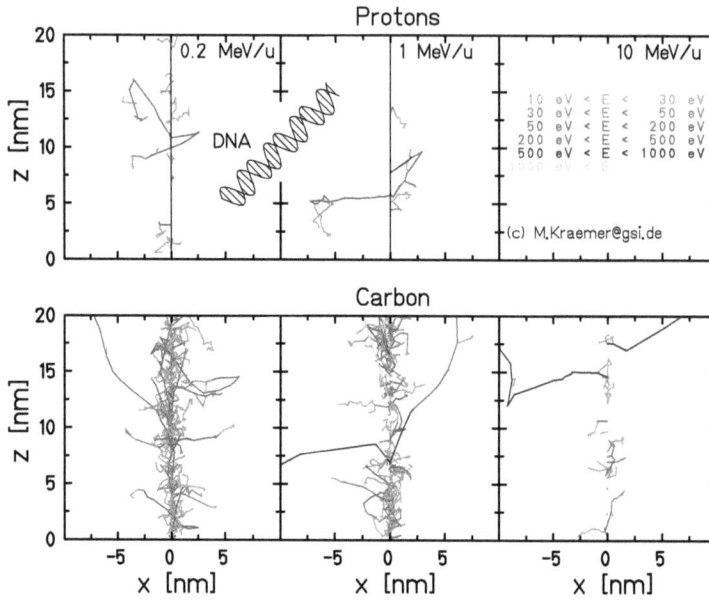

**Figure 18.2**   TRAX computed particle tracks for protons and carbon ions of different energies.

The simulation geometry is specified and included from an external file. These geometries can be combinations of different volumes (boxes, spheres, cylinders), composed by all the possible target materials compatible with TRAX, which can be atomic, molecular or a mixture of them. The different media are described by their physical properties, e.g., their density and information on their shell structure (including binding energies, number of electrons in a specific shell and corresponding kinetic energy). Parameters are taken from experimental values as far as possible. In the simulation dedicated to biological targets, water is considered as a tissue equivalent material.

The update of many available cross sections in TRAX, for different materials, and the comparison of simulations to experiment results (see Figure 18.3) is one of the most important recent advances of the code. In the next section, a brief overview of the cross sections for different interaction models implemented in TRAX is presented.

## 18.2   CROSS SECTIONS

In a track structure code, the availability of robust and trustworthy cross section models is of primary importance. The reliability and the accuracy of the whole simulation depend on the capability of reproducing all the possible interaction events, and thus on the selection of the cross section set. In particular, cross sections for electron interaction play a very important role. While the cross sections for ions are needed only to describe the interaction of the primary projectile, the electron cross sections are used also to simulate all the interactions of secondary and higher order electrons generated along the primary radiation trajectory, which make up the large majority of the final energy deposition.

TRAX supports cross sections for electron and (positive) ion projectiles, photons are envisaged for a future extension. As a surrogate, their secondary electron spectrum can be used as a source distribution [10]. Both projectile and target properties are specified via an external collection of plain text files, thus offering a high degree of flexibility without the necessity to rebuild the code. Target properties include shell structure and associated data such as Auger emission probabilities and fluorescence yields and may include excited states as well. TRAX so far considers the interactions

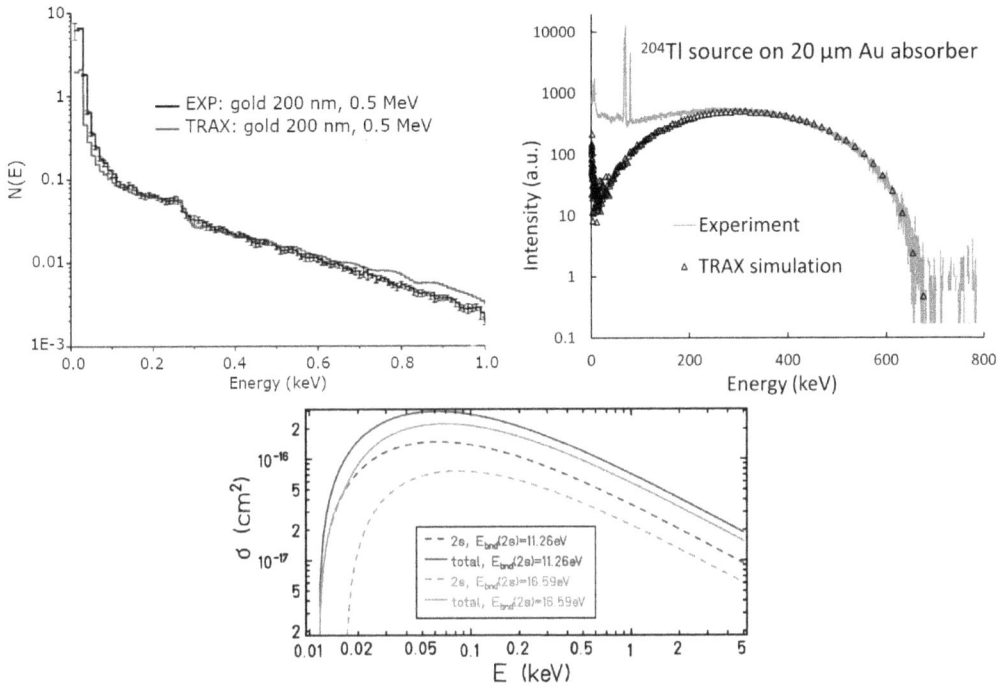

**Figure 18.3** Examples for TRAX cross section validation studies for different particles and absorbers: Upper left, comparison of experimental electron energy spectra with TRAX simulations for a gold foil irradiated with protons, adapted from [7]. Upper right, emission spectra from Tl-204 irradiation on a gold absorber from experiment (photons and electrons) and TRAX calculation (electron spectra), data from [8]. Lower panel, dependence of shell-specific electron ionization cross section values for a carbon target on binding energy, from [9].

elastic scattering, ionization, electronic, subelectronic and plasmon excitation. Bremsstrahlung is neglected for the time being. Nuclear fragmentation is implemented in the forthcoming version, for the purpose discussed here it is neglected since its cross sections are about eight orders of magnitude lower than the electromagnetic cross sections.

When the corresponding input data are available, both ionization and excitation can be treated in a shell-specific manner. This is a prerequisite for the simulation of Auger electron emission and for the determination of specific radical yields in water targets. Cross sections can be total (TCS), single differential (in energy or emission angle, SDCS) or double differential (in energy and emission angle, DDCS). These dimensionalities can exist in parallel for the same interaction. As an example, if a TCS is believed to be more accurate than a SDCS/DDCS, the overall interaction probability can be taken from the TCS, whereas the distribution is derived from the SDCS/DDCS. Cross sections can either be read from precompiled base data sets or created internally using a variety of models. In either case, interactions can be switched on or off by the user.

### 18.2.1  ELECTRON IONIZATION

Total electron induced ionization cross sections are obtained by the binary encounter Bethe (BEB) model [11]. This approach is based on a combination of the Mott theory, for hard collision processes, with the dipole interaction between the incident particle and the target electrons, for soft collisions. BEB provides shell specific electronic cross section without the need of empirical or fitting parameters. The model parameters are easily available for a large range of atomic materials: the electron shell occupation $N$, the shell specific binding energy $B$ and the kinetic energy of each bound electron $U$. The shell specific cross section then is:

$$\sigma(T) = \frac{S}{t + (u+1)/n} \left[ \frac{\ln(t)}{2} \left( 1 - \frac{1}{t^2} \right) + \left( 1 - \frac{1}{t} - \frac{\ln(t)}{t+1} \right) \right] \tag{18.1}$$

where T is the energy of the incident electron and $t = T/B$ and $u = U/B$ are dimensionless quantities. With the Bohr constant $a_0$=0.52918 Å and the Rydberg constant R=13.6057 eV, $S = 4\pi a_0^2 N (R/B)^2$. TRAX also provides a relativistic version of the BEB model, derived in [12].

## 18.2.2  ION IONIZATION

The Binary Encounter Approximation (BEA) is the basic method to obtain cross sections for ion induced ionization.

This approach treats the interaction of an incident, light and structureless, ion and the electron as a binary encounter between two free classical particles of velocity respectively $v_p$ and $v_e$ [3]. This condition is well met for small impact parameters between the incident and the target electron.

The mean kinetic energy of secondary electrons predicted by the BEA method is in the order of 50 to 100 eV with a maximum energy transferred in the case of forward scattering [3]. The approach allows the calculation of the ionization cross section for all possible combination of target and projectile but its range of application is restricted to light and structureless ions and is known to underestimate the backward emission at high energy, [3].

An empirical hybrid approach is available for selected materials. It implements the Rudd model [13] for TCS and SDCS, whereas the BEA is still used for the angular distribution. The Rudd model is derived from experimental data and thus it is available only for a restricted set of targets (He, Ne, Ar, Kr, $H_2$, $N_2$, $O_2$, $H_2O$, $CO_2$, $CH_4$, $C_3H_8$, $C_2H_4$ and C). Appropriate scaling procedures, however, allow approximations also for other targets.

For heavy projectiles with nuclear charge $Z_0$, an effective projectile charge $Z_{\text{eff}}$ is assumed according to the Barkas formula [14], in order to account for the effect of electron capture at low energy:

$$Z_{\text{eff}} = Z_0 \left[ 1 - exp\left( -125\beta Z_0^{-2/3} \right) \right]; \tag{18.2}$$

with $\beta = v/c$ where $v$ is the ion velocity and $c$ is the speed of light.

## 18.2.3  ELECTRONIC EXCITATION

Electron induced excitations play a major role in energy losses for electrons at energies lower than 100 eV. Recently the set of TRAX electronic excitation cross sections has been updated to support a broader range of target materials and to handle individual electronic transitions. This is important e.g. to simulate dissociation of excited molecules.

The angular deflection of an electron after an electronic excitation process is considered to be negligible. The excitation is thus considered to be an interaction where only an energy loss occurs, and the projectile electrons keep their propagation direction. The justification for this assumption comes from experimental results for electronic excitation in $N_2$, where a strongly forward peaked distribution of the electrons exciting molecular levels has been shown [15, 3].

### 18.2.3.1  Water targets

Water is often used as a proxy for biological systems, therefore a particular focus is here given to the model used to simulate it in the TRAX code. Excitation cross sections for electrons incident on water are calculated channel-specific and include single excited states [16, 17, 1]. In particular the

8 major excitation modes of $H_2O$ are considered: five molecular excitations ($A^1B_1$, $B^1A_1$, Rydberg A+B, Rydberg C+D and diffuse bands) and three dissociative channels ($H^*$ Lyman $\alpha$, $H^*$ Balmer $\alpha$ and $OH^*$). The energy losses required to reach these excited states range from 7.4 eV to 21.0 eV, detailed information can be found in [5].

In order to describe the transport of sub-excitation electrons, i.e. electrons having kinetic energies below the first excitation level of water, a set of cross sections down to the very low energies has been included in the TRAX cross section database, according to measurements in amorphous ice [18]. These cross sections include 9 possible channels of excitation leading to a certain vibrational, librational, translational, bending or stretching modes of the molecule and allow to reduce the cut off energy for electrons to 1.7 eV. In the latest extension of the TRAX code, these processes are treated as additional excitation channels. It should be noted, however, that the experimental data have an estimated uncertainty of 30-40% [1, 18].

Even though the contribution of the sub-excitation cross sections to the total stopping power is very small, the introduction of this additional channel results to be important for the implementation of the chemical extension of the code. It provides, indeed, information on the displacement of the sub-excitation electrons, when they are very close to their thermalization.

### 18.2.3.2 Gold targets

Among the different materials of particular interest for radiation biophysical modeling, gold targets gained importance as high Z nanoparticles were studied as possible local dose enhancers and sensitizers (for further details, see chapter 12). The electronic excitation cross sections for gold targets are obtained via measured collision strengths for the three most important electron transitions: from the ground state to the $(5d^{10}6p)^2P_{1/2}$ state with an energy transfer of 4.6 eV, from the ground state to the $(5d^{10}6p)^2P_{3/2}$ state ( $E = 5.1$ eV) and from the ground state to the $(5d^96s^2)^2D_{3/2}$ state with an energy loss of 2.7 eV [19, 20]. Since experimental data are available only up to certain energies, for higher energies the cross sections are extrapolated according to the Bethe-Born approximation [21].

Theoretical approaches exist to calculate the contribution of further transitions, however, it has been shown that these methods are able to reproduce the measured energy dependency but not the absolute cross section value: theoretical cross sections are larger than the measured values by approximately a factor two [19]. Thus, considering also that the higher lying electron shells are not expected to contribute significantly to the total excitation cross section, further transitions are neglected [21]. Recently a large part of the implemented cross section in TRAX have been revised and extended [21, 4, 22].

### 18.2.3.3 Excitation by ions

Ion excitation cross section are obtained by scaling the cross sections for electrons traveling at the same velocity. This latter approach is, strictly speaking, valid only for high-energy ions: in the case of protons for energies larger than 500 keV [23]. In the low-energy regions different approaches, such as the semiempirical model developed by Miller [24] based on the electron impact excitation, might yield more accurate results, but are currently not implemented.

### 18.2.4 ELASTIC SCATTERING

Elastic scattering processes do not contribute to dose deposition, however, they contribute significantly to the spatial distribution of energy and secondary chemical species around the primary particle trajectory. Especially in the low-energy region (few eV), they may well be the dominant interaction [3].

Screened Rutherford electron cross sections are the easiest way to calculate elastic cross sections, for a nucleus of charge $Z \cdot e$ [25]:

$$\frac{d\sigma}{d\Omega}(E, \theta) = \frac{Z^2 \cdot e^4}{4E^2(1 - cos\theta + 2\eta)^2}. \tag{18.3}$$

The screening parameter, $\eta$, accounts for the screening of the nuclear charge by the orbital electrons and can be calculated as suggested by Berger [25] : $\eta = Z^{2/3} \cdot 1.7 \times 10^{-5}\eta_c(1/\beta^2 - 1)$, where $\eta_c{}^1$ is a semi-empiric parameter [26].

The range of validity of the screened Rutherford cross sections is restricted to high projectile energies and low Z target material, according to the Born approximation ($v/c >> Z/137$, with $v$ being the particle velocity and Z the atomic number of the target).

For high Z material, PWA cross sections, often denoted as Mott cross sections, should provide a more realistic description. Unfortunately they are difficult to calculate because of the need of a correct description of the scattering potential and the summation of partial terms up to infinity. For selected materials and energies, PWA cross sections are available from the ELAST database. The latest version of TRAX uses precalculated single differential cross sections as a combination of screened Rutherford and PWA cross sections, the cross-over point e.g. for gold targets being 20 keV [21].

For some targets, e.g. water and $N_2$, empirical cross sections fitted to experimental data can be selected. In any case, screened Rutherford serves as a fallback approximation. For ion projectiles so far only screened Rutherford cross sections are implemented. For these projectiles, however, their elastic scattering is less important on the length scales discussed here.

### 18.2.5 AUGER ELECTRONS

Auger electrons are electrons which can be emitted during the relaxation process taking place after an ionization event. They play a significant role in the irradiation of high-Z material nanoparticles. The vacancy created by ionization is filled by an outer shell electron and the excess energy can be transferred either to a fluorescence photon (characteristic X-ray emission) or to another shell electron. This so-called Auger electron has a discrete energy corresponding to the difference between the binding energies of the shells involved and is emitted isotropically. The competing fluorescence probability depends on the atomic number and, for a K-shell ionization, it is approximately proportional to $Z^4$. For low Z materials, the photon production can be almost neglected while for high-Z atoms, such as gold, the probability of fluorescence emission after an ionization process in the K-shell reaches 97%. However, in high Z materials Auger electron cascades can occur: if an inner shell of these materials is ionized, Auger electrons are emitted until the vacancy has moved to the outermost shell. In TRAX, the production of Auger electrons, including cascades, has been implemented as described in Waelzlein [21]. The probability for different Auger transitions and fluorescence photons for atomic targets are taken from the Livermore Evaluated Atomic Data Library [27]. For water targets, Auger emission probabilities according to experimental data from [28] are used.

### 18.3 RADIATION CHEMISTRY SIMULATION WITH TRAX-CHEM

In the case of biological systems, the radiation effect extends also to the chemical stages, characterized by the production of radiation-induced free water radicals, which are considered to be the

---

[1]the formulation of the semi empirical screening parameter, $\eta_c$, in the original version of the code was incorrect, with little impact on the simulation results. However, recently the correct formulation of the $\eta_c$ parameter has been implemented and, in the present work, all the calculation have been performed with the revised elastic cross sections.

main responsibles of the so-called indirect effect of radiation. These radicals are produced as a consequence of water radiolysis and can be followed through their production, diffusion and interaction with dedicated track structure codes.

For simulating water radiolysis until chemical equilibrium is reached, Monte Carlo approaches normally follow the standard paradigm of radiation damage which classifies the chemical interactions into three stages characterized by a typical time scale.

- The physical stage corresponds to the direct effect of radiation and provides the spatial distributions of the ionized and excited water molecules and sub-excitation electrons. This stage is supposed to be complete $10^{-15}$ s after the particle passage through medium and it is the core part the standard version of the TRAX code as described above.
- The pre-chemical stage, consists in the dissociation and thermalization process of all ionized and excited water molecules and electrons produced during the physical stage. This stage lasts until approximately $10^{-12}$ s from the passage of radiation. This time point corresponds to the time needed for the longitudinal relaxation of water and represents an estimation to the time required for the hydration of an electron[2] in the lower sub-excitation energy range.
- The chemical stage, where the newly produced chemical species diffuse and react with each other and with the solvent until reaching an equilibrium at $\sim 10^{-6}$ s after the irradiation. At this time the chemical track development is typically finished and the radical yields can be assumed to be constant.

In the following sections, a more detailed description is provided on the methods used for modelling the pre-chemical and chemical stages in the chemical extension of TRAX: TRAX-CHEM [5, 6],

### 18.3.1  SIMULATION OF THE PRE-CHEMICAL STAGE

The pre-chemical stage of radiation consists in the dissociation and thermalization process of all the products generated during the physical stage of radiation: $H_2O^+$, $H_2O^*$, $e^-$. An accurate description of this stage, including the determination of the initial yield of the radiolytic products and the positions / mutual initial distances between nearby chemical species, is critical to properly simulate the time evolution and kinetics of the chemical track. Due to the lack of experimental data in this spatio-temporal time frame, this stage is subject to large uncertainties. For this reason in TRAX-CHEM dissociation and thermalization models are loaded by external tables making the code flexible to modification and updates of the implemented models. In the following, the methods used to describe the molecular dissociation and thermalization of hot fragments and the thermalization process of electrons will be shortly reviewed.

#### 18.3.1.1  Molecular dissociation and thermalization of hot fragments

The probability of ionized and excited water molecules to relax to the ground state or to dissociate following a specific dissociation channel depends on the particular ionization type or excited state. In a liquid environment, virtually all ionized water molecules can be considered to effectively dissociate according to reaction (a):

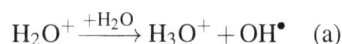

$$H_2O^+ \xrightarrow{+H_2O} H_3O^+ + OH^\bullet \quad (a)$$

---

[2]A aqueous or hydrated electron, $e_{aq}$, is a free electron in a water solution. It is the smallest possible anion and is the primary reducing radical formed upon water radiolysis. The thermalized electron occupies an excluded volume in the structure of liquid water, where, thanks to its negative charge, it forms hydrogen bonds with four to six water molecules, resulting in a cluster. In this form the aqueous electron acts as a molecular species.

For the case of excited water molecules, there is only fragmented experimental evidence about the quantitative differential production of chemical species from each excited state. In the TRAX-CHEM code, four possible dissociation patterns are included: auto-ionization (b), two dissociative decays (c) and (d) and relaxation to the ground state (e).

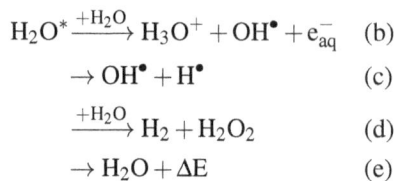

$$H_2O^* \xrightarrow{+H_2O} H_3O^+ + OH^\bullet + e_{aq}^- \quad (b)$$
$$\rightarrow OH^\bullet + H^\bullet \quad (c)$$
$$\xrightarrow{+H_2O} H_2 + H_2O_2 \quad (d)$$
$$\rightarrow H_2O + \Delta E \quad (e)$$

The dissociation scheme adopted is compatible with the information currently available when combining the experimental findings reported.

During the dissociation process, a small amount of energy is transferred to the dissociation fragments as kinetic energy. Only after releasing this energy and thermalizing with the medium the hot dissociation fragments start to behave as chemical species. In TRAX-CHEM this process is described as a single displacement of the radiolytic fragment with respect to the original position of the ionized or excited water molecule. Due to the absence of experimental observation able to provide quantitative information on the picosecond time resolution, thermalization distances have to be estimated and are usually validated by comparison to experimental yields of the species at later stages.

In TRAX-CHEM, the spatial relocation of the hot fragment is estimated based on measurements of the translational energy transferred to the hot fragment, during the dissociation process, $E_k$.

The thermalization distance for the different molecules is calculated representing the excess energy of the fragment as a thermal equivalent energy. A local increase in the system temperature will affect the diffusion coefficient and, consequently, the distance traveled in a fixed amount of time. For a system at temperature $\tau$, the diffusion coefficient, $D_\tau$, can be calculated according to the relationship $\frac{D_\tau}{\tau} = \frac{D}{T}$ with $D$ being the diffusion coefficient at room temperature $T$. The equivalent temperature $\tau$ of the dissociation fragment can then be calculated from $E_k = \frac{3}{2}k_B\tau$. The mean square displacement, $\lambda_\tau^2$, of a species after a time interval $\Delta t$ is obtained by applying the Einstein-Smoluchowski equation:

$$\lambda_\tau^2 = 6D_\tau \Delta t. \quad (18.4)$$

### 18.3.1.2 Thermalization and displacement of sub-excitation electrons

Sub-excitation electrons deposit their remaining energy through a series of vibrational excitations including librational, bending or stretching modes until they reach thermal equilibrium with the surrounding medium ($\sim 25$ meV). Once they are thermalized they form aqueous electrons, which behave similarly to a chemical species. The distance traveled by the sub-excitation electrons before thermalization depends on the initial electron energy.

The spatial distribution of the aqueous electrons plays a fundamental role in the simulations of the dynamics of chemical species along an ion track and extensive studies have been carried out using theoretical, stochastic and experimental approaches [29]. However, because of the scarce experimental information and the uncertainties on low-energy cross sections in liquid water, there is no general agreement between the different methods [30].

In TRAX-CHEM this process is described as a single step in a random direction. According to the initial energy, the mean free path of the sub-excitation electron before thermalizing is sampled from a 3D Gaussian distribution with mean value and FWHM selected following the energy dependent thermalization ranges suggested by [31].

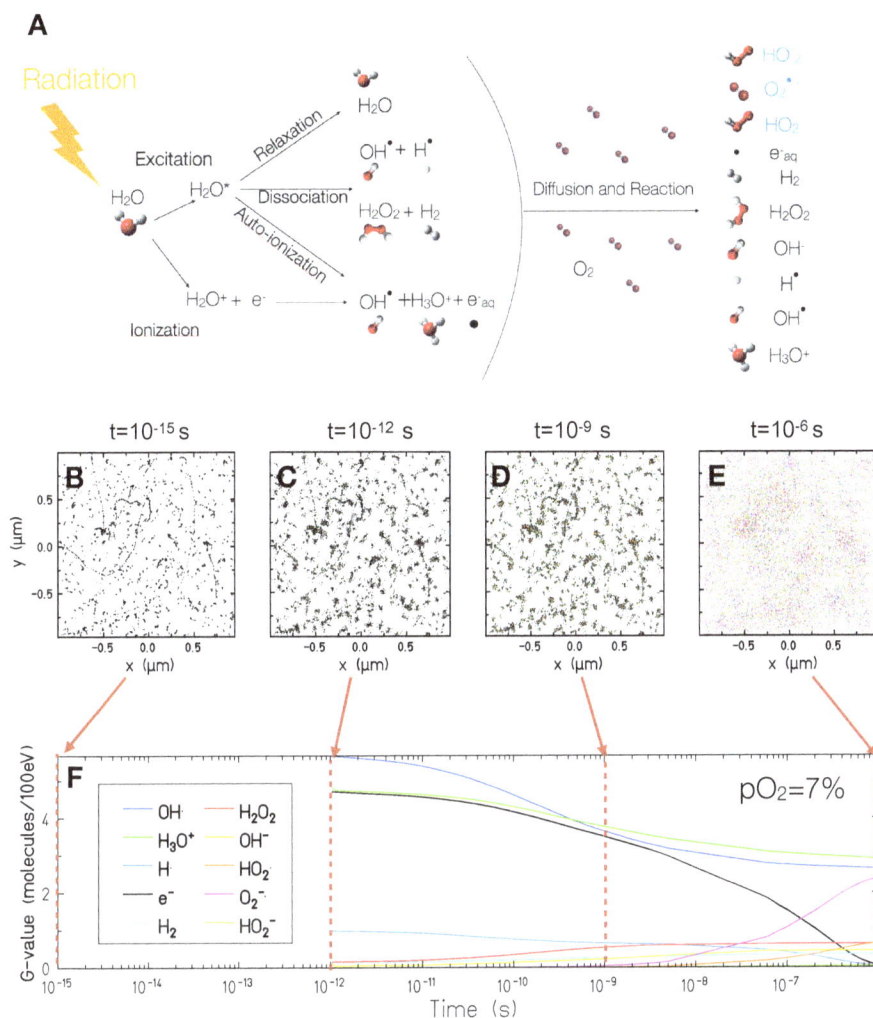

**Figure 18.4** Schematic of the main parts of the chemical track evolution until the end of the heterogeneous chemical stage (1 μs). The example corresponds to 1 MeV electrons.

## 18.3.2   SIMULATION OF THE CHEMICAL STAGE

During the chemical stage (Figure 18.4), all the radiolytic products start to diffuse and interact with each other until the track evolution is concluded. Two main approaches exist for Monte Carlo codes to describe the chemical track evolution: the so-called independent reaction time (IRT) technique and the step by step approach. The IRT approach is based on the initial separation of pairs of chemical species and the time evolution of their mutual (pair-wise) distance obtained from localization distribution functions, to give reaction times. This method is computationally fast, but does not allow to track the position of all the molecules as a function of time. In the step by step approach all the chemical species and their reactions are followed one by one during each simulation time step. This approach is more accurate but it is computationally heavier and can be up to hundred times slower than IRT methods. In TRAX-CHEM, this second method is used: the simulation time is divided into defined short simulation steps $\Delta t$ for which all the chemical species undergo two main processes: the radical diffusion and the chemical reactions.

The diffusion process is modeled as a jump in a random direction where step size is sampled from a 3D Gaussian distribution with root mean square displacement given by $\lambda = \sqrt{6D\Delta t}$. Reactions are described by a proximity parameter $a$, the reaction radius. The reaction takes place if the distance between the reactants at a given time step is smaller then $2a$. For diffusion-controlled reactions the reaction radius $a_{AB}$ for two species $A$ and $B$ is calculated based on the species diffusion coefficients $D_A$ and $D_B$ respectively, according to the Smoluchowski theory, as

$$a_{AB} = \frac{k_{AB}}{4\pi(D_A + D_B)}. \tag{18.5}$$

When a reaction takes place, the two reactants are removed from the simulation and replaced by the corresponding reaction products.

### 18.3.3  SIMULATION IN OXYGENATED TARGETS

Additionally to the possibility of simulating the particle chemical track evolution in water, the TRAX-CHEM code can also include reactions with solute molecules dissolved in the target material, e.g. molecular oxygen which is particularly relevant for studying important radiobiological effects such as the oxygen radiosensitization effect or the influence of reactive oxygen species e.g. in FLASH applications.

Differently from the other species, which are explicitly included in the code and treated with the step by step approach, mentioned above, the molecular oxygen can be assumed to be homogeneously distributed in the target and is treated as a continuum. This approximation, proposed by [32, 33], is necessary to limit the computational cost of the simulations. Under the assumption that the global oxygen concentration does not change during the track evolution (i.e., the amount of oxygen consumed during the track evolution is small compared to the total molecular oxygen dissolved in the simulation volume), the interaction probability is sampled based on the initial oxygen concentration. Given a certain solute concentration $c_s$, the probability $\Omega(t)$ that a molecule will not have interacted with the solute molecules can be described by the rate equations:

$$\frac{d\Omega(t)}{dt} = -k(t)c_s\Omega(t) \tag{18.6}$$

where $k(t)$ is a time dependent rate coefficient depending on the diffusion coefficient and reaction rates of the analyzed molecule and solute material.

## 18.4  OUTLOOK

For many applications (see Figure 18.5) that aim to connect radiation chemistry to a biological effect, simulations in pure or oxygenated water and concluding at $1\,\mu s$ after physical irradiation can become a limiting aspect. While the current ab initio method links heterogeneous stage effects successfully to relevant macroscopic, experimental results such as radiolytic oxygen depletion of sealed targets [34], additional features could significantly enhance the applicability of TRAX-CHEM to living cells or tissues. Water is a convenient target medium for simulations and a necessary basis to be validated, but a biological target is different in many ways, e.g. the existence of cellular targets sensitive to chemical damage, reactions of radiolytic species with target molecules competing with those in water, the buffered pH condition, and the presence of small-molecule or enzymatic scavengers for removing cytotoxic species. Even primary radical interactions can change in presence of high concentrations of competing biomolecular species and form organic radicals $R^\bullet$, which in turn react with dissolved oxygen producing $ROO^\bullet$.

A meaningful quantification of these and other relevant reactions at longer times in the chemical track evolution is however more conveniently performed with a simulation based on the homogeneous species concentrations instead of explicit single molecules. In a biochemically more realistic

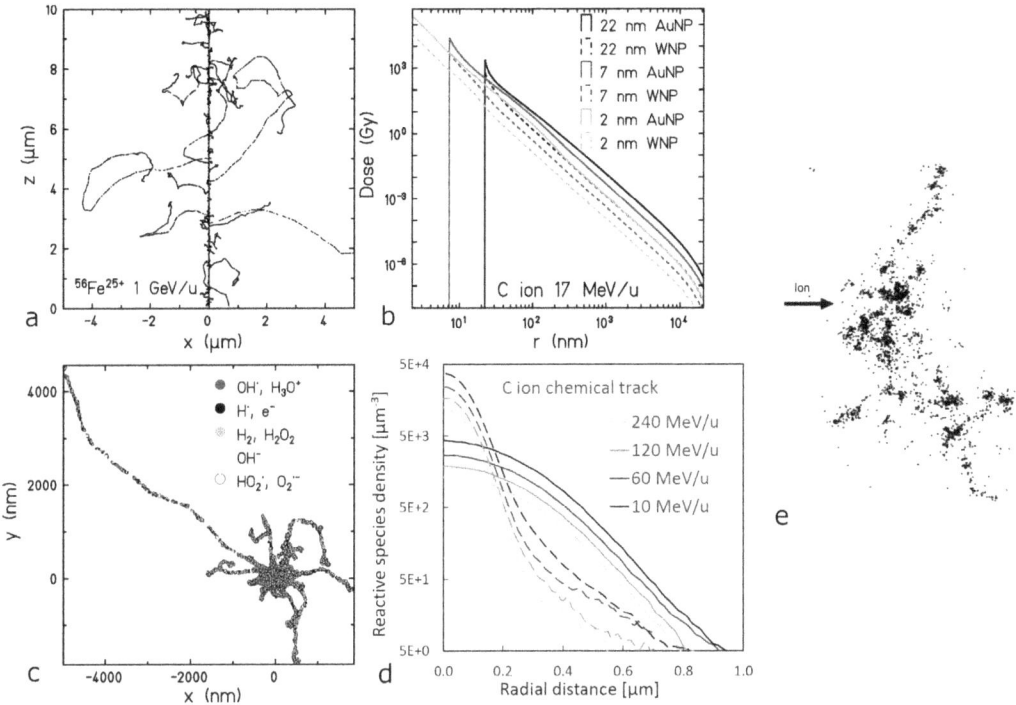

**Figure 18.5** Examples of recent applications of the TRAX and TRAX-CHEM codes. (a) Physical track of a 1 GeV/u Fe ion and its secondary electrons; (b) radial dose around different sizes of gold (AuNP) or water (WNP) nanoparticles hit by a 17 MeV/u C ion; (c) chemical track of a 10 MeV/u C ion at 10 ns into the diffusion-reaction evolution; (d) radial distributions of reactive chemical species around C ions at different energies at 1 ns and 10 ns; (e) visualization of radiolytic radicals produced around an ion-irradiated gold nanoparticle.

model, it is also desirable to extend the radiation chemical simulations until longer time scales, e.g. a few ms where the oxygen effect becomes effective biologically. The mentioned functionalities are currently under evaluation and development for a future extension.

## REFERENCES

1. H. Nikjoo, S. Uehara, D. Emfietzoglou, and F.A. Cucinotta. Track-structure codes in radiation research. *Radiation Measurements*, 41(9):1052–1074, 2006. Space Radiation Transport, Shielding, and Risk Assessment Models.

2. Michael Krämer and Marco Durante. Ion beam transport calculations and treatment plans in particle therapy. *The European Physical Journal D*, 60(1):195–202, 2010.

3. M. Krämer and G. Kraft. Calculations of heavy-ion track structure. *Radiation and Environmental Biophysics*, 33(2):91–109, Jun 1994.

4. C Wälzlein, M Krämer, E Scifoni, and M Durante. Advancing the modeling in particle therapy: from track structure to treatment planning. *Applied Radiation and Isotopes*, 83:171–176, 2014.

5. D Boscolo, M Krämer, M Durante, MC Fuss, and E Scifoni. Trax-chem: A pre-chemical and chemical stage extension of the particle track structure code trax in water targets. *Chemical Physics Letters*, 698:11–18, 2018.

6. Daria Boscolo, Michael Krämer, Martina C Fuss, Marco Durante, and Emanuele Scifoni. Impact of target oxygenation on the chemical track evolution of ion and electron radiation. *International Journal of Molecular Sciences*, 21(2):424, 2020.

7. F Hespeels, S Lucas, T Tabarrant, E Scifoni, M Krämer, G Chêne, D Strivay, H N Tran, and A C Heuskin. Experimental measurements validate the use of the binary encounter approximation model to accurately compute proton induced dose and radiolysis enhancement from gold nanoparticles. *Phys. Med. Biol.*, 64:065014, 2019a.

8. A Williart, A Muñoz, D Boscolo, M Krämer, and G García. Study on tl-204 simultaneous electron and photon emission spectra and their interaction with gold absorbers. Experimental results and Monte Carlo simulations. *Nucl. Instrum. Meth. A*, 927(435–442), 2019.

9. Cathrin Wälzlein. *Nanometer scale description of electron transport and damage in condensed media using the TRAX Monte Carlo Code*. PhD thesis, TU Darmstadt, 2014.

10. Tamara Buch, Emanuele Scifoni, Michael Krämer, Marco Durante, Michael Scholz, and Thomas Friedrich. Modeling Radiation Effects of Ultrasoft X Rays on the Basis of Amorphous Track Structure. *Radiation Research*, 189(1):32–43, 01 2018.

11. Yong-Ki Kim and M. Eugene Rudd. Binary-encounter-dipole model for electron-impact ionization. *Physical Review A*, 50:3954–3967, Nov 1994.

12. Yong-Ki Kim, José Paulo Santos, and Fernando Parente. Extension of the binary-encounter-dipole model to relativistic incident electrons. *Physical Review A*, 62(5):052710, 2000.

13. M E Rudd. Differential cross sections for secondary electron production by proton impact. *Phys. Rev. A*, 38:6129–6137, 1988.

14. Walter H Barkas. *Nuclear Research Emulsions*, volume 1. Academic Press, 1963.

15. Sandor Trajmar, David F Register, and Ara Chutjian. Electron scattering by molecules II. Experimental methods and data. *Physics Reports*, 97(5):219–356, 1983.

16. Herwig G Paretzke. *Simulation von Elektronenspuren im Energiebereich 0, 01-10 keV in Wasserdampf*. Gesellschaft für Strahlen-und Umweltforschung mbH München, 1988.

17. AES Green and RS Stolarski. Analytic models of electron impact excitation cross sections. *Journal of Atmospheric and Terrestrial Physics*, 34(10):1703–1717, 1972.

18. M. Michaud, A. Wen, and L. Sanche. Cross sections for low-energy (1-100 eV) electron elastic and inelastic scattering in amorphous ice. *Radiation Research*, 159(1):3–22, 2003.

19. M. Maslov, M. J. Brunger, P. J. O. Teubner, O. Zatsarinny, K. Bartschat, D. Fursa, I. Bray, and R. P. McEachran. Electron-impact excitation of the $(5d^{10}6s)^2S_{1/2} \rightarrow (5d^{10}6p)^2P_{1/2,3/2}$ resonance transitions in gold atoms. *Physical Review A*, 77:062711, Jun 2008.

20. O Zatsarinny, K Bartschat, Maxim Maslov, Michael James Brunger, and PJO Teubner. Electron-impact excitation of the $(5d^{10}6s)^2S_{1/2} \rightarrow (5d^96s^2)^2D_{5/2,3/2}$ transitions in gold atoms. *Physical Review A*, 78(4):042713, 2008.

21. C Wälzlein, E Scifoni, M Krämer, and M Durante. Simulations of dose enhancement for heavy atom nanoparticles irradiated by protons. *Physics in Medicine & Biology*, 59(6):1441, 2014.

22. C Wälzlein, M Krämer, E Scifoni, and M Durante. Low-energy electron transport in non-uniform media. *Nuclear Instruments and Methods in Physics Research Section B: Beam Interactions with Materials and Atoms*, 320:75–82, 2014.

23. Michael Dingfelder, Mitio Inokuti, and Herwig G Paretzke. Inelastic-collision cross sections of liquid water for interactions of energetic protons. *Radiation Physics and Chemistry*, 59(3):255–275, 2000.

24. JH Miller and AES Green. Proton energy degradation in water vapor. *Radiation Research*, 54(3):343–363, 1973.

25. Martin J Berger et al. Monte Carlo calculation of the penetration and diffusion of fast charged particles. *Methods in Computational Physics*, 1:135–215, 1963.

26. S Uehara, H Nikjoo, and DT Goodhead. Cross-sections for water vapour for the Monte Carlo electron track structure code from 10 eV to the MeV region. *Physics in Medicine & Biology*, 38(12):1841, 1993.

27. ST Perkins, DE Cullen, MH Chen, J Rathkopf, J Scofield, and JH Hubbell. Tables and graphs of atomic subshell and relaxation data derived from the LLNL Evaluated Atomic Data Library (EADL), Z= 1–100. Technical report, Lawrence Livermore National Lab., CA (United States), 1991.

28. H Siegbahn, L Asplund, and P Kelfve. The auger electron spectrum of water vapour. *Chemical Physics Letters*, 35(3):330–335, 1975.

29. Jintana Meesungnoen, Jean-Paul Jay-Gerin, Abdelali Filali-Mouhim, and Samlee Mankhetkorn. Low-energy electron penetration range in liquid water. *Radiation Research*, 158(5):657–660, 2002.

30. F. Ballarini, M. Biaggi, M. Merzagora, A. Ottolenghi, M. Dingfelder, W. Friedland, P. Jacob, and H. G. Paretzke. Stochastic aspects and uncertainties in the prechemical and chemical stages of electron tracks in liquid water: a quantitative analysis based on Monte Carlo simulations. *Radiation and Environmental Biophysics*, 39(3):179–188, Sep 2000.

31. M. Zaider, M.G. Vracko, A.Y.C. Fung, and J.L. Fry. Electron transport in condensed water. *Radiation Protection Dosimetry*, 52(1-4):139–146, 1994.

32. Simon M. Pimblott, Michael J. Pilling, and Nicholas J.B. Green. Stochastic models of spur kinetics in water. *International Journal of Radiation Applications and Instrumentation. Part C. Radiation Physics and Chemistry*, 37(3):377–388, 1991.

33. N. J. B. Green, M. J. Pilling, S. M. Pimblott, and P. Clifford. Stochastic modeling of fast kinetics in a radiation track. *The Journal of Physical Chemistry*, 94(1):251–258, 1990.

34. D Boscolo, E Scifoni, M Durante, M Krämer, and M C Fuss. May oxygen depletion explain the FLASH effect? A chemical track structure analysis. *Radiother. Oncol.*, 2021.

# 19 Machine learning for Monte Carlo simulations

*Tommaso Boccali*
Istituto Nazionale di Fisica Nucleare (INFN) Section of Pisa, Pisa,
Italy

*Carlo Mancini Terracciano*
Sapienza University of Rome, Rome, Italy
National Institute for Nuclear Physics (INFN) Section of Rome,
Rome, Italy

*Alessandra Retico*
Istituto nazionale di Fisica Nucleare (INFN) Section of Pisa, Pisa,
Italy

## CONTENTS

Computing techniques loosely based on mimicking the behavior of the human brain are becoming more and more important in a vast range of applications. Their utilization is not new, with studies based on simple Neural Networks (for example, [1, 2, 3]) dating back at least to the 80s; what is instead quite recent is the possibility to deploy efficient computing architectures, often specifically built to be optimal for such tasks.

At the same time, the capability to deploy larger and larger system has triggered theoretical studies, driving to more solid bases and to the definition of more complex and specialized models.

In these chapter we will start with an introduction to the models most relevant for Monte Carlo simulations, followed by a selection of applications. In the last part of the chapter, we will review strong and weak points about the utilization of Neural Networks applications for Monte Carlo simulations.

## 19.1 INTRODUCTION TO NEURAL NETWORKS

Neural Networks are a specific branch of the Artificial Intelligence (AI) domain in Computer Science. They get their inspiration from the fact that humans are evidently able to fulfill complex tasks; hence, by replicating the low-level mechanisms of the human brain on computing systems, one can potentially construct high level algorithms with similar capabilities.

### 19.1.1 THE HUMAN BRAIN

Neglecting any functional description, the human brain can be described as an organ composed by neurons, glial cells, neural stem cells and blood vessels. In our current understanding, the neurons are the units performing basic "operations" within the human brain, and their aggregated response is responsible for the high-level behavior typical of humans. A neuron is composed of three main units: a number of dendrites, the soma (the cell body), and an axon; the total size largely varies between different types of neurons; the neurons used for cognitive functions (as those in the grey matter of the brain) are usually short, of the order of 10 mm [4]. Functionally, a neuron is able to generate an electric response on the axon (*output*), depending on the electrical potential present at the synapses (*inputs*) on the dendrites. Neurons can be chained by connections between axons and dendrites, generating a configuration in which N neurons are connected via M synapses. The high-level response of the human brain to stimuli is understood to come from the complexity of such connections, with a standard human brain featuring $\sim 10^{11}$ neurons each with 7000 synapses, for a total of $\sim 10^{15}$ synapses; as we will see in the following, the brain can be interpreted as a complex mathematical system with $10^{15}$ degrees of freedom.

In literature various models of the neuron behavior have been proposed [5, 6]; here, we will focus on the simplest yet most simple to implement in computer systems [7] (see Figure 19.1): in

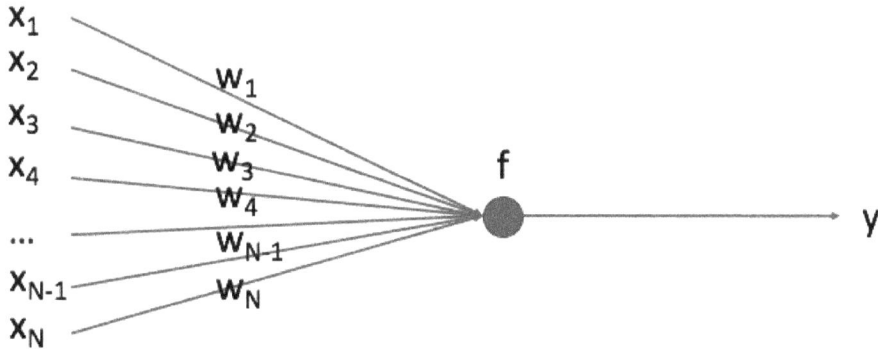

**Figure 19.1** The artificial neuron.

this model, the *output* y signal at the axon is assumed to be a function of the *inputs* $x_i$ via

$$y = f\left(\sum_{i=1}^{N} w_i x_i\right) \tag{19.1}$$

where $w_i$ are weights modeled after the chemical potentials at the synapses, and the function $f$ wants to model the non linearity of response of biological neurons with the *inputs*; on top of this, the function $f$ is needed in the mathematical model in order to allow the description of non linear phenomena [8]. The perceptron [9], one of the first models used in literature to model Neural

Networks, uses a very similar model, with a simplified $f$ function which is simply

$$f(\mathbf{x}) = \begin{cases} 1 & \text{if } \sum_{i=1}^{N} w_i x_i > 0 \\ 0 & \text{otherwise} \end{cases} \tag{19.2}$$

In modern systems, two modifications are typical when using Neural Networks:

- the addition of a further synapse $x_0$ which is always 1, used as a bias to the system; its weight is referred to as $x_0$ or $b$ (as in *bias*).
- the use of continuous $f$ non linear functions, as logistic or hyperbolic [10] functions, in order to model non binary signals.

Neural networks are designed by combining multiple neurons in *networks*, usually in a layered structure: one layer is used to map the inputs, a few/many layers are *hidden*, and a single layer is used to to map the outputs. On top of that, more complex neurons can be used, for example including a "memory" cell, or presenting a recurrent behavior by reusing its output as one of the inputs. A full description of all the type of neurons and networks is beyond the scope of this chapter; in the following, the ones most relevant to Monte Carlo simulations will be presented with more detail. For reference, still, a quite complete classification of currently relevant neural networks is shown in Figure 19.2.

As visible there, some network topologies have a high number of hidden layers. While the Universal Approximation Theorem [8] states that, under quite generic conditions, a single hidden layer between inputs and outputs should be enough in all cases, networks used in science during the last decade tend to be "deep" (i.e. with many hidden layers) [11]. This has multiple motivations: on one side, the theorem states that it is possible to have just one hidden layers, but does not state with how many neurons (and it tends to be a very large number); on the other side, a deep structure tend to be better human readable, with cascade sub networks with identifiable and logical roles. Hence, relevant networks in today's science tend to be deep.

The typical utilization pattern for a majority of network topologies is to feed them as input a large set of data representing the problem of interest, be it a medical image, a set of features or any output from the instrumentation, and at the same time provide the "expected output" from a so-called training set.

In the simplest type of networks, the responses from the neurons in the hidden and the final layers are considered in sequence (inputs to outputs), with each layer *feeding* the following layers; hence the name Feed Forward Neural Networks (FFNNs).

During the training, the network adjusts its internal free degrees of freedom (the weights $w_i^j$ in equation 19.1, extended to the $j$ neurons in the various layers) to better reproduce the desired answers, via minimization procedures which can be either numerical or analytical and involve the definition of a loss function to be explicitly minimized. Typical loss function can be simple weighted differences between the networks results and "expected results," but functional forms like cross entropy and mean square errors are more typical [12].

What has just been described is the training process for *supervised* Neural networks, which rely on an externally provided "truth" to adjust for optimal performance, without having any a-priori knowledge or description of the physical process they want to reproduce. Other topologies describe instead *unsupervised* Neural Networks, in which the training process just implies the utilization of datasets without the need to provide the correct answers (which can be unknown). Examples of such networks will be provided in Section 19.1.4.1.

## 19.1.2 CONVOLUTIONAL NETWORKS

Convolutional networks (CNNs) are a useful subset of neural networks, which exhibit peculiar characteristics of showing response space invariant with respect of the inputs.

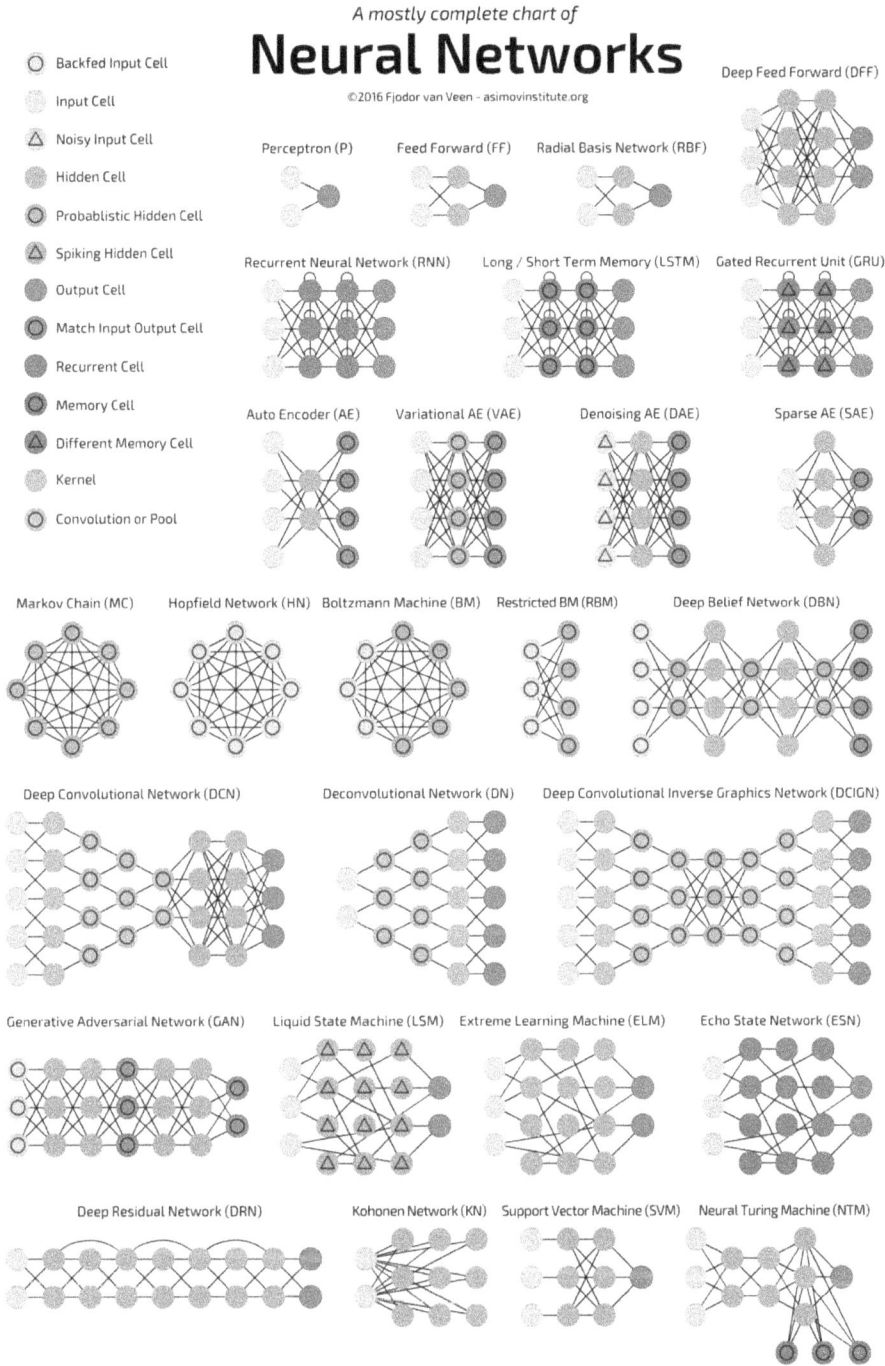

**Figure 19.2** Types of neurons and neural networks currently relevant in literature (Copyright F. van Veen 2016).

CNNs use basic neurons as explained in Section 19.1.1, with those in the hidden layers fed by small portions of the inputs per iteration, thus realizing spatial independence. As depicted in Figure 19.3, multiple application of several convolutional layers and pooling layers drive to an overall analysis on the inputs, and to the final outputs. Inputs can be either one dimensional (e.g. vectors of features), two dimensional (e.g. images) or multidimensional arrays. CNNs are used with success in categorization problems, where specific structures, must be discovered into a set of input data: a typical example is the identification of images with lesions in medical imaging, where CNN classifiers are trained on reported images by clinicians [13].

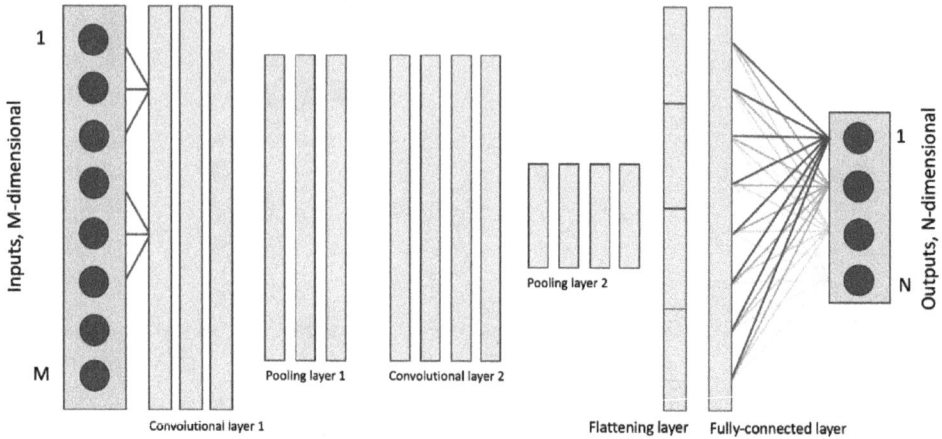

**Figure 19.3**   Basic structure of a CNN.

CNNs are particularly interesting in the realm of Monte Carlo simulations, since the space invariance is a valuable characteristics: the energy deposition of a particle into a material does not depend on the specific entry point nor on its direction.

### 19.1.3   RECURRENT NETWORKS

The CNNs above described are a type of *stateless* network, in which the output depends only (given a static set of weights) on the inputs presented on the first layer. In Recurrent Neural Networks (RNNs), the response to a specific input feature set also depends on the history of the network, i.e. the inputs presented at prior times; as such, the network presents a "memory," which can be used to correlate multiple inputs in sequence. A typical utilization pattern is in the presence of inputs of variable length, which cannot be estimated *a priori*, like in the analysis of text or speech sequences. In simulation processes, the feature is often utilized when the signals from a non fixed number of inputs (i.e. the incoming particles to a volume) must be piled up in a coherent way: the inputs per each particle are presented to the network, with a specific input pattern which may or may not be used to signal the end of the sequence.

### 19.1.4   GENERATIVE MODELS

The networks popular up to 10 years ago were mostly useful during decision processes, such as categorizing inputs (signal vs background, for example) or counting and defining specific regions inside it (segmentation, counting of lesions, etc.).

In order to be applied to Monte Carlo simulations, instead, the capability to produce ("generate") an output as close as possible to reality, or to a more standard algorithm is essential. In order to do this, different network topologies and strategies for training are relevant.

### 19.1.4.1 Auto-encoders and variational auto-encoders

The autoencoders are a family of unsupervised Neural Networks designed to learn a lower dimensional representation (say N dimensions) out of a set of data (with M dimensions, M > N). The N dimension representation ("latent space") can be seen as coming from an "understanding" of internal patterns and correlations in the initial data.

The easiest form of autoencoder has the number of inputs and outputs equal to M, and an internal hidden layer at dimensionality N. The training is obtained by forcing the network during training to reproduce as close a possible the input features at the output layer, thus requesting the N-dimension space to be as perfomant as possible when representing the M-dimension inputs (see Figure 19.4).

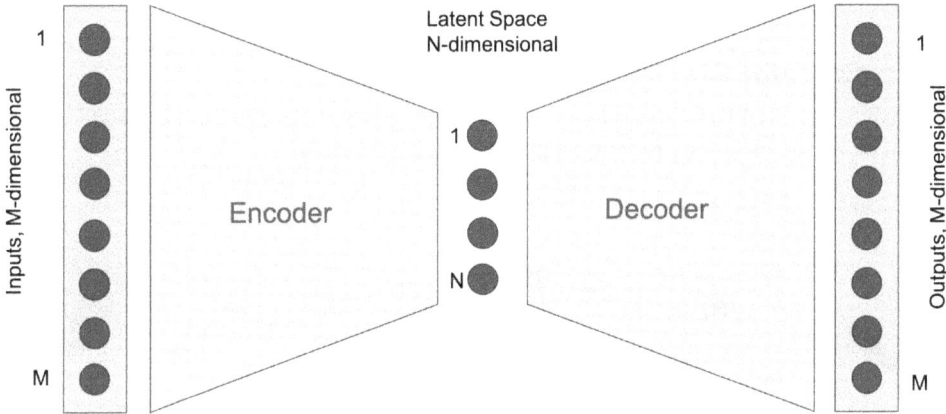

**Figure 19.4** An autoencoder in its simplest form.

Autoencoders in such form are used for two distinct purposes:

* auto-discover in the inputs hidden symmetries or underlying correlations, which can be used, for example, in lossy compression [14] or to drive understanding on the inputs themselves;
* since the network is trained on a specific data sample, it will minimize the difference outputs vs inputs on that specific dataset. Once the same network is presented with "different" data, it is expected to fail to reproduce the inputs at the outputs; hence, it can be used to detect anomalous inputs, such as corrupted input samples in medical imaging analysis pipelines [15] or not expected events in High Energy Physics [16].

Auto-Encoders are only able to reproduce the elements of the training set but not to interpolate among them; Kingma and Welling [17] introduced the Variational Auto-Encoder (VAE) class of algorithms, or more correctly "Auto-Encoding Variational Bayes" methods as they are more related to Variational Bayesian methods then to Auto-Encoders. The main differences of VAEs with respect to AEs is that VAEs encodes the input into a probability density function (PDF) rather than a point in the latent space; in this way, close points in the latent space generate events similar to each other. This is essential if willing to use VAEs as generators, as in Monte Carlo simulations: a sampling of the latent space "close" to the training configurations can be used to generate "valid" output configurations. In standard AEs, instead, only the precise points in the latent space where the the training set inputs have been encoded can be safely used to generate outputs.

As said, VAEs, once trained to generate elements from points sampled nearby the latent space position where the training set events are encoded, can be used to *generate* realistic data, interpolating or extrapolating from the training set events; this make them very useful for the generation of Monte Carlo simulations.

The loss functions of AEs is a "distance" between the input element and the one generated in output; in VAEs there is another term, typically a Kullback-Leibler (KL) [18] divergence, that measures the distance between the encoding PDF and a reference PDF, usually a Normal distribution.

There is no guarantee that the latent space gets optimally organized with respect to the input features. However, it has been shown [19] that increasing the coefficient of the KL term in the sum of the two loss function addenda, increases the probability that the VAE learns a disentagled representation of the input. This hyper parameter is usually referred as $\beta$ and this modification of the VAE, $\beta$-VAE.

VAEs tend to produce outputs blurred with respect to inputs, however, they have the great advantage that it is possible, especially with $\beta$-VA, to control the features of the generated output and to interpolate with continuity between two input samples.

### 19.1.4.2   Generative adversarial networks

Generative Adversarial Networks (GANs) are a recent [20] class of networks designed to reproduce the behavior of complex systems without an explicit programming.

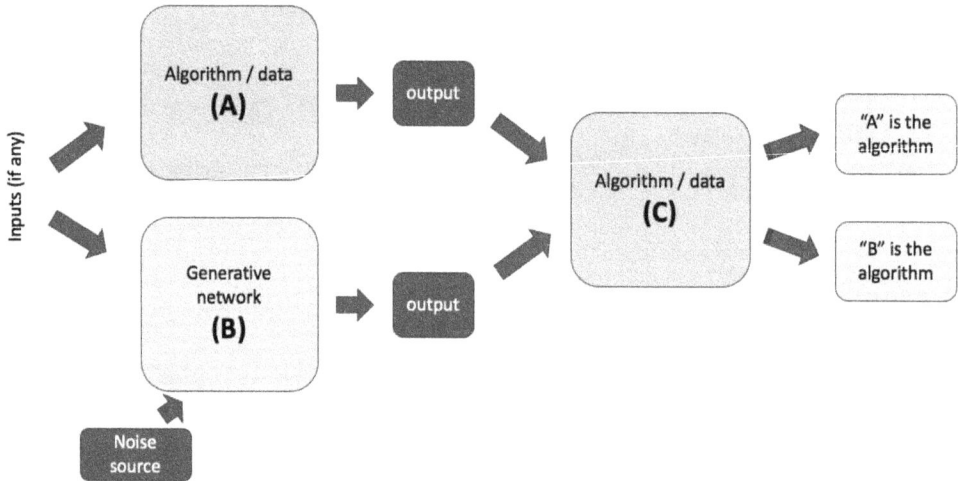

**Figure 19.5**   The structure of a simple GAN.

The method (see Figure 19.5) implies putting in competition a reference algorithm (or real data, A) with a generative network (B), which produces an output with the same structure and whose response, initially, is sampled from a random space. A second network (C) is trained on the capability to distinguish between the algorithm's output and the generated one. The two networks are put in competition (hence the term *adversarial*), with B "winning" if it can convince C that its response is the real one; in the opposite case, C wins. The tension between the two networks pushes the network B to generate outputs which are indistinguishable from the real data / the output of the algorithms. B and C are generic networks, with convolutional neural structures mostly used.

GANs are more and more used when in the need for replicating the behavior of a known data source, with improved computing performance. Upon successful training, in fact, the network B has the typical speed of (say) a CNN, and is able to reproduce the output of A, which can be a complex and time consuming algorithm. Successful examples are the famous generation of realistic faces [21], the capability to reproduce the showering of particles in calorimeters [22], or for for beam source modelling in Radiation Therapy linacs [23].

### 19.1.4.3 Graph networks

In a quite general category of problems, the task is to discover the relations between objects; in the segmentation of medical images, for example, there is the need to understand whether certain areas are part of a specific organs. Clusterization algorithms in many science realms is another example [24]. The most used network architecture for these use cases is a Graph Neural Network (GNN, [25]). In a GNN, nodes (representing objects) and edges (representing connections between nodes) are the basic entities, and the training process aims to correctly categorize the nodes, via an assessment of the strength of each connection. GNNs are finding large applications in cases where one wants to replace a complex, combinatorial algorithms with a Neural Network: typical examples in literature are jet clustering in High Energy Physics [26], and tracking in dense particle environments [27].

## 19.2 EXAMPLES OF APPLICATIONS FOR MONTE CARLO SIMULATIONS

### 19.2.1 EMULATION OF RADIATION-MATTER INTERACTIONS

One of the most complex tasks in Monte Carlo simulations involving the use of detectors (medical apparatuses, particle physics detectors) lies in the dual need of being able to optimize the design before detector construction, and to simulate the behavior under working conditions after the setup has been prepared. In both cases, unless the setup is very similar to existing detectors, extensive Monte Carlo simulations of the expected detector capabilities are the widely used solutions. Various such tools exist (Geant4 [28], Fluka [29], MCNPX [30]), with different application regimes and specific utilization patterns. As a general rule, these implement iteratively basic radiation-matter low-level processes to a knowledge of the detector setup, including materials, geometry and other experimental conditions; as such, they incur into two general limits:

- a scarce capability to be tuned to experimental results, by changing the basic modelling of the processes;
- a large to very large need for computational resources, given the iteration oriented approach and the need to increase the level of iterations in order to obtain a better precision and adherence to data.

Both limitations can in principle be surpassed via the use of Artificial Intelligence oriented tools. In presence of experimental data, the response of the AI system can be tuned to that without any explicit modelling of the physics processes; speed can be vastly improved by the change from iteration-based computations to standard Deep Learning matrix algebra, with its intrinsic capabilities for high performance processing on, for example, GPU systems.

As an example, we want to consider here CaloGan [22], an attempt to reproduce the details of radiation-matter interactions in the complex setup of segmented (3 layers) electromagnetic calorimeters. A Generative Adversarial Network, as those presented in Section 19.1.4.2, is used in conjunction with an as-accurate-as-possible Geant4 simulation of the same experimental setup. The generator side accepts in input particles' 4-momenta, and, after the passage through quite standard convolutional (matching the detector response as 2-D images) and dense layers, the output is compared with detailed Geant4 simulations of particles with the same parameters. The training optimizes the energy deposition per layer and per 2-D transverse cell, in a way in principle suited also for using real data in input. Results are very encouraging, even in an extreme detector scenario: not only the quantities of direct training are well reproduced, but also secondary and derived quantities like shower shapes are in most cases well described.

Results are shown in Figure 19.6 for the explicit targets of the calculation (2-D layered images of the energy deposits, in the specific case of incoming positrons).

Interestingly, one can look into quantities derived from shower shapes, but not directly targeted by the GAN training step, like for example the energy weighted shower depth. As we will see in

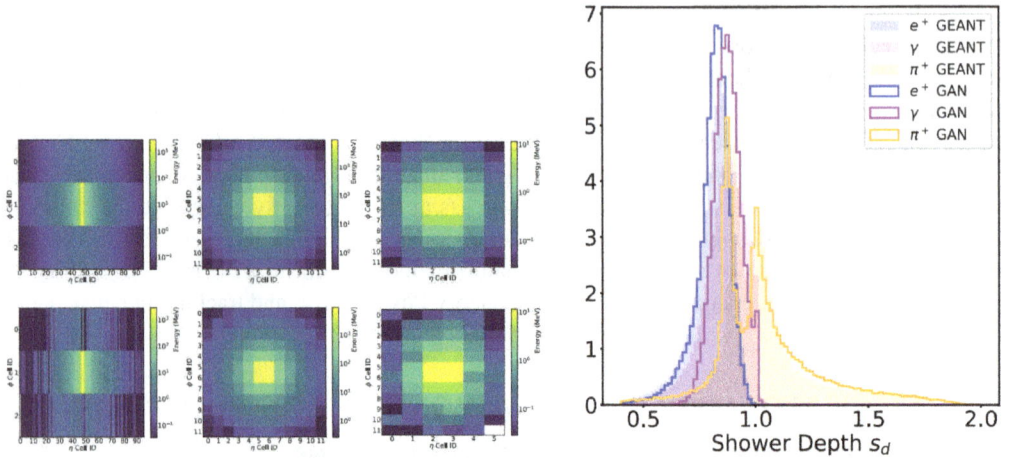

**Figure 19.6** (left) Average e$^+$ Geant4 shower (top), and average e$^+$ CALOGAN shower (bottom), with progressive calorimeter depth (left to right). (right) Energy weighted shower depth (in a.u.) from CaloGan and Geant4 detailed simulations. (From [22]).

Section 19.3.1, in general one cannot assume these quantities will be perfectly reproduced; in this specific case, though, the agreement level is quite impressive.

A second similar attempt, applied to the not-yet existing CLIC proposed electromagnetic and hadronic calorimeter, is presented in [31], with the goal to directly reproduce 3-D signals in a highly granular calorimeter. The reference dataset, in absence of real data, has the form of Geant4 generated showers sampled in a 25x25x25 cells around the impinging particle. Figure 19.7(left) shows the longitudinal shower shapes for 100 GeV electrons in the electromagnetic part of the calorimeter compared with detailed Geant4 simulations. The level of agreement is very satisfactory. Figure 19.7(right) shows a pictorial rendering of the expected energy deposit by a 100 GeV electron in the calorimeter.

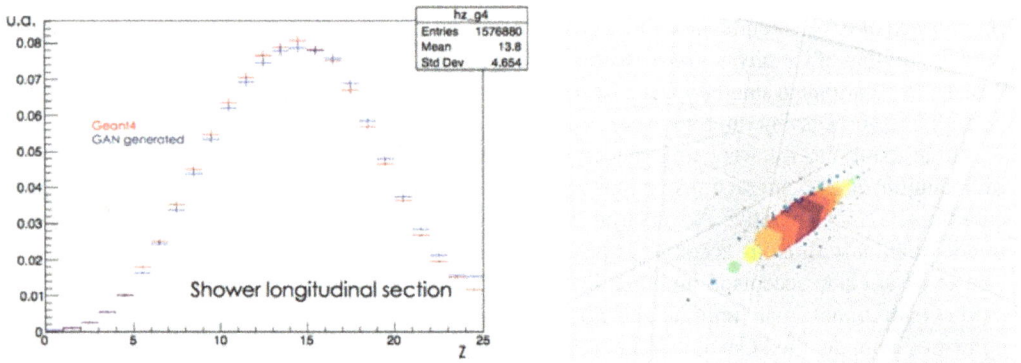

**Figure 19.7** (Left) Longitudinal shower shapes for 100 GeV electrons: GAN result is compared to full Geant4 simulation. The Z coordinate indicates the bin index in the longitudinal direction. (Right) The three-dimensional representation of an energy shower created by a 100 GeV electron as generated by the GAN, using particle type as conditioning information. (From [31]).

In sections 19.3.1 and 19.3.2 we will discuss about the speed gain with respect to standard methods, and solutions and needs to prevent unphysical results.

The last two examples are related to High-Energy particle Physics, however, a similar approach can be used also to emulate the energy deposition in a voxel geometry, such as the CT of a patient.

In the field of hadron therapy, strong requirements are imposed on the accuracy in predicting the range of the treatment field in patients, and the development of patient specific dose verification methods is highly desired. Positron Emission Tomography (PET) imaging can be used to monitor the activity generated in the body tissues by the interaction with the therapeutic hadronic beams. Attempt to establish the correlation between the activity measured with a PET detector and the dose released to tissues have been carried out by utilizing machine learning techniques based on RNN in the study by Hu et al. [32] and on GAN in the study by Ma et al. [33]. Imaging the prompt gamma radiation is another approach to dose monitoring in hadron therapy. A deep learning based conversion of the prompt gamma information into proton dose distribution has been proposed by Liu et al. [34].

### 19.2.1.1 Emulation of detector responses

Monte Carlo tools like Geant4 are designed to simulate, as accurately as possible, the energy deposition (in keV, for example) due to the passage of particle / radiation in the material of a detector. In real life, what a scientist measures is instead the response, as analog or digital signals, of a measuring device in which energy deposition is read and processed by some electronic boards. In classical systems, the simulation of radiation-matter must be followed by an ad-hoc simulation of the electronic readout system, in order to be compared with actual readings from a detector. In the case of AI inspired tools, this can be avoided by completely bypassing the "energy deposition" output results, and training the system directly with real or realistic (from the above ad-hoc simulation) signals from the electronic back-end (see Figure 19.8).

MC simulations are also frequently used to estimate the efficiency and the geometrical acceptance of a detector, or a system of detectors. The simulation of a Single Photon Emission Computed Tomography (SPECT) is usually done in two steps: the first one simulates the interactions of the produced photons with the patient, producing as output the emerging photons; and the second one simulates the response of the collimator-detector system to the emerging photons. This second step is called Angular Response Function (ARF). Sarrut et al. [35] used a GAN to emulate the ARF. The DL algorithm takes as input the incidence angles of the photon and its energy and gives back the probability of detecting it in one of the possible energy windows. In summary, the DL algorithm emulates the detector system, including the collimators.

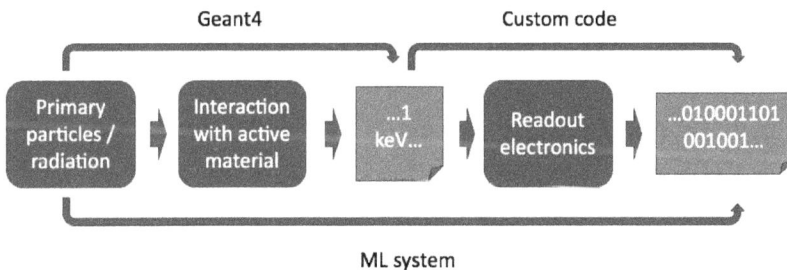

**Figure 19.8**  Difference between classical and AI inspired simulation of experimental setups.

### 19.2.2  EMULATION OF NUCLEAR INTERACTION MODELS

Nuclear reactions models are one of the most demanding part of a MC simulation in terms of running time. Despite the large running time, the models already available in toolkits made to develop MC simulation, such as Geant4, have shown severe limitations in reproducing experimental data below 100 MeV/u [36]. Models developed by theoreticians for this energy domain can be interfaced with Geant4 with good results [37], however their running time is even larger. Ciardiello et al. [38] obtained encouraging preliminary results in emulating one of the state-of-the-art models for low-energy nuclear reactions with a VAE. The model in question is BLOB ("Boltzmann-Langevin One Body") [39], which simulates the first part of the nuclear reaction, i.e. from the contact of the two nuclei until the energy of the nucleons composing the fragments is balanced among them. The BLOB output is a PDF of finding a nucleon in a given position of the phase space. The authors trained a VAE in reproducing the BLOB prediction in the interaction of two $^{12}$C nuclei at 62 MeV/u. For this purpose, they discretized and reduced the dimensionality of the BLOB output to use 3D convolutional layers. In detail, the dimensionality reduction uses the fact that in the reaction in exam BLOB predicts at most three large fragments, i.e. larger than one nucleon. Therefore, they divided the PDF produced by BLOB in three PDFs, one per large fragment, and associated all the nucleon emitted in the first part of the reaction to one of these three large fragments. In this way they used the three color channels of convolutional layers to represent each of the possible large fragments. In spite of controlling the generative part, they trained a classifier for the event impact parameter ($b$) jointly with the VAE itself. This joint training helps the VAE in learning a the task, given the large sparsity of the input, and forces the latent space in being organized with respect to the impact parameter. Moreover, it will be possible to sample from the latent space deciding the impact parameter of each generation. Figure 19.9 shows that the VAE is able to generate PDFs very similar to the input one when sampling a point nearby the position in the latent space where the input has been encoded.

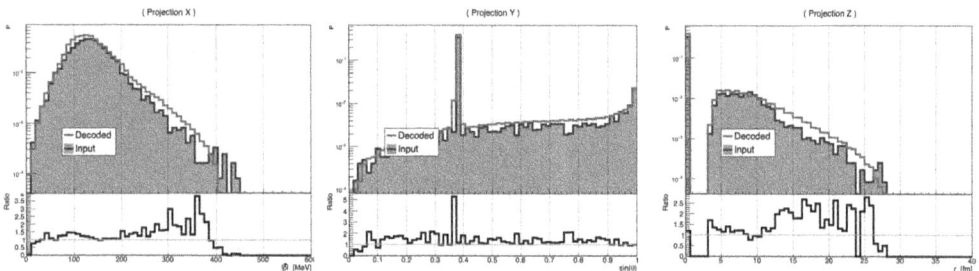

**Figure 19.9**   Example of results obtained in generating with the VAE a distribution, represented by a line, starting from a point sampled from the neighborhood of the point where the input distribution, the filled area, is encoded. The three distributions are the projections on the three axis of 3D PDFs. Plot from [38].

### 19.2.3  A POSSIBLE APPLICATION OF GRAPH NEURAL NETWORKS

To date, no specific study on Monte Carlo simulations of radiation / matter interactions using Graph Networks can be found in literature; still, it is clear from studies in other scientific domains suggest the potential of the technique. We want to cite here a study simulating the mechanical behavior of a fluid system, which shows capabilities of rendering the physics behind a complex system such as an ensemble of water small volumes [40]; we expect similar GNN systems to become available for our research fields in short time.

**Table 19.1**

**Geant4 vs GAN performance under various setups, as extracted from [22] and [31].**

| System | Software | Speed |
|---|---|---|
| Intel Xeon E5-2683 | Geant4 | 1 min |
| Nvidia RTX 1080 | 3d-GAN | 0.04 msec |
| AWS p2.8xlarge | Geant4 | 1.7 sec |
| AWS p2.8xlarge | CaloGan | $O(10)$ msec |
| AWS p2.8xlarge + Nvidia K80 | CaloGan | $O(0.01)$ msec |

## 19.3 STRONG AND WEAK POINTS ABOUT NEURAL NETWORKS APPLICATIONS FOR MONTE CARLO SIMULATIONS

Different AI based techniques for Monte Carlo simulations have been presented in literature, as shown in Section 19.2; their level of maturity varies between proofs of concept, advanced tests and production systems. Still, while we may be convinced that Neural Networks can be a reasonable substitute for classical algorithms, that would not be enough in absence of clear advantages in other areas.

### 19.3.1 SPEED, ACCURACY AND RELIABILITY

As described in Section 19.2.1, one of the main expected advantage of AI inspired systems, when compared to more standard simulation algorithms, is a potential speed-up without necessarily impacting performance. The improvement comes from the nature of feed-forwards Neural Networks used at inference time, which are described as a series of matrix multiplication of fixed length[1], without access to any data structure apart from the inputs and the weights. Today's processors, from CPUs to GPUs to TPUs, are very efficient in processing matrix algebra calculations; this reflects directly to short processing times. In order to give quantitative examples, we can refer to the two complex GANs described in Section 19.2.1, which are fed by Geant4-processed events in the training phase. Table 19.1 reports on the absolute time needed to process Geant4 vs the GAN for events with similar input; the speedups are of order 100x using CPUs, and an additional factor 100x with GPUs[2].

So, speed-wise there is a clear advantage; but what about the accuracy of the simulations? We can refer back to Figures 19.6 and 19.7 to compare the reference (detailed simulations) with AI predictions. In general, a perfect agreement is not to be expected, but in many applications a $O(10)\%$ agreement at the much reduced cost is a viable solution, also because even the detailed simulation is not expected to be perfectly describing the data. A different problem is present when one wants to use the AI system beyond the quantities explicitly used in the training phase: while these can be accurately reproduced, there is no guarantee that derived or different quantities are, since these are not explicit target of the minimization procedure. In these case, as discussed in [22], an accurate check should be done *a posteriori* on all the quantities used from the system; if any of them turns out to be unsatisfactory, the standard solution is to include them explicitly in the GAN training as an additional target.

An item which recently has gained a lot of attention is the capability to explain results from Machine Learning systems: the high number of degrees of freedom combined with the non-linearity

---

[1]This is not strictly valid for some types of recurrent networks, where the recurrence can introduce an indetermination in the sequence of mathematical operations.

[2]It can be said that it is an unfair comparison since Geant4 cannot currently use GPUs; still, it shows how AI inspired tools offer a path to the use of more performing technologies.

of response makes to difficult to justify results from first principles. While this is not a priori a problem in most applications, it becomes worrying when mission critical and potentially dangerous systems are driven by AI decisions (think of treatment plans for radiotherapy, or the assessment of radiation damages in industrial environments). Explainability of ML results is not a solved problem; still, tools and procedures exist in order to identify typical problems and effects. This is beyond the scope of this chapter, and a review can be found in [41].

### 19.3.2   UNPHYSICAL RESPONSES AND HOW TO IMPOSE PHYSICAL CONSTRAINTS

AI inspired tools are a mathematical solution to problems we have problems solving algorithmically, either because too difficult or too slow. An important difference with respect to standard "human-written" code is the impossibility to impose at algorithmic level precise conservation laws, such as the conservation of energy and momentum. There is no guarante a ML system will conserve them, since their validity is not implemented in any explicit form but should be recognized as an emergent behavior of the system.

In most of the cases shown in Section 19.2 the strict conservation (for example) of energy in particle showering into calorimeters does not need to be exact, since in the transfer between the energy in the impinging particle and the final products is in any case approximate due to effects of leaking, and smoothed by the detector resolution. In cases like this, while the training tries to match the "cell by cell" energy deposition, there is no explicit request that the total energy deposited in the calorimeter matches the precise simulation. In principle, a loss function designed to have the minimum when all the cells have the "expected" energy would suffice, but experience (and somehow common sense) shows that by adding to the loss function an explicit term tending to the conservation of total energy, like in Eq. (2) in [22], constrains can implemented even if not in exact form. This solution is called "soft" precisely due to this. The relative weight of the various terms in the loss functions are somehow arbitrary, and an higher weight to the part tending to the constraint (not really imposing it!) represents the developer desire to have it more precisely maintained, even if never exactly.

A different approach, as presented in [42], tries to implement instead "hard" and exact constraints on the outputs during the training phase; though, the mathematical complexity and the time needed increase, such as to advice the use of (eventually up-weighted) "soft" constraints in any case.

### REFERENCES

1. R. Barate, D. Decamp, and P. Ghez et al. Measurement of the $e^+e^- \to ZZ$ production cross section at centre-of-mass energies of 183 and 189 GeV. *Physics Letters B*, 469(1-4):287–302, dec 1999.
2. Berkman Sahiner, Heang Ping Chan, Nicholas Petrick, Datong Wei, Mark A. Helvie, Dorit D. Adler, and Mitchell M. Goodsitt. Classification of mass and normal breast tissue: A convolution neural network classifier with spatial domain and texture images. *IEEE Transactions on Medical Imaging*, 15(5):598–610, 1996.
3. Moshe Ben-Bassat, Karin L. Klove, and Max H. Weil. Sensitivity analysis in bayesian classification models: Multiplicative deviations. *IEEE Transactions on Pattern Analysis and Machine Intelligence*, PAMI-2(3):261–266, 1980.
4. Transmitting fibers in the brain : Total length and distribution of lengths - AI IMPACTS, https://aiimpacts.org/transmitting-fibers-in-the-brain-total-length-and-distribution-of-lengths/.
5. A. L. Hodgkin and A. F. Huxley. A quantitative description of membrane current and its application to conduction and excitation in nerve. *The Journal of Physiology*, 117(4):500–544, aug 1952.
6. Wulfram Gerstner and Werner M. Kistler. *Spiking Neuron Models*. Cambridge University Press, aug 2002.

7. Artificial neuron - Wikipedia https://en.wikipedia.org/wiki/Artificial_neuron.

8. Kurt Hornik. Approximation capabilities of multilayer feedforward networks. *Neural Networks*, 4(2):251–257, jan 1991.

9. F. Rosenblatt. The perceptron: A probabilistic model for information storage and organization in the brain. *Psychological Review*, 65(6):386–408, nov 1958.

10. Logistic function - Wikipedia https://en.wikipedia.org/wiki/Logistic_function.

11. Yann LeCun, Yoshua Bengio, and Geoffrey Hinton. Deep learning. *Nature*, 521(7553):436–444, may 2015.

12. Qi Wang, Yue Ma, Kun Zhao, and Yingjie Tian. A Comprehensive Survey of Loss Functions in Machine Learning. *Annals of Data Science*, pages 1–26, apr 2020.

13. Syed Muhammad Anwar, Muhammad Majid, Adnan Qayyum, Muhammad Awais, Majdi Alnowami, and Muhammad Khurram Khan. Medical Image Analysis using Convolutional Neural Networks: A Review, nov 2018.

14. Tong Liu, Jinzhen Wang, Qing Liu, Shakeel Alibhai, Tao Lu, and Xubin He. High-Ratio Lossy Compression: Exploring the Autoencoder to Compress Scientific Data. *IEEE Transactions on Big Data*, 2021.

15. Elisa Ferrari, Paolo Bosco, Sara Calderoni, Piernicola Oliva, Letizia Palumbo, Giovanna Spera, Maria Evelina Fantacci, and Alessandra Retico. Dealing with confounders and outliers in classification medical studies: The Autism Spectrum Disorders case study. *Artificial Intelligence in Medicine*, 108(July):101926, 2020.

16. O Knapp, O Cerri, G Dissertori, T Q Nguyen, M Pierini, and J R Vlimant. Adversarially Learned Anomaly Detection on CMS open data: re-discovering the top quark. *Eur. Phys. J. Plus*, 136:236, 2021.

17. Diederik P. Kingma and Max Welling. Auto-encoding variational bayes. In *2nd International Conference on Learning Representations, ICLR 2014 - Conference Track Proceedings*. International Conference on Learning Representations, ICLR, dec 2014.

18. S. Kullback and R. A. Leibler. On Information and Sufficiency. *The Annals of Mathematical Statistics*, 22(1):79–86, mar 1951.

19. Diederik P. Kingma and Max Welling. An introduction to variational autoencoders. *Foundations and Trends in Machine Learning*, 12(4):307–392, nov 2019.

20. Ian Goodfellow, Jean Pouget-Abadie, Mehdi Mirza, Bing Xu, David Warde-Farley, Sherjil Ozair, Aaron Courville, and Yoshua Bengio. Generative adversarial networks. *Communications of the ACM*, 63(11):139–144, oct 2020.

21. This Person Does Not Exist, https://thispersondoesnotexist.com/.

22. Michela Paganini, Luke de Oliveira, and Benjamin Nachman. CaloGAN: Simulating 3D high energy particle showers in multilayer electromagnetic calorimeters with generative adversarial networks. *Physical Review D*, 97(1):014021, jan 2018.

23. D Sarrut, N Krah, and J M Létang. Generative adversarial networks (GAN) for compact beam source modelling in Monte Carlo simulations. *Physics in Medicine & Biology*, 64(21):215004, oct 2019.

24. Jonathan Shlomi, Peter Battaglia, and Jean-Roch Vlimant. Graph neural networks in particle physics. *Mach. Learn.: Sci. Technol*, 2:21001, 2021.

25. F Scarselli, M Gori, A Chung Tsoi, M Hagenbuchner, G ; F Monfardini, and G Monfardini. The graph neural network model. *This journal article is available at Research IEEE TRANSACTIONS ON NEURAL NETWORKS*, 20(1):61–80, 2009.

26. Xiangyang Ju and Benjamin Nachman. Supervised jet clustering with graph neural networks for Lorentz boosted bosons. *Physical Review D*, 102(7):075014, oct 2020.

27. Xiangyang Ju, Steven Farrell, Paolo Calafiura, Daniel Murnane, Prabhat, Lindsey Gray, Thomas Klijnsma, Kevin Pedro, Giuseppe Cerati, Jim Kowalkowski, Gabriel Perdue, Panagiotis

Spentzouris, Nhan Tran, Jean-Roch Vlimant, Alexander Zlokapa, Joosep Pata, Maria Spirop-ulu, Sitong An, Adam Aurisano, Jeremy Hewes, Aristeidis Tsaris, Kazuhiro Terao, and Tracy Usher. Graph Neural Networks for Particle Reconstruction in High Energy Physics detectors. *arXiv*, mar 2020.

28. S. Agostinelli, J. Allison, and K. Amako et al. GEANT4 - A simulation toolkit. *Nuclear Instruments and Methods in Physics Research, Section A: Accelerators, Spectrometers, Detectors and Associated Equipment*, 506(3):250–303, jul 2003.

29. T. T. Böhlen, F. Cerutti, M. P.W. Chin, A. Fassò, A. Ferrari, P. G. Ortega, A. Mairani, P. R. Sala, G. Smirnov, and V. Vlachoudis. The FLUKA Code: Developments and challenges for high energy and medical applications. *Nuclear Data Sheets*, 120:211–214, jun 2014.

30. H. G. Hughes, M. B. Chadwick, R. K. Corzine, H. W. Egdorf, F. X. Gallmeier, R. C. Little, R. E. MacFarlane, S. G. Mashnik, E. J. Pitcher, R. E. Prael, A. J. Sierk, E. C. Snow, L. S. Waters, M. C. White, and P. G. Young. Status of the MCNPX Transport Code. In *Advanced Monte Carlo for Radiation Physics, Particle Transport Simulation and Applications*, pages 961–966. Springer Berlin Heidelberg, 2001.

31. F. Carminati, A. Gheata, G. Khattak, P. Mendez Lorenzo, S. Sharan, and S. Vallecorsa. Three dimensional Generative Adversarial Networks for fast simulation. *Journal of Physics: Conference Series*, 1085(3):032016, sep 2018.

32. Zongsheng Hu, Guangyao Li, Xiaoke Zhang, Kuangkuang Ye, Jiade Lu, and Hao Peng. A machine learning framework with anatomical prior for online dose verification using positron emitters and PET in proton therapy. *Physics in Medicine & Biology*, 65(18):185003, sep 2020.

33. Saiqun Ma, Zongsheng Hu, Kuangkuang Ye, Xiaoke Zhang, Yuenan Wang, and Hao Peng. Feasibility study of patient-specific dose verification in proton therapy utilizing positron emission tomography (PET) and generative adversarial network (GAN). *Medical Physics*, 47(10):5194–5208, 2020.

34. Chih Chieh Liu and Hsuan Ming Huang. A deep learning approach for converting prompt gamma images to proton dose distributions: A Monte Carlo simulation study. *Physica Medica*, 69(December 2019):110–119, 2020.

35. D. Sarrut, N. Krah, J. N. Badel, and J. M. Létang. Learning SPECT detector angular response function with neural network for accelerating Monte-Carlo simulations. *Physics in Medicine and Biology*, 63(20), 2018.

36. P. Arce, D. Bolst, M. C. Bordage, J. M.C. Brown, P. Cirrone, M. A. Cortés-Giraldo, D. Cutajar, G. Cuttone, L. Desorgher, P. Dondero, A. Dotti, B. Faddegon, C. Fedon, S. Guatelli, S. Incerti, V. Ivanchenko, D. Konstantinov, I. Kyriakou, G. Latyshev, A. Le, C. Mancini-Terracciano, M. Maire, A. Mantero, M. Novak, C. Omachi, L. Pandola, A. Perales, Y. Perrot, G. Petringa, J. M. Quesada, J. Ramos-Méndez, F. Romano, A. B. Rosenfeld, L. G. Sarmiento, D. Sakata, T. Sasaki, I. Sechopoulos, E. C. Simpson, T. Toshito, and D. H. Wright. Report on G4-Med, a Geant4 benchmarking system for medical physics applications developed by the Geant4 Medical Simulation Benchmarking Group. *Medical Physics*, 48(1):19–56, jan 2021.

37. C. Mancini-Terracciano, M. Asai, B. Caccia, G. A.P. Cirrone, A. Dotti, R. Faccini, P. Napolitani, L. Pandola, D. H. Wright, and M. Colonna. Preliminary results coupling "Stochastic Mean Field" and "Boltzmann-Langevin One Body" models with Geant4. *Physica Medica*, 67:116–122, nov 2019.

38. A. Ciardiello, M. Asai, B. Caccia, G. A.P. Cirrone, M. Colonna, A. Dotti, R. Faccini, S. Giagu, A. Messina, P. Napolitani, L. Pandola, D. H. Wright, and C. Mancini-Terracciano. Preliminary results in using Deep Learning to emulate BLOB, a nuclear interaction model. *Physica Medica*, 73:65–72, may 2020.

39. P. Napolitani and M. Colonna. Bifurcations in Boltzmann-Langevin one body dynamics for fermionic systems. *Physics Letters, Section B: Nuclear, Elementary Particle and High-Energy Physics*, 726(1-3):382–386, oct 2013.

40. Alvaro Sanchez-Gonzalez, Jonathan Godwin, Tobias Pfaff, Rex Ying, Jure Leskovec, and Peter W Battaglia. Learning to Simulate Complex Physics with Graph Networks. *http://arxiv.org/abs/2002.09405*, Feb 2020.

41. Pantelis Linardatos, Vasilis Papastefanopoulos, and Sotiris Kotsiantis. Explainable ai: A review of machine learning interpretability methods. *Entropy*, 23(1):1–45, 2021.

42. Pablo Márquez-Neila, Mathieu Salzmann, and Pascal Fua. Imposing Hard Constraints on Deep Networks: Promises and Limitations. *http://arxiv.org/abs/1706.02025*, Jun 2017.

# 20  Speed-up Monte Carlo in charged particle applications

*Angelo Schiavi*
Sapienza Università di Roma, Rome, Italy
Istituto Nazionale di Fisica Nucleare (INFN) Section of Rome I,
Rome, Italy

## CONTENTS

Numerical simulations of particle-medium interaction are of fundamental importance in many clinical applications involving charged particle radiation. Among others, they are used in developing new treatment protocols in cancer therapy, to plan patient treatment using particle beams, to design new detectors for online treatment monitoring, and to validate and commission beam models at treatment centers.

Monte Carlo (MC) simulations are the most accurate tool for reproducing direct effects of human tissue irradiation, e.g. dose deposition, and also indirect effects, such as emission of secondary radiation and nuclear activation. This is possible thanks to the detailed description of the fundamental processes through which a charged particle interacts with the traversed medium.

In order to meet clinical requirements for accuracy and precision, MC simulations have to be preformed at high statistics, i.e. by transporting a significant fraction of the particles actually delivered in a treatment. In this chapter we will address the performance requirements for MC simulations to meet the timescale of clinical practice, and we will discuss possibile hardware and software solutions that can speed up MC calculations.

DOI: 10.1201/9781003023920-20

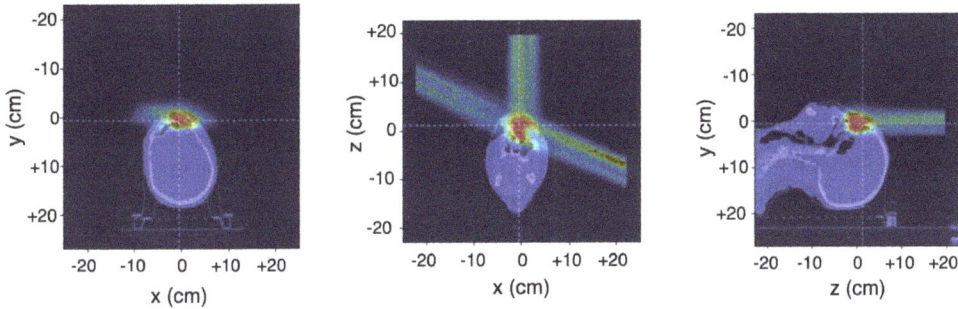

**Figure 20.1**    Three-field superficial pediatric treatment with proton beams.

## 20.1    SPEED-UP OF MONTE CARLO FOR THE INTRODUCTION IN THE CLINIC

The stochastic nature of the interaction is simulated in MC algorithms by sampling distributions obtained from theoretical models and confirmed by experimental data.

A large number of particles need to be simulated in order to reduce statistical fluctuations in the scored quantities, e.g. the dose deposited inside the patient. In order to meet the requirements for clinical applications, MC simulations are much expensive in terms of computational resources with respect to simplified interaction models (see MC and analytical codes analysis by A. Mairani in this book).

Introduction in the clinic requires high accuracy and short simulation times. We will analyze the problem of speeding-up MC simulations, and we will identify a few strategies and guidelines for developing and using MC codes in the clinical practice.

### 20.1.1    CASE STUDY: HEAD AND NECK 3-FIELDS TREATMENT IN PROTON THERAPY

In order to discuss about accuracy and performance of MC simulations, we need a reference case. In fact different treatment districts and different radiation beams can lead to substantial differences in terms of particle tracking rate and overall simulation time. We chose for our case study a Head&Neck treatment with protons using 3 fields, see Figure 20.1. The total number of protons to be delivered by the accelerator is about $7 \cdot 10^{10}$. In the clinical practice for proton therapy, recalculation at 1% of total primary protons is typically needed in order to reduce dose fluctuations below the desired level. All in all, this leads to a workload for the MC simulation of $7 \cdot 10^8$ complete histories.

In this scenario, the metric for defining the speed of an MC code is the *tracking rate*, i.e. the number of completed particle histories per unit time. It can be easily computed by measuring the time spent by the code in tracking the particles, and dividing it by the total number of simulated primaries. Hence we will use *primary/s* as our MC performance metric.

### 20.1.2    MOTIVATION: CLINIC VS RESEARCH PERFORMANCE REQUIREMENTS

Until recently, treatment planning was carried out using analytical pencil-beam algorithms, and only in some selected cases, the so-called *difficult* cases, an MC recalculation was performed. The cases were *difficult* for the pencil-beam algorithm, which was typically remapping a dose distribution of a pencil beam in water into a 3D reconstruction of the patient using a water-equivalent model. Hence the analytical algorithm was sometimes failing in reaching the desired accuracy in presence of large density gradients inside the patient anatomy. In those cases, an MC recalculation at high statistics was (and still is) performed in order to check the outcome of the TPS, and eventually correct the treatment strategy. In that framework, even if a single MC simulation could take a few days on a single core, or a few hours on a dedicated cluster, it was not a problem for the clinical workflow, since planning and checking was typically carried out several days before irradiation.

On different grounds, MC simulations performed for research purposes (e.g. for proof-of-principle of a given protocol, or for *a posteriori* analysis of a database of patient treatments) do not have significant time constraints with respect to the clinical routine. These technical studies can also benefit from the possibility of being run on large HPC clusters, an option that is rarely available to treatment centers as will see in the following .

In the last decade, great effort has been spent in bringing the superior accuracy of MC simulation to various aspects of everyday practice, corresponding to different temporal *windows*. For instance, we could identify the following cases

- offline plan recalculation: half an hour
- dose verification with patient on the couch: couple of minutes
- on-line dose monitoring: a few tens of ms

### 20.1.3  AVAILABLE SOFTWARE SOLUTIONS (GENERAL PURPOSE MC TOOLS, HOMEMADE SIMULATION CODES)

Having identified the task and the calculation time, we have to choose a tool for performing the simulation. Two main options are available: to *use* or to *develop*.

The first option corresponds to adopt one of the long-standing general-purpose MC codes, such as FLUKA, Geant4, MCNPX. Those MC codes are the result of decades of development, testing and upgrading. They are considered the *de facto* standard for MC radiation transport. Originally developed mainly for high-energy particle physics experiments, these tools have been refined in the last twenty years in order to better reproduce experiments and commissioning data in the therapeutic energy range for charged particle therapy.

The second option is that of developing a new code, usually starting from scratch. The main motivation is to reach the highest tracking rate possible using new computing hardware that was not available at the time general-purpose MCs were originally developed. New hardware, as we will see, demands for rethinking the structure of an MC code. Memory constraints impose limitations on the data structures that can be held in memory at once. Dynamic memory allocation might not be supported by new devices, so that modular codes based on object-oriented programming (e.g. Geant4 toolkit) cannot be easily ported to new hardware.

Therefore in developing new codes, the journey is very long and demands for significant manpower. The best strategy is to identify the project goals depending on the final application. For instance, if we are interested in a dose engine (i.e. a tool for fast and accurate recalculation of energy deposition), it makes sense to rebuild the minimal software infrastructure that can deliver the result. We call this family of MC tools as *fast-MC* codes. They share with the standard MC codes, the so-called *full-MC* codes, the same core strategy of MC particle tracking and the same fundamental description of particle-medium interactions. But *fast-MCs* are somehow trimmed-down and simplified implementations with respect to standard full-fledged codes.

### 20.1.4  AVAILABLE BUDGET AND AFFORDABLE HARDWARE

Another key element is the available budget that can be dedicated to running MC simulations. For instance, one can speed-up calculations by running a large number of independent simulations on a distributed cluster of nodes, and then combine all output together. This solution demands for at least driving 100 to 1000 nodes, in order to reach clinical routine timeframe. Buying such a cluster could easily cost in the 100 k\$ range and above. If the hardware is proprietary (i.e. not shared with other institutions), the treatment center has to provide also money for paying the electricity bill, the yearly maintenance costs, and the salary of dedicated staff for managing such a complex hardware.

On one hand, rewriting MC codes for new hardware (such as GPUs), requires a long and costly investment in terms of manpower dedicated to code development . On the other hand, the possibility of exploiting GPUs can reduce the budget for acquiring the simulation computer to less than 10 k$, with no need for dedicated IT staff and a significantly reduced electricity bill.

Hence *fast-MCs* appear to be a very interesting solution for treatment centers, wanting to bring MC simulations to the clinic. This option is not only cheep with respect to buying a dedicated HPC cluster, but it could also guarantee service continuity by hardware redundancy, e.g. by replicating the simulation hardware.

## 20.1.5   ISSUES CONCERNING PATIENT DATA PROTECTION

A important issue to take into consideration is data security. A typical treatment center can examine and cure a few 100 patients per year. All patient information has to be managed by assuring data protection, privacy and security, as this is very sensible data. The common solution is to keep all patient data within a private Local Area Network (LAN). Therefore using shared and/or distributed computing resources over the Internet is usually not an option for the clinical routine. It would require anonymization on the fly before sending data outside the LAN: a task that can be non trivial and not reliable.

Also to consider is the problem of running on a distributed cluster were jobs are executed using a queue manager. In order to have results in the clinical timeframe, i.e. half an hour or less, a high-priority queue has to be used (and possibly paid for).

All in all, what it clearly emerges is that they are two main different scenarios. The *research* scenario, where existing full-MC codes can be easily used: here it is possible to used large HPC centers with many thousands of nodes and perform high-statistics MC simulations for which the execution time is not a critical issue.

The *clinical* scenario, where the best option would be to use fast-MC tools that can provide on-demand results on dedicated and proprietary hardware.

## 20.1.6   CORE STRUCTURE OF AN MC CODE FOR CHARGED PARTICLE TRACKING

Having identified the need for speeding up MC simulations, we can now address the characteristic features of an MC charged particle tracking code. The task to be performed is that of advancing a charged particle, e.g. a proton, through a virtual geometry representing the treatment room with the last part of the accelerator beamline. Particles are produced typically in the form bunches or pulses inside the *gun*, namely the first part on an accelerator device. Then particles are accelerated, filtered in space and energy, and transported by the active components of a beamline to the treatment room. In the of Intensity Modulated Proton Therapy, for instance, the beam is then deflected by the steering magnets, sent through the beam monitoring section, and eventually delivered to the patient.

In a simulation, the features of the beam at the steering point are condensed in an effective model called *virtual source*. From the source, particles are extracted by sampling a phase-space distribution, whose parameters are usually finely tuned using commissioning data for each beamline and each treatment room.

Accurate MC simulations require to track the generated particles thorough the final passive elements of the beamline (e.g. monitoring ionization chambers, energy degraders, exit windows, range shifters) until they reach the patient. The patient morphology is usually obtained from imaging diagnostics such as CT or NMR scans. The patient *slices* are stacked up along the scanning direction (typically from head to toe) combining them into a 3D rectangular grid. To each element of the grid, called *voxel*, a value in HU is assigned, taken from the CT image. The MC codes have built-in models that convert HU values into material properties of the corresponding human tissue, such as density and chemical composition. The conversion from HU to medium properties is typically carried out using a look-up table (LUT) called *calibration curve*.

The *treatment plan* is the set of instructions that a Treatment Planning Software (TPS) produces combining together patient morphology, irradiation directions, dose prescription and accelerator properties. The treatment plan is generated and optimized for each patient by the medical physicists of a treatment center using the TPS. The information is usually structured in *fields* or treatment directions, corresponding each to a given gantry position and couch position. Then a field is composed of *pencil beams* or beamlets, corresponding to a steering magnets deflection and a given energy. Finally each pencil beam is carrying a given amount of particles, usually expressed in terms of Monitoring Units (MU) that can be readily used by the accelerator delivery system to control the beam.

The treatment plan is hierarchically parsed, and particles to be tracked are generated for each pencil beam using the aforementioned virtual source. MU values are converted into actual number $N_p$ of particles carried by each pencil beam. This is actually the main parameter that is optimized by the TPS in order to obtain the best compromise between a highly conformal dose to the PTV and the minimum dose delivered to OARs or healthy normal tissue. The number of MC histories $N_h$ to be simulated is equal to $N_p$ times the recalculation percentage. As said before, a recalculation at 1% is considered as a large enough statistics for clinical use. At that level, for instance in proton therapy, the final dose uncertainties due to reduced MC statistics are well below the dose level in the regions of interest, namely the PTV and the OARs.

Eventually we are left with the task of tracking the particles through the geometry and score, for instance, the dose or the LET on a given spatial grid of interest. The core of a MC code is called the *tracking kernel*. The kernel takes a particle, and advances it step by step through the geometry setup until the particle exits the room, or its energy goes below a user-prescribed tracking threshold. At each step, the particle interacts with the traversed medium in many different ways described by the physics interaction models. The main interactions of a charged particle are usually divided into *continuous* and *discrete* processes. Continuous processes are those interactions that can be parametrized by the step length, such as the energy loss, the energy straggling, and the Multiple Coulomb Scattering (MCS). Discrete processes are those that occur on a very tiny scale (typically sub-nuclear) and that can be described as a point-like process. Nuclear elastic and inelastic scattering, for instance, are discrete processes.

The stepping of the particle, i.e. the length of each step, is controlled by the *step limiter*, an algorithm that determines the longest possible step taking into consideration the geometry boundary crossing between regions and the limitations imposed by each interaction model.

As the result of an interaction, a given particle can generate other particles. These particles can be neglected or they can be queued to the tracking kernel. During the simulation then we observe the creation and evolution of different particle generations. Particles extracted from the source are called *primary* particles, and are first generation. Then we have *secondary* particles, that can be second, third or higher generation.

### 20.1.7 PARALLELIZATION OF MC TOOLS FOR CHARGED PARTICLE TRACKING

As seen in the description above, an MC simulation can be segmented into three main blocks: initialization, tracking, writing output. Coming back to our case study, the time needed for initialization and for writing simulation output is usually not very long, let's say of the order of a couple of minutes even using serial execution. Most of the time is spent in tracking a large number of particles. For instance, the patient case shown in Figure 20.1 requires 7 solid days of computation (170 hours) on a single CPU core using a standard full-MC.

The MC tracking is a sequence of independent tasks, since each particle evolves independently of other particles, interacting with the underlying medium only, and not with other particles of the beam. If the simulation domain can fit in the memory of each computing instance (e.g. node

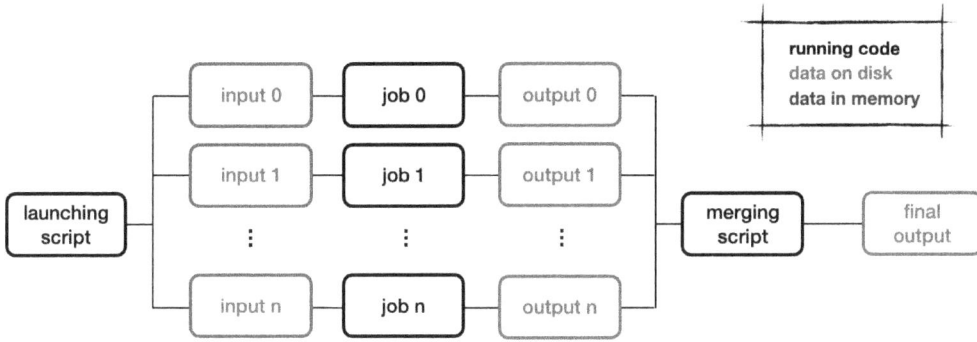

**Figure 20.2** Queueing multiple independent jobs and merging results at the end.

or GPU), then the problem is somehow *embarrassingly* parallel. No communications are needed between computing instances and the tasks can just be distributed to the available computing resources.

The problem we are discussing is that of reducing the calculation time of a constant-size problem. This means that we have to compute as fast as possible in our case $N_h = 7 \cdot 10^8$ independent tasks. In parallel programming, this is called strong-scaling speed-up. The reference case takes about 170 hours on a high-end CPU core, corresponding to a tracking rate of roughly 1000 primary/s.

If we want to bring this calculation time to the clinical timeframe, i.e. 30 min, then the overall tracking rate we need is $7 \cdot 10^8 / 1800 \simeq 4 \cdot 10^5$ primary/s. Hence the speed-up we need to achieve has to be larger than 400 times.

### 20.1.8 REPLICATING SIMULATIONS USING SCRIPTS AND QUEUES

The first solution we present is that of running existing MC codes on a cluster of CPU nodes. The most trivial attempt is queueing $n$ independent jobs, each one with a workload of $N_h/n$ primaries to track. A key-point to consider is that all jobs have to be statistically independent. This can be accomplished using a script that generates a sequence of random seeds for the $n$ jobs. Each job will then start its own pseudo-random sequence at a different point. This will guarantee that particles extracted from the source, and the sequence of events in each particle history are uncorrelated among the different jobs.

Once all the jobs have ended, a script can be used to merge all $n$ scorers into a single one. For instance, one could obtain in this way the dose delivered inside the patient as shown in Figure 20.1. The corresponding workflow is presented in Figure 20.2.

Bottleneck of this approach is the speed of the distributed filesystem. In fact, we need to create a file-tree with a directory for each job containing a copy of the input files and receiving the output of each simulation job. A dose map in the patient CT resolution is typically 100-500 MiB in size. Hence, using $n = 500$ jobs, we could expect to generate at least 100 GiB of dose maps that then we have to merge into a single one. If this task is not parallelized using consecutive parallel reduction on chained MPI jobs, the merging operation can easily take longer than the MC simulation time on the cluster.

### 20.1.9 MPI WRAPPERS (PORTING IS NOT NEEDED)

For some MC tools (e.g. Geant4) it is possible to write a simple skeleton code, called a *wrapper*, that integrates the tracking code with a communication library for massive parallel computers. The Message Passing Interface (MPI) is the *de facto* standard protocol in this field. Each computing

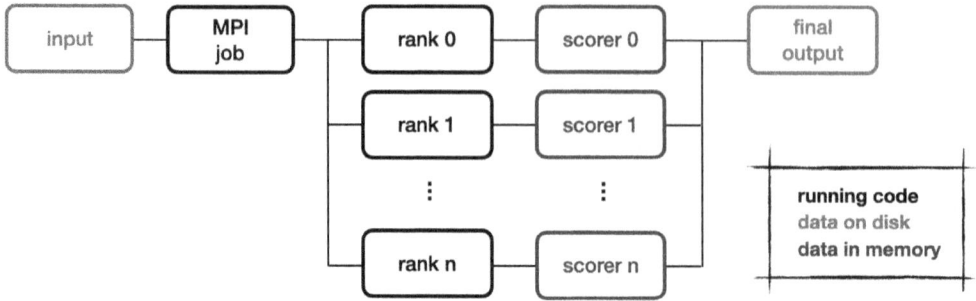

**Figure 20.3**  Running an MPI job and merging scorers using parallel reduction operations.

entity is named *rank*. Using the *master-slaves* paradigm, a single job can drive $n$ simultaneous and statistically independent simulations.

A single input file can be parsed by the master, and shared with $n$ running ranks using MPI broadcasting operations in memory. The master can generate the series of random seeds for all ranks. At the end of the simulation, all scorers can be merged into one using the MPI reduction operations, which are purposefully developed and optimized for massive parallel jobs, i.e. $n \gg 1000$.

This solution requires minimal coding, and it can guarantee almost perfect linear parallel scaling with the number $n$ of computing processors. Porting of existing code is not needed. Just a simple layer of processor communications needs to be implemented combining well-defined and already developed solutions. Disk input and output is not a significant issue, and just the final relevant results are actually stored, preventing clogging up the filesystem. See Figure 20.3 for a schematic representation of the MPI workflow.

### 20.1.10   ONBOARD HARDWARE ACCELERATORS (PORTING IS NEEDED)

Another option for speeding-up MC calculations is to exploit special hardware components called onboard accelerators. Examples of what is nowadays available are Graphical Processing Units (GPU), Field Programmable Gate Arrays (FPGA) or integrated manycore processors (Intel Phi co-processor). We will focus our attention here on GPUs. In the last two decades, driven by the huge market of video gaming industry, the GPUs have seen a steady increase in peak performance (measured in GFLOPS) and memory capacity, see Figure 20.4. They are presently the most interesting hardware solution for scalable massive parallel computers, thanks also to their energy saving design. In fact, they presently offer the best ratio of computing performance over consumed electric power. This is becoming very important for scaling-up the number of computing nodes, since not only the power consumption increases with the number of nodes, but also the cooling system is a non-trivial task in designing super-computers.

At the time of writing, a single GPU card can offer tens of TFLOPS and more than 10 GB of memory at the cost of 1 k$. The power consumption of such a GPU is about 300 W, the same as a high-performing multi-core CPU.

Standard full-MC codes are not running out-the-box on GPU. Existing code has to be adapted to the new technology. The typical GPU architecture differs significantly from a typical CPU. Understanding the differences in design and resources distribution can help in guiding an efficient and effective rewriting of an MC code. On one hand, a Central Processing Unit (CPU) is designed for serial execution of a handful of highly complex independent tasks. It has a few computing cores (1–10), a large data cache, and is designed for low latency access to memory. Each core has its own Arithmetic and Logic Unit (ALU) and a dedicated double-precision Floating-Point Unit DP-FPU (see Figure 20.5). On the other hand, a GPU is designed for parallel execution of simple tasks. It

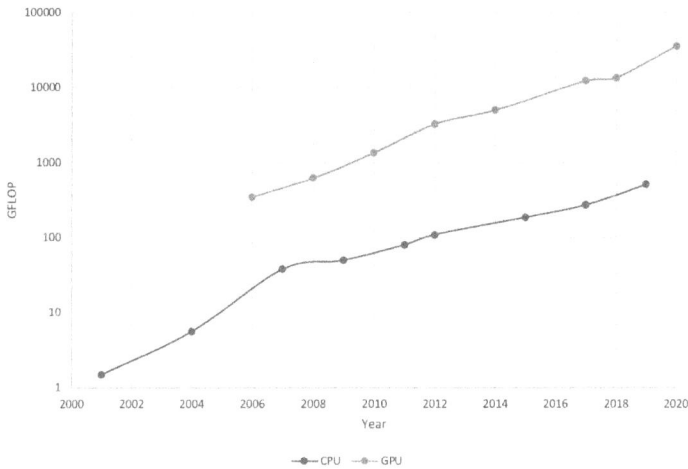

**Figure 20.4** Theoretical peak performance of multicore CPUs and GPUs in the last 20 years.

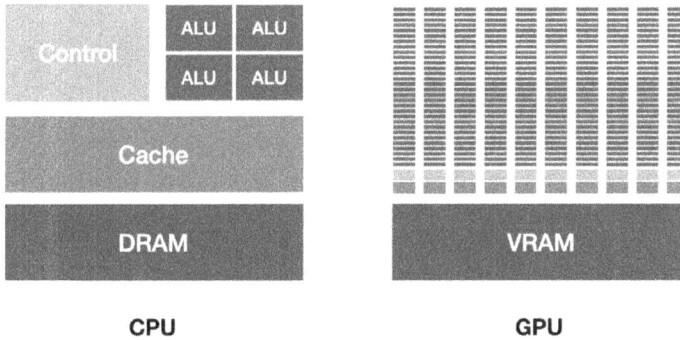

**Figure 20.5** Breakdown representation of CPU and GPU using logical blocks.

has thousands of cores, sharing several data caches and the memory bus. As such, a GPU has a large latency compared to CPU cores, and this latency is only partially mitigated by the memory manager and the task scheduler.

The GPU cores are hierarchically grouped both logically and in hardware. The GPU core is the fundamental unit at the lowest level, and it has the capability of executing instructions and performing calculations. The core is not a completely independent unit. In fact the fundamental processing block is the *partition*, namely a bundle of cores that share the same program counter and scheduler. The partition presently corresponds to 32 cores, a *warp* in GPU jargon. The warp is the hearth of a GPU, adopting the execution model named Single Instruction Multiple Threads (SIMT). The part of code that is executed on a GPU is called *kernel*. In an MC code, we can imagine a front-end code running on the CPU, which is responsible for input and output, for setting up the simulation environment (geometry, materials, primary particles to track) and calling GPU kernels for tracking particles, i.e. the most computationally intensive part of an MC simulation.

Two main limitations in GPU kernels have been identified. A kernel is said to be *memory bound*, when data transfer from cores and main memory is the most demanding part of the algorithm. A kernel is said to be *compute bound*, when most of the time is spent in performing calculations at the core level. In particle tracking MC codes, which limitation is the most severe one depends on the strategy adopted in parallelising the main execution loop.

In *history-based* transport algorithms, as in traditional full-MC codes, each particle is assigned to a GPU core, which follows it step-by-step from particle generation until its removal from simulation. In this case, particle information is retrieved only once from main memory. Particle status has to be kept in local private memory, i.e. in the *registers*. Excessive use of registers can lead to underusage of computing resources of the GPU: the number of tasks that can run at once is less than the physical number of cores, and part of the card just stays idle. In this case the achieved *occupancy* on the GPU is just a fraction of the theoretical 100% available resources.

Low occupancy is usually related to large and complex tracking kernels. It can easily happen in kernels that are able to transport a set of different particles with several interaction processes, e.g. energy loss, multiple scattering, point-like interactions. An alternative strategy is to split the stepping algorithm and the interaction processes in smaller kernels, i.e. adopting the *event-based* transport model. Here particles a split among different buffers and kernels are launched repeatedly for each elementary step of the MC algorithm. The clear advantage is that lightweight kernels allow to fill completely the GPU, achieving almost 100% occupancy. The price to pay is that at each kernel invocation information on tracked particles has to be retrieved from global memory and stored back. Hence the pressure is moved from the computing resources (cores) to the memory bus (bandwidth). In order to achieve high tracking rate, a lot of effort has to be put in studying the data flow during execution, which makes the event-based solution much similar to linear algebra algorithms, where tiling, interlacing and memory access patterns are crucial keypoints to address in order to achieve high performance.

### 20.1.10.1   Single vs double precision

For typical graphics applications, 3D scene rendering does not need double precision floating point operations (FP64), hence GPUs are mainly built for top performance using single precision (FP32). On the contrary, most scientific codes developed in the last 40 years are based on FP64 calculations. It is usually safe to compile legacy FP32 code in double precision, but viceversa is not true. Numerical overflow and underflow can easily occur, and numerical algorithms can become unstable and unreliable.

Double precision FPUs are a scarce and expensive resource in GPU world. On a consumer card ($\sim 1$ k\$) the FP64 performance is typically 1:32 or 1:64 with respect to FP32 performance. Top-of-the-line cards ($\sim 10$ k\$) especially built for HPC applications have many more 64-bit FPUs, reaching a performance ratio of 1:2.

In order to fully exploit the GPU computing power, it is mandatory to reduce the use of FP64 operations to a minimum. Revisiting legacy code and rewriting it for single precision is a necessary step to take into account when porting code to GPU. Clearly this has a significant cost in terms of skilled manpower and development time, but it will allow to run efficiently the MC simulation on non-expensive hardware.

### 20.1.10.2   Scorers

The results of a MC simulation are usually stored on disk in the form of 3D maps. For instance, the most important clinical parameter is the deposited dose. Usually the dose is scored on a cartesian grid of voxels which have the same resolution of the planning CT or coarser. At each energy deposition event (e.g. continuous energy loss along the track, or local energy deposition by recoiling nuclei) the *scorer* updates the voxel occupied by the particle by adding a small contribution. This operation is very frequent (almost at every step), and the access to the 3D map is sparse and unpredictable. When thousand of particles are traced at the same time by the GPU, it frequently happens (especially in the entry channel of a treatment beam) that many threads want to score the same location. As such, *atomic operations* have to be used to avoid data race conditions. These functions are serialising memory write operations, and are nowadays available on most GPU cards. The penalty to pay for their use is small, and depends heavily on the irradiation geometry and delivery strategy.

An important point to stress is that the scorers are one of the part of a GPU code that actually requires **double precision**. Hundred of thousands of small increments to the dose in a voxel can easily lead to floating point underflow in single precision, producing therefore a completely wrong dose map. Therefore, to keep it simple, double precision is mandatory for scoring purposes.

### 20.1.10.3  Special hardware on GPU

In this overview of GPU porting strategies for MC codes, it is important to mention the presence on the GPU of special hardware that can be used in MC algorithms, and that can lead to significant increase of overall tracking performance. Each *warp* has access to dedicated *texture units*, which can be efficiently used to linearly interpolate look-up tables (LUT). Most particle-medium interaction processes depend on a cross sections that are typically function of kinetic energy. Evaluation of all cross sections is required at each step. Texture units have a dedicated memory path and independent data cache. Using them can reduce the evaluation of a single cross section from several hundred of card clock cycles to just a couple of cycles, resulting in a significant speed-up of this repeated task.

Other dedicated units can be found (e.g. tensor units or ray-tracing units) on recent GPUs: finding a part of the MC algorithm that can benefit from such hardware it is for sure a winning strategy.

### 20.1.11  FINAL CONSIDERATIONS

From the discussion, two main alternatives are emerging for speeding up MC simulations. The first one is to use *de facto* standard MC codes running on multicore CPU nodes (CPU clusters). The second one is to use fast-MC tools especially written for GPU hardware.

An example of an in-house solution is the double CPU cluster at CNAO (about 60 CPUs in total), where a typical recalculation at 1% statistics using FLUKA takes a few hours depending on the number of fields and on the radiation beam (proton or Carbon ions) [*priv. comm.*].

Motivated largely by the increasing number of proton treatment facilities, the development of GPU-accelerated fast-MC tools has been mainly focused in recent years on tracking proton beams. Examples of research and academic solutions presently available are gPMC (MGH, Boston, USA), Fred (URLS,Rome, Italy) and a tool by Tseung et al. (Mayo Clinic, Rochester, USA). All these codes, although different in implementation details, compare very well with dose predictions by standard full-MC codes. The reported performance depends on the tested GPU hardware, but it is always well in excess of 500.000 primary/s, hence meeting well our estimated tracking rate of $4 \cdot 10^5$ primary/s for bringing MC simulations into the clinical timeframe. It is worth mentioning that in time the capabilities of fast-MC codes are expanding from the prediction of just the physical dose inside the patient, to include also estimates of the LETd maps for radiobiological effectiveness models, and nuclear activation upon proton beam irradiation.

As commercial TPS vendors are also moving to GPU-based MC dose engines, it is expected in the next few years an increase in fast-MC solutions for time-critical applications in the clinical routine. In this scenario, the full-MC codes will surely retain their superior capabilities for innovative research and proof-of-principle investigations, where the best physical models are needed to identify successful solutions that could be later on re-implemented in fast-MC tools.

**primary:**  A *primary* particle is extracted by a source (e.g. an accelerator device) and introduced in the simulation geometry at the beginning of the tracking kernel.

**history:**  The complete history of the interactions of a given *primary* particle from its birth (in the accelerator machine, or in a source) to its death (e.g. thermalization or exit for simulation domain), together with all the sub-histories of secondary particles produced by the primary itself.

**kernel:** The program code executed on the GPU.

**warp:** The GPU partition corresponding to a fixed number of cores that are forced to run together by a single instruction scheduler and dispatcher.

**full-MC:** A standard general-purpose MC code. It is a tool developed for maximum accuracy in particle-medium interaction models.

**fast-MC:** A trimmed-down implementation of an MC code. It is a tool developed for maximum tracking rate using simplified particle-medium interaction models.

## FURTHER READING

1. [MPI] MPI: A Message-Passing Interface Standard, www.mpi-forum.org
2. [GPGPU programming] Engel, W. (Ed.). (2018). GPU Pro 360: Guide to GPGPU (1st ed.). A K Peters/CRC Press.
3. [GPGPU programming] NVIDIA OpenCL Best Practices Guide , 2009, www.nvidia.com
4. [review of MC simulations in clinical practice] "Challenges in Monte Carlo Simulations as Clinical and Research Tool in Particle Therapy: A Review", S. Muraro, G. Battistoni and A.C. Kraan, Frontiers in Physics, **8**, 567800 (2020)
5. [full-MC in clinical practice] "Integration and evaluation of automated Monte Carlo simulations in the clinical practice of scanned proton and carbon ion beam therapy", J Bauer et al. 2014 Phys. Med. Biol. **59** 4635, doi: 10.3389/fphy.2020.567800
6. [full-MC] "The FLUKA Code: Developments and Challenges for High Energy and Medical Applications", T.T. Böhlen, F. Cerutti, M.P.W. Chin, A. Fassò, A. Ferrari, P.G. Ortega, A. Mairani, P.R. Sala, G. Smirnov and V. Vlachoudis, Nuclear Data Sheets 120, 211-214 (2014), www.fluka.org
7. [full-MC] "Recent developments in Geant4", J. Allison et al. Nuclear Instruments and Methods in Physics Research Section A, **835** (2016) 186-225, geant4.web.cern.ch
8. [full-MC] "MCNP Users Manual - Code Version 6.2", C.J. Werner(editor), Los Alamos National Laboratory, report LA-UR-17-29981 (2017). mcnp.lanl.gov
9. [GPU fast-MC] "GPU-based fast Monte Carlo dose calculation for proton therapy", Jia X, Schümann J, Paganetti H and Jiang S B 2012 *Phys. Med. Biol.* **57** p 7783–7797, doi:10.1088/0031-9155/57/23/7783
10. [GPU fast-MC] "A fast GPU-based Monte Carlo simulation of proton transport with detailed modeling of nonelastic interactions", Wan Chan Tseung H, Ma J and Beltran C 2015, *Med. Phys.* **42** p 2967–2978, doi:10.1118/1.4921046
11. [GPU fast-MC] "Fred: a GPU-accelerated fast-Monte Carlo code for rapid treatment plan recalculation in ion beam therapy", Schiavi A., Senzacqua M., Pioli S., Mairani A., Magro G., Molinelli S., Ciocca M., Battistoni G., Patera V. 2017, *Phys. Med. Biol.* **62** p 7482–7504, doi:10.1088/1361-6560/aa8134

# 21 Monte Carlo and analytical codes for dose planning and recalculation: limits and differential advantages

*Andrea Mairani*
Heidelberg Ion-Beam Therapy Center (HIT), Heidelberg,
Germany
National Centre of Oncological Hadrontherapy (CNAO), Pavia,
Italy
Clinical Cooperation Unit Radiation Oncology, German Cancer
Consortium (DKTK) Core-Center Heidelberg, National Center for
Tumor Diseases (NCT), Heidelberg University Hospital (UKHD)
and German Cancer Research Center (DKFZ), Heidelberg,
Germany
Heidelberg University, Heidelberg, Germany

*Mein Stewart*
Division of Molecular and Translational Radiation Oncology,
Heidelberg University Medical School, Heidelberg Institute of
Radiation Oncology (HIRO), National Center for Radiation
Research in Oncology (NCRO), Heidelberg, Germany

## CONTENTS

The debate on usage of Monte Carlo (MC) codes versus analytical engines in particle therapy has persisted for the last decade [1] and boils down to three main areas of discussion – computational complexity, calculation times, and limits in accuracy. With increased complexity of physics engines making their way from purely research oriented efforts to fast-paced clinical environments, particularly for proton beams with the advent of GPU-ported MC codes, the limits and differential advantages of analytical versus Monte Carlo codes are outlined in this chapter for dose planning and recalculation.

## 21.1 ANALYTICAL DOSE OPTIMIZATION IN PARTICLE THERAPY

Dose optimization in particle therapy tries to maximize the dose to the tumor, while sparing healthy tissue and organs at risk. By minimizing an objective function ($\chi2$) that includes the aims of the treatment e.g. target coverage and normal tissue dose, a plan can be inversely derived. A basic objective function including target dose difference and organ at risk dose was given by [2] and [3]:

$$\chi^2 = \int_{i=1}^{N} g_i(P_i - D_i)^2 + \int_{k=1}^{L} \tilde{g}_k (O_k - D_k),$$

where P$i$ is the prescribed dose to dose grid point i, D$_i$is its calculated dose, $g_i$ is an importance factor for the grid point and N is the number of such grid points. L, $\tilde{g}_k$ and $O_k$ refer to the organ at risk part of the cost function.

The dose in voxel i (D$_i$) is the convolution of the dose from a pencil beam in a voxel (which combined forms the dose influence matrix) with the weights w$j$ of the in individual pencil beams (d$_{ij}$):

$$D_i = \int_{j=1}^{M} w_j \, d_{ij}$$

M represents the total number of pencil beams contributing to making up dose D$i$.

The above reported cost function is minimized with respect to the individual weights to yield an acceptable treatment plan. Because of the complex particle track structure and high LET, for particle therapy with particles with Z > 1, the dose optimization algorithms must also be able to optimize the biologically weighted dose as well as physical dose. The biological weighted dose is normally defined as RBE times dose where RBE is the relative biological effectiveness.

The biological dose in every voxel is then calculated by

$$D_i = RBE(w,d) \int_{j=1}^{M} w_j d_{ij}$$

while the objective functions remain the same. In clinical practice analytical algorithms are primarily used for treatment plan generation, leading to multiple ways to minimize the objective function. Recent works have used interior point optimization methods [4], while others employed derivatives of Newtonian optimization schemes [5, 6]. Especially for fast optimization with GPUs the latter is preferred, as the algorithm structure is highly parallelizable and can therefore be efficiently adapted to GPU programming to achieve high calculation speeds [5]. Furthermore, although simplistic, the Newtonian methods can also be employed to optimize for complex secondary biophysical endpoints, such as RBE for multi-ion particle therapy [7, 8].

Regardless of the optimization algorithm, the dose influence matrix determines the overall accuracy of the dose optimization. Consequently, errors and uncertainties that derive from the dose calculation carry over to the dose optimization itself and directly affect the patient treatment. Therefore, also the dose calculation algorithm plays a big role in dose optimizations as its the basis information.

## 21.2   MONTE CARLO AND ANALYTICAL CODES

Analytical dose calculation engines usually follow a similar calculation schema best described by Hong et al. Dose in a voxel at position (x,y,z), $D(x,y,z)$, is calculated by:

$$D(x,y,z) = \int \int dx' \, dy' \, \Phi_0(x',y') \, C(x',y',z) \, \Omega(x'-x, \, y'-y, \, z),$$

where $\Phi_0(x',y')$ is the intensity profile, $C(x',y',z)$ is the central axis term of the beam and $\Omega(x' - x, \, y'-y, \, z)$ is the lateral beam shape at depth z [9]. The integral is over the lateral area of the beam and dose contributions from all pencil beams are considered. As $\Phi_0(x',y')$ is fixed from the treatment plan and $C(x',y',z)$ is usually derived from measurements, $\Omega(x'-x, \, y'-y, \, z)$ is a key aspect in dose calculation. Next generation GPU dose calculation engines, such as FRoG or Da Silva et al. approach, can employ up to triple gaussian approximations [10, 11].

## 21.2.1 PERFORMANCE ASSESSMENT: DOSIMETRIC ACCURACY

Tissue heterogeneities are one of the main sources of calculation errors in analytical dose engines that consequently influence the dose optimization and recalculation capabilities of a TPS. Calculation capabilities are normally challenged using ad-hoc *in-silico* scenarios such as a monogenetic proton pencil beam traversing a homogeneous material (e.g., water) and at a depth of half of the beam range, impinges on two-medium interface of different compositions and/or density. In a purely homogenous setting, the pencil beam would continue its penetration unaffected; however, in reality, pencil beam deformation will occur, since the high-density material incorporates a change in beam physics for nearly half of the traversing particles (i.e. higher electron density yielding increased stopping power and reduced range). Ideally, 3-dimensional measurement of the exact shape of this pencil beam deformation would take place, however, absolute 3D dosimetry for particle beams is still a precarious subject and therefore, sequence of 2D array ion chamber measurements or validated Monte Carlo simulation provide the "best" evidence of altered dose deposition in heterogeneous material. For Monte Carlo prediction of beam deformation, the accuracy limitation is dictated by the comprehensiveness of the inherent physics models and validity of the digitized geometry/how representative the voxelized heterogeneity of the patient anatomy. Analytical approaches to the pencil beam algorithm will handle heterogeneity effects on the dose distribution with a varying degree of accuracy [12]. Performance of these models are dependent on location and severity of the heterogeneity.

Several independent works investigating different clinical and/or research-based treatment planning/dose calculation systems found varying degrees of accuracy when compared with reference measurements and Monte Carlo simulations. Particularly for proton beams, evaluations of analytical algorithm performance in treatment of thorax identify two main drawbacks in clinical application. First, analytical approaches may substantially underestimate lateral spread of protons due to beam divergence differences between water-approximated beam profiles and that of low-HU (density) compositions like lung tissue [13]. Similar problems arise in air cavities within the thorax as well as sinuses within the skull and daily variation of air pockets in proximity to abdominal treatment sites. Although negligible for most clinical cases, beam degradation effects in lung treatments that arise from alternating low- and high-density tissues have been shown to cause so-called "pencil-beam degradation," which effectively causes Bragg-Peak "smearing," similar to additional range straggling [14]. In effect, this will cause underdosage of the target volume due to overestimation in the TPS since these effects are not explicitly considered in the clinical practice. Furthermore, algorithm performance tests also indicate potential deficiencies in proton dose calculation for field characteristics such as small fields in the presence of tissue heterogeneity. Lastly, handling beam modifiers in challenging patient cases, for example range shift and particularly with large air gaps (modifier to patient surface distances) may lead to clinically relevant dose deviations when performing computations analytically as opposed to Monte Carlo [15]. This is a particular issue that is well explored within the literature for clinical proton algorithms and suggests either dose correction factors [16] or inevitably transitioning to Monte Carlo may provide the most reliable calculation.

Nevertheless, using correction factors or different beam models (Kopp et al. 2021, Choi et al. 2018), the effects of range modifiers on the beam shape in air can be to an extent also be well described with analytical dose calculation engines.

Few works present comparisons of multiple analytical codes in the context of measurements and Monte Carlo in highly heterogeneous regions. Investigation of analytical and Monte Carlo calculation performance demonstrated that in a skull anthropomorphic phantom, dose calculation using state-of-the-art analytical algorithms achieve similar accuracy for both clinical and research ion beams. This was particularly true for helium, carbon and oxygen ions within the target regions and towards the distal end, while for proton beams, the ray casting approach showed substantial deviations from measurements and Monte Carlo predictions, particularly within the target and towards the distal edge, where pencil beam deformation with grossly overestimated. Both ray-casting

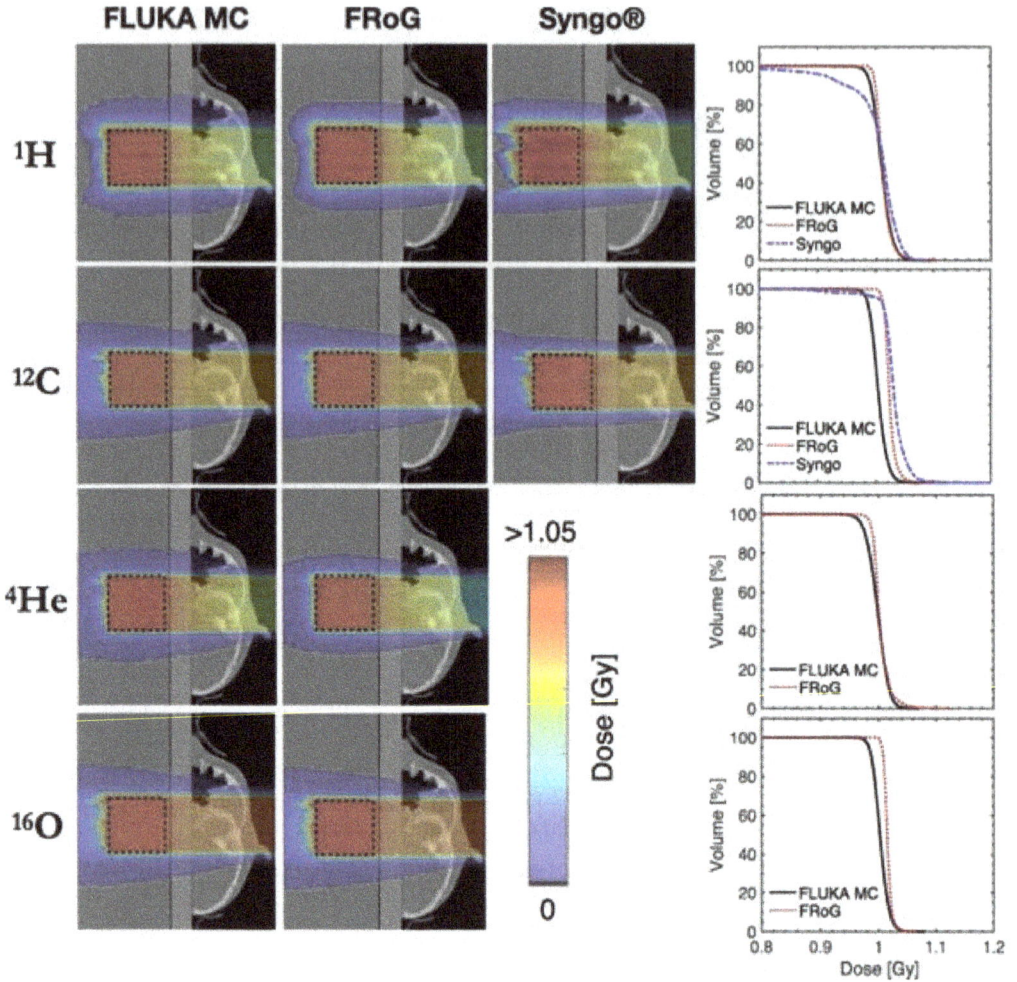

**Figure 21.1** SOBPs in a homogeneous target after traversing an anthropomorphic head phantom calculated with a recently used clinical TPS, MC simulation and a state-of-the-art GPU based analytical code. Current clinically and experimentally applied ion beams at the Heidelberg Ion-Beam Therapy Center facility have been used. For proton beams, high variations are seen to the MC simulation at the distal edge and the target coverage for the recently used clinical TPS. Figure taken from [17].

and pencil beam splitting (fluence-dose model) have their own unique architecture for handling heterogeneity effects on pencil beam deformation and accordingly, will perform differently when encountering either superficial or deep-seated heterogeneities. For instance, the Syngo ® TPS consists of a unique ray-casting algorithm, also referred to as "point-of-interest," and can provide sufficient estimations of pencil beam deformation for brain cases where the beam impinges on the skull and no severe heterogeneities are encountered before or within the target volume. However, performance between splitting and ray-casting can substantially differ for base of skull or nasopharynx, similar to the investigation in [17] shown in Figures 21.1 and 21.2. Comparison of dose maps and dose volume histograms for three investigated computation approaches (Monte Carlo, FRoG [pencil beam splitting] and Syngo ® ["point-of-interest"]) clearly demonstrates a more clinical-like scenario of how anatomic heterogeneity can greatly distort whole treatment fields. Using the

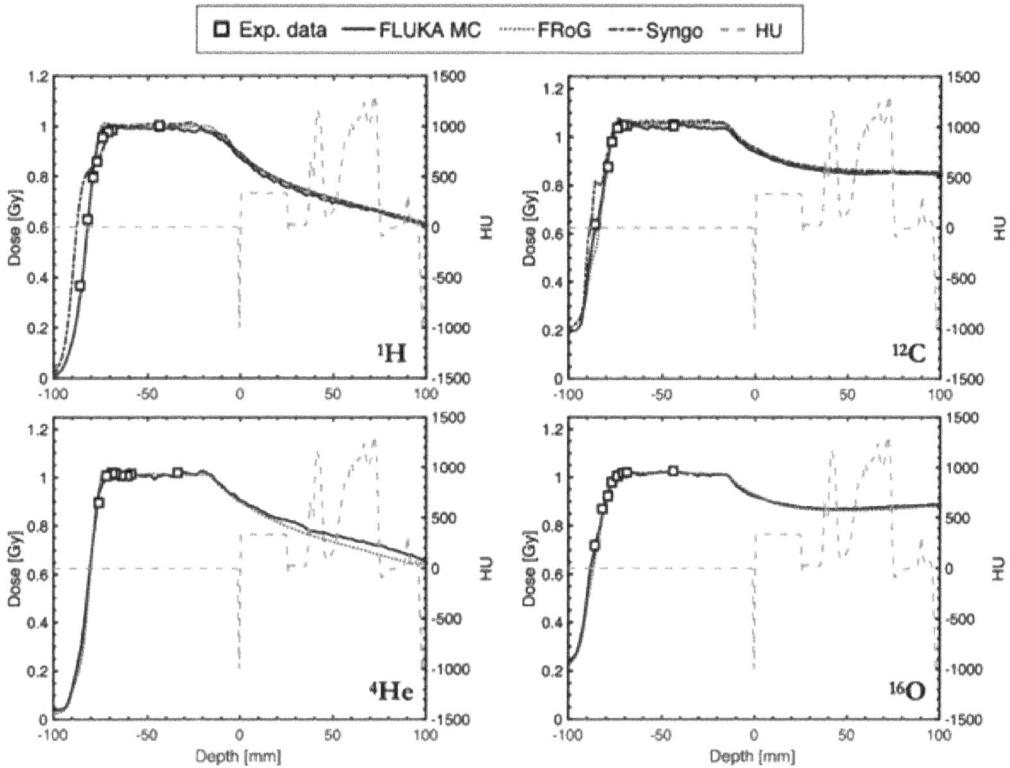

**Figure 21.2**   Line profiles of SOBPs in a homogeneous target after traversing an anthropomorphic head phantom calculated with a recently used clinical TPS (Syngo), FLUKA MC simulation and a state-of-the-art GPU based analytical code (FRoG). Dose predictions are compared to 24-pin point ionization chamber measurements that are submerged in a water tank. Figure taken from [17].

half-head phantom and Monte Carlo treatment optimization, beam traversal through the skull base involves consideration of various bone/soft-tissue/air cavity interfaces proximal to the $6x6x6cm^3$ target volume delineation in a homogenous water region. For protons, Monte Carlo (FLUKA MC) and GPU-accelerated pencil beam splitting algorithms (FRoG) exhibit similar results while the clinical TPS (Syngo®) overestimated the degree of pencil beam "warping," most notable in the jagged feature within in the target volume and distal end and underdosage in the target volume shown in the DVH (dose-volume-histogram). For carbon ions, all three calculation types exhibited similar field distortion features with again a slight overestimation of sharpness in range modulation in the ray-casting inspired algorithm. Overestimations of target dose on the order of 1–5% were found for both analytical approaches, owing to difficulty in analytical modeling of the low-dose halo caused by nuclear-interaction and changes in lateral evolution of this mixed radiation field in the presence of complex heterogeneities. The surveyed pencil beam splitting and ray-casting approaches implement a triple and double Gaussian model, respectively, for lateral beam evolution [18, 19] and propagation of these models in heterogeneous structures should be a subject of scrutiny. As performed for facility specific beam model characteristics such as integral depth dose, these models are determined for homogeneous water-equivalent settings only and therefore are known to have limitations even in homogeneous media, especially when considering the analytical propagation methods of lateral beam evolution. Nonetheless, this test presented in [17] provides baseline performance results for a head-based treatment sites and demonstrated that at least for heavier ions (helium, carbon and oxygen), agreement between Monte Carlo and GPU-accelerated high-order PB splitting methods like FRoG, which subdivide each spot in the raster-scanning plan by approximately 400 sub-pencil beams for handling heterogeneity, may provide satisfactory results. This is further supported by comparison with dosimetric ion chamber measurements in Figure 21.2, which present representative profiles along the beam path.

The discussed results in [17] is a single study from one facility which has unique proton beam characteristics and beam application and monitoring systems composed of high Z material (e.g., tungsten) compared to modern systems with short nozzle to isocenter distances. Therefore, performance of various analytical techniques should be expected to produce varying degrees of accuracy compared with Monte Carlo and measurements. However, the reliability of an engine's methodology for propagating the dose distribution and mathematical assumptions for handling beam distortions in heterogeneous anatomy. Since the publication of these results, installation and commissioning of GPU-accelerated Monte Carlo dose calculation took place using RayStation (RaySearch Laboratories, Stockholm) and therefore the clinic is no longer relying on analytical treatment planning methods for proton therapy. Results from other aforementioned studies as well as several others not particularly discussed or referenced in this chapter provide sufficient testimony to suggest that clinical practice will greatly benefit from fast MC proton. However, there is no overwhelming evidence yet for the heavier ions using conventional delivery techniques in particle therapy that analytical dose calculation approaches are insufficient. Therefore, for the time being, analytical approaches to dose calculation and optimization will continue to be used in clinical particle therapy for ions heavier than protons. Developments of fast Monte Carlo codes may however improve clinical practice using heavy ions and may bolster reliability of treatment planning in anatomically heterogenous sites which are typically avoided due treatment delivery complexity.

## 21.2.2 PERFORMANCE ASSESSMENT: SPEED AND EFFICIENCY

One key feature of analytical dose calculation engines are quick calculation speeds that arise from the simplification of the multi-dimensional physics description often yielding highly parallelizable algorithms. Often, GPUs are used to achieve high computation throughputs when a task is completely parallelizable, i.e., one can build on the GPUs ability to parallelize (SIMT technology). Through its high number of computational cores compared to a standard CPU, GPUs achieve very fast computation times in dose calculation. Fast calculation enables many computational expensive methods such as:

*Online Dose Calculation:* Here, dose consistency to the prescribed plan is verified online during the patient treatment for all (or selected) fractionations, delivering an interlock when the deviation of delivered to prescribed dose plan is not acceptable. In online dose calculation, the information on the current beam position and current particle number is fed to the calculation engine directly from the delivery machine information. To this end, fast (sub-second) calculation times are necessary to calculate the dose in real time as otherwise latency issues could apply the interlock too late. Online dose calculation is already feasible with current hardware, as an online dose calculation using GPUs has been developed and experimentally verified in recent works [21].

*Adaptive radiotherapy* is a combination of *online dose calculation* with fast dose optimization. Similar to *online calculation*, the machine delivery parameters are fed to the calculation engine that calculates the dose in real time. Instead of interlocks, the treatment plan is updated after every pencil beam (or optionally isoenergy layer) is delivered i.e., intra-fractional, minimizing the already delivered dose and the prescribed dose. Adaptive therapy requires both, fast dose and optimization speeds but together with live imaging information enables very conformal dose delivery for moving tumors, such as in lung or the thorax region. Furthermore, with onboard imaging, organ movement, volume and other anatomical/physiological changes could also be considered.

Using an analytical dose calculation engine combined with an GPU based optimization, treatment plans can nowadays already be calculated and optimized within 10 seconds. There are also big scale projects underway to enable adaptive and online dose calculation within clinical settings.

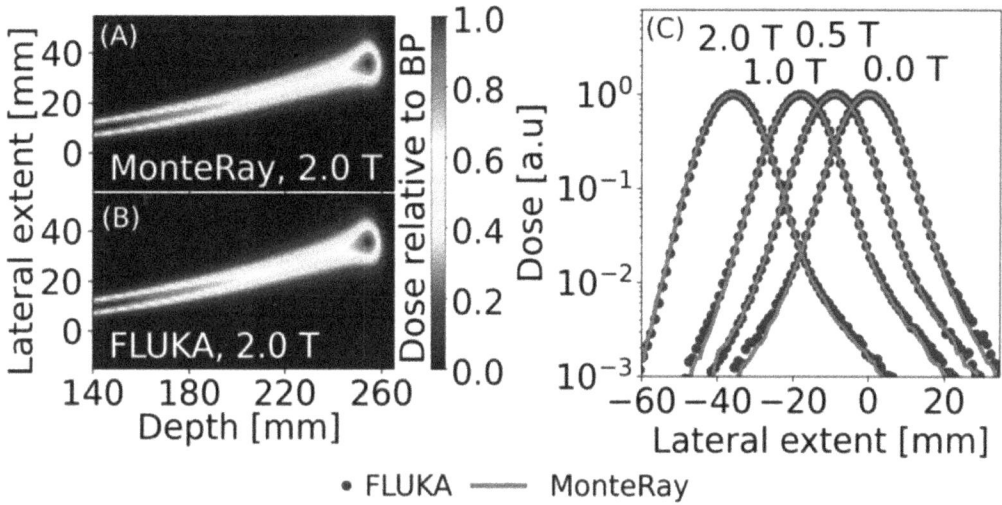

**Figure 21.3** Depiction of beam distortion of high energy protons (250 MeV) traversing a 0T, 0.5T, 1.0T and 2.0T homogeneous magnetic field (Taken from [20]), computed via MonteRay, a framework for fast Monte Carlo calculations.

There does exist an advantage worth noting in terms of convenience in analytical codes for implementation and testing of novel treatment planning, delivery and monitoring techniques as opposed to Monte Carlo engines. For example, MR-guided radiotherapy is gaining interest and focus in R&D both in academic settings and industry. For example, TPS can implement analytical approaches to prediction of the degree/magnitude at which a low to mid strength (e.g., 0–3 T) magnetic field would impact particle beam paths in various materials for proton beams [22]. On the other hand, fast Monte Carlo codes are already under development for modeling MR guided particle therapy using proton and helium ions (Lysakovski 2021, 2022) and demonstrated good agreement with other gold-standard Monte Carlo methods. Figure 21.3 depicts the MonteRay MC code versus FLUKA calculations for predicting pencil beam dose depositions of high energy proton beams in water for various magnetic field strengths. Both fast Monte Carlo and analytical algorithms may in some circumstances serve as a sand-box environment for testing preclinical models and/or approaches to treatment which are otherwise computationally challenging or impractical from a developmental standpoint [23]. Eventually, updates to clinical computation frameworks may occur and for best accuracy, make their way to Monte Carlo codes given speed is sufficient.

Monte Carlo simulations offer highly accurate dose calculations in particle therapy but were usually too slow to be employed for dose calculation and optimization in clinical practice. However, only recently have Monte Carlo simulations been commercially available for treatment planning and dose calculation, often employing GPUs for improved calculation times [24, 25, 26, 27, 28] (Shiavi et al. 2017). However, compared to full scale MC simulations such as FLUKA/Geant4 the decrease in calculation time in fast Monte Carlo engines comes at a cost in physics description and reduction of capabilities. This reduces the use cases for these MC simulations specific for clinical particle therapy. Furthermore, with the exception of one of the latest GPU MC codes MonteRay [20], magnetic fields which are necessary for adaptive therapy using MRI are also neglected. Lastly, the primary focus of fast Monte Carlo engines has been on protons due to the larger proton community and simplicity. To date, there exist two fast Monte Carlo engine for carbon ions and one for helium [29].

## REFERENCES

1. Lomax, Antony; van Herk, Marcel, et al. "Monte Carlo or bust? Are Monte Carlo calculations a must in proton therapy?" Oral Talk PTCOG58 Physics slam, 13th June 2019
2. Lomax, Antony. "Intensity modulation methods for proton radiotherapy." Physics in Medicine & Biology 44.1 (1999): 185.
3. Bortfeld, Th, et al. "Methods of image reconstruction from projections applied to conformation radiotherapy." Physics in Medicine & Biology 35.10 (1990): 1423.
4. Wieser, Hans-Peter, et al. "Development of the open-source dose calculation and optimization toolkit matRad." Medical physics 44.6 (2017): 2556-2568.
5. Matter, Michael, et al. "Intensity modulated proton therapy plan generation in under ten seconds." Acta oncologica 58.10 (2019): 1435-1439.
6. Böhlen, Till Tobias, et al. "A Monte Carlo-based treatment-planning tool for ion beam therapy." Journal of radiation research 54.suppl_1 (2013): i77-i81.
7. Böhlen, Till Tobias, et al. "Investigating the robustness of ion beam therapy treatment plans to uncertainties in biological treatment parameters." Physics in Medicine & Biology 57.23 (2012): 7983.
8. Kopp, Benedikt, et al. "Development and validation of single field multi-ion particle therapy treatments." International Journal of Radiation Oncology* Biology* Physics 106.1 (2020): 194-205.
9. Hong, Linda, et al. "A pencil beam algorithm for proton dose calculations." Physics in Medicine & Biology 41.8 (1996): 1305.
10. Mein, Stewart, et al. "Fast robust dose calculation on GPU for high-precision 1 H, 4 He, 12 C and 16 O ion therapy: the FRoG platform." Scientific reports 8.1 (2018): 1-12.
11. Da Silva, Joakim, Richard Ansorge, and Rajesh Jena. "Sub-second pencil beam dose calculation on GPU for adaptive proton therapy." Physics in Medicine & Biology 60.12 (2015): 4777.
12. Schaffner, Barbara, Eros Pedroni, and Antony Lomax. "Dose calculation models for proton treatment planning using a dynamic beam delivery system: an attempt to include density heterogeneity effects in the analytical dose calculation." Physics in Medicine & Biology 44.1 (1999): 27.
13. Taylor, Paige A., Stephen F. Kry, and David S. Followill. "Pencil beam algorithms are unsuitable for proton dose calculations in lung." International Journal of Radiation Oncology* Biology* Physics 99.3 (2017): 750-756.
14. Titt, Uwe, et al. "Degradation of proton depth dose distributions attributable to microstructures in lung-equivalent material." Medical physics 42.11 (2015): 6425-6432.
15. Kern, A., et al. "Impact of air gap, range shifter, and delivery technique on skin dose in proton therapy." Medical Physics 48.2 (2021): 831-840.
16. Zhang, Yang, et al. "Dose calculation for spot scanning proton therapy with the application of a range shifter." Biomedical Physics & Engineering Express 3.3 (2017): 035019.
17. Mein, Stewart, et al. "Dosimetric validation of Monte Carlo and analytical dose engines with raster-scanning 1H, 4He, 12C, and 16O ion-beams using an anthropomorphic phantom." Physica Medica 64 (2019): 123-131.
18. Parodi, Katia, Andrea Mairani, and Florian Sommerer. "Monte Carlo-based parametrization of the lateral dose spread for clinical treatment planning of scanned proton and carbon ion beams." Journal of radiation research 54.suppl_1 (2013): i91-i96.
19. Hirayama, Shusuke, et al. "Evaluation of the influence of double and triple Gaussian proton kernel models on accuracy of dose calculations for spot scanning technique." Medical physics 43.3 (2016): 1437-1450.
20. Lysakovski, Peter, et al. "Development and benchmarking of a Monte Carlo dose engine for proton radiation therapy." Frontiers in Physics (2021): 655.

21. Giordanengo, S., et al. "RIDOS: A new system for online computation of the delivered dose distributions in scanning ion beam therapy." Physica Medica 60 (2019): 139-149.

22. Fuchs, Hermann, et al. "Magnetic field effects on particle beams and their implications for dose calculation in MR-guided particle therapy." Medical physics 44.3 (2017): 1149-1156.

23. Mein, Stewart, et al. "Spot-scanning Hadron Arc (SHArc) therapy: a study with light and heavy ions." Advances in radiation oncology 6.3 (2021): 100661.

24. Jia, Xun, et al. "GPU-based fast Monte Carlo dose calculation for proton therapy." Physics in Medicine & Biology 57.23 (2012): 7783.

25. Giantsoudi, Drosoula, et al. "Validation of a GPU-based Monte Carlo code (gPMC) for proton radiation therapy: clinical cases study." Physics in Medicine & Biology 60.6 (2015): 2257.

26. Ruciński, A., et al. "GPU-accelerated Monte Carlo code for fast dose recalculation in proton beam therapy." Acta Phys. Polon. B 48.10 (2017): 1625.

27. Deng, Wei, et al. "Integrating an open source Monte Carlo code "MCsquare" for clinical use in intensity-modulated proton therapy." Medical physics 47.6 (2020): 2558-2574.

28. Tian, Zhen, et al. "A GPU OpenCL based cross-platform Monte Carlo dose calculation engine (goMC)." Physics in Medicine & Biology 60.19 (2015): 7419.

29. Lysakovski, Peter, et al. "Development and benchmarking of the first fast Monte Carlo engine for helium ion beam dose calculation: MonteRay." Medical Physics (2022): DOI: 10.1002/mp.16178.

30. Bueno, M., et al. "An algorithm to assess the need for clinical Monte Carlo dose calculation for small proton therapy fields based on quantification of tissue heterogeneity." Medical physics 40.8 (2013): 081704.

31. Schiavi, Angelo, et al. "Fred: a GPU-accelerated fast-Monte Carlo code for rapid treatment plan recalculation in ion beam therapy." Physics in Medicine & Biology 62.18 (2017): 7482.

# Appendix: Chemical reactions

Reaction rate constants ($k_{obs}$), reaction radii ($\sigma$), and probability of geminate recombination ($P_{React}$) for type I reactions. (*) These are reactions with spin statistical factor (type V).

**Table A.1**

**Type I reactions**

| Reaction | $k_{obs}$ ($10^{10}$ M$^{-1}$s$^{-1}$) | $\sigma$ (nm) | $P_{React}$ |
|---|---|---|---|
| H. + H. $\rightarrow$ H$_2$ | 0.503 | 0.38 | 0.25* |
| H. + e$^-_{aq}$ $\rightarrow$ H$_2$+ OH$^-$ | 2.50 | 1.11 | 0.25* |
| H. + O($^3$P) $\rightarrow$ .OH | 2.02 | 0.29 | 1.00 |
| H. + O.$^-$ $\rightarrow$ OH$^-$ | 2.00 | 0.29 | 1.00 |
| .OH + O($^3$P) $\rightarrow$ HO$_2$. | 2.02 | 0.63 | 1.00 |
| HO$_2$. + O($^3$P) $\rightarrow$ O$_2$+ .OH | 2.02 | 0.62 | 1.00 |
| O($^3$P) + O($^3$P) $\rightarrow$ O$_2$ | 2.20 | 1.45 | 1.00 |

Reaction rate constants ($k_{obs}$, $k_{dif}$ and $k_a$), reaction radii ($\sigma$), probability of geminate recombination, and $\alpha$ for type II reactions. The rate constant $k_{dif} = 4\pi\sigma D$ (see text) in nm$^3$s$^{-1}$ can be converted to M$^{-1}$s$^{-1}$ by multiplication by the factor $10^{-24}N_0$, where $N_0$ is Avogadro's number.

Reaction rate constants ($k_{obs}$), reaction radii ($\sigma$), Onsager's radii ($r_c$), effective radii ($\sigma_{eff}$), and probability of geminate recombination ($P_{React}$) for type III reactions. (*) Reaction with a spin statistical factor (type V).

Reaction rate constants ($k_{obs}$, $k_{dif}$ and $k_a$), real and effective reaction radii ($\sigma$ and $\sigma_{eff}$), and probability of geminate recombination ($P_{React}$) for type IV reactions. For all reactions, the Onsager's radius is 0.71 nm multiplied by the product of the charges of the reactants.

Reaction rate constants ($k_{obs}$) for first-order reactions and scavenging power ($k_{obs}$[B]) for reactions with H$_2$O, H$^+$ and OH$^-$. [B] is the concentration of species present in the background.

DOI: 10.1201/9781003023920-A

## Table A.2
## Type II reactions

| Reaction | $k_{obs}$ $(10^{10}$ $M^{-1}s^{-1})$ | $\sigma$ (nm) | $k_{dif}$ $(10^{10}$ $M^{-1}s^{-1})$ | $k_a$ $(10^{10}$ $M^{-1}s^{-1})$ | $P_{React}$ | $\alpha$ $(nm^{-1})$ |
|---|---|---|---|---|---|---|
| $H. + .OH \rightarrow H_2O$ | 1.55 | 0.41 | 2.86 | 3.40 | 0.33 | 5.34 |
| $H. + H_2O_2 \rightarrow H_2O + .OH$ | 0.0035 | 0.40 | 2.82 | 0.0035 | 0.00 | 2.50 |
| $H. + OH^- \rightarrow H_2O + e^-_{aq}$ | 0.00251 | 0.52 | 4.84 | 2.51 | 0.00 | 1.92 |
| $H. + O_2 \rightarrow HO_2.$ | 2.10 | 0.36 | 2.56 | 11.7 | 0.67 | 15.4 |
| $H. + HO_2. \rightarrow H_2O_2$ | 1.00 | 0.40 | 2.82 | 1.55 | 0.19 | 3.88 |
| $H. + O_2.^- \rightarrow HO_2^-$ | 1.00 | 0.41 | 2.72 | 1.58 | 0.20 | 3.86 |
| $.OH + .OH \rightarrow H_2O_2$ | 0.550 | 0.44 | 0.732 | 2.21 | 0.55 | 9.14 |
| $.OH + H_2O_2 \rightarrow HO_2. + H_2O$ | 0.00288 | 0.43 | 1.46 | 0.00288 | 0.00 | 2.33 |
| $.OH + H_2 \rightarrow H. + H_2O$ | 0.00328 | 0.36 | 1.91 | 0.00329 | 0.00 | 2.78 |
| $.OH + e^-_{aq} \rightarrow OH^-$ | 2.95 | 0.72 | 3.87 | 12.5 | 0.49 | 5.87 |
| $.OH + OH^- \rightarrow O.^- + H_2O$ | 0.630 | 0.55 | 3.12 | 0.790 | 0.08 | 2.28 |
| $.OH + HO_2. \rightarrow O_2 + H_2O$ | 0.790 | 0.43 | 1.4 | 1.72 | 0.33 | 5.05 |
| $.OH + O_2.^- \rightarrow O_2 + OH^-$ | 1.07 | 0.44 | 1.32 | 5.76 | 0.64 | 12.2 |
| $.OH + HO_2^- \rightarrow HO_2. + OH^-$ | 0.832 | 0.47 | 1.28 | 2.38 | 0.42 | 6.08 |
| $.OH + O.^- \rightarrow HO_2^-$ | 0.100 | 0.47 | 1.49 | 0.107 | 0.03 | 2.28 |
| $.OH + O_3.^- \rightarrow O_2.^- + HO_2.$ | 0.850 | 0.42 | 1.34 | 2.34 | 0.42 | 6.55 |
| $H_2O_2 + e^-_{aq} \rightarrow OH^- + .OH$ | 1.10 | 0.71 | 3.87 | 1.54 | 0.11 | 1.97 |
| $H_2O_2 + OH^- \rightarrow HO_2^- + H_2O$ | 0.0471 | 0.54 | 3.11 | 0.0478 | 0.01 | 1.88 |
| $H_2O_2 + O(^3P) \rightarrow HO_2. + .OH$ | 0.160 | 0.41 | 1.33 | 0.182 | 0.05 | 2.77 |
| $H_2O_2 + O.^- \rightarrow HO_2. + OH^-$ | 0.0555 | 0.46 | 1.50 | 0.0576 | 0.01 | 2.26 |
| $H_2 + O(^3P) \rightarrow H. + .OH$ | $4.77 \times 10^{-7}$ | 0.34 | 1.75 | $4.77 \times 10^{-7}$ | 0.00 | 2.94 |
| $H_2 + O.^- \rightarrow H. + OH^-$ | 0.0121 | 0.39 | 2.01 | 0.0122 | 0.00 | 2.58 |
| $e^-_{aq} + O_2 \rightarrow O_2.^-$ | 1.74 | 0.67 | 3.70 | 3.23 | 0.22 | 2.79 |
| $e^-_{aq} + HO_2. \rightarrow HO_2^-$ | 1.29 | 0.71 | 3.87 | 1.92 | 0.13 | 2.11 |
| $OH^- + HO_2. \rightarrow O_2.^- + H_2O$ | 0.630 | 0.54 | 3.11 | 0.791 | 0.08 | 2.32 |
| $OH^- + O(^3P) \rightarrow HO_2^-$ | 0.0420 | 0.53 | 2.93 | 0.0426 | 0.01 | 1.91 |
| $O_2 + O(^3P) \rightarrow O_3$ | 0.4.00 | 0.37 | 1.23 | 0.592 | 0.18 | 4.00 |
| $O_2 + O.^- \rightarrow O_3.^-$ | 0.3.70 | 0.42 | 1.40 | 0.503 | 0.13 | 3.24 |
| $HO_2. + HO_2. \rightarrow H_2O_2 + O_2$ | $9.80 \times 10^{-5}$ | 0.42 | 0.731 | $9.80 \times 10^{-5}$ | 0.00 | 2.38 |
| $HO_2. + O_2.^- \rightarrow HO_2^- + O_2$ | 0.00970 | 0.43 | 1.32 | 0.00977 | 0.00 | 2.34 |
| $HO_2^- + O(^3P) \rightarrow O_2.^- + .OH$ | 0.530 | 0.45 | 1.16 | 0.977 | 0.25 | 4.10 |

## Table A.3
## Type III reactions

| Reaction | $k_{obs}$ $(10^{10}$ $M^{-1}s^{-1})$ | $\sigma$ (nm) | $r_c$ (nm) | $\sigma_{eff}$ (nm) | $P_{React}$ |
|---|---|---|---|---|---|
| $e^-_{aq} + e^-_{aq} \rightarrow H_2 + 2OH^-$ | 0.636 | 1.00 | 0.71 | 0.67 | 0.25(*) |
| $H^+ + OH^- \rightarrow H_2O$ | 11.3 | 0.58 | −0.71 | 1.01 | 1.00 |
| $H^+ + O_3.^- \rightarrow .OH + O_2$ | 9.00 | 0.61 | −0.71 | 1.04 | 1.00 |

## Table A.4
## Type IV reactions

| Reaction | $k_{obs}$ $(10^{10}$ $M^{-1}s^{-1})$ | $\sigma$ (nm) | $\sigma_{eff}$ (nm) | $k_{dif}$ $(10^{10}$ $M^{-1}s^{-1})$ | $k_a$ $(10^{10}$ $M^{-1}s^{-1})$ | $P_{React}$ | $\sigma''_{eff}$ (nm) |
|---|---|---|---|---|---|---|---|
| $e^-_{aq} + H^+ \rightarrow H.$ | 2.11 | 0.75 | 1.16 | 12.6 | 2.53 | 0.04 | 0.194 |
| $e^-_{aq} + O_2.^- \rightarrow H_2O_2 + 2OH^-$ | 1.29 | 0.72 | 0.42 | 2.12 | 3.35 | 0.39 | 0.258 |
| $e^-_{aq} + HO_2^- \rightarrow O.^- + OH^-$ | 0.351 | 0.75 | 0.45 | 2.14 | 0.420 | 0.07 | 0.074 |
| $e^-_{aq} + O.^- \rightarrow 2OH^-$ | 2.31 | 0.75 | 0.45 | 2.35 | 153. | 0.96 | 0.443 |
| $H^+ + O_2.^- \rightarrow HO_2.$ | 4.78 | 0.47 | 0.91 | 7.74 | 12.5 | 0.27 | 0.563 |
| $H^+ + HO_2^- \rightarrow H_2O_2$ | 5.00 | 0.50 | 0.94 | 7.71 | 14.5 | 0.29 | 0.612 |
| $H^+ + O.^- \rightarrow .OH$ | 4.78 | 0.50 | 0.94 | 8.13 | 11.6 | 0.24 | 0.551 |
| $O_2.^- + O.^- \rightarrow O_2 + 2OH^-$ | 0.06 | 0.47 | 0.20 | 0.57 | 0.0671 | 0.06 | 0.021 |
| $HO_2^- + O.^- \rightarrow O_2.^- + OH^-$ | 0.035 | 0.50 | 0.23 | 0.581 | 0.0372 | 0.03 | 0.014 |
| $O.^- + O.^- \rightarrow H_2O_2 + 2OH^-$ | 0.01 | 0.50 | 0.23 | 0.342 | 0.0103 | 0.02 | 0.007 |
| $O.^- + O_3.^- \rightarrow 2O_2.^-$ | 0.07 | 0.45 | 0.18 | 0.558 | 0.08 | 0.08 | 0.023 |

## Table A.5
## Type VI reactions

| Reaction | $k_{obs}$ or $k_{obs}$[B] $(s^{-1})$ | Reaction | $k_{obs}$ or $k_{obs}$[B] $(s^{-1})$ |
|---|---|---|---|
| $HO_2. \rightarrow H^+ + O_2.^-$ | $7.15 \times 10^5$ | $OH^- + H^+ \rightarrow H_2O$ | $1.11 \times 10^4$ |
| $O_3.^- \rightarrow O.^- + O_2$ | $2.66 \times 10^3$ | $HO_2^- + H^+ \rightarrow H_2O_2$ | $4.98 \times 10^3$ |
| $H. + H_2O \rightarrow e^-_{aq} + H_3O^+$ | 5.94 | $O.^- + H^+ \rightarrow .OH$ | $4.73 \times 10^3$ |
| $e^-_{aq} + H_2O \rightarrow H. + OH^-$ | 15.8 | $O_3.^- + H^+ \rightarrow .OH + O_2$ | $8.91 \times 10^3$ |
| $O_2.^- + H_2O \rightarrow HO_2. + OH^-$ | 0.15 | $H. + OH^- \rightarrow H_2O + e^-_{aq}$ | $2.49 \times 10^3$ |
| $HO_2^- + H_2O \rightarrow H_2O_2 + OH^-$ | $1.36 \times 10^6$ | $.OH + OH^- \rightarrow O.^- + H_2O$ | $6.24 \times 10^2$ |
| $O(^3P) + H_2O \rightarrow 2.OH$ | $1.90 \times 10^3$ | $H_2O_2 + OH^- \rightarrow HO_2^- + H_2O$ | $4.66 \times 10^2$ |
| $O.^- + H_2O \rightarrow .OH + OH^-$ | $1.36 \times 10^6$ | $HO_2. + OH^- \rightarrow O_2.^- + H_2O$ | $6.24 \times 10^2$ |
| $e^-_{aq} + H^+ \rightarrow H.$ | $2.09 \times 10^3$ | $O(^3P) + OH^- \rightarrow HO_2^-$ | $4.16 \times 10^1$ |
| $O_2.^- + H^+ \rightarrow HO_2.$ | $4.73 \times 10^3$ | | |

# Index

Note: Page numbers in bold and italics refer to tables and figures, respectively.

For Product Safety Concerns and Information please contact our EU
representative GPSR@taylorandfrancis.com
Taylor & Francis Verlag GmbH, Kaufingerstraße 24, 80331 München, Germany

www.ingramcontent.com/pod-product-compliance
Lightning Source LLC
Chambersburg PA
CBHW080912220326
41598CB00034B/5555

* 9 7 8 1 0 3 2 5 6 2 7 4 2 *